This book, both in its preparation and in its publication, has been made possible through the interest and the generosity of the Mayo Association of Rochester.

THE PEOPLE'S HEALTH

A HISTORY

OF PUBLIC HEALTH

IN MINNESOTA

TO 1948

By Philip D. Jordan

MINNESOTA HISTORICAL SOCIETY   SAINT PAUL 1953

Copyright 1953 by the MINNESOTA HISTORICAL SOCIETY, *St. Paul*

Preface

CURIOUSLY enough, public health is a vague and shadowy thing to many Minnesotans who, when asked what a health department does, shake their heads and mutter something about quarantine signs; or fidget nervously and guess that health officers now and again examine school children. It is the exceptional citizen who has even a relatively comprehensive knowledge of the functions of local and state public health programs.

This lack of knowledge stems from several sources. The Minnesota State Board of Health, although the fourth oldest health board in the Union, never has developed an over-all public relations policy designed to reach out and capture the imagination and support of the rank and file.[1] Local boards and officers have been equally reluctant. The Minnesota legislature frequently has curtailed public health activities by trimming appropriation requests. And the people of the state, except in rare instances, have not called for explanations of policies and activities. They are equally unaware of the relationships between state programs and federal programs, not realizing, for example, that the present United States Public Health Service is the outgrowth of an act passed in 1798 for the relief of sick and disabled seamen. This act resulted in the establishment of the Marine Hospital Service, whose title was changed in 1902 to the Public Health and Marine Hospital Service and a decade later to the United States Public Health Service.[2]

Although it is obvious that a public health program on any governmental level costs money, few residents of the North Star State know how much is spent for the state program and where the money comes from. What does Minnesota's public health program cost? Data reported in an analysis made by the Minnesota Institute of Governmental Research, Inc., indicate that state expenditures for activities

[1] Robert G. Paterson, ed., *Historical Directory of State Health Departments in the United States of America*, 61 (Columbus, Ohio, 1939).
[2] Ralph C. Williams, *The United States Public Health Service, 1798–1850* (Washington, D.C., 1951).

broadly classified as conservation of health and sanitation, exclusive of the financing of tuberculosis sanatoriums by the state, accounted for 0.8% of total state expenditures in 1939 and 0.9% in 1948. The per capita state appropriations for health services are lower in Minnesota than the average of all states. On the basis of the 1950 federal census, which gave Minnesota a population of 2,982,482, the total funds of $1,184,714 from all sources represent a per capita expenditure of $0.38. The total appropriations from the state legislature for all aspects of public health services administered by the state health department for 1951–52 and 1952–53 were approximately $0.38 per capita. The per capita state appropriations to the Minnesota Department of Health for the fiscal year 1948, exclusive of hospital care and sanatoriums, was $0.293, making the state thirty-second in rank. The average per capita appropriations for all states for 1948 was $0.504, according to figures compiled by the United States Public Health Service. For 1949 and 1950, the United States Public Health Service reported that Minnesota was below the average per capita of all states both in general appropriations for health purposes and in appropriations for hospital care and sanatoriums; for the year 1950, the Minnesota public health appropriations from state revenues for general purposes, including those for the University of Minnesota and the division of public institutions programs, was $0.43 per capita, as compared with $0.48 for the median state and $0.63 for the all-states combined average.

Until recently, public health authorities have estimated that an expenditure of approximately $1.00 per capita was required to maintain a minimum standard of community public health service. More recent estimates of the cost of minimum services have been raised to $1.50 per capita and over. It has been pointed out that there are very few areas in Minnesota where expenditures for public health services by the state health department and by the local governments approach these so-called standards of expenditure for minimum services. It has been said also that Minnesota as a state should provide for adequate fundamental public health services; that the state should not rely overmuch on federal appropriations, because funds of this nature vary from year to year and may even be discontinued; and that the state should encourage the development of public health services through local health departments, with the state providing not more than half of the cost of standard local health services.

This informal history of the people's health does not concern itself primarily with finances nor with organization and administration, although necessarily these subjects are included. Nor does it explore exhaustively intergovernmental relations in public health.[3] Rather, the volume is the story of the beginnings and unfolding of public health with emphasis upon social aspects and upon the roles that persons, as well as organizations, have played. Unfortunately not everything could be included and not everything that is included could always receive as much space and attention as it deserved. Almost every major topic discussed could justly have been elaborated to book length; many lesser areas deserve monographic treatment. In some instances, persons and events have been omitted, not because they were unimportant, but because a general account cannot possibly include everything. Selection is, indeed, difficult, and each author applies selective criteria differently.

It is bromidic, of course, to say that a book is the product of many minds and hands, but the truism of this commonplace cannot be denied. *The People's Health* could not have been written as it is without the co-operation from such a variety of agencies and such a large number of persons that it is virtually impossible to enumerate all of them and thank each one. The Mayo Association of Rochester provided two generous grants that made research and publication possible. A grant from the Graduate School of the University of Minnesota enabled me to spend a summer in research. Librarians, who seldom are praised sufficiently, guided me to sources, secured scarce titles, and helped check citations. I would be most ungrateful if I failed to acknowledge the constant friendly assistance of Miss Eleanor C. Barthelemy, librarian of the Minnesota Department of Health. Others in the department who invited me to accompany them on trips, ferreted out information, explained procedure and policy, or read portions of the manuscript (although they have no responsibility for the final draft) include H. S. Adams, Dr. R. N. Barr, H. M. Bosch, J. W. Brower, O. E. Brownell, Dr. A. J. Chesley, Dr. D. S. Fleming, Mrs. Marie Ford, William Griffiths, Dr. H. G. Irvine, Dr. W. A. Jordan, Dr. Paul Kabler, Anne Kimball, Dr. Helen L. Knudsen, Dr. Hilbert Mark, G. S. Michaelsen, Dr. C. B. Nelson, Ann S. Nyquist, Dr. N. O. Pearce, H. G. Rogers, Dr. A. B. Rosenfield, Harry Smith, Dr. P. T. Watson, Professor H. A. Whittaker, Mrs. Netta Wilson, and F. L. Woodward. Dr. Orianna McDaniel, Professor Frederic H. Bass, O. C. Pierson, and Dr. Hibbert W.

[3] On this subject, see Laurence Wyatt, *Intergovernmental Relations in Public Health* (Minneapolis, 1951). This is *Research Monograph No. 4* in a series entitled *Intergovernmental Relations in the United States as Observed in the State of Minnesota* and edited by William Anderson and Edward W. Weidner.

Hill all gave graciously of their time in interviews. The city health departments of Minneapolis, St. Paul, and Duluth furnished information relative to municipal programs. Superintendents of waterworks in smaller cities took time to guide me through their plants; Indian agents on several reservations explained aspects of Indian health; visiting nurses in many communities explained duties and procedures; hotel inspectors took me on a tour of restaurants, resorts, and summer camps; state and local laboratory workers explained techniques. All these and others have helped to determine the matrix of this book.

Professor A. C. Krey has demonstrated a sustained interest during the progress of the book, and Dean Theodore C. Blegen, who was largely responsible for the inception of the project, has supported it warmly and generously. Dr. Robert Rosenthal of St. Paul always could take time from a busy practice to answer professional questions baffling to a layman. The person whom I relied on the most during the days of digging and putting-together was Clodaugh Neiderheiser. My debt to her is a real one, and mere mention of my appreciation for her work and loyalty discharges it only in part. I have the greatest admiration also for the editorial skill of Mrs. Mary Wheelhouse Berthel, associate editor on the staff of the Minnesota Historical Society, where the bulk of the research and all the writing for this volume was accomplished. Competent, tactful, and knowledgeable, Mrs. Berthel through her editing has improved the book so much that I feel fortunate indeed to have had the benefit of her wisdom and talent.

Despite the many helping hands, I, of course, assume responsibility for the selection, organization, and interpretation of materials. It is hoped that the people of Minnesota will take pride in what the state has accomplished through its public health program and will lend aid and encouragement to the end that this program may be steadily expanded and made more effective.

PHILIP D. JORDAN

University of Minnesota
  Minneapolis

Table of Contents

1. Salubrious Minnesota 1
2. A Doctor Goes to War 17
3. The Shoulder Straps Come Off 30
4. With Probe and Microscope 44
5. The End of an Era 61
6. Years of Growth 77
7. The Fight for Pure Water 99
8. With Pump and Pipe 125
9. Toward Better Food and Drink 148
10. Moving Toward Modernity 176
11. Epidemics in the North Woods 197
12. Health Officer *vs.* Medicine Man 220
13. Control of Venereal Disease 243
14. The White Plague 266
15. Streams That Run Filth 286
16. Keeping Workers Fit 308
17. Eternal Vigilance 331
18. Blue Cap and Black Bag 352

19. Health of Mother and Child	373
20. Old Plagues Don't Die	394
21. Adding Life to Years	418
22. Wanted: More Hospital Beds	436
23. The Mentally Ill	454
24. Patterns for Tomorrow's Health	474

List of Illustrations

Surgeon Hewitt and "Fan"	48
Dr. Justus Ohage, St. Paul Health Officer, in His Office	48
Secretaries of the State Board of Health	49
Hibbert W. Hill, Orianna McDaniel, Oscar C. Pierson, Frank F. Wesbrook, Harold A. Whittaker, Louis B. Wilson	80
Minnesota Department of Health Laboratory in the 1890s	81
How Pollution May Enter a Poorly Constructed Well	112
How Flies May Spread Disease	112
The Public Drinking Cup	113
The Mississippi River Before and After Construction of the Twin Cities Sewage Treatment Plant	144
Old Type Water Pipes	145
Rats Are a Menace to Health	145
How Not To Serve Butter	208
How Not To Wait on Table	208
A Modern Milk Plant with Pasteurization Equipment	209
A Lumber Camp Kitchen	240
A Lumber Camp "Sitting Room"	240

An Indian Diphtheria Immunization Clinic 241

Posters Used in a Campaign Against Venereal Disease . . . 272

Effect of Stream Pollution on Fish 273

Pollution of Rainy River from Paper Mill Wastes 304

A Sand Blaster Protected According to Public Health
Standards 305

E. B. Hoag Examining School Children 368

Therapy for Youngsters 368

Modern Care for the Aged 369

St. Luke's Hospital, Duluth, in the 1880s 400

A Visiting Nurse of Yesterday 400

Crowded Conditions in a State Hospital 401

Mortality Rates, Tuberculosis and Typhoid Fever 432

Mortality Rates, Diphtheria and Smallpox 433

Mortality Rates, Diarrheal Diseases and Infants 464

Sanitation Notices Issued by the Eveleth Board of Health . 465

For

A. C. MOERKE, M.D.

GEORGE J. PEARSON, M.D.

ROBERT ROSENTHAL, M.D.

The People's Health

1

Salubrious Minnesota

I REGARD Minnesota as a very desirable country to migrate to," wrote a New Englander in 1852, "on account of its healthful climate." He spoke of thousands of Easterners who were prevented from going to the rich lands of the West because of the prevalence of bilious fevers and malaria. But in Minnesota immigrants would be free from disease. Minnesota, he continued, possessed a climate which for purity and salubrity was not equaled by any other area east of the Rocky Mountains.[1]

Buoyant enthusiasm for Minnesota's climate was widespread. From early days travelers had commented upon its bracing air, its healthful scent of pine and spruce, and its ability to make a sick man well and a well man better. A settler at St. Anthony's Falls exclaimed joyfully that he experienced no lassitude and prostration of energy so common in other sections. "We have more sunshine than in any country I ever saw," he wrote pridefully. Guidebooks and private letters sang praises of a health-giving region. They told of a dry, pure atmosphere full of electricity, which gave strength to sufferers. They told of consumptives — poor, pale, haggard, and weak — who, after living in Minnesota one or two years, became hale and hearty, fat and strong. They said that no one in Minnesota thought of catching cold. They extended their arms in welcome: "And now, ye poor, pale coughing weak ones, God has made this country for you; come out here, and may God keep you all out of Heaven these many years yet, to labor and to bless the world."[2]

In all corners of the nation the invitation was heard and answered. After the Civil War the state looked forward to an annual migration of invalids, who settled in hotels and boardinghouses, determined to

[1] *Northampton* (Massachusetts) *Courier*, September 28, 1852.
[2] *Northampton Courier*, November 30, 1852, April 26, 1853.

gain their health. At St. Anthony the Winslow House took them in. This famous ordinary, eager to capitalize on the prevalent water-cure fad, became the Western Hygiean Home for Invalids after the Civil War. There patients ran the gamut of baths, from total immersion to wet packs. Manasseh Pettengill, shrewd businessman, opened the mineral waters of the Chalybeate Springs at St. Anthony for public use. Attractive benches dotted landscaped grounds, where health seekers walked leisurely when not quaffing medicinal waters guaranteed to be good for a variety of diseases, including diabetes and tuberculosis. Band concerts and dances attracted the not-too-sick, and ice-cream parlors and cigar stands beckoned to others. Both White Bear Lake and Lake Minnetonka were ideal health resorts. At Lake Elmo the Park Palace Hotel sought to make invalids comfortable, and near Cedar Lake the fashionable Oak Grove House strove for its share of business. The Dalles of the St. Croix, St. Croix Lake, and Frontenac, known as the "Newport of the Northwest," paid particular attention to the wants of the unhealthy.[3]

Stillwater, Winona, and Duluth were hosts to hundreds of unfortunates. Their newspapers advertised scores of nostrums, and druggists dispensed patent medicines guaranteed to cure. Braces, therapeutic corsets, and magnetic rings were all advertised. Consumptives put down gallons of whisky and cod-liver oil. Early in the 1870s both St. Paul and Duluth gained fame as havens for hay-fever victims. Camps and inns offered locations where no city dirt fouled the air and cigar makers advertised tobacco that, it was promised, could not stimulate a single sneeze.

There was real reason why Minnesota sought eagerly for the trade of the sick. In the first place, many residents firmly believed that the climate did restore health. Moreover, the state wanted the profits that came from visitors searching for improvement. Competition between states also complicated the picture. Florida and Minnesota, together with other states, were making strenuous efforts to attract consumptives, pledging immediate benefits. The air was balmy and kind in Florida and California. Patients could fill their injured lungs with ozone, kind to tissues. They could be out of doors more than in frigid Minnesota. Those were the arguments that attracted the sick away from Minnesota. On the other hand, the north country pointed out

[3] Helen Clapesattle, "Florida's Rival," in *Northwest Life*, 16:24 (October, 1943); Bertha L. Heilbron, "Health and Recreation in Minnesota," in *Minnesota Alumni Weekly*, 33:276 (January 13, 1934).

that Florida's warm climate was enervating and Minnesota's weather was stimulating. Florida had a sedative climate, but Minnesota had a tonic atmosphere. Even physicians disagreed as to which was the better. Both regions captured their share of the invalid business.

Distinguished persons journeyed either to the northland or to the sunny south. A few tried both regions. Some were benefited and others were not. To Minnesota in quest of health came Schuyler Colfax, once vice-president of the United States. He found what he sought, and his testimony undoubtedly influenced others to come.[4] Artemus Ward, the great humorist, was advised to go to Minnesota, but he preferred England. Edward Eggleston, Hoosier author, and Thoreau, New England lover of the out-of-doors, sampled Minnesota climate. Clara Barton, founder of the American Red Cross, and Horace Greeley, New York newspaperman, visited the state and commented upon its healthfulness. The list of distinguished visitors was long. Scores of other men and women, with little wealth and no claim to fame, laboriously arrived.

For many, only gravestones marked their exertions. There was Gilbert Horton, of Elizabeth, New Jersey, who spent a year in Minnesota before he died; and Stephen Case, from Pennsylvania, who returned home swearing the climate had not helped him; and James A. Fisher, of Connecticut, who died after three years' residence. With each death, newspapers explained that Minnesota's climate still was effective, but that the deceased had not lived in it long enough.

The truth was hard to face. Minnesota was not "a land where Nature has lavished her choicest gifts and where sickness has no dwelling."[5] No amount of wishful thinking could guarantee health. Not even the state's much-touted climate was potent enough to effect a cure when tissues were permanently destroyed or when smallpox struck. Hay-fever victims were relieved, but not cured. Tuberculosis patients, if they submitted to prolonged rest and followed an adequate diet, might improve. Some recovered, but others died. Probably a regimen of rest and diet did more for them than climate. An infected body could not be made well by a salubrious climate alone. It was absurd to boast that Duluth residents did not feel the cold, just as it was ridiculous to assert that overcoats were left at home when the thermometer stood at sixteen degrees below zero. Many a patient had

[4] *St. Paul Daily Press*, January 23, 1872.
[5] Henry H. Sibley, "Description of Minnesota," in *Minnesota Historical Collections*, 1:42.

lost faith in Dr. Brewer Mattocks' *Minnesota as a Home for Invalids* after he had failed to find health in the North Star State.

Even the medical profession, in 1874, attempted to explain why the state's climate seemed to be failing. Dr. J. E. Finch, chairman of the State Board of Health committee on epidemics, climatology, and hygiene, reported that the weather of 1873 had an unfavorable effect on consumption and catarrh. He deplored the lack of an Indian summer, said that lake currents were unfavorable to health, and regretted a lack of electricity in the air.[6]

So exaggerated became defenses of Minnesota's salubrious climate that a series of tales developed to poke fun at the state's health claims. Essentially they were a people's wit, crude and pungent, yet devastatingly pointed. A testy invalid from Detroit inquired of a fine-looking young man whether he had come to Minnesota for his health. The youth replied that when he arrived he could not control his arms or legs, that he could not command a single muscle or make use of a single faculty. He said that he was toothless, unable to speak, and was completely deprived of all power to help himself. But, he continued, he commenced to gain immediately upon his arrival and had scarcely experienced a sick day since.

"My limbs soon became strong," he said, "my sight and voice came to me slowly, and a full set of teeth, regular and firm, appeared."

"Remarkable, miraculous!" exclaimed the invalid. "Surely, sir, you must have been greatly reduced in flesh?"

"Madame," answered the lad, "I weighed but nine pounds. I was *born* in Minnesota."[7]

Such good-humored bunkum, of course, delighted natives, but it was relished little by patients who had been victimized into coming to Minnesota. The scores of honest enthusiasts who sincerely believed in the health-giving properties of the climate were not to blame. The nineteenth century itself was at fault. In all times, the sick have followed fads and all too frequently have endorsed with equal impartiality mumbo jumbo and science. They clamored for heroic doses until Oliver Wendell Holmes satirized their abnormal appetites; they purged and puked themselves with the *lobelia inflata* of the botanic schools; and they followed the dubious teachings of the hydropathists and Grahamites. They petitioned the spirit world to prescribe for them. Their faith was pinned to Old World practices — a sharp ax un-

[6] *St. Paul Daily Press*, February 4, 1874.
[7] *Pioneer-Press* (St. Paul), June 25, 1875.

der the bed to cut labor pains or a deer's heart worn under the vest to ward off the plague.

Weather and climate, of course, since classical times had been believed to influence the health of man. The belief grew with the centuries, gaining credence during the Middle Ages and influencing the thought of nations colonizing the New World in the sixteenth century. By then, scientists as well as laymen thought of climatology as a respectable discipline. The great plagues of eighteenth-century America were explained in part by climatic conditions. After the nation became free and began to spread westward, typical frontier illnesses were blamed on climate. Pioneer doctors spoke knowingly of evil vapors that rose from swamp lands, said that the American Bottoms near St. Louis had a fever-and-ague climate, and described southern states as possessing a climate that was enervating. Most medical colleges instructed their students in the relationship of weather to health, basing their lectures upon principles laid down in James Johnson's famous *The Influence of Tropical Climates on European Constitutions.*

Both Cincinnati, Ohio, and Lexington, Kentucky, were centers of medical instruction during the early decades of the nineteenth century. Dr. Daniel Drake, known as the West's most distinguished medical researcher and lecturer, imposed an elaborate structure of climatic doctrines upon young students in his classes. They, in turn, spread the gospel up and down the Ohio and Mississippi rivers. Even Samuel Thomson, establishing his botanic publishing house in Columbus, Ohio, paid particular attention to the relationship between weather and health. Scores of frontier physicians kept careful computations of temperature, rainfall, and aridity. From New Orleans to St. Paul, doctors advised their patients to seek a change of climate. Military surgeons, stationed in far-flung wilderness posts, spoke knowingly of the effect of climate upon troops and sometimes recommended that a soldier be transferred to a more salubrious climate.

Scores of "home doctor" books, as dear to emigrants as the family Bible, told plainly where a pioneer should settle if he wished to enjoy health and warned him against "sick-bringing" miasma. Miasma, the frontiersman learned, was poisonous material or noxious effluvium floating above putrid swamps or even over prairie lowlands. Sometimes it meant a contaminated atmosphere. The miasma-minded settler slept with his windows shuttered and permitted his children to go abroad at night only if their mouths were covered. It was but natural, then, that Minnesota should fall heir to a nation-wide concept and that its physicians should endorse ideas that could not be proved false until a new science brought its enlightenment.

Climatotherapy, possessing some merit, had its vogue and had to run out its course. Competent men, laboring to do their best with what knowledge they possessed, had long been anxious about the state's claim of a climate that would help anybody. They were skeptical of purple passages maintaining that the "climate of Minnesota is one of the healthiest in the world." Hard, dry statistics do not always spell truth, but frequently they sketch out a trend or show tendencies. Medical men knew that deaths totaled 6,061 in Minnesota in 1875, and of these 621 were credited to tuberculosis. The greatest number of deaths from consumption occurred in March, and Hennepin County reported the largest number. Health officers, studying these figures, worried.[8]

A group of physicians in 1874 set about to investigate as scientifically as possible the beneficial values of Minnesota's climate. "It has come to the minds of intelligent observers," they said, "that important questions relating to the actual benefits to be derived from our climate by different classes of invalids, as well as what, if any, may be the prevailing disease tendency to be guarded against by our people, may now be studied and answered — that now such means of investigation exist as may afford conclusions in a measure satisfactory. It cannot be doubted that it is the duty of the state, not only for the information and benefit of its own citizens, but also in response to a general public inquiry of vast importance, to answer questions pertaining to this subject as soon as intelligent and reliable answers can be made from actual observation and a collation of facts." [9]

Every thinking man knew, of course, that Minnesota never had been free from disease. But some believed that diseases, including cholera and consumption, had never originated in the state; that they had been imported by soldiers, trappers, settlers, and immigrants. As early as 1849, the very year that Minnesota became a territory, the steamer "Cora" docked at St. Paul with cholera aboard. Two lumberjacks came down the gangplank and died shortly thereafter. Later that year Winnebago Indians at Sauk Rapids were afflicted with smallpox. Cholera continued to come up the Mississippi on the "Lamartine" and other river boats, and smallpox continued to strike down Indians. At Stillwater scarlet fever swept through the youthful population in

[8] Frederick B. Goddard, *Where to Emigrate and Why*, 237 (New York, 1869); *Pioneer Press*, December 27, 1876.
[9] Minnesota State Board of Health, *Annual Reports*, January, 1876, p. 58.

1848. The editor of a St. Paul paper commented in 1862 that diphtheria was becoming prevalent. The next year "spotted fever" appeared to mar Minnesota's salubrious climate. Physicians reported considerable sickness among children in 1868, and whole families of little ones were said to be suffering from scarlet fever, scarletina, or a "low" form of typhoid fever. Severe colds also were widespread. At both Anoka and Ottawa sickness increased. The majority of patients at St. Joseph's Hospital in St. Paul were typhoid victims.[10]

From pioneer days, then, to 1876 the state looked upon a pageant of ills that seemed to be increasing with every decade and appeared to give the lie to careless claims that Minnesota, in general, was without sickness. Even Henry H. Sibley, staunch supporter and builder of the commonwealth, admitted that malaria, or fever and ague, commonly believed never to have visited the state, appeared along the Mississippi and lower Minnesota rivers soon after he arrived at Mendota. Sibley also testified, over his signature, that "Rapid consumption, caused by pneumonia, has always found victims in the Indian villages and camps." Ole Rynning, after an American tour, wrote that an unaccustomed climate usually caused some kind of sickness among new settlers during the first year.[11]

It was to sift observations like these and to come to fact regarding the climate that the group began its investigation. First, it placed Minnesota in its proper geographic setting and compiled tables of atmospheric pressure and rainfall. Then a long series of questions was sent to physicians. Their replies seemed inclusive, but their voluntary notations were more revealing. Some clung to the notion that Minnesota was healthful "no matter what," and others tempered their enthusiasm with caution. A few specified that, in their practice, they had seen tuberculosis patients improve, but went on to admit that the same benefits might have been just as pronounced in other sections of the nation.

Finally, the committee concluded that the "climate of Minnesota is stimulating and curative to most chronic diseases of the lungs and air passages, except certain forms of catarrhal diseases of an inflammatory nature." But, the report continued, such beneficial results "are due largely to influences exerted directly or indirectly upon the func-

---

[10] *Minnesota Pioneer* (St. Paul), June 7, August 23, 1849; *Messenger* (Stillwater), December 14, 1858; *St. Paul Press*, January 3, 1862; *St. Paul Pioneer*, January 28, 1863, December 9, 1870; *Minneapolis Tribune*, February 6, 1868.

[11] State Board of Health, *Annual Reports*, 1876, p. 61; Theodore C. Blegen, ed., *Ole Rynning's True Account of America*, 90 (Northfield, 1926).

tions of nutrition." Its conclusion — objective and fair in the light of the knowledge of the times — was that, "while the climate of our State, in common with that of all others, has its imperfections, its disadvantages to some classes of invalids, as well as its great advantages to others, an intelligent discrimination should be exercised on the part of the medical profession of the country, and of invalids themselves, concerning who should come and when they should come to Minnesota; and, finally, that it is easier to preserve health than to restore it, whether by climatic influence or artificial hygienic means." [12]

Although early physicians put some faith in Minnesota's salubrious climate, they found it a great hindrance in their practice. The pioneer doctor fought swollen streams in the spring, beat off swarms of angry, buzzing mosquitoes in June, sweltered under scorching heat during the summer, and pitted his strength against snow and ice throughout a long winter. Only during beautiful Indian summer did the physician feel that the weather was ideal for his practice. Then rivers no longer rolled roisterously, the bugs were gone, and summer's heat had softened to a balmy beatitude. But always he was aware of the shortness of Minnesota's most ideal season and of winter's rapid approach.

No matter what the weather, the frontier doctor was expected to answer calls. He never knew what baffling problem faced him when he lifted a cabin latch to step into a settler's log home. Most people waited to call the doctor until they had exhausted all domestic remedies. By then, the patient was apt to be sick indeed. Relatives cooled a sick man in summer with a fan of leaves; in winter, piles of faggots were fed into clay-and-stick fireplaces to provide warmth that seemed stifling. Clusters of medicinal herbs hung from rafters, their pungent odors stronger because of the intense heat. The doctor noticed drying roots of the white pond lily, rolled bundles of birch bark, clusters of sumac berries, and bark carefully slit from the balsam. Pond-lily tea was believed useful in bowel complaints and as a gargle; birch bark flavored medicines; sumac-berry tea cleansed the mouth of fever's horrid taste; and a plaster of balsam was applied to burns and scalds.

Tucked carefully away in a dry spot was the family medical book. Frequently it was wrapped in a square of tanned deerskin for protection. Sometimes it reposed in a place of honor in the corner cupboard or the dower chest. From Quebec to Minnesota and from New York to the first crude bookshops of St. Paul, domestic medical texts were sold. After the Civil War peddlers hawked them through the north

[12] State Board of Health, *Annual Reports*, 1876, p. 80.

country. Translated in foreign tongues, they were as necessary to the frontiersmen as rifle or plow. John C. Gunn advertised his domestic medicine as the "poor man's friend." *The Botanic Physician*, carefully prepared by Elisha Smith, not only indicated the therapeutic uses of native plants, but also instructed the wilderness Martha in the arts of making soap, baking saleratus biscuits, and dyeing cloth without the use of a mordant. Many a physician not only endorsed the use of these volumes, but also based his own practice upon them. Morris Mattson's *The American Vegetable Practice* and John Kost's *Domestic Medicine* were both extensively relied upon in Minnesota.

The doctor did what he could with his limited resources. Frequently he wished that he might be called upon before disease struck and not afterward. "An ounce of prevention," the wise ones said, "is worth a pound of cure." But preventive medicine was practically unknown before Minnesota became a state, and it was commonly believed to be the physician's task to treat the sick, not to keep a well man well. The major task of Dr. Edward Purcell, the surgeon at Fort Snelling, was to bring a sick trooper back to health. Purcell had not been tutored in the arts of preventing disease. Indeed, he, unlike some healers, went to Fort Snelling to make money. "You may think it strange," he wrote to his brother in March, 1819, "that I have consented to go with the Regiment out of the world, as you may call it, but the fact is I go, not because I like it, but because I think I can make money." Unfortunately Purcell left few accounts of medical practice at the Minnesota military post.[13]

In 1849 President Zachary Taylor set aside a reservation at Fort Ripley, and Assistant Surgeon J. Frazier Head was ordered there. Well trained and a discriminating observer, Dr. Head was not overly impressed with the salubrity of Minnesota's climate. "Fires are necessary to comfort," he said, "during a part of every month in the year except, occasionally, July and August; and cattle must be foraged from seven to nine months." The post itself was no picturesque place, for it was built upon a sandy plateau, partially drained by shallow ravines. Above and below the fort, Head continued, the river skirted a narrow belt of swampy land, usually partially inundated in spring. The sense of desolation was completed by the ravages of a forest fire, "leaving hundreds of scorched and decaying pines still standing, or encumbering the ground." Head enumerated carefully and vividly the fruits

[13] John M. Armstrong, "Edward Purcell: The First Physician in Minnesota," in *Annals of Medical History*, 7:169 (March, 1935).

and wild flowers and inventoried local animals and birds. He saw the golden eagle, the golden plover, and the green heron and watched the spring and autumn migrations of ducks — mallards, teal, bluebills — that frequented the rice beds.

Yet, naturalist that he was, Head was more interested in the health of troops and of immigrants whom he saw slowly moving toward the village of Crow Wing. Malarial fevers were prevalent and cases of cholera, diarrhea, dysentery, and catarrh were numerous. At the same time that Minnesota was beginning to be advocated as a healthful place, Head was writing: "The three summers during which the post has been occupied have been marked by the prevalence of dysentery and diarrhoea — to a greater extent among civilians employed at the post, and residents in the neighborhood, than among the troops." Then he came to a cautious conclusion: "Although the sudden variations of temperature, particularly the alternation of hot days with cold nights, might be considered amply sufficient to account for this tendency, these diseases are said not to have prevailed extensively in the Territory previous to the year 1849; and their frequency of late years should probably be referred to the epidemic influence which seems to have extended more or less over the whole continent, rather than to any local causes." He believed that residents of Minnesota were temperate, industrious, and healthy.[14]

Three years after Fort Ridgely was established in 1853 another military doctor recorded his impressions of climate and health. Assistant Surgeon Alexander B. Hasson, an accomplished practitioner, treated both soldiers and civilians, laboriously making his way over frozen prairies to treat the sick. "On one occasion, during the present winter," he reported to the surgeon general in 1856, "when the mercury was six degrees below zero, the atmosphere was so thick with drifting clouds of snow, borne onward by a furious northwest wind, that at three o'clock in the afternoon a house could not be seen at the distance of forty yards; and it was almost impossible to keep one's eyes open, even for a single moment, in the face of the storm." One night he amputated both legs of a woman whose feet had been frozen in a storm. He used chloroform for all surgery, except a urethrotomy, when he tried a local application of ice and salt.[15]

[14] F. Paul Prucha, "Fort Ripley: The Post and the Military Reservation," in *Minnesota History*, 28:205–224 (September, 1947); Richard H. Coolidge, comp., *Statistical Report on the Sickness and Mortality in the Army of the United States, Compiled from the Records of the Surgeon General's Office, January, 1839, to January, 1855*, 61 (34 Congress, 1 session, Senate Executive Documents, no. 96 — serial 827).

[15] Coolidge, *Sickness and Mortality in the Army, 1839–55*, 72.

Even more pertinent observations were made by Hasson's successor, Dr. N. S. Crowell, who reported in 1857 that about November first diseases of the throat and respiratory organs began to appear. "Many cases of these disorders," Crowell continued, "occurred simultaneously, and from the universality with which it afterwards prevailed, not only among the troops and others exposed to the inclemency of the weather, but also among children, it is probable that the origin of the disease was due to some peculiar condition of the atmosphere." He noted that, although the weather was unusually mild, it also was exceedingly damp and unwholesome.[16]

Civilian physicians coped with the identical diseases that troubled military surgeons. They had to be prepared to pit their skills against not only native ills, but also imported maladies. "In such a variety of climates and exposures," wrote a layman describing health in the Mississippi Valley, "in a country alternately covered in one point with the thickest forests, and in another spreading out into grassy plains — in one section having a very dry, and in another a very humid atmosphere — and having every degree of temperature, from that of the Arctic regions, to that of the West Indies, there must necessarily be generated all the forms and varieties of disease, that spring simply from climate." Cholera, smallpox, diphtheria, typhoid, and venereal diseases kept doctors busy.[17]

Perhaps a majority of Minnesota pioneer physicians were not graduated from a medical school. No more than fifteen medical schools were in existence in 1832, but the number was to increase rapidly. Faculties were small and course offerings limited. Daniel Drake was convinced that every medical college ought to have eight professors, and he recommended instruction in institutes of medicine, anatomy, practice of medicine and clinical cases, surgery, materia medica, chemistry and pharmacy, obstetrics, and medical jurisprudence. Drake was not enthusiastic over the age-old system of learning medicine by becoming an apprentice to the practitioner. He thought, too, that short courses could not possibly prepare a student to heal adequately.[18]

The medical student, striving earnestly to train himself, was handicapped on every hand before the Civil War. Instruments to measure climactic conditions were crude and expensive, as were surgical tools.

[16] Coolidge, *Statistical Report on the Sickness and Mortality in the Army, January, 1855, to January, 1860*, 44 (36 Congress, 1 session, Senate Executive Documents, no. 52 — serial 1035).
[17] Timothy Flint, *The History and Geography of the Mississippi Valley*, 1:35 (Cincinnati, 1832).
[18] Daniel Drake, *Medical Education and the Medical Profession in the United States*, essay 3 (Cincinnati, 1832).

A few surgical manufacturers in the East were producing superior instruments, yet the frontier physician in Minnesota before 1850 was fortunate if he possessed a pocket kit. The clinical thermometer had not been perfected. In its place some men substituted a curious contraption consisting of a glass tube filled with liquid in which a tiny naked figure floated. The patient held the tube, and the heat of his body, it was believed, caused the figure to rise. The higher the fever, the higher climbed the miniature in the tube.

Prepared drugs were scarce in the north country, although, as time went on, St. Paul pharmacists imported crude and prepared drugs up the Mississippi from Cincinnati and overland from Philadelphia and New York. The student even found it difficult to secure anatomical specimens for dissection. Public sentiment had long been opposed to the mutilation of corpses. Few states made legal provision for supplying anatomical materials. Most students resorted to grave-stealing. So great were their depredations that frequently guards were stationed over new graves. A special grave bomb was used in the 1840s. Buried directly above the casket, about eighteen inches under ground, the bomb exploded when the resurrectionist's long, iron grave probe touched it. A "doctor's riot" was touched off in New York in 1788 because of a dissectionist at work. At least one Ohio school closed its doors because of public opposition to grave-robbery. The body of John Scott Harrison, son of President William Henry Harrison, was pilfered from a Cincinnati cemetery in 1878, causing a nation-wide scandal and resulting in the revision of an Ohio statute to make anatomical specimens easier to secure.[19]

The problem was acute in Minnesota. The territorial legislature had passed an act to prevent violation of the sepulchre, but it was not until 1872 that provision first was made to legally supply anatomical specimens for scientific research. Between 1849 and 1872 students and physicians had to procure bodies as best they could. It is related that doctors exhumed the bodies of the Indians hanged at Mankato and carried them off for dissection. Dr. William J. Mayo's father secured the body of Cut Nose, and young Will and his brother learned their osteology from it. Dr. Charles N. Hewitt kept the body of an Indian pickled in brine in a hogshead in his barn.

Somehow or other student problems were mastered and young

---

[19] A. G. Ross, "The Fine Art of Body Snatching," in *Medical Economics*, 21:64–68, 103, 107, 109 (March, 1944); "Scenes in a Medical Student's Life — Resurrectionizing," in the *Scalpel* 7:93–100 (April, 1855); *Cincinnati Enquirer*, May 31, 1878, June 1, 2, 3, 4, 1867.

physicians followed the frontier to hang crude shingles outside new offices. Yet, even in 1872, many Minnesotans were without resident doctors. In that year thirty-five miles separated Otter Tail City from the nearest physician. The country doctor found roads almost impassable because of mudholes, stumps, rocks, ruts, and heavy snowbanks. When he finally succeeded in fighting his way to a primitive cabin, he found "absolute ignorance of the simplest sanitary principles." Dr. P. A. Walling of Grand Rapids remembered graphically what happened when he asked for clean water and towels: "I have had a wash dish brought to me with a rim of dirt at the water line, two or three rags drawn in at the bottom, and a towel at the sight of which a printer would die of envy." [20]

The earliest Ramsey County practitioners learned that climate salubrious for patients was difficult for the doctor, who had to brave the elements. Drs. John Jay Dewey and William C. Renfro, the former a graduate of New York's Albany Medical College and the latter possessed of no formal training, arrived at St. Paul in 1847. Dewey opened the town's first drugstore and prospered, but Renfro was frozen to death. Two years later seven men were practicing. One of them, Dr. N. Barbour, advertised "a good assortment of Drug Medicines, Paints, and Dye Stuffs and will also Prescribe Medicines for all those who wish it according to the Eclectic practice, as taught in the Cincinnati Reformed College of Medicine." [21]

An old settler at St. Anthony left a vivid picture of Dr. John H. Murphy at work. His office on Front Street, a short distance below the mill, was the focal point for residents in ill health, who frequented his primitive establishment for advice and medication. St. Anthony boasted nearly a hundred buildings, with a sawmill, a lathe, five stores, and a grocery when Murphy hung out his shingle. He, too, had to face Minnesota's rigorous climate.

"The morning of April 30, 1851," remembered Colonel John H. Stevens, "was the coldest for the season ever known in the country. The wind was blowing from the north like a hurricane. The air was full of snow. The river bank was full and the waves were high. It was deemed almost impossible to cross the river either in a bateau, skiff, or canoe. It was necessary that I should have communication with

[20] *St. Paul Daily Press*, January 7, 1872; Constant Larson, *History of Douglas and Grant Counties, Minnesota*, 277 (Indianapolis, 1916); P. A. Walling, "The Country Doctor and Aseptic Surgery," in *Northwestern Lancet*, 18:443 (November 1, 1898).
[21] John M. Armstrong, "History of Medicine in Ramsey County," in *Minnesota Medicine*, 27:701 (October, 1938); *Minnesota Pioneer*, May 12, 1849.

Saint Anthony, for the services of Dr. Murphy, who resided there, were required in my family. The aid of three as good boatmen as ever swung an oar, with Captain Tapper, at their head, was secured. The question was anxiously discussed: Can any water craft at our command withstand the fierce wind, high waves and swift current? Captain Tapper thought one large bateau could weather the storm, but we were short of hands. Fortunately Rev. C. A. Newcomb, of the Methodist church, on the east side, joined us. . . . With much difficulty and some danger the crossing was made, and they safely returned with Dr. Murphy. About noon on that bleak, cold, eventful day my first child and the first-born white child on the west bank of the Falls, was added to my happy household." [22]

Murphy, like many of his nineteenth-century colleagues, wore a Prince Albert coat. A spool of silk thread rested in an ample pocket. When Murphy needed to suture, he fished for the spool, snipped off a length, sharpened his pocketknife on his boot heel, and said: "This is going to hurt and hurt like Hell, but I can't help it, so look out." Yet many preferred his rough, but kind, manner to the slick tricks employed by some physicians. These men of medicine were not averse to stealing one another's patients, and so developed the saying: "Physicians with the fastest horses always have the most patients." [23]

Winona, formerly called Wabasha Prairie, testified eloquently in 1852 that Minnesota's climate was far from healthful. Its early practitioners — one of whom ran a livery stable to supplement his income while another managed a general store — knew of the "sickly season," when hot, dry weather stirred clouds of miasma from drying sloughs and marshes. Malaria and bilious diseases assumed epidemic form. But settlers blamed the climate rather than the presence of the anopheles mosquito.[24] Newcomers, pitting their strength against land and climate, saw the doctor doing his utmost to alleviate pain and cure disease in a land that overenthusiastic zealots claimed was healthful.

The organization of each new county, whether in prairie regions, the Big Woods, or amid the majestic beauty of the ore country, found the immigrant and his doctor facing difficult problems. Even in the days of the fur companies, when pelts were wealth, the chill of northern woods ate into men's bodies and brought them to the doctor. For many years Dr. Charles William Wulff Borup was the only physician

[22] Arthur S. Hamilton, "History of Medicine in Hennepin County," in *Minnesota Medicine*, 22:785 (November, 1939).
[23] Hamilton, in *Minnesota Medicine*, 22:785, 838 (November, December, 1939).
[24] "History of Medicine in Winona County" and "Malaria Threat in Minnesota," in *Minnesota Medicine*, 23:252, 585 (April, August, 1940).

west of the Sault Ste. Marie and north of Fort Snelling. With headquarters at La Pointe, Borup traveled with his primitive kit of instruments along the south shore of Lake Superior and as far west as Leech Lake. In 1835 he ordered from the New York office of his employer, the American Fur Company, a pound of camphor, two ounces of quicksilver, and a pint of spirits of pennyroyal. He needed also a good tooth-drawer and two gross of assorted vials with corks.[25]

After the heyday of the trapper, the lumberjack moved out from Duluth. And after the woodcutter came the miner to loosen the hard ores near Vermilion Lake and to scoop up the dirt and coarse pebbles of the Mesabi Range. Ore explorers were urged to take with them "two or three simple remedies for biliousness, colds, and dysentery." The trail from Duluth to Vermilion led through swamps and forests, over mountains and through gorges, and the explorer must submit himself to disease-carrying effluvia from interminable swamps infested with insects. Among the early arrivals in Tower was Dr. Isaac van Dusen, a homeopath. The Minnesota Iron Company, however, soon brought its own physicians and in 1889 established a company hospital at Soudan. Dr. W. E. Harwood from Illinois was placed in charge. Harwood had had previous experience with mining practice at Ishpeming, Michigan.[26]

Frequently physicians from the ore country, coming to St. Paul on business, met doctors employed by lumber interests. The St. Croix Lumber Company engaged the professional services of a Dr. Fitch in 1838. At Stillwater, a German — Dr. Christopher Carli — ministered to private patients as well as to lumberjacks. The Thomsonians, who believed in vegetable drugs, were represented by a Mrs. Page, who practiced at Hudson. After 1850 the number of doctors along the St. Croix increased rapidly. Like their brothers on the range, lumber company doctors faced one emergency after another. Shafts and saws both are dangerous. Frequently a laborer's hands so stiffened in Minnesota winter weather that he handled his tools clumsily and an accident resulted. When that happened the climate was blamed.

Lumbermen also put upon the climate the responsibility for the periodic epidemics of typhoid, scarlet fever, and diphtheria. Tuberculosis and cholera were also present in the camps. Captain Stephen Hanks was rafting logs down the St. Croix in the early 1850s when

[25] Richard Bardon, "The Background of Medical History for Northeastern Minnesota and the Lake Superior Region," in *Minnesota Medicine*, 21:127 (February, 1938).
[26] Newton H. and Horace V. Winchell, *Iron Ores of Minnesota*, 169 (Geological and Natural History Survey of Minnesota, *Bulletins*, no. 6 — Minneapolis, 1891); Owen W. Parker, "Pioneer Physicians of the Vermillion and Missabe Ranges of Minnesota," in *Minnesota Medicine*, 21:332 (May, 1938).

cholera struck. Four of his crew died. "Two were taken ill in the evening and were dead in the morning," said Hanks. "We stopped at the sand point between Willow River and Catfish Bar and I furnished the wood for coffins and Bowles made them. We buried them about a mile and a half above Catfish Bar on the top of the bluff. The rest of my crew deserted at Willow River." [27]

No physician believed that Minnesota's salubrious climate could cure cholera. Few doctors, as a matter of fact, pinned much faith to a fresh air cure. Perhaps it might have been better if they had. On one occasion a practitioner purchased calomel and strychnine and placed them in unmarked packets in opposite pockets. Then, forgetting what was in each packet, he mistakenly gave a patient the poison in place of the calomel. But patients dosed themselves with every conceivable remedy and frequently came to grief because of their own ministrations. Opium was used in large quantities in the Twin Cities and in Duluth during the 1870s. A standard gargle was an ounce of camphorated oil and five cents' worth of potash. "Whiskey," reported an editor seriously, "if given in sufficient quantities, is an infallible cure for lockjaw." Then he added waggishly: "You must have your lockjaw before you take your whiskey." From Mankato came news that the diphtheria patient could be cured if only he would gargle with water in which gunpowder had been dissolved.[28]

Even children, sturdy youngsters who enjoyed Minnesota's winters on skis and sleds, were told of innumerable remedies for frostbite and warned against the climate. Their practice of eating snow was said to be a frightful cause of catarrh, and snow- and ice-eating boys and girls "almost always have colds in the head and running noses." [29]

It was not until after a physician returned from the Civil War to inaugurate a public health program in the state that it was learned that not only climate, but also water supplies, sewerage systems, pure food, and sanitation in general determined the pattern of the people's health.

[27] "Medicine in Washington and Chisago Counties," in *Minnesota Medicine*, 21:504 (July, 1938).
[28] George E. Warner and Charles M. Foote, eds., *History of Washington County and the St. Croix Valley*, 471 (Minneapolis, 1881); *Minneapolis Tribune*, December 27, 1874, March 9, 1880; *Pioneer Press*, January 9, 1877.
[29] *Stillwater Gazette*, February 25, 1880.

2

A Doctor Goes to War

WAR CLOUDS hung heavily over the trim village of Geneva, New York, in April, 1861. All America was excited over Lincoln's call for volunteers, and Geneva was no exception. The grim threat to the nation finally had become a reality with the firing upon Fort Sumter. A thousand chattering telegraph keys were clicking in red depots and city railway stations. In a score of state capitols lights burned brightly while harassed adjutant generals girded a country for conflict. Great mass meetings, complete with burning oratory and impassioned gestures, were stirring the North to action. Before long the recruiting sergeant, with fife and drum, would be setting up office, and New York farm boys and clerks would exchange overalls or starched cuffs for Federal blue.

Regiment after regiment received standards of colors from loyal ladies and marched away. In a few years they would return as weary veterans and within measurable decades would be known only as "old soldiers." At Geneva a twenty-six-year-old physician, hardly yet initiated into the maturity of private practice, packed his hardwood box of instruments and put away his few texts. Lincoln needed doctors as well as plowboys. Charles Nathaniel Hewitt, who was later to play an important role in the advancement of public health in Minnesota, was willing to minister to those who shouldered rifles or heaved at heavy artillery wheels. Hewitt knew many of the men in the Fiftieth New York Volunteers when he was mustered in at Elmira as assistant surgeon on August 16, 1861.[1] He had treated them for coughs and burns; he had bound up their cuts and sprains; and he had carried their wives safely through childbirth. They spoke to him in friendly

[1] New York Adjutant General, *A Record of the Commissioned Officers, Non-Commissioned Officers and Privates of the State of New York*, 2:311 (Albany, 1864).

fashion and called him "Doc," the way men do when they like and respect their physician. Hewitt was friendly, too, but for all his informality a streak of stubbornness ran through him. When it came to professional matters, Dr. Hewitt could be both dour and strict.

When the regiment arrived in Washington, D.C., on September 22, Hewitt's duties began in earnest. Glitter and braid were forgotten in the humdrum tasks of everyday soldiering. Regimental activities centered at Camp Lesley, near the Navy Yard. The responsibilities of keeping the men healthy rested heavily upon the young surgeon. For a young man to take charge of a regimental hospital — two tents fourteen by sixteen feet and a small house with five rooms and three fireplaces — was no easy matter. Hewitt selected five men to serve as nurses and saw to it that neatness and cleanliness prevailed. That in itself was unusual. After a medical inspector looked through the wards, he turned to Hewitt: "Doctor, I am happy to tell you that you have the best arranged and managed Camp Hospital in the Army of the Potomac as far as I know." [2]

Hewitt took his praise lightly enough, for his training for years had emphasized thoroughness. His father, Henry Hewitt, was a medical man and early had instructed his son in preciseness. The young surgeon had been born in Vergennes, Vermont, on June 3, 1835, but had spent much of his childhood in Potsdam, New York. The senior Hewitt, a graduate of Yale Medical College, soon began instructing his son in medical practice. The boy dissected all animals that came under his hands. On one occasion he chose his father's razor to open a calf's head. For once the elder Hewitt forgot his scientific objectivity and laid a bigger strop across his son's backside than he used to sharpen the blunted razor. Then he relented and soon invited the lad to assist with an autopsy. Thirteen-year-old Charles had to push his courage to the sticking point, but he succeeded in dissecting out the heart.[3]

The knowledge of heart action and blood flow gained from the postmortem soon came in handy. The lad was visiting on a farm when a laborer was carried in hemorrhaging from a main leg artery. Charles

[2] William W. Folwell to Sarah Heywood, March 20, 1862, and Dr. Charles N. Hewitt to Dr. Henry Hewitt, December 14, 1861, February 28, 1862, Folwell Papers, boxes 66, 71. The letter of December 14, 1861, as transcribed by Folwell, is headed "Camp Lesley, Elmira," but Hewitt at that time was at Camp Lesley, Washington, D.C. The Folwell Papers are in the possession of the Minnesota Historical Society.

[3] Notes for a speech delivered in 1908, in the Hewitt Papers, in the possession of the Minnesota Historical Society. If Hewitt's own word is accepted, Folwell is incorrect in his statement of the year (1836) of Hewitt's birth. See Hewitt's Diary, June 3, 1853, with the Hewitt Papers.

correctly applied a tourniquet made from handkerchief, pebble, and stick, and bleeding stopped. That evening he went to the injured man's house to inquire about his condition. There he found his father and another physician in attendance. The senior Hewitt asked his son what he had done, and Charles told him.

"What is your fee, doctor?" inquired Dr. Hewitt gravely.

"Five dollars," answered the lad promptly.

His father plunged a hand into his pocket and turned over to the delighted "doctor" a crumpled five-dollar bill.[4]

Such an alert boy deserved competent schooling, and Charles was sent to Cheshire Academy in Connecticut and then to the Geneva Grammar School in New York, where he was a good, but not an outstanding, scholar. No grind, he edited his school paper and was president of the Geneva Grammar School Union, a debating society. He found time also to tramp the valleys and to dangle a line in fishing streams. In the autumn of 1853 Charles was admitted as a sophomore to Hobart Free College. The institution was not large, but it enjoyed real distinction. Unfortunately the newly arrived boy found the college permeated with religious skeptics. "Nothing," he wrote in his crabbed scribble, "so degrades a young man in my estimation and I think in the opinion of every thinking person as to see him come out boldly and avow his disbelief of the immortality of the soul, and consequently of the Bible, in fact of God." The Hobart debating society also displeased him, for he said he found only "three good debaters." A member of the Episcopal church, Hewitt sang at chapel and observed daily devotions.[5]

Good luck came to Charles in his junior year. He became a student assistant to Dr. Hazard Potter and began a long friendship that continued during later military days. Preceptor and student jounced along together in Potter's carriage making house calls. Sometimes Charles made a follow-up call alone and, in emergencies, did the best he could until his tutor arrived. Charles also served as operating assistant, ligating arteries and handling instruments. The boy must have earned the respect of his superiors, for in his junior year he also became prosector for Hobart's professor of anatomy, helping to prepare and dissect bodies. Frequently dissection material was obtained illegally. One evening excited men arrived and asked permission to search the dissecting room. The professor agreed, but politely requested that they wait a moment while he went to light the room. Swiftly the doctor amputated

[4] Notes for 1908 speech.
[5] Hewitt Diary, January 1, 1854.

the head from the body being sought, tucked it under his arm beneath a long cloak he was wearing, and went back to guide the search party. He showed them everything, and they found nothing. He accepted their apologies, bade them good-by, closed the door, and returned the head. Young Hewitt chuckled over that episode.[6]

After his graduation from Hobart in 1856, Hewitt entered Albany Medical College. He continued as a demonstrator in anatomy and served as assistant surgeon in the Albany Hospital. His course of study, like most medical curricula of his day, included healthy and morbid anatomy, physiology, pathology, organic and inorganic chemistry, and prognosis and treatment of disease. No passive student who meekly accepted what he saw in classroom and ward, Hewitt was critical of physicians who practiced medicine as they would "take a trade or saw wood." He considered medicine a profession both elevated and ennobling.[7]

When Hewitt stepped on the platform to receive his degree of Doctor of Medicine on December 22, 1857, gathering clouds of war already were in the air. The ominous slavery issue and the controversy over secession were dark signs of coming conflict. But the young physician could not know, as he read the class valedictory, that within a few short years he would change the black frock coat of his profession for the army blue. The *Albany Evening Transcript* hailed Hewitt's address as "one of the most brilliant valedictories ever issued from the worthy Institution [from] which he has graduated with such high honor."[8]

With the freshly lettered initials "M.D." after his name, Hewitt set himself up in practice in Geneva. His apprenticeship to Potter had resulted in an invitation for him to go into Potter's office. The two men were an ideal combination; the older man contributed the maturity that comes only after long practice, and the younger man enthusiastically introduced the newer techniques of his day. Their practice was divided between town and country, and their office was filled with farmers, tradesmen, and local businessmen. Hewitt had many friends who remembered him as a student and some of them recommended him. Perhaps Potter became jealous of the young doctor, or perhaps Hewitt found Potter's old-fashioned ways a bit antiquated. It may be that Hewitt himself was at fault, for he could be most dog-

[6] Notes for 1908 speech.
[7] Hewitt Diary, September 16, 17, 1856, October 6, 1858.
[8] *Albany Evening Transcript*, December 22, 1857.

A DOCTOR GOES TO WAR

matic and uncompromising. Before long he left Potter to associate himself with Dr. G. N. Dox. But when Hewitt entered the army, he was to serve as assistant to Potter, who was senior surgeon of the regiment.

Army life, even during dull days at Camp Lesley, stimulated Hewitt, who matured rapidly. Responsibility frequently ages a man. A thick Grant beard with long sideburns and bushy mustache gave Hewitt the appearance of a man of forty-five. As he strode through wards, soldiers saw a not-too-tall individual, broad across the shoulders, with deep-set eyes beneath heavy brows. Surgeon Hewitt wore the uniform more like a civilian than a soldier. In the field his light fatigue trousers were unpressed and his unbuttoned coat flopped over a dark vest that buttoned to the neck beneath his black beard. A campaign hat sat precariously on unruly hair and was yanked down a tilt to shade his eyes. Even when he was photographed in dress uniform, Hewitt's brass-buttoned coat appeared full of creases and wrinkles over the shoulders and across the front.[9]

Hewitt marched with his regiment from Washington on March 19, 1862, and went into camp near Alexandria, Virginia. A month later the Fiftieth Engineers took part in the siege of Yorktown. Hewitt's baptism of fire came at the battle of Williamsburg on May 7. "I have been in a real live battle," he wrote to a friend, "where shot and shell whizzed harmlessly over my head. Our ambulance was in advance, and we worked all the afternoon in the open air on wounded men of other regiments. It was a fearful and horrible spectacle." [10]

Wounded streamed into Yorktown's general hospital. The engineers had been under enemy fire while throwing pontoons across rivers, and some had been hit in the brief engagement at Williamsburg. Most Civil War military hospitals were overcrowded, and the one at Yorktown was no exception. Men lay on bare floors, and it was virtually impossible to supply them with necessities. Hewitt's wounded occupied the second floor of a private home. He heard that this house was the same one in which Cornwallis had signed his surrender in 1781.

When the Confederates retreated, Hewitt followed with his regiment. He could leave no doctor with the wounded, but he was able to assign them a hospital steward and a small store of food and medi-

[9] Francis T. Miller, ed., *The Photographic History of the Civil War*, 7:265 (New York, 1911). The photograph captioned "Surgeon Hawkes, Fiftieth New York Engineers," actually is of Hewitt. The photograph of Hewitt in dress uniform is in the Hewitt Papers.
[10] Hewitt to Mrs. Charles O. Tappan, May 8, 1862, Folwell Papers, box 71.

cines.[11] The hospital steward was Mahlon B. Folwell, brother of William Watts Folwell, first president of the University of Minnesota.

War's tempo increased, with the engineers trading rifles for axes and felling southern timber to lay pontoons across a score of meandering creeks and flowing rivers. Hewitt noted the equipment which burdened the soldier-engineer: rifle, forty rounds of ammunition, ax, spade, knapsack, and three days' rations. Frequently advance details of engineers were so far ahead of a supply line that they were forced to forage from the land. Even when the regiment rested behind the lines, Hewitt observed that an engineer's life never was quiet. Details constantly were throwing up defenses around the camp, opening new roads wide enough to accommodate creaking, ponderous supply wagons, and repairing bridges. Gradually the young physician realized that the corps of engineers was more than unsung pick-and-shovel men. To him the engineers were as important as infantrymen or even artillerymen, those brash cannoneers who flaunted red cords as if the distinguishing color of the artillery outshone the blue of the infantry and the yellow of the cavalry.

On June 7, 1862, Potter resigned from the service. His abrupt departure two days later left Hewitt as senior surgeon of the regiment. As he glanced at his map, he saw that the Fiftieth was scattered over some sixteen miles of country. In mud and water, day after day, too many men answered to sick call. The Chickahominy swamplands finally affected Hewitt's health. He was losing weight, and his breath came in asthmatic wheezes. He, too, toyed with the idea of leaving the service. But when, on June 19, his appointment as regimental surgeon came through, Hewitt decided to stick with the troops.

This was no easy decision. Some sixty to seventy men daily were reporting for medical care. Four nonbattle deaths had occurred in four weeks.[12] Scurvy, that ancient scourge of armies, plagued Hewitt's men. Their diet lacked eggs, vegetables and fruit, butter and milk. Only a few potatoes and onions were available.

From the Chickahominy the regiment moved into camp at Harrison's Landing. By then the men were well on their way toward becoming veterans. But Hewitt believed that even seasoned troops should be protected by sanitary quarters. He prepared the new camp carefully: underbrush was cleared away; streets were policed daily; and

---

[11] Hewitt to Sarah Heywood, May 12, 1862; W. W. Folwell's notes on Mahlon B. Folwell's Diary, May 11, 1862. Folwell Papers, box 66.
[12] Hewitt to Mrs. Tappan, June 22, 1862, Folwell Papers, box 71.

clean latrines were established on slopes that drained away from living quarters. Quartermasters freighted up quantities of fresh potatoes and onions. Hewitt saw to it that the men received sufficient rest and relaxation. Writing to his father, he said that army camps, if properly tended, were healthful, adding that diseases were largely the result of scurvy and exhaustion.[13]

Soon Hewitt was riding hard to take part in the battle of Fredericksburg. Drs. Michael Hillary and A. Clark Baum accompanied him along twisting paths and roads clogged with brigades on the march. After the battle was joined, Hewitt set up a temporary hospital. A sergeant with a fractured arm staggered in. He had steadfastly refused to permit other surgeons to amputate. In Hewitt's hospital the sergeant saw a soldier with a similar wound that had been dressed and splinted.

"Could you save my arm too?" the sergeant asked Hewitt.

"I think I can; lie down there on the straw."

Chloroform was dripped slowly onto a gauze pad over the man's nose. Then Hewitt set to work. Three days later the arm was healing. Extraction of bone in the field was forbidden by regulation, but Hewitt violated that order three times and each time he was successful. Strangely enough, his first commendation came as the result of this disobedience of orders. Dr. Jonathan Letterman, medical director, thanked him for his conduct.[14]

The Fiftieth New York Regiment was widely scattered during the early months of 1863. Hewitt welcomed the New Year at Aquia Creek, regimental headquarters. With two friends he spent the evening telling stories, drinking whisky punch, and eating oysters and lemon snaps.[15] His guests returned to quarters in a "charming" moonlight. Other units were located at Harper's Ferry, Belle Plain, and White Oaks Church. By late January, Hewitt had moved to Camp Falmouth near Falmouth, Virginia.

"Back in old quarters except the pontoon train," he wrote somewhat wearily. "Divided trains, one sent to Bank's Ford, the other at United States Ford on the 18th. Located two hospitals. Spent 19th finding road to U.S. Ford. Hospitals all ready on the 20th. Trains hitched up all day waiting orders. Came at sundown to move both to Bank's Ford.

[13] Hewitt to Henry Hewitt, July 29, 1862, Folwell Papers, box 71.
[14] Hewitt to Henry Hewitt, undated; Folwell to Sarah Heywood, December 25, 1862. Folwell Papers, boxes 66, 71.
[15] Ben W. Woodward to George Gordon Brooks, January 9, 1863, Folwell Papers, box 61.

Began to rain at seven P.M. Roads in horrible condition. Got my train through and into camp at 8 P.M. Tents up and sick provided for. Rained all day and all night. Wagons sank in up to hubs. Artillery stuck in mud. Couldn't get into position. I took Colonels, Majors, Brigadiers into my hospital sick and no medicines, doctors or porters. A medical director shared my tent — regimental surgeons all without stores or tents — criminal neglect entailed suffering awful." [16]

Evil condition of the roads that sucked at wheels and made horses pant with exertion retarded Hewitt's tours of inspection. To reach outlying units he was forced to travel on horseback or in light ambulances. The weather was cold and damp, alternating between light snowfalls and damp, drizzling, freezing rain. Fevers struck savagely and sick rosters mounted alarmingly.

Hewitt did his work as well as he could. He was rewarded on April 18, 1863, when he became senior surgeon of the engineer brigade.[17] This brigade consisted of the Fifteenth and Fiftieth New York regiments and a detachment of regular army engineers, all assigned to the Army of the Potomac. Hewitt found his new assignment a great responsibility. Not only was he charged with the health and welfare of his own regiment, but he was also accountable for the entire brigade organization.

As regimental surgeon Hewitt was responsible for the general health of the regiment and the care of the sick, as well as for keeping on hand adequate medical and hospital supplies. Then, too, he supervised the enforcement of the sanitary and hygienic regulations. Paper work was immense. Weekly reports of sick and wounded had to be compiled and checked. As brigade surgeon he received both daily and weekly reports. All medicines and supplies were charged to him. It was his duty to see that regimental surgeons were thorough and conscientious, that they maintained adequate supplies, that they properly checked cooking, clothing, and cleanliness in camp, and that they knew how and where to locate disposal pits and latrines. In addition, Hewitt had general supervision over the training of hospital attendants and ambulance men. He collected the reports of the regimental surgeons, endorsed them, and forwarded them to the medical director. Within twenty-four hours after an enemy engagement, Hewitt was to submit in writing to the medical director the "name, rank, and regiment of each of the wounded; the situation of the wound, and the surgical

---

[16] Hewitt to Henry Hewitt, January 17, 1863, Folwell Papers, box 71.
[17] Hewitt Diary, April 18, 1863.

means adopted in the case."[18] He found himself more and more a general clerk and less and less a practicing physician.

No doubt army red tape fretted him; but to offset reams of regulations, there was a rather lively social life open to regimental and brigade surgeons. Visits back and forth among officers were common. During long evenings in winter quarters, little groups of friends knotted pleasantly before log fires to talk of home, exchange army gossip, and speculate on current campaigns. Hewitt frequently visited the Folwells. William Watts Folwell and his brother Mahlon both were serving in the Fiftieth New York. With them Hewitt perched on a camp stool or lounged in an armchair confiscated from the "seceshes." Will Folwell drew enthusiastically upon a pipe presented him by a Confederate officer. He thought Hewitt a "very active, energetic officer, equally unpopular and indifferent to popularity."[19]

Hewitt received a pipe too. It happened this way. After a skirmish, a flag of truce appeared on the Confederate line, and a message asked for a physician to attend a seriously wounded officer. Hewitt volunteered. Led blindfolded through the lines, he was taken to a desolate jerry-built shack. Hewitt spread his instruments out and operated swiftly. When his patient came out of the anesthetic, he presented Hewitt with a fine meerschaum pipe. The doctor treasured it for many years and later brought it to Minnesota with him.[20]

Despite all his preoccupation with clerical details, Hewitt personally supervised many surgeons under him. He was apt to appear on unannounced inspection trips, his sharp eyes taking in the slightest hospital blemish. An innovation of his was the establishment of a convalescent camp for men not sick enough to warrant hospitalization, but not well enough for active duty. They received wholesome food, good beds, and clean clothes. In Washington he set up a brigade hospital at the engineers' depot, to which he sent his seriously sick and wounded.

Yet his first love was the regimental hospital of the Fiftieth New York, and he considered it the best in the Army of the Potomac. "All seriously sick are comfortable on beds with ticks filled with hay, feather pillows, cotton pillow-cases, and white blankets," he wrote proudly. "We have a full supply of underclothing of cotton and wool. Each pillow has its mosquito net and little bedside table and today one of

[18] Joseph K. Barnes, comp., *The Medical and Surgical History of the War of the Rebellion*, 1 (part 1):59, 60 (Washington, 1870).
[19] Folwell to Sarah Heywood, May 24, 1863, Folwell Papers, box 66.
[20] Rough notes of Edwin Hewitt, Hewitt Papers.

our ingenious Yankees has built a tiptop easy chair. I have a full supply of potatoes and onions, fresh bread, lemons and oranges, ice and fresh beef. Today I have obtained from the Sanitary Commission a supply of domestic and sherry wine and brandy."[21] His routine duties frequently took him to the nation's capital, where he made his reports and invested savings from his pay in current war bonds.

The Fiftieth, during the summer of 1864, occupied trenches at the siege of Petersburg. Hewitt remained at the regimental hospital six miles from Petersburg and near City Point, Virginia. As the tedious siege wore on, sickness increased rapidly. More and more men lined up at sick call, complaining of fever or chronic diarrhea. Hewitt said, on August 20, that there were "nearly two hundred on sick report and over three hundred at the Surgeon's Camp Report."[22]

A few weeks earlier Hewitt had described graphically an army on the march, commenting on its health and saying: "I feel a growing repugnance to witnessing surgical operations and yet feel no hesitation [to perform] such as fall to my lot." Then he added: "There is still a great deal of bungling surgery here and large numbers of incompetent men." He was annoyed also by the great striving for promotion by men in the medical department.[23]

Shortly thereafter Hewitt sent his father a detailed picture of the army organization of which he was a part. "You are under a false impression," he began, "as to the status of this Regiment in the Army. The Engineer Brigade is an independent Command like a Corps. This regiment is for the present on duty independent of the Brigade. Two Companies under the command of the Lieutenant Colonel are attached to General Meade's headquarters. This Command is called the Reserve Battalion. I have my headquarters and the Regimental Hospital with it. There are three other battalions of three Companies each one with the second Corps, one with the 5th Corps one with the 6th Corps."

The picture became clearer as Hewitt continued. "The Reserve Battalion has a canvas pontoon train with each Company. In each of the other battalions one Company has a wooden pontoon train. The other two Companies do duty as sappers and miners. All sick and wounded are immediately sent to me. I have been very busy fitting up the hospital. We have a fine location in a hardwood grove with plenty of water."[24]

[21] Hewitt to Henry Hewitt, June 30, 1864, Folwell Papers, box 71.
[22] Hewitt to Tappan, August 19, 1864, Folwell Papers, box 71.
[23] Hewitt to Tappan, June 9, 1864, Folwell Papers, box 71.
[24] Hewitt to Henry Hewitt, June 30, 1864, Folwell Papers, box 71.

In another letter he wrote admiringly of a new brick oven sufficiently large to bake forty loaves of bread at once, mentioned having a vegetable cellar dug, and requested his sister to send him a few good recipes for rice tapioca and farina puddings. When, in August, an alarming increase in sick call drastically reduced the number of men fit for duty, Hewitt personally inspected living quarters. He began a "searching examination of camp, food, clothing, police of the men, the kind and amount of work they were doing." But that was not all. He "procured fresh vegetables of the Sanitary Commission and distributed them personally," and "obtained a large force for police duty and cleaned the camp, digging drains, covering sinks, drawing off rubbish, etc." Within ten days his sick call was reduced by half.[25]

If he drove his men hard to achieve sanitary results, Hewitt also watched their personal comfort. Just before Christmas of 1864 he sent to Washington, D.C., for twenty turkeys, forty chickens, a half bushel of cranberries, fifty pounds of nuts, ten pounds of raisins, and a barrel of cider. "My bakers and cooks," he wrote gleefully, "are busy getting ready 600 biscuits nice and light and tomorrow a force of men will go to work to fit up the convalescent ward with cedar and holly and pine for Christmas Eve." Hewitt saw that presents were distributed — "an assortment of odd and ridiculous knick knacks" — and he ordered the brigade band to play appropriate holiday airs. "I am now able to provide for my sick better than any other Regimental Surgeon," he scribbled in a Christmas letter, "and I am bound that they shall profit by it." [26]

Yet the watchful army surgeon was no softhearted individual who permitted his men undue liberties. William Folwell, who admired the doctor but was utterly frank about his personality, said that Hewitt, in one instance, at least, certified soldiers' deaths as debility induced by "deliberate and persistent malingering." The strain of responsibility no doubt preyed upon Hewitt, manifesting itself in bursts of temper and even in physical illness. Hewitt was far from well during early autumn of 1864. His weight fell to 136 pounds, a loss that worried Folwell. Folwell long had told stories of the young doctor who was making a name for himself as one of the best sanitarians in the army. After traveling with Hewitt on the "Sally Ann" en route to Washington in July, 1863, he told the following story: " 'Give my respects to your wife,' says the Dr. who comes down to fish a matchbox from his coat pocket with which to light another cigar. He is a great

---
[25] Hewitt to Tappan, July 24, August 19, 1864, Folwell Papers, box 71.
[26] Hewitt to Tappan, December 20, 1864, Folwell Papers, box 71.

smoker. I read him what I write, without removing his cigar he tries to say, That's the *ide augh*. [*That's the idea, grunt.*] Off he shoots to resume his observations upon a fresh-water bloodsucker, which has occupied his professional curiosity for many minutes." [27]

Hewitt's intentness and capacity for long hours of grueling work won him the professional respect of his superiors, who, even though they sometimes were annoyed by the doctor's uncompromising attitude, nevertheless realized his great desire to improve the health of the sick. On April 11, 1865, Hewitt received a citation and was recommended for promotion to lieutenant colonel by brevet for gallant and meritorious services at Fredericksburg in December, 1862. The citation further spoke of Hewitt's "careful and skillful treatment of the wounded of his own and other regiments on that occasion, for the same good conduct at the construction of the bridges at Franklin crossing, below Fredericksburg, on the 5th of June, 1863, for the able and skillful manner in which he has managed the affairs of his department since the crossing of the Rapidan in the spring of 1864, for his untiring zeal and energy in searching out all the men of his regiment sent to general hospitals, and having them as well as the men in his own hospital returned to duty as soon as they are able, as shown in his reports to the medical director of the army, and especially for the able manner in which he has managed his department since the commencement of the late movements of the army." [28]

Although Lee's surrender early in April, 1865, put a dramatic stop to Hewitt's field activities, the weary wounded still needed care. Reams of paper work had to be completed before Hewitt could be mustered out. His desk was piled high with reports. As his pen perfunctorily scratched his characteristic signature, perhaps Lieutenant Colonel Hewitt remembered the day when General Grant arranged a field inspection in honor of Lincoln. Twenty-five thousand men or more, in rigid company front, swept across the field before Grant and the President. Near Lincoln sat Hewitt on his favorite horse, Fan. He remembered Lincoln as a pathetic figure on horseback. As the president watched his troops, he removed his beaver hat, crushing it down hard upon the pommel of his saddle. Tears coursed down his deeply lined cheeks. [29]

[27] Folwell Diary, July 21, 1864; Folwell to Sarah Heywood, July 28, 1863, and to Sarah Heywood Folwell, December 19, 1864. Folwell Papers, boxes 66, 69.
[28] War Department, *The War of the Rebellion: A Compilation of the Official Records of the Union and Confederate Armies*, series 1, vol. 46, part 3, p. 705 (Washington, 1894).
[29] Edwin Hewitt, typescript dated July 23, 1937, Hewitt Papers.

Finally his clerical work and his administrative duties were over, and Hewitt, astride Fan, watched the magnificent parade of the Grand Army of the Republic up Pennsylvania Avenue on May 23, 1865. Sherman's troops quickstepped in patched but proud uniforms. A group of gay young folks clustered in front of a handsome residence. In the group was a beardless lad in the fresh, new uniform of a cadet. Hewitt saw the veterans eye the boy balefully as they swung past. Finally a seasoned soldier broke from the ranks, ran up to the cadet, and held out his musket, saying: "Would you like to snap a cap in this war, Sonny?" Hewitt was mustered out with his regiment on June 13.

3

The Shoulder Straps Come Off

BRAVE in a spick and span uniform, with the new shoulder straps of a lieutenant colonel gleaming on his shoulders, Hewitt returned to his father's home in Potsdam.[1] He took with him his horse Fan and Uncle Hart, the old Negro servant who had brushed his clothes and cooked for him throughout the war. It was good to be home again with friends and relatives whose daily humdrum of life was determined by peaceful chores and not by the bugle's strident call. Unpacking his few books and instrument cases, Hewitt laid aside a flat, wooden kit of amputating knives and bone saws and put his field notes away safely. The blue uniform with its high-standing collar and double rows of brass buttons was replaced by the more somber black of the private physician.

The change from army surgeon to town doctor was not easy. Like many another veteran, Hewitt felt a deep restlessness that frequently brought him up short and made him wonder just what he should do with his life. The war years had left a deep impression which could not be shrugged off easily. Military discipline had come naturally to him, for he was dogmatic and enjoyed the exercise of authority. He found, however, as he resumed practice that patients did not relish abrupt, unexplained instructions. He could not order them, as he had soldiers, out of unsanitary homes into clean tents, where the sun and fresh air helped heal. Neither could he force villagers to fill in reeking garbage pits and to police littered streets. Potsdam seemed to oppress him, and he began to consider the idea of leaving the East and starting afresh elsewhere.

As Hewitt pondered, a letter from an old school friend reached him. From Red Wing in far-off Minnesota, Dr. Augustine B. Hawley wrote

---

[1] Notes for 1908 speech, Hewitt Papers.

THE SHOULDER STRAPS COME OFF

of the glorious opportunities open to professional men in the North Star State. Hewitt read Hawley's letter with great attention. He knew that Hawley was a competent physician and a discerning observer. The two men had kept in touch with one another for years, even during the middle 1850s when Hawley had studied in the great clinics of Edinburgh, London, and Paris. Urged by the Presbyterian minister at Red Wing to come there, Hawley had migrated to Minnesota in July, 1857.[2] Hewitt knew how delighted Hawley had been with that Mississippi River village. He learned also that his friend's practice was a flourishing one.

Yet, as Hewitt read Hawley's letter inviting him to take over the Red Wing practice, he was undecided. Why should Hawley wish to abandon a prosperous business? Should Hewitt risk giving up everything at home in exchange for a career on a western frontier? Minnesota in 1866 was a relatively new state. Perhaps a man would have a better chance there. Certainly a physician would be welcome in many a small town struggling toward maturity. On the other hand, Hewitt knew he already had established a reputation for himself. To make a definite decision was difficult. Finally Hawley wrote suggesting that Hewitt come out for a visit. He need not commit himself until he had surveyed Minnesota for himself. The idea appealed to Hewitt and within a few weeks his carpetbags and instruments were packed and he was on his way to the Mississippi.

Hewitt broke his trip at Venice in northern Ohio, where he visited with his old army friend Will Folwell, who after the war had become a clerk in his father-in-law's milling business. As soon as Folwell heard that Hewitt was coming west, he wrote the doctor urging him to stop. "Arrange so as to spend some time with us," said Folwell, "if you find it agreeable. If you will make your appearance abt. March 15th–25th, I will give you some professional employment. 'I might as well *tell*' — We expect a *boy* this time."[3] The two friends had a delightful time reliving war experiences and discussing the advisability of Hewitt's settling in Minnesota. Soon after Mrs. Folwell gave birth to a daughter, Hewitt continued his trek westward.

Red Wing looked its best that bright spring day in 1867, but even

[2] Augustine B. Hawley, "Record of Things Seen and Heard during My Stay Abroad, from August 18th, 1855, to October 17, 1856"; Hawley's smaller Diary, London and Paris, Glasgow and Dublin, 1855–56; Anne MacDonald Hawley, "Augustine Boyer Hawley, M.D., Pioneer of Minnesota," 18. These typewritten manuscripts are in the possession of the Minnesota Historical Society.
[3] Folwell to Hewitt, February 5, 1866, Folwell Papers, box 71.

its best could not conceal its essential crudity. Yet the town had made startling progress since early claims had been staked out in 1852 by John Bush and Calvin Potter on a site that for generations had been Indian camping grounds. Hewitt learned that the opening of navigation in 1853 had brought a veritable flood of settlers to seize town lots and to build stores, hotels, and mills. A United States land office attracted so many cunning speculators that a vigilance committee was formed to protect honest men. When Hewitt arrived, Red Wing was known as a wheat center, it boasted a fine brick building that housed Hamline University, and it was convinced that it should have been the state capital.

Beneath this cultural veneer the rough life of a frontier people pulsed with energy that spilled tipsy settlers from tavern doors, fighting and whooping it up when the Fenians gathered to work for Irish freedom or when the Tanner's Club campaigned for U. S. Grant. Until the railroad arrived at Red Wing, contact with the outside world was by river steamer during open-water season and by lurching stage when the Mississippi was frozen.

Hewitt gazed wide-eyed at this flourishing community of some three thousand persons as Hawley guided him to his moderate-sized frame house on Main Street. After he had washed the grime of travel away, Hewitt came down to a pleasant parlor to hear at first hand of the prospects of practice. Hawley had done well in Red Wing and Goodhue County. There was no doubt of that. The constant flow of immigration through town kept a physician busy, while permanent residents provided a steady income from the treatment of accident wounds and disease. Cholera, typhoid, dysentery were all present. Children's diseases — whooping cough, measles, diphtheria — were as annual as the wheat crop. Hawley had built up an obstetrical practice, too, sometimes riding far into the country to deliver a Swedish woman whose squalling son would grow into a sturdy builder of Minnesota. There was satisfaction, Hewitt learned, in a frontier practice. A man felt that his skill and medicines were playing a vital role in helping a people to make a wilderness into a state.

As Hewitt walked the streets, his sharp eyes picked out piles of decaying rubbish. He saw butchers casually slaughtering hogs and cattle with disregard for cleanliness. Behind homes stood squalid lines of privies. Sometimes a well stood perilously close to refuse pits. Farmers came in with gashes on hands and arms, which had been smeared with mud or manure. It seemed to Hewitt that people were far more intent

THE SHOULDER STRAPS COME OFF

upon taking up land and working it than upon sanitation and careful treatment of their bodies. He decided to take over Hawley's practice.

The beginning was not easy. Fortunately Hawley had purchased a half interest in a drugstore and thus was able to refer patients to the new doctor. At first they resented his brusque manner, but soon they realized that behind Hewitt's directness lay skill and sympathy. Gradually town activities absorbed his energies. He took an active part in the affairs of Christ Episcopal Church, where another Hobart friend, Edward Randolph Welles, was rector. He helped to establish a parish library and reading room and was appointed to the building committee. A few years later he organized a vested choir of boys. He also found himself much in demand as a public speaker.

Public attention was drawn to Hewitt dramatically in the summer of 1868. Up the Mississippi came a boat with cholera victims aboard. The captain unceremoniously dumped them on the Red Wing levee. Horrified citizens refused to give aid. Hewitt immediately hurried to minister to them, making arrangements for their isolation in a house on an island opposite the city and securing money from the city to care for them.[4] This incident gave Hewitt another opportunity in a public speech to crusade for public health. He felt strongly that effective prevention of disease could come only if county physicians banded together in societies to exchange experiences and to profit by one another's cases. He also favored the organization of a state medical association.

Late January of 1869 found Hewitt on his way to St. Paul. The weather was bitter cold and a penetrating wind whipped across Lake Pepin. Although the country was drab and cheerless, Hewitt's heart sang. He was riding to attend the reorganization meeting of the Minnesota State Medical Society. A small group of physicians assembled in the International Hotel on February 1. There were distinguished-looking Dr. Samuel Willey of St. Paul and Dr. A. E. Ames of Minneapolis. Hewitt was introduced to Dr. E. J. Davis from Mankato and Dr. S. B. Sheardown of Stockton. From Stillwater came Dr. J. C. Rhodes, who knew the rough antics of lumberjacks, and from Carver, Dr. E. C. Roger, most of whose patients were farmers. Dr. W. W. Mayo arrived from Rochester. Hewitt was pleased to meet these men, many of whom were to be his close friends for years. From them he learned that, although the state society had been organized in December, 1853,

[4] Joseph W. Hancock, *Goodhue County, Minnesota, Past and Present*, 237 (Red Wing, 1893).

no regular meetings had been held. The old society really was defunct. Hewitt was appointed one of three delegates to attend the meetings of the American Medical Association in May at New Orleans and also was invited to read an essay at the next session of the state group.[5]

Returning to Red Wing, Hewitt thought hard about his coming trip to New Orleans. Suddenly the idea came to him, canny New Englander that he was, that perhaps he might combine a professional trip with a honeymoon. Helen Hawley, a cousin of Dr. Hawley, had arrived in Red Wing in 1868 to teach in the parish school of Christ Church. The daughter of a New York physician, Helen understood the rigors of practice and was drawn to Hewitt by his devotion to medicine and his interest in people. They were married by Bishop Henry B. Whipple on April 22, 1869, and left immediately on the steamer "Tom Jasper" "with a gentle rain and a rainbow spanning the boat till she shoved out."

The American Medical Association, organized in 1847, was meeting in New Orleans for a very special purpose. Physicians hoped that sessions in a southern city would help heal the bitterness of war days, and also might soften the hard, cruel reconstruction program imposed on the South by a radical Republican Congress. Hewitt noticed that Northern and Southern physicians generally ignored sectional controversy to devote themselves to strengthening their national organization. As he listened to papers and reports with that vital intentness so peculiar to him, he speculated on American medical education. He agreed with Dr. William O. Baldwin that "Almost any body of medical men may obtain a charter for a medical college in most of the States of this Union, with pretty much such regulations and privileges as they may agree upon among themselves and ask for." [6] Hewitt endorsed also a proposal to publish a weekly medical journal.

Preoccupied as he was by his duties as a delegate, Hewitt found time to investigate New Orleans' winding, dirty streets, its above-ground cemeteries, and its famous cafes. He gallantly squired his bride to the wharf district and together they visited quaint curio shops and patches of park. They could not fail to notice what war had done to the South. The evidence was apparent everywhere — in the attitude of freed Negroes, in high prices, and in the lack of spirit among some natives. Brash Yankees swaggered through New Orleans streets, en-

---

[5] Minnesota State Medical Society, *Transactions*, 1869, p. 3.
[6] Quoted in Morris Fishbein, *A History of the American Medical Association, 1847 to 1947*, 78 (Philadelphia, 1947).

gaged in loud bar talk, and told how they picked up fine plantations for a song. These things impressed Hewitt deeply and, although he never had believed in slavery, he felt genuine sympathy for Southerners who still were being punished long after the war was over.

The Hewitts were glad to return to Red Wing. They had gone by boat from New Orleans to New York and, after a short visit, had left for Minnesota. Their spirits rose with each mile put behind them and, when at last Red Wing came into view, they felt like cheering. Hewitt plunged immediately into his practice, and his wife unpacked wedding presents and set the house to rights. Within a few years this rambling frame structure, with additions for the Hewitts' children, was to be known for its charm of intimacy and hospitality. Later a pipe organ stood in a library corner and a small conservatory brightened the house.

At his office Hewitt treated patients, kept case records, and made big plans for the progress of Minnesota medicine. He was inordinately fond of his medical library, the rows of calf-bound books that gave off the musty odor of good leather and were imprinted with the distinguished names of London, New York, and Philadelphia publishers. There was John Baptist Morgagni's outstanding *Seats and Causes of Diseases Investigated by Anatomy*, published in three volumes in London in 1769, and Jean Cruveilhier's *Anatomy of the Human Body*, published in New York in 1844. Hewitt was proud of his copy of William Benjamin Carpenter's *The Microscope* and of a shelf of volumes on public health, among them Charles B. Coventry's famous *Epidemic Cholera* and Henry H. Porter's *Account of the Origin, Symptoms, and Cure of the Influenza, or Epidemic Catarrh*. He owned, too, a first edition of William Beaumont's epoch-making *Experiments and Observations on the Gastric Juice, and the Physiology of Digestion*, published at Plattsburgh in 1833. A much-read book was Benjamin Rush's *Essays, Literary, Moral and Philosophical*.[7]

Perhaps Hewitt's unusual library was one reason why the members of the Goodhue County Medical Society enjoyed meeting in his office, although sometimes they came together in the Christ Church reading room. Hewitt enjoyed his duties as secretary and frequently suggested policy. After his trip to New Orleans his mind turned more and more to public health, and on July 11, 1871, he proposed that the county society try to determine the relative prevalence of epidemic and en-

[7] Thomas E. Keys, "The Medical Books of Dr. Charles N. Hewitt," in *Minnesota History*, 21:357–371 (December, 1940).

demic diseases in different parts of Goodhue County. A committee of three, which included Hewitt, was appointed to prepare a topographic map.[8]

Plunging into this work with characteristic vigor, Hewitt soon realized that a county survey was not enough. Disease has little regard for artificial boundaries and it sweeps casually across township and county lines. What was really needed was a state-wide program of investigation and prevention. Yet Hewitt at first was none too confident that support of a state plan would be forthcoming. For many years he had been critical of both the medical profession and the new science, although he was not antagonistic to either. "There is so little fact & so much theory," he confided to his diary in 1856, "that I am sometimes tempted to think that a medical practice founded upon the honest experience of *one* practitioner of sterling common sense would be safer and more successful than a practice based on what is vauntingly called 'the united experience of centuries.'" Two years later he wrote: "Practice never will be correct till the practitioner *knows* what he is about. Such a proposition may seem very plainly true — it is so — but plain as it is it expresses what I think is the great fault among those who are honored with the title M.D." Of course this was a young man speaking, but Hewitt could never endorse physicians unqualifiedly. This was emphatically true if a doctor disagreed with him. Indeed, it was one of his wife's constant social obligations to see that her impulsive husband did not irritate dinner guests. Hewitt's manner of being in the right was frequently such as to put him virtually in the wrong.

Yet with all his trifling faults, in Red Wing Hewitt was considered an honest man and a competent physician. Local opinion swung stanchly behind him in 1875 when he was sued for malpractice by a youth whose hand the doctor had amputated. The initial surgery had been performed in December, 1868, when a gun had exploded in the boy's hand. Afterwards, however, the lower arm withered, and suit was instituted against Hewitt. When the case came to trial, so many physicians were on hand to testify in Hewitt's behalf that the prosecuting attorney not only withdrew the suit, but also expressed his regret that it ever had been commenced. What might have happened had the case gone to a jury no one knows, but an editor commenting upon the trial credited Daniel Webster as saying "that God Almighty knew almost everything; but one thing he didn't and never could

[8] *Weekly Republican* (Red Wing), April 15, 1869, July 20, 1871.

know, and that was what a jury of twelve men would do in almost any given case." [9]

Much too busy to worry long about a lawsuit, Hewitt continued his usual practice of starting a dozen projects at once and completing only a few. Sometimes, his friends said, he completely forgot pet investigations and was surprised when asked about them. His energies piled up so many uncompleted, half-completed, and finished plans that frequently he neglected to write in his diary for weeks on end. He had a habit of using odds and ends of paper for notes, filling endless scraps with such crabbed script that acquaintances scarcely could make out the meaning. Many of his speeches were written on ruled paper and then tied loosely together with string; others were only pages of assorted sizes carelessly tied with red ribbons.

But whatever the appearance of his notes, Hewitt's thinking was consistent. In a talk before the Minnesota State Medical Society in 1870 on the relationship of the medical profession to the people, he asked: "What are the duties of the profession in the education of the people?" Here he laid down fundamental public health precepts that were to guide him in later years.[10]

Meanwhile, in every minute he could spare from a rapidly growing practice, Hewitt was working frantically on a survey of the climate and epidemics of Minnesota. Members of the county society assisted him, as did physicians in St. Paul and Minneapolis. When he rode through the country he questioned patients persistently, and no farmer grubbing in the field was safe from the doctor's inquiries. Finally the first rough draft was completed and revised. Then the revision was combed for errors, and only after Hewitt was sure he had been as meticulous as possible did he send it off for publication in the *Transactions* of the American Medical Association. Later it was reprinted as a nineteen-page pamphlet, and he proudly distributed copies to friends in the East and in Minnesota.[11]

This little publication gave stature to Hewitt's already growing reputation. Critics found it objective and well balanced, with no attempt to go beyond evidence that its author had at hand. And Hewitt candidly observed: "Opinions as to change in climate are the results of ordinary experience and observations, rather than of scientific ex-

[9] *Pioneer-Press*, August 29, December 25, 28, 1875.
[10] The talk, delivered in St. Paul on February 3, 1870, was entitled "What Are the Relations of the Profession of Medicine to the People and What Are the Duties of the Profession in the Education of the People Growing Out of Those Relations?" A copy is in the Hewitt Papers.
[11] *Report on the Climatology and Epidemics of Minnesota* (Philadelphia, 1871).

periment." Then he made four general comments concerning Minnesota's population:

1. There are but few white natives of the State twenty years of age.
2. There is a large and constant influx of foreign immigration. They bring with them not only existing contagious and infectious disease, but, in many cases, constitutions broken by the hardships and privations of peasant life abroad, and the cachexia and diatheses, the result of generations of such life and influence. Add to these causes the influence of acclimatization, and the exposure to the hardships incidental to pioneer life, and we have a list of morbific agencies which would explain a much greater prevalence than actually exists.
3. The reputation of Minnesota as a health resort for sufferers from pulmonary disease has for many years induced a constant addition to our resident American population, not only of individuals, but whole families, those having incipient or developed disease, and those with known or suspected predisposition.
4. The rapid subjugation of the soil to wheat culture on the prairies; the settlement of the valleys along the bluffs which line our great watercourses; the removal of the timber from the river bottom land; the diminution of paludal accumulations by floods, sunlight, and the operations of domestic animals, with the consequent improvement of the river drainage, and other admitted influences of which it is very difficult to estimate the character and power.

Jogging across country with horse and buggy, Hewitt saw immigrants pouring in by the thousands. He soon realized that the state's health problem was affected by two groups: immigrants who brought disease with them and settlers who became ill after they had reached the state. Red Wing, located as it was on the Mississippi, was an excellent spot from which to watch the flow of new people. Standing on the wharf with his hat pushed forward a little to shade his eyes, Hewitt quickly inventoried travelers from the Old World as they struggled ashore loaded down with quaint luggage and shawl-tied bundles. He saw the marks of malnutrition, the flush of fevers, the deep pits of smallpox. His professional journals kept him in touch with the tribulations of the ocean voyage to America.

All too frequently the emigrant ship was a floating pesthouse and its sailors were persistent carriers of disease. Indeed, some vessels were so poorly repaired that their "fastenings and knees could be seen working between decks in the cabin." Ships were carriers of disease, and Hewitt learned that sailing vessels in the immigrant trade reported more illness than did steamships. The death rate among steerage passengers in both sailing ships and steamships between 1864 and 1873 was 2.78 per thousand. Although Hewitt enthusiastically endorsed

THE SHOULDER STRAPS COME OFF 39

stricter inspection of immigrant ships, he felt there was slight possibility that those coming to America could have sanitary accommodations. Even before the United States Marine Hospital Service undertook the inspection of immigrants at the Port of New York, Hewitt felt that the states themselves should provide supervision. He believed thoroughly in immigrant inspection at principal distributing centers, such as Wheeling, Cincinnati, Detroit, and Chicago, and thought instructions to inspectors were adequate, but he held strongly that medical examinations should follow the foreigner to his ultimate destination.[12]

Railroads, booming toward Minnesota during the 1870s and 1880s, were also suspect. Hewitt found plenty of opportunity to see the nation's railways hauling wheat from Minnesota and settlers to Minnesota. The railroad, of course, gave rise to a more immediate problem for the state than did ocean vessels, and Hewitt noted carefully articles discussing these new sanitary problems. He thought that quarantine regulations and baggage disinfection were imperative. When, during a threatened cholera epidemic, Hewitt learned that immigrants having a clean bill of health in Chicago were said to need no further inspection, he exploded: "Oh, I'll have no such nonsense as that. Chicago is a large distributing point where an immigration train from the East is broken up and the immigrants in small lots then scatter here and there over the West. Now there is just as much danger of infection from a lot of three immigrants as there is from 100 immigrants. . . . The railway companies have cars which are one-half baggage and one-half passenger, and can be used for these small lots of immigrants." An avid newspaper reader, Hewitt read everything he could on railroads. He noted city celebrations when the railroad first came to town, and he poured over official reports.[13]

[12] John M. Woodworth, "Some Defects in the Immigration Service" and "The Safety of Ships and of Those Who Travel in Them," in *Public Health*, 1:442; 3:83 (New York, 1875, 1877); Heber Smith, "Sailors as Propagators of Disease," in *Public Health*, 1:447 (New York, 1875); Albert J. Gihon, "The Need of Sanitary Reform in Ship-Life," in *Public Health*, 3:97 (New York, 1877); A. N. Bell, "Marine Hygiene on Board Passenger Vessels," in *Public Health*, 3:99 (New York, 1877); T. J. Turner, "Air and Moisture on Shipboard," in *Public Health*, 4:105 (Boston, 1880); H. R. Mills, "The Immigrant Inspection Service of the National Board of Health at Port Huron, Michigan, and Its Bearing on Public Health of the West and North-West," in *Public Health*, 8:102 (Boston, 1883); United States National Board of Health, *Annual Reports*, 1879, pp. 295–297; 1882, p. 34; United States Marine-Hospital Service, *Annual Reports*, 1890, p. 55.

[13] Thomas J. Dunott, "Sanitary Safety in Railway Traveling — Suggestions in the Interest of Travelers and Carriers," in *Public Health*, 4:127 (Boston, 1880); S. S. Herrick, "Railroad Sanitation, Its Objects and Advantages," in *Public Health*, 7:218 (Boston, 1883); *Minneapolis Tribune*, September 16, 1892; *Saint Cloud Times*, March 18, 1871; *Willmar Republican*, November 28, 1871; Minnesota Railroad Commissioner, *Reports*, August 31, 1872.

Yet, with all his mounting interests, Hewitt did not neglect his practice. Early in his work at Red Wing he felt it necessary to keep a few patients under close observation. He hired local carpenters to construct a small building in the yard near his house. This he fitted up as a simple hospital of three or four beds. Here were his office and later his laboratory. The ground sloped away to the rear, and in the well-lighted hospital basement the doctor kept rabbits and guinea pigs.[14] Hewitt's military training exerted itself here. The little building was policed as carefully and supervised as rigorously as the hospitals he had charge of in the Army of the Potomac. He had enjoyed his army experiences, and he was perfectly willing to accept an appointment as government medical examiner for pensions. He kept his Civil War records at his hospital and thus was able to establish a veteran's right to a pension or to save the government money by proving that an applicant's disability was not the result of military service.

Each successive season found Hewitt busier. He darted at new projects like an energetic hummingbird swooping on an insect. There was a real love of the soil in the doctor, and he liked to pull his team to a halt to watch wheat sowers in the fields; he relished harvest time, when pumpkins grew big and yellow corn was in the shock; and he learned to love Minnesota winter, the silent season, when deep drifts covered roads. Then he guided his team by sighting tops of fence posts jutting up through the snow. He chuckled over the antics of farmers who, having disposed of their wheat at a profit, celebrated with so much drink that the tavern keeper would toss them into the wagon bottom, slap the horses, and send team and wagon careening homeward. On a lonely road in the late night Hewitt learned to stop frequently to listen. If he heard madly thudding hoofs and the jangle of harness, he drove off the road to wait until the wagon hurtled past. Then the road once more was safe for a tired and sober country doctor.[15]

On Sunday afternoons, after he had attended church service, Hewitt took his boys' nature club to wander through fields, stopping to catch butterflies and to lock green frogs in stoppered bottles. He taught the lads some simple anatomy and, more important, he instilled in them a love for growing and living things. Eventually he opened a boys' reading room which was in charge of the youngsters themselves. Of course the choir continued to meet in the doctor's home at 828 Third Street. Hewitt's copy of the Episcopal hymnbook was well worn.

[14] Edwin Hewitt, undated notes, Hewitt Papers.
[15] Edwin Hewitt, undated notes, Hewitt Papers.

The project that Hewitt held dearest, however, was the organization of a state board of health. Every time the county or the state medical society met, he informally urged his proposal. He could point to precedent. In 1850 a special legislative committee had made an exhaustive sanitary survey of Massachusetts and had reported a general plan for the promotion of public and personal health.[16] This plan was the basis for the organization of the Massachusetts State Board of Health in 1869. Hewitt knew also that both Virginia and California had state boards.

By 1872 Hewitt felt that Minnesota was ready to approve his carefully conceived proposal. Then, at a meeting of the Minnesota State Medical Society on February 6, he proudly introduced the following: "Resolved, That a Committee of five members be appointed by the Chair, to take into consideration all matters upon which legislation is asked by any member of the Society: said Committee to systematize them as far as possible, and present them to the Society at the present session, with drafts of bills which they may advise this Society to ask of the Legislature." The resolution was adopted and a committee, consisting of Dr. A. B. Stuart, chairman, and Drs. Hewitt, C. Hill, S. D. Flagg, and A. E. Ames, was appointed. Hewitt breathed a sigh of relief, for Stuart was a member of the American Medical Association's committee on state boards of health and could be counted upon to press the Minnesota plan. Stuart ran true to Hewitt's predictions and brought in a memorial and a bill to establish a state board. This was accepted and ordered printed.[17]

The next hurdle, of course, was to convince the legislature. This was not too difficult, but even so Hewitt spent long hours explaining why he felt a state board of health would make Minnesota a better place to live in. Every sick man made well and every person prevented from becoming ill would save man power that the state needed so desperately to forge ahead in agriculture, business, and commerce. Public health was a program of human economy; it was a vast plan of conservation. Hewitt knew that the first key to health was sanitation. His army experiences had taught him that, and he never forgot the lessons learned at Harrison's Landing and Petersburg.

How Hewitt and his colleagues must have rejoiced when the bill establishing the Minnesota State Board of Health became law on March 4, 1872. Most physicians thought the law was a good one, and

[16] Commonwealth of Massachusetts, *Report of a General Plan for the Promotion of Public and Personal Health* (Boston, 1850).
[17] Minnesota State Medical Society, *Transactions*, 1872, pp. 30, 36.

Hewitt knew most of its provisions by heart, for he had helped draft it. It stemmed from the police powers of the state, and it stipulated that the board should place itself in touch with local boards of health and with hospitals, asylums, and public institutions and that it should "take cognizance of the interests of health and life among the citizens generally." Hewitt was particularly pleased with the section reading: "They [*the board*] shall make sanitary investigations and inquiries respecting the causes of disease, especially of epidemics, the source of mortality and the effects of localities, employments, conditions and circumstances on the public health; and they shall gather such information in respect to these matters as they may deem proper for diffusion among the people."

The board was charged also with devising some scheme by which medical and vital statistics could be collected, with acting as an adviser in all hygienic and medical matters, and with supervising all matters pertaining to quarantine. The board's secretary was to administer these and other functions, and a report was to be made annually to the legislature. Other members of the board were to act in an advisory capacity and to handle emergencies in their own areas.

Dr. A. B. Stuart of Winona became the board's first president, and Hewitt was named secretary, a position he was to hold for a quarter of a century.[18] The secretaryship carried a meager salary — two hundred dollars a year paid in quarterly installments — but involved a multitude of duties as yet undefined. Its potentialities were limited only by the vision and energies of the incumbent. Hewitt was eminently fitted for the post. He had the broad, fundamental knowledge of the careful scholar and an alertness to changing conditions. He possessed common sense. In addition, he was thoroughly convinced of the importance of the work to be done and of the necessity for accomplishing as much as possible immediately. He believed the next step was an intensive educational campaign to prepare the way for further reforms. When necessity compelled, he had a singleness of purpose and a stubborn tenacity that brooked no interference.

Although, in the main, the new secretary was kindly and genial, he could, when displeased, be brusque and censorious. In his own mind he knew what the board could and should do, and he proposed to attain that end. "The Governor has selected seven physicians, residents of different parts of the State," he wrote, "not for personal, local, or

---

[18] Other members of the board were Drs. Daniel W. Hand, St. Paul; Nathan B. Hill, Minneapolis; Asa W. Daniels, St. Peter; Vespasian Smith, Duluth; and George D. Winch, Blue Earth City.

partisan ends, but honestly and sincerely in the spirit and path of science, to search out the causes of disease among us, and to warn us how much easier and better it is to prevent disease than to await its onslaught before attending to it. Their purpose is to diffuse information to this end among the people; to stimulate the practical study of the science of health in the colleges and schools of the State; to investigate carefully and thoughtfully, the sanitary condition of our public institutions, our cities, towns and villages; to ward off the attacks of epidemics and pestilence, and, (if they receive, for their work's sake, the cordial assistance and support of thinking citizens), to vindicate to and for us, as similar Boards have elsewhere done, the wisdom and necessity of their organization." [19]

Hewitt imposed the secretarial duties on top of his private practice at Red Wing, flinging himself into the work with his usual enthusiasm. He corresponded with city officials and physicians throughout Minnesota, for he wished, if possible, to co-ordinate the health activities of the state with the work of the board. He was determined, in his impetuous manner, to keep his finger on the pulse of all Minnesota. He soon found, however, that local officials were unresponsive and lethargic. He had not yet learned that interference and compulsion by the state board were almost a sure way of losing community and municipality support. Later he realized that the soft approach and the offer of a helping hand would do more than military brusqueness. The straps had been removed from his shoulders, but they had left a deep imprint upon his character.

[19] "Letter from the Secretary of the State Board of Health to the Public," in the *St. Paul Daily Press*, September 3, 1872.

4

With Probe and Microscope

THREE major activities ate into Hewitt's energies during his early years as secretary of the State Board of Health. He campaigned to bring local boards of health closer to the state board, he waged war almost singlehanded against smallpox, and he developed a publication program with himself as editor. Innumerable other problems plagued him. Indeed, he sometimes felt that no sooner had one baffling situation been solved than a dozen new ones sprang up. Moreover, his old techniques and points of view were being challenged by the dramatic revelations of a new science, which, stemming from Europe's great reseach centers toward the close of the nineteenth century, took him across the Atlantic for study in London, Berlin, and Paris.

Although Hewitt was inclined to attack all his problems simultaneously, he soon learned to concentrate on only a few at a time. He began with a program to force local health agencies to co-operate with the state board. The village health officer, he knew, was age-old in American life. Paul Revere had once headed Boston's town board. After the colonies gained independence most communities set up some sort of health organizations, which were independent of the state and were fiercely jealous of their privileges. Hewitt found this true in Minnesota. The territorial code had authorized justices of the peace, village trustees, and city councils to exercise control over the maintenance of the sick and the poor, over nuisances injurious to health, and over quarantine.[1]

As Hewitt thumbed the health acts, he noticed a statute providing for the punishment of offenses against the public health. Originally passed by Wisconsin, this act automatically became law in the Terri-

[1] Minnesota, *Revised Statutes*, 1851, pp. 124–126.

tory of Minnesota. Undoubtedly the first public health law of Minnesota, the act provided penalties for the sale of "diseased, corrupted, or unwholesome" provisions, for the adulterating of foods and liquors and of drugs and medicines, and, finally, for the deliberate inoculation with smallpox in order to "cause the prevalence or spread" of this infectious disease.[2]

Shortly after the Civil War town supervisors assumed jurisdiction over health matters. A supervisor, in Hewitt's opinion, was an improper person to trust with the health of citizens. Traveling through the state, Hewitt found supervisors too busy with political affairs to give the necessary attention to sanitary regulations. Some frankly snubbed the secretary, and others made only a thin pretense of cooperating. Yet, despite Hewitt's resentment, the earlier acts and the work of supervisors had accomplished much. Local newspapers showed this. A St. Paul woman was fined for permitting too much filth to accumulate in her back yard, and a Miss Ellen Grant was penalized for keeping pigs within the city limits. Health officers were raiding tanneries where green hides were treated.[3]

Despite these efforts, Hewitt concluded that any locally elected health official was at a disadvantage, and he determined, if possible, to keep the state board free from political manipulation. Perhaps he also developed an exaggerated respect for the importance of law, believing that a legislative statute itself would solve evils. He failed to realize that the personal equation was quite as important as the law. As he became mellower, however, he learned that, while law was necessary, men were imperative if the law was to be administered successfully. Co-operation was more efficient than compulsion.

Nevertheless, in 1873 Hewitt persuaded the legislature to pass an act destined to have far-reaching consequences in the protection of the health of the average citizen. It provided for boards of health in all incorporated towns, villages, boroughs, and cities. It stipulated that health officers be appointed, and advised that physicians assume the duties of health officers. Sanitary officers, under this act of March 10, 1873, were to make "once in every three months and oftener if necessary, a thorough sanitary inspection" and "present a written report of such inspection at the next meeting of the board of health." Hewitt was delighted with the next clause, which read: "and all local boards

[2] *Republication of Important General Laws of Wisconsin, Now in Force in the Territory of Minnesota, by Provision of the Organic Act*, chapter 56 (St. Paul, 1850).
[3] Minnesota, *General Statutes*, 1866, p. 145; *St. Paul Daily Press*, July 4, 8, August 1, 28, 1872.

of health and health officers shall make such investigations and reports, and obey such directions as to infectious diseases as shall be directed by the state board of health."[4]

Backed by this authority, Hewitt inaugurated his attack upon contagious diseases. By 1877 local boards were sending him reports of scarlet fever, diphtheria, and smallpox cases. All were fearful diseases, and each took its toll of Minnesota lives annually. Newspapers reported smallpox cases almost casually, so common had they become. Hewitt, slaving in Red Wing under a score of tasks, thought that the disease might be prevented. There was no real reason why an immigrant woman should bring smallpox to Shakopee with her; there was no excuse for travelers to arrive at St. Paul with the disease and cause four deaths; and there was no excuse for Winona having to fear the disease. Hewitt would not shut his eyes to the dreadful fact that "the pestilence is abroad in the land"; but he also would not tolerate the idea that smallpox epidemics could not be avoided. Far too many persons, young and old, were walking the streets scarred for life with smallpox's deep pits.[5]

Innumerable Minnesota communities sought to avoid contagion by instructing their citizens how to behave when smallpox entered the home. Hewitt helped to formulate some of these instructions, and he approved most of them. Printed as handbills or published in the daily press, they usually emphasized seven points:

1. On the first appearance of the disease the patient should be placed in a separate apartment, as near the top of the house as possible, from which curtains, carpets, bed-hangings and other needless articles of furniture should be removed, and no persons except the medical attendant and the nurse or mother be permitted to enter the room.

2. A basin containing a solution of chloride of lime, or carbolic acid, should be placed near the bed for the patient to spit in.

3. Handkerchief not to be used, but pieces of rag employed instead for wiping the nose of the patient. Each piece, after being used, should be immediately burned.

4. A plentiful supply of water and towels should be kept for the use of the nurse, whose hands, of necessity, will be soiled by the secretions of the patient. In one hand basin the water should be impregnated with Condys fluid of chlorid, by which the taint on the hands may at once be removed.

5. Outside the door of the sick room a sheet should be suspended so as to cover the entire doorway; this should be kept constantly wet

[4] *General Laws*, 1873, p. 116.
[5] *General Laws*, 1877, p. 232; *St. Paul Daily Press*, January 5, 11, 21, 1872; *Minneapolis Tribune*, January 27, 1872.

with a solution of lime. The effect of this will be to keep every other part of the house free from infection.

6. The discharge of the bowels and kidneys of the patient should be received into vessels charged with disinfectants, such as the solution of carbolic acid, or chloride of lime, and immediately removed. By these means the poison thrown off from internal surfaces may be rendered inert, and deprived of the power of propagating disease.

7. The thin skin or cuticle which peels off from the hands, face and other parts of the body in convalescent patients is highly contagious. Baths should be continued every day for four times, when the disinfectation of the skin may be regarded as complete. This, however, should not be done without first consulting the medical attendant.[6]

These pointers probably were adequate enough after smallpox struck, but Hewitt was much more concerned with prevention. The old adage, "An ounce of prevention is worth a pound of cure," was a rule he lived by. Vaccination was the ounce of prevention that he emphasized constantly. Again and again he explained that vaccination really was nothing new; but all too frequently his patients, arriving in Minnesota from the Old World, carried with them a deep repugnance to the scratch of the virus-covered knife. Sometimes folk superstitions, handed down for generations, stood in the way; at other times religious beliefs prevented foreigners from being vaccinated. Hewitt used persuasion and force to combat superstition and church prejudice.

On one occasion, so the story goes, Hewitt arrived at a Minnesota monastery on a bitter winter evening to urge vaccination of the clergy. He had heard that the monks had refused to be scratched and he was determined, in his forthright manner, to show them the error of their ways. He was shown into a cold hall and told that the abbot would see him soon. The doctor waited. Hungry, chilled, and not too patient normally, he grew more irritated by the moment. After an hour that seemed like ages, he was ushered into the presence of the abbot, whose frigidity was exceeded only by that of the hall Hewitt had just left.

"I want to tell you," Hewitt exploded, "that I am familiar with the rules of your order, and I know that one of its main tenets is hospitality to strangers. You have grossly disobeyed that rule! You kept me waiting in a cold hall for over an hour!"

Abashed, the abbot apologized and promised the doctor that he would be made comfortable. The next day Hewitt walked into a large room where the monks had assembled. To his amazement, they told him that one of the clergy would read a paper proving that vac-

[6] *St. Paul Daily Press*, March 1, 1873.

cination was not only wrong but useless. Hewitt was totally unprepared and listened uneasily. Suddenly an idea struck him, and he settled down in his high-backed chair to listen complacently. At the paper's conclusion, the monks nodded their satisfaction and approval.

Then the abbot turned to Hewitt, who slowly rose to his feet. "This," he said, "has been very interesting. I, a physician, have listened to a paper on medicine written by a theologian. Now I propose that you, theologians, listen while I, a physician, address you on a matter of theology. There is one of your doctrines which I, as a physician, know to be impossible, and I can prove it." The humor of the situation struck them all and, led by the abbot, the monks rolled up their cassock sleeves and were vaccinated, down to the youngest novice.[7]

Control of smallpox seemed impossible, but Hewitt doggedly went ahead giving directions for the care of the sick, mailing circulars which he had written and had printed, keeping in touch with local health officers, and dispensing vaccine. On January 10, 1878, he received a letter from Dr. E. J. Davis telling him that smallpox had appeared in Mankato. Then began a typical Hewitt routine, which he had worked out and which he followed, with necessary variations, for years. He replied to Dr. Davis immediately, requesting particulars and asking for the names of reliable physicians near Mankato who could aid in vaccination. He rushed to the town a hundred circulars on contagious diseases. They were written so that the average person could understand them and they had been worked out well in advance. They urged the vaccination of the entire population, for "in this way we can with the greatest certainty prevent an epidemic of this dreaded disease." Hewitt emphasized that vaccination was a simple process and free from danger, saying that all that was necessary was to have fresh and pure virus carefully introduced into the little wound. Most circulars ended with the following: "Should small pox appear anywhere in the State this Board requests that any one, knowing the fact, give notice of it immediately to the Secretary, at Red Wing, that we may co-operate with the local authorities in limiting it to the place where it occurs."[8]

In addition to sending circulars to Mankato, Hewitt, as a matter of routine, notified health officers of St. Paul, Minneapolis, and Winona. On January 17 Dr. Davis reported six cases of variola, or true smallpox, and one of varioloid, a mild form of the disease. Davis also sub-

---

[7] Charles Lewis Slattery, *Certain American Faces*, 154 (New York, 1918).
[8] A typical smallpox circular was pubished in the *Pioneer Press*.

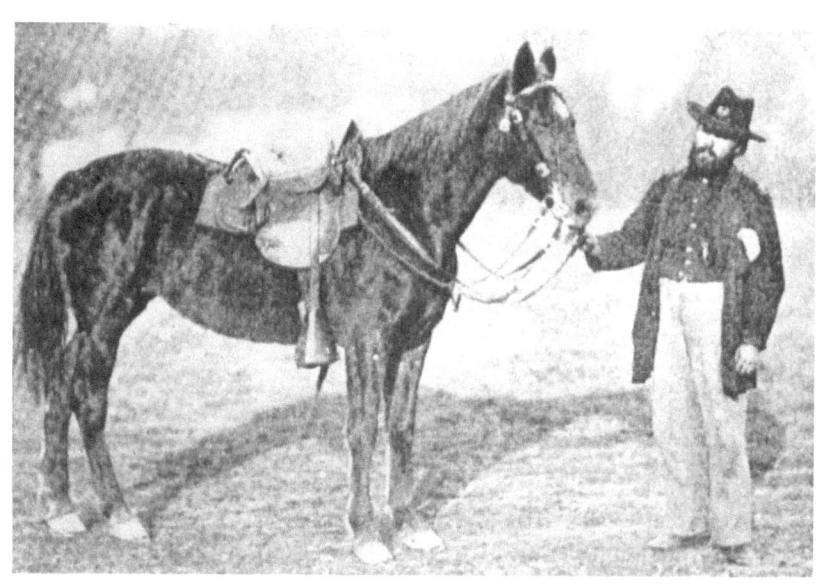

SURGEON HEWITT AND "FAN"
From F. T. Miller, ed., Photographic History of the Civil War, vol 7 (New York, 1911)

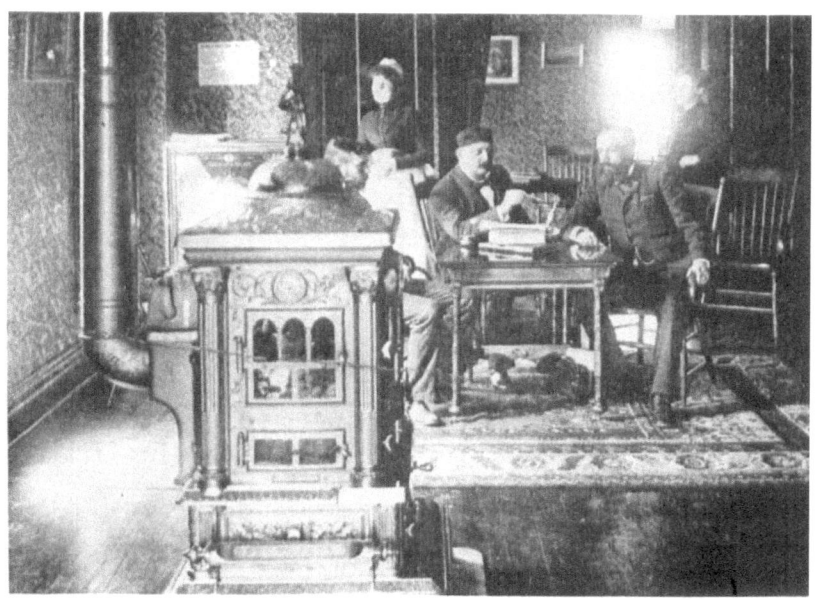

DR. JUSTUS OHAGE, ST. PAUL HEALTH OFFICER, IN HIS OFFICE
Courtesy Ramsey County Medical Society

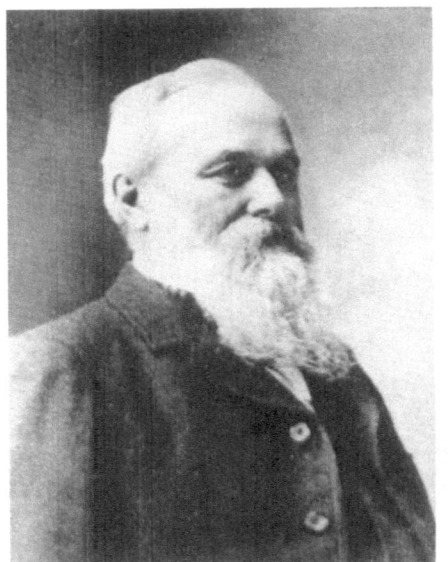
CHARLES N. HEWITT, 1872–97

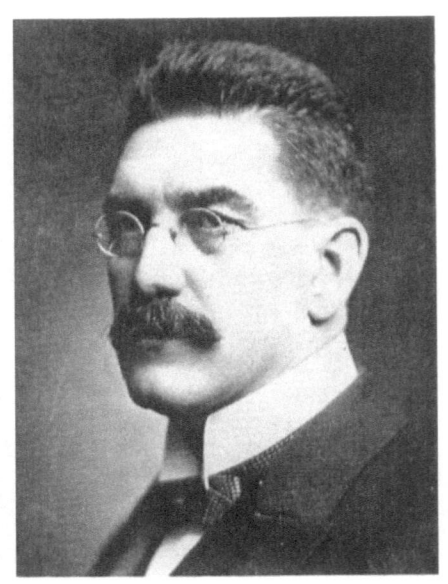
HENRY M. BRACKEN, 1897–1919

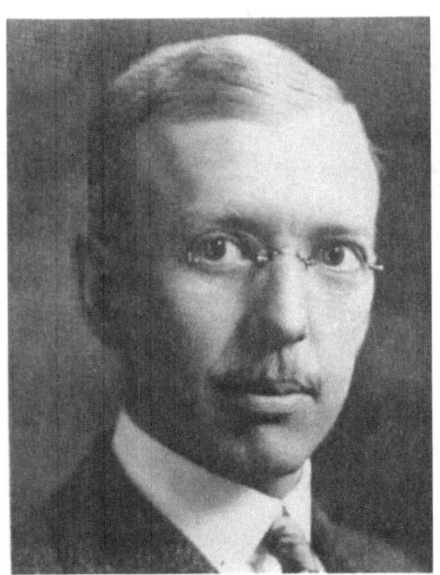
CHARLES E. SMITH, 1919–21

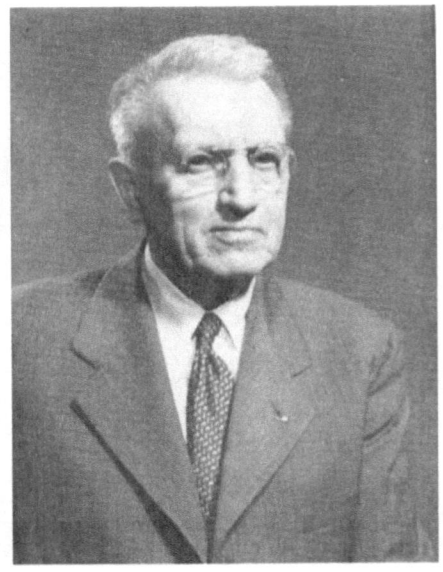
ALBERT J. CHESLEY, 1921–

SECRETARIES OF THE STATE BOARD OF HEALTH
Courtesy Minnesota Department of Health

mitted a list of physicians. To them Hewitt wrote immediately, requesting their assistance.

Then he began tracing the source of the disease. His detective work was not too difficult, for he soon learned that a woman and her two children had brought smallpox with them when they returned to Mankato from a visit in Wisconsin. Fearing that the train crew of the St. Paul and Sioux City Railroad might have become infected, Hewitt wrote to the general manager, explaining the circumstances and requesting that trainmen be vaccinated. He also asked that no sick person be admitted to a train at Mankato without a medical certificate which showed him free of smallpox.[9] The railroad complied with Hewitt's first request, but refused the second because it was without warrant in law.

Soon Hewitt's mail was heavy with letters from physicians throughout the Minnesota Valley. They invariably asked for further information and requested that vaccine be sent them. Hewitt was securing the board's supply of vaccine from Dr. Ezra Griffin at Fond du Lac, Wisconsin, and then selling it at cost to Minnesota physicians. By the close of the first week of February, he had dispensed at least two hundred points of vaccine. Many persons had been vaccinated in Mankato and Blue Earth County.[10]

Before the epidemic ended, with thirty-eight cases in Blue Earth County, twenty-seven in Mankato, and a total of seven deaths, Hewitt was faced with one of the great tribulations of the health officer. Misinformation and rumor seeped through the state, with falsehoods increasing with each retelling. Even Dr. A. A. Ames, Minneapolis health officer, stated publicly that smallpox existed in Chicago, Milwaukee, and Albert Lea. At once Hewitt checked this report, and then denied it officially. "The Pioneer Press," wrote the editor, "hasn't heard of any such rumor, but takes pleasure in stamping it as a base fabrication. Whatever Secretary Hewitt says about it we will swear to." [11] This was not an unusual reaction.

Hewitt did not close a file on an epidemic until he had received a complete report from local health officers. Always interested in the source of infection, he urged physicians to try to establish where and how epidemics started. He stressed the importance of tracing the in-

[9] State Board of Health, *Annual Reports*, 1879, p. 17; Hewitt Diary, January 12, 1878.
[10] State Board of Health, *Annual Reports*, 1879, p. 25. A "point" was the vaccine serum collected on the point of a splinter of ivory or wood and permitted to dry for use later, usually up to a period of three months.
[11] Hewitt Diary, 1878; *Pioneer Press*, January 19, 20, 1878.

fection's source in each individual case. As early as 1871 he was paying serious attention to the germ theory, and he took every opportunity to gather evidence that either would support or deny the idea that microbic agencies were responsible for illness. Local epidemics, such as the one at Mankato, were searched for clews. He reported to the Minnesota State Medical Society two theories as to the cause of disease — the germ and the physical theories — without stating his own opinion. Speaking of the treatment of wounds, he mentioned deodorants which remove "noxious gases," but "cannot arrest decomposition or fermentation, or, more exactly speaking, cannot kill *disease germs*." He continued: "Antiseptics act by destroying all sources of decay in producing the death of *organic living germs*." [12]

Hewitt also abandoned the idea that pus formation was the natural sequel to any operation or wound. "Union direct, or by first intention, should be the first aim," he said. "That impossible, come as near to it as may be by imitating its conditions. Removal of blood clots, coaption of surfaces, thorough drainage of discharges, as little dressing and as few ligatures as possible, torsion of blood vessels, when practicable, and the thorough exclusion of morbific poison from without, by the mechanical, chemical, and vital means already indicated." [13]

Vaccination, however, remained among Hewitt's primary interests. Yet he did not neglect the development of bacteriology and the discoveries of Koch and Pasteur. Hewitt had established a small, primitive laboratory in 1877, where tests of food and water were begun. In 1888 he became the proud possessor of a Zeiss microscope and shortly thereafter wrote: "I'm spending all the time I can spare in my cozy little bacteriological laboratory and enjoying it hugely." [14]

As the years moved swiftly, Hewitt realized more and more that working alone in his crude laboratory brought him neither the knowledge nor the proficiency that he wanted. A great drama was being enacted abroad, and he wanted a place where he might watch it unfold. He believed that one of the major functions of a health program was to furnish laboratory service. If physicians could have specimens examined by skilled technicians, they would be in a vastly better position to serve patients. The more Hewitt pondered, the more he came

---

[12] State Medical Society, *Transactions*, 1872, pp. 84, 86.
[13] Mechanical means were a layer of cotton wool as a filter to keep out foreign material, and adequate and correct suturing; chemical means were deodorizers, disinfectants, and antiseptics; vital means were fresh air, sunshine, and cheerful surroundings.
[14] Hewitt Letter Book, November 28, 1888, Hewitt Papers.

to the conclusion that it would be beneficial for him to get additional laboratory training.

His eyes naturally turned to Europe, and in the fall of 1889 he left on a five-months leave of absence to familiarize himself with foreign methods of vaccine production and bacteriological research. The doctor and Mrs. Hewitt landed in Ireland in late November. At Dublin, a town of dirty tenements and scores of poor, Hewitt visited the vaccine department of the local board and learned, to his gratification, that vaccination against smallpox was compulsory for all children over three months old. The strain of virus in use, he was told, had been continued since 1802.[15]

Hewitt found London health officers enthusiastic advocates of vaccination, doing their utmost to prevent smallpox and receiving public support, although a "persistent and noisy" minority made difficulty. After visiting vaccine stations and watching health officers at work, Hewitt sent home a complete description of what he saw. "I have seen such virus collected and stored for distribution and watched it from the arm of the child into the glass tube used for its collection — seen the tubes sealed and watched the process of their microscopic examination at the office of the Local Government Board before they are accepted or issued for use, and the methods of recording the results there," he wrote, "and it is but justice to say that we have nothing approaching to the painstaking labor which is here given to secure the most perfect lymph and to protect it from all possibility of admixture and to bring it to the person upon which it is to be used in the most perfect condition."

"The name of every child vaccinated at these public stations," he continued, "is recorded with the age, sex, residence and physical conditions. It is brought back to the vaccinator on the eighth day, and the results of the operation are carefully recorded. Any unfavorable appearance is carefully recorded, too, and another examination is requested if anything untoward should happen afterward. . . . The Local Government Board spares no pains or expense needed to get the true history of all cases found to present any unfavorable symptoms and promptly investigates all complaints as soon as received."

Then, in his usual meticulous manner, he described postvaccination procedure. He wanted his Minnesota colleagues to know exactly what was going on. "Perfectly typical eighth-day vesicles on healthy children

[15] "Correspondence of the Secretary," in *Public Health in Minnesota*, 5:104 (December, 1889).

who are carefully examined and found free of abrasion, pimple or rash are used for supplying lymph," he wrote. "Only such lymph as flows without pressure and free of blood is collected in delicate glass capillary tubes which are immediately sealed at each end in a flame. They are put into separate envelopes and marked with the number corresponding to the record of the child from which they are taken. These tubes are immediately sent to the office of the Local Government Board where each is again recorded and carefully examined with a microscope. If clear, free from blood or any opacity, they are returned to their proper envelopes as fit for distribution. When called for they are again examined, and if still clear are sent out in the original envelope so that results can be traced from the person upon whom they may be used directly back to the child from which each one was taken. So much in brief as to humanized vaccine virus." [16]

When Hewitt learned that Sir Robert Corey was directing a calf-vaccine station, he made arrangements to visit it. Corey welcomed the Minnesota secretary graciously, giving him detailed plans of the organization, expenses, and methods in use and furnishing him with plans of operating tables and a set of instruments. Hewitt photographed calves in position for operation and their appearance 96 and 120 hours later. He also took pictures of children's arms after inoculation with calf lymph. He was amazed at the mild reactions; they "are no greater than we have very often with humanized virus," he wrote.[17]

Concerned as he was with the problem of vaccination, Hewitt found time for a variety of experiences. He worked with Dr. E. Klein, distinguished English bacteriologist, on the etiology of diphtheria. Klein also showed him slides of streptococci isolated from the sputum of influenza patients, which he believed to be the cause of this disease. Hewitt traveled through southern England, visiting York, Hull, Bradford, Manchester, and Leicester, to observe water supplies, sewerage systems, garbage disposal, and housing. The housing of English laborers bothered him, and he wrote rather bitterly that there was scarcely proper place for man, or even pig, pony, or cow; "almost total destruction" must take place, he wrote, before "decent reconstruction" would be possible.[18]

On his return to London, Hewitt developed a mild influenza, which left him weak and a little dispirited. By the time he arrived in Berlin

---

[16] *Public Health in Minnesota*, 5:117 (February, 1890).
[17] *Public Health in Minnesota*, 5:119 (February, 1890).
[18] *Public Health in Minnesota*, 5:120 (February, 1890).

he had lost forty pounds. In April, 1890, the Hewitts were in Paris, staying at the Hotel d'Angleterre. If the doctor had been disappointed in his hope to study with Koch in Berlin, he was charmed by an opportunity to become Pasteur's pupil. He was assigned a laboratory and received instruction from Drs. Emile Roux and Alexandre Yersin, who just then were developing their diphtheria antitoxin.

Hewitt's first meeting with Pasteur lingered long in his memory. A mutual friend introduced the two. Pasteur greeted him kindly in broken English and listened attentively while Hewitt outlined his interest in learning the Pasteur treatment for rabies, the bacteriology of diphtheria, more about tuberculosis in both men and animals, and general bacteriological technique.[19]

The Pasteur Institute, in which Hewitt spent his happiest days abroad, was a large brick building standing back from the street. Between it and a high iron fence a flower garden rioted in color. Scattered throughout spacious grounds were stables, rabbit houses, and, wrote Mrs. Hewitt in her diary, a "pretty little house for the gardener."[20] The large reception room was filled with patients of all ages awaiting treatment. Children pointed out pictures hung on light, cheerful walls. Down a short hall was the inoculating room. Here was a flat-topped desk holding fourteen wine glasses, each containing the virus solution and each successive glass attenuated one day longer than the preceding one. Mrs. Hewitt noticed a tad come from Ireland for treatment and an Algerian wearing a Turkish fez. A little girl of six sobbed violently. Pasteur, who could not resist the cries of a child, came into the room, lifted the little one in his big arms, and said with tender pity, "Ma pauvre petite fille." Not even a paralyzed hand could keep him from tending children. Mrs. Hewitt described Pasteur as a "little old man with a strong face, anxious but vivid."

Although Hewitt hated to leave the excitement of Pasteur's laboratory, he was eager to return to Red Wing where he could inaugurate techniques he had acquired. Again at home, he set to work enthusiastically. His vaccine station was shaped in his mind before carpenters began pounding special stalls together in the spacious barn. They added a small, boxlike room containing a stove and boiler. This was the doctor's working office. It was supplied with artesian well water. The winter of 1890 found all in readiness, and Hewitt made arrangements with a retired dairyman to furnish young calves. On December 13 — a day Hewitt never forgot — he inoculated his first calf with vac-

[19] Hewitt Diary, April 12, 1890.
[20] Mrs. Charles N. Hewitt Diary, April, 1890, Hewitt Papers.

cine obtained from the Massachusetts State Board of Health. Fifty of the sixty-four inoculations worked. The first production of vaccine in Minnesota had begun.

Five days later Hewitt inoculated a second calf, "a very fine nursing bull," from the best three pustules of the first calf. Later he started another strain of vaccine obtained from Sir Robert Corey in London. Hewitt wanted to compare the two resulting vaccines. He wrote glowingly to Corey on January 23, 1891, that there had been no bad reaction in any of the calves and that none had shown "any variation of temperature, appetite or any other evidence of ill-effects." Then he added another significant sentence: "I have not ventured to use the vaccine on children yet, but shall as soon as I have applied every test of its purity." [21]

Hewitt estimated that from fifty to seventy-five per cent of Minnesota's children were not vaccinated, and he was extremely anxious to protect them if possible.[22] He must be sure before he started work, however, that he possessed an absolutely safe and reliable vaccine. Early morning and late evening found him in his stable workroom, testing and rechecking until he convinced himself that his vaccine would work no harm. Only then did he begin using it. By August he had vaccinated two thousand persons with good results. He had even sent samples of the lymph to England to be tested against the original strain. The two corresponded perfectly.

His station at Red Wing supplied vaccine free to state health officers. Private practitioners were sent five points gratis for a first trial. Printed directions were enclosed, as well as a postal card to be returned as a report to the station. The canny Hewitt also designed a certificate of vaccination to be presented to children who reported to their physician on the seventh day after vaccination. These certificates, properly signed by health officers and physicians, were presented to little ones who boasted their scratches had "took." [23]

The Red Wing station was for the "propagation of pure calf vaccine," and Hewitt made that perfectly plain. He took pains also to indicate to the medical profession exactly what the secondary objectives of his work were. As usual, he listed them neatly: [24]

1. To answer professional and popular objection to humanized vaccine by furnishing one of natural origin which has never entered a human body, is cultivated on healthy, nursing calves, who drink the

---
[21] Hewitt Letter Book, 1889–93, p. 139.
[22] Hewitt Letter Book, 1889–93, p. 157.
[23] *Public Health in Minnesota*, 8:40 (May–June, 1892).
[24] *Public Health in Minnesota*, 8:39 (May–June, 1892).

milk from our own cows, selected for the purpose, and whose bodies are examined after slaughter for any evidence of disease.

2. To maintain a constant supply of calf vaccine.

(a) For the free vaccination of children in Minnesota under proper restrictions, and under the direction of the Local Boards of Health.

(b) To be prepared for the emergency of a sudden outbreak of small pox in the State.

(c) To supply physicians, what they have long asked, reliable calf-lymph at reasonable prices.

(d) To be able to offer to other State and Local Boards of Health the same facilities as to our own.

(e) In the above and other helpful ways, to do our share to restore vaccination to its rightful place as the surest protection against small pox.

Professional response was so enthusiastic that the station became self-supporting in 1894. Three years later it had furnished 26,240 points of vaccine to the state board, local boards, and state institutions. Hewitt maintained his interest in the station after his connection with the state board had ceased. It was one of the enduring activities of his life. In his final report he urged "the need for vaccination in the schools, and for infants" and he recommended the products of his Red Wing station.[25]

Editorship was farthest from his thoughts when Hewitt accepted the secretaryship of the state board, but it was not long before circumstances forced the blue pencil into his hand. He was not unwilling to edit the board's publications, even though he knew that work would multiply the demands upon his already crowded schedule. His primary obligation was the preparation and editing of the annual report. This he found to be an arduous task, for it not only must contain the secretary's report, but also should carry health statistics, results from questionnaires, reports of the sanitary investigations of public institutions, and directions and instructions. It was Hewitt's duty also to edit special articles received for publication.

The first annual report of the State Board of Health, printed under legislative authority, was brought out by Hewitt in 1873. It contained, in addition to the secretary's report, several general articles. Dr. A. B. Stuart contributed a study of the causes of disease with special reference to epidemics; Dr. D. W. Hand, a paper on the causes

---

[25] Minnesota State Board of Health and Vital Statistics, *Biennial Reports*, 1895–96, p. 77. The Minnesota State Board of Health became the "Minnesota State Board of Health and Vital Statistics" in March, 1887. At first, reports were issued annually, but beginning with the eighth report, that for 1879–80, they appeared biennially. In following citations of its publications, the board will be named in abbreviated form as "State Board of Health."

of mortality and another on tapeworm; and Dr. Charles Gronvold, lengthy remarks on Norwegian leprosy. Hewitt himself wrote on "The Duty of the State in the Care and Cure of Inebriates." He also described inspections of state institutions, including the prison at Stillwater and the Normal School at Mankato.

In his first official report as secretary Hewitt, as was his custom, spoke frankly. The man was never anything but direct. He said that when "this Board was authorized by the Legislature, and appointed by the Governor, the idea of public health, as a science to be studied by a body of medical men under State authority and at public expense, for the practical benefit of the State and its inhabitants, was almost entirely new to the people at large, and even to the educated classes. As you are aware, doubt was freely expressed by intelligent citizens. Many thought our State not sufficiently advanced to justify such an attempt at the scientific study of our sanitary condition, and questioned whether the benefit to come of it, would repay the labor and expense which it involved." [26]

Hewitt's desk at Red Wing was littered with notes when he prepared his manuscript. Brought together and published, they outlined the secretary's conception of the board's program. "The future work of the Board," wrote Hewitt in this first report, "is indicated by what has already been done." Then he enumerated four points:

1st. To use every effort to make the registration of births, marriages and deaths accurate and reliable.

2d. To encourage, steadily, the study of the science and art of public health in the university, colleges, and schools.

3d. To continue the careful inspection of the public institutions with the object of improving their sanitary condition, and to enable the Board to act intelligently as the advisor of the State in this regard.

4th. To carry out fully the study of the sanitary condition of our centres of population, and to stimulate local boards of health to the performance of this important part of their duties.

He also listed special problems of research, arranging them as neatly as the others in a group of three:

1st. (a) The number of sufferers from all forms of scrofulous diseases who come to Minnesota for *prevention and cure,* their condition on coming here, and the effect of climate, etc., upon the disease.

(b) The operations of scrofula as a disease cause on our resident population.

2d. The etiology and history of zymotic disease in the State, especially typhoid and eruptive fevers.

[26] State Board of Health, *Annual Reports,* 1873, p. 14.

3d. The influence of climate, residence and occupation in inducing or aggravating non-specific disease of the air passages.

As Editor Hewitt read what Secretary Hewitt had written, he nodded with satisfaction and, striking pen boldly in ink, came to his conclusion: "The work of the Board is so much of it in the office and library, that little else than the *results* of it come under direct popular observation. It is quiet, persistent research into the causes of sickness and mortality influencing our population, to discover and apply the means whereby their life and health may be preserved and prolonged. . . . Let us hope that legislative and popular co-operation and support will lighten the burden and facilitate the labors of those whose duty it is to guard the interests of public health." [27]

Year by year, as the activities of the board developed, Hewitt edited larger volumes. Even after he was given clerical assistance, he continued to pass on manuscripts and to take home with him long strips of galley proof. He even conceived ideas for articles, passing these along both to associates and private practitioners. Dozens of suggestions flitted through his own head, but most of them never came to print. His notes were stubbed with problems which should be investigated and the results printed. He was interested in the adulterations of foods, in infant mortality, and in the proper heating and ventilation of schools. After exhaustive labor he compiled and interpreted vital statistics of an average Minnesota population of ten thousand for an "average" year. Hewitt reasoned that "in our supposed population of 10,000 persons" thirty-five would die from zymotic diseases (typhoid fever, cholera infantum, whooping cough); eighteen, from some "local" disease (inflammation of the lungs, convulsions, heart disease); fourteen, from a constitutional disease (consumption, hydrocephalus, scrofula); and ten, from such developmental disease as premature birth and infantile debility. Five would be killed accidently.[28]

As editor of the annual reports, Hewitt also planned and wrote a sanitary water survey of Minnesota, paying special attention to the Red River Valley. In this he was assisted by S. F. Peckham, state chemist. At the same time Hewitt wrote a long report on the relations of scholastic methods to the health of public school children. Yet, with all his other interests, he did not forget his preoccupation with smallpox and vaccination. He wrote that he had never before encountered so many outbreaks nor faced more opposition to vaccination among Minnesota farmers. In a forceful paper entitled "Vaccination:

[27] State Board of Health, *Annual Reports*, 1873, p. 18.
[28] State Board of Health, *Annual Reports*, 1876, pp. 57–64.

What It Is and What It Has Accomplished in Minnesota in 1881–'82," he repeated once again what he had said so many times before: "Finally, it is my duty to call upon all intelligent people to come up to the measure of their responsibility as respects the loathsome and fatal disease small pox; a work easily done if heads of families, mothers particularly, will insist upon the vaccination of children in early infancy, and that it be carefully and thoroughly done. By that is meant to secure at least, three perfect vesicles upon each child. Unless they are obtained, repeat the operation until they are. If mothers will be careful to insist upon this, they will find their family physicians ready and glad to co-operate with them. Do not wait for a 'small pox scare' before doing this." [29]

In 1885 Hewitt added another editorial responsibility to his already crowded program. This was the establishment of a monthly magazine designed to be the official communication between the state board and local boards and health officers and to inform the public of current health news and practices. In addition, said Hewitt, "there will be given a brief of current sanitary discovery and news; excerpts from foreign and American journals; and other matter pertaining to the general subject." [30]

The first issue of *Public Health in Minnesota* appeared in March, 1885. Now Hewitt's desk at Red Wing was littered with additional manuscripts and proof. He lengthened his working day to crowd in his new editorial responsibilities, for *Public Health* was the child of his own brain and he was anxious for it to flourish. Two thousand copies were printed, and the subscription price was set at fifty cents a year. The venture proved successful almost from its beginning. As Hewitt had predicted, its monthly appearance, together with the freshness of its news, brought the state board and local boards closer.

Hewitt generally wrote the first two or three pages himself, commenting in short paragraphs and in popular language upon sanitary inspections, health conferences, and proposed legislation. He devoted his August, 1885, issue largely to school health, saying to the teachers of Minnesota: "This number of *Public Health* is largely addressed to you. You are directly concerned in the sanitary survey of schools and school buildings to be made by the Local and State Boards of Health." He asked teachers to sketch their buildings, showing dimensions, heating equipment, and condition of outhouses, and to report illness

[29] State Board of Health, *Annual Reports*, 1878, pp. 57–64, 71–108; *Biennial Reports*, 1881–82, pp. 182–192.
[30] *Public Health in Minnesota*, 1:1 (March, 1885).

among pupils. He urged them to read his article on the teaching of hygiene and then to try his plan. "Write to us," he said, "for any explanation or advice we can give, and tell us of your success." [31]

As issue followed issue, Hewitt broadened the scope of his journal and increased the number of its pages. He wrote with satisfaction at the end of the first year of publication that *Public Health* had received cordial approval at home and abroad and that both health officers and physicians had sent him "a series of fresh and original papers upon topics of the greatest interest." His pleasing informality — an editorial trait which must have been difficult for the blunt secretary to acquire — not only made *Public Health* enjoyable, but also brought him unsolicited manuscripts written, in many instances, in an easy style. He published, for example, Dr. B. J. Merrill's account of a vaccinating trip to lumber camps near Stillwater and printed Dr. W. A. Hunt's report of diphtheria in Dodge County. Hewitt's own contributions were numerous, ranging from a semihumorous recital of his experiences as a speaker at the Women's Club of Wisconsin to his letters from abroad, which appeared in 1889 and 1890.[32]

Despite Hewitt's attempt to create popular interest in *Public Health*, the little journal appealed more and more to the medical profession and less and less to the ordinary citizen. Not even all public officials approved it, for Hewitt wrote in 1889 that each month copies were returned by the Post Office Department from chairmen of county boards. A Norwegian chairman returned his copy, said Hewitt, with a card "written in the Norwegian language, in which he expressed himself very forcibly that he could not pay for the journal, and he did not want to read anything he could not pay for." [33] Hewitt replied angrily that his journal was sent free of charge to the fifteen hundred boards of health in Minnesota through their health officers or chairmen and said that it should be read and carefully filed.

By 1892, when *Public Health* was in its eighth volume, Hewitt sensed that his publication was no longer the effective medium it had been. He himself could no longer spend the time to make it as readable as he wished. Then, too, he was growing weary of endless disputes with printers and with authors who objected to having their manuscripts altered. Hewitt's editorials began to lack spark and showed the speed under which he labored. Now and again he issued

[31] *Public Health in Minnesota*, 1:45 (August, 1885).
[32] *Public Health in Minnesota*, 1:79 (December, 1885); 2:93 (February, 1886); 4:52–54 (August, 1888); 5:13 (April-May, 1889).
[33] *Public Health in Minnesota*, 5:90 (November, 1889).

a double number "because the work of the Secretary's Office has been so great as to prevent the regular issue." A professorship in public health at the University of Minnesota took time that might otherwise have been devoted to his journal. A hundred and fifty students were listening to Hewitt's lectures in 1893, and more than seventy-five had requested laboratory instruction.[34]

Soon after Hewitt removed his office from Red Wing to St. Paul in 1894, he determined to suspend publication. Undoubtedly the opening of new quarters in Room 515 of the Pioneer-Press Building influenced his decision, for upon him fell the responsibility of arranging correspondence and reports, of opening a reading room, and of enlarging the activities of the state board. The last issue of *Public Health* — a double one — was issued from Red Wing for May and June, 1894. It then had a circulation of four thousand. True to his nature, Editor Hewitt sent the final issue to press without a line of explanation. He was more concerned with his last article in *Public Health*, an appeal to public school teachers to know the principles of public health and to use them for the "instruction and benefit of their pupils and themselves."[35]

Hewitt hated to leave Red Wing with its charming river view. His home was there, and there his children had prattled through babyhood. His study, with its rows of calf-bound books and its littered desk, had been the battleground for victories and defeats. The vaccine station, where he had thrilled to success, would be hard to leave behind. He would miss, too, the little Episcopal Church and the friends he had made as a vestryman. But he knew as well as anyone that a state capital was a better location for a state agency than was a pleasant village town. There he would be nearer important officials and would be closer also to the rapidly growing University of Minnesota, in which he took so much interest.

He struggled with the decision. The advantages of each balanced nicely, but so did the disadvantages. Finally he made up his mind. He would not give up Red Wing and all it meant, but would keep his home and family there and commute to and from St. Paul. For years he had commuted, and it was no novelty. The decision made, he brushed it aside. Other problems fretted him more.

[34] *Public Health in Minnesota*, 8:97 (January–February, 1893); 9:64 (September 1893).
[35] *Public Health in Minnesota*, 10:24–27 (June, 1894).

5

End of an Era

COMMUTING from Red Wing to St. Paul, Hewitt found opportunity to write up case notes, jot down ideas for speeches, and prepare public health lectures for his classes at the University of Minnesota. He had been invited by President Folwell in 1873 to become a nonresident professor of public health. In his letter of July 13, Folwell explained the situation fully:

"I have the honor to inform you," he wrote, "that at the last meeting of the Board of Regents there was erected a 'department of instruction' of Public Health with the subjects Anatomy & Physiology associated, to be in charge of a nonresident professor. It was further resolved that the said department be put in charge of the Secretary of the State Board of Health. Permit me to express the wish that you will not decline to assume this task although it will add to your burden. I do not need to remind you of the importance of the department." [1]

Hewitt accepted promptly. He already was giving two lectures a week on hygiene to university students and was glad to extend this program to include courses in public health. The general physical condition of students had troubled him for some time, for he feared development of the mind at the expense of the body. The Board of Regents was pleased to adopt his recommendation that a system of physical examinations and a careful program of student health records be established. Although no student was to be required to submit to a physical examination, most undergraduates seemed pleased to avail themselves of the new health service. After Hewitt concluded his examinations for 1878, he wrote in his diary: "Am glad to notice a decided disposition to abandon the corset among the young ladies." [2]

[1] Folwell Papers, box 73.
[2] December 4, 1878.

Within a few years Hewitt was forced to discontinue physical examinations for lack of official support.

His public health courses, however, developed rapidly. Not until 1882 did Hewitt bring them to a point where he believed they were fairly complete. By then he had divided the work, delivering lectures on personal hygiene to subfreshmen and new students and offering work in sanitary science to university seniors. The upper-class course included instruction in sewerage, heating, lighting, and ventilation of private homes and public buildings, and epidemic diseases. In addition, Hewitt gave public lectures at the university on public health and its problems.

Concerned with administering the state board and busy with his university duties, Hewitt nevertheless found time to take an active role in the organization at the university of a College of Medicine, which was to examine applicants and grant diplomas, but was not to instruct. Provision was made even for a special examination to be given graduates in medicine who wished to become health officers. President Folwell and Hewitt planned carefully before Folwell presented Hewitt's plans to the Board of Regents on June 29, 1882. The first step, approved by the regents, was the appointment of Folwell, Hewitt, and Dr. William Leonard of Minneapolis to draw up definite organizational plans and to prepare an examination syllabus for medical students. This committee of three recommended to the regents that a nine-man faculty be appointed, each individual being a specialist in a particular branch of medicine. The program was approved on January 5, 1883, and five appointments were made. Dr. Franklin Staples was named professor of the practice of medicine; Dr. D. W. Hand, professor of surgery; Dr. William Leonard, professor of obstetrics; Dr. Perry H. Millard, professor of anatomy and physiology; and Dr. Hewitt, professor of preventive medicine. All these men were at one time or another members of the State Board of Health, and each was considered unusually competent in his specialty.

Meanwhile, the Minnesota legislature passed an act which regulated the practice of medicine and conferred upon the university the functions of an examining board, "with power to approve and accept diplomas of recognized medical colleges, as evidence of fitness to practice, or to require the applicant for license to be examined by the board." This was known as the "diploma law," and it represented Minnesota's first attempt to regulate medical practice.

President Folwell called the first meeting of the medical faculty for April 23, 1883. The men met in his office to organize the State Medical

Examining Board. Hewitt acted as chairman and, for all practical purposes, as dean, for he not only supervised administrative details but also prepared examinations in pathology, materia medica, and medical chemistry. He was at a loss to know just how difficult to make these examinations. For days he debated with himself and sought advice from others. Finally he decided to shape his questions practically "in the sense of relating to the actual business of a medical man's life & 'elementary' as the law requires by making them relate to the most common & ordinary work of a practitioner." [3]

This was no easy task, but on October 11, 1883, the date of the first examination, he was ready. This was to be a very formal occasion. The examining faculty marched single file into the Capitol's Senate Chamber. Behind followed thirteen candidates for licenses. President Folwell explained the function of the State Medical Examining Board and Hewitt outlined the order of procedure. Then the questions that had been so carefully prepared were passed out, and the chamber settled down to a quiet broken only by the scratching of pens on paper. After the written questions had been corrected and the oral answers weighed, it was announced that only three candidates had failed.[4]

Hewitt, however, was not convinced that Minnesota should only examine and pass on a candidate's fitness to practice. That was good enough as far as it went, but it did not go far enough. Both Folwell and Hewitt hoped for the establishment of a medical teaching department at the university. They believed that the university's medical school should be built around a department of public health. This argument was put forcibly to President Cyrus Northrop, Folwell's successor. "The matter of medical & associated work at the University is constantly on my mind as it has been for years," wrote Hewitt. "If we can develop systematically and as proper occasion offers a grand future is before us. My plan includes not only medical higher education, but the resting [of] that & all other associated work on development in the Department of Public Health which is more & more the admitted foundation of Practical Medicine. 'Prevention first, cure if you must; capacity *to do* in both directions.' Around Preventive Medicine are grouped the education & work of the Health officer, the Sanitary engineer & the Plumber, the Pharmacist, the Water Engineer, &c." [5]

No doubt Hewitt's ideas were out of line with the times. Perhaps

[3] Hewitt Diary, October 9, 1883.
[4] Hewitt Diary, October 11, 1883.
[5] Hewitt to Folwell, June 14, 1886, and to Cyrus Northrop, May 22, 1886, Folwell Papers, boxes 33, 71.

he was overly impressed, as the result of his own enthusiasm for public health, with the belief that medical training should center around a core of training in preventive medicine. Some physicians objected to his insistence upon the importance of training health officers, sanitary engineers, and plumbers. Perhaps they even objected to the public school teaching of hygiene, feeling that physicians would lose income if children were too well. But Hewitt believed that children who were properly instructed in public health would demand better medicine when they grew up.

Hewitt's plans for superior medical education and service called for a laboratory, a recitation room, a library, and a sanitary museum. He wished medical students to have laboratory instruction in original experimentation, and research in sanitary science and in biology and chemistry.[6] His medical school was not to ignore the basic sciences, even if it was to revolve around public health. He did not reckon, however, upon both the source and the strength of the opposition.

Apparently Dr. Millard led the fight against Hewitt. Resigning from the examining board, Millard supported a new medical practice act, which was passed by the legislature in 1887 despite Hewitt's objections. This act created a Board of Medical Examiners to be appointed by the governor and to be independent of any medical school. The result was obvious: Hewitt's examining committee immediately lost its authority and significance. The new examination law, from every point of view, was much better than the old one, even though Hewitt failed to admit this. Indeed, it was the first act of its type to be placed upon the statute books of any state, and it became the model for other commonwealths to follow.[7] It placed Minnesota among the most progressive states in the nation.

Millard continued to push his campaign, urging the faculties of the Minnesota Hospital College and the St. Paul Medical College to petition the Board of Regents to establish a teaching department of medicine at the university. The Minnesota College of Homeopathic Medicine followed the trend. All three institutions offered to surrender their charters and tender their property to the state for the temporary use of the new university department.

This was the plan that ultimately prevailed, although the university chose to use the facilities of the Minnesota Hospital College. In October, 1888, the first entrance examinations were held under the

[6] Hewitt to Northrop, May 22, 1886, Folwell Papers, box 71.
[7] Hewitt to Folwell, February 14, 1887, Folwell Papers, box 33; Richard O. Beard, "The History of Medical Education in the State of Minnesota," in *Northwestern Lancet*, 29:32 (January, 1909).

supervision of Dr. Millard, who had then become dean. Hewitt found himself squeezed out in the reorganization. The reasons for his exclusion are not too difficult to determine. First of all, he still was a dogmatic, determined individual, who shunned compromise. Moreover, his friendship was not as close with President Northrop as it had been with President Folwell. In the third place, critics felt that Hewitt overemphasized the public health aspect of medical education. Finally, the homeopaths were Hewitt's bitter enemies. He had spoken of homeopaths as "little pills" and had raged against any merger with them. Certainly the homeopaths wanted no part of an organization which would be dominated by Hewitt.[8]

Then, too, there was growing opposition on the part of younger men to submitting to domination by a single individual. They thought Hewitt had become too powerful. As executive secretary of the State Board of Health and Vital Statistics, he controlled that board; he had been dean of the examining faculty of medicine at the university; he was a past president of the Minnesota State Medical Society and was one of its most influential leaders; and, in 1888, at the time of the reorganization, he was president of the American Public Health Association. Perhaps Hewitt was preoccupied with too many duties to give sufficient time to the new medical school. If a place was not made for him in the medical school, he at least was able to keep his professorship in public health.

Folwell was disappointed in the new organization. He wrote Hewitt on April 10, 1888, saying, with a trace of rancor: "My impression is that the Pres. [*Northrop*] and regents have a bigger job on hand than they thought in getting the Med. Dept. into shape. My expectation is that some of them will be sorry enough that they did not let things alone as you, with my feeble assistance, had arranged them. Your plan was the only one by which real service could be done at once to the public and to the profession."

When Hewitt journeyed to Milwaukee in the cold November of 1888 to deliver his presidential address before the American Public Health Association, he had perhaps reached the climax of his career. During his busy years in Minnesota he had held almost every important medical office the state had to offer. He was known as a skilled planner and organizer. He had become a popular lecturer to both lay and professional groups, and he was respected by health authorities in the United States and Canada. Even his enemies acknowledged

[8] Hewitt to Folwell, July 4, 1872, Folwell Papers, box 71; Hewitt to Daniel W. Hand, April 9, 1888, Hewitt Letter Book.

the man's abilities, although they were willing enough to differ with him.

Hewitt prepared his Milwaukee speech carefully, rejecting scores of titles and tossing aside stacks of notes until finally he decided exactly the approach he considered best. Taking as his title "Public Health a Public Duty," he spoke for more than an hour, shaping each sentence carefully and developing every paragraph logically. He meant this address to be the high spot of his career, a document that would lay the sturdy foundation for continued progress in public health. It was meant to epitomize his entire thinking on health. He had less desire to entertain the delegates than to instruct them. "I wish I dare limit myself to the saying of pleasant things," he told his large audience, "or to such topics as make up the average of public addresses, and which compose, flatter, amuse, soothe, help to pass a pleasant hour, and leave nothing but a pleasant memory. But I dare not, nor do you expect it. We are here for business."

The speech really was praiseworthy, not merely because it traced briefly the development of public health activities in Minnesota and the nation, but chiefly because it set forth a series of propositions and problems that Hewitt felt were essential if preventive medicine were to expand into the importance he felt it deserved. He defined the first essential of sanitary authority as executive power which must be used systematically in the regular and scrupulous performance of everyday duty; he called for a better classification of causes of death; he urged changes in isolation techniques to insure "more thoroughness with the least interference with the liberty of the family"; and he asked for better apparatus for disinfecting sickrooms. He deplored the large mortality from noninfectious disease in children under five, and suggested more investigation. In connection with this, he recommended greater attention to home sanitation. A long paragraph was devoted to city sanitation, including water supply and sewage disposal. He spoke, too, of controlling offensive trades and of the protection of public and private water supplies.

As he approached his conclusion, Hewitt talked of the duties of a state board of health within a commonwealth, but hastened to say that a properly constituted state board of health had equally important duties outside the state. "The causes of ill-health, sickness, and premature death, and infectious diseases of men and domestic animals," he pointed out, "are no more limited by state than by township lines; nor are the most important of the other sanitary problems so restricted, but relate to interests and dangers common to more than one state; so that if it were not an imperative duty, the union of our states, defensive and offensive, against the enemies of public health, would pay in a purely commercial sense, as a mutual benefit insurance company pays, in the legitimate returns of the business."

But even state boards having due regard for national problems, said Hewitt, were not sufficient to provide adequate public health. A national board of health was imperative to protect the nation:

First, by a thorough knowledge of the character, location, and movements of diseases abroad.

Second, by preventing, by the best known methods, the shipping to this country of infected persons, animals, or things.

Third, by insisting upon competent sanitary service on board ship, with the best facilities for preventing, controlling, and crushing out any form of infection discovered on the passage out.

Fourth, by providing that the sanitary authority at the port of entry shall be fully informed of what is known of the sanitary history of the ship and her lading, up to the date of arrival, with later telegraphic report from the American consul and health officer at the port of departure, if necessary.

Hewitt's concluding remarks not only reflected his own enthusiasm for public health work, but also pointed the way for a more efficient national organization: "Let us unite, then, more thoroughly than ever, in pushing on to our common end and aim, by making every sanitary organization, from the least to the greatest, the best possible, for the duty it has to perform. Then, sooner than we expect, out of our honest and faithful labors, and our disagreements, too (always inevitable in every real advance — I had almost said, essential to it), shall come the crown of our common work, a national organization coordinate in all essential details with the state boards, and their representatives abroad. Standing in the same intimate and dignified relation with the government as did the old National Board, it will be the seal and the pledge of our union, disturbing no relations, rights, or duties of the state or local boards, but supplying another and essential help to the ideal of what it ought to be, which is, for the earnest health officer, the ambition of his professional life, and the truest gauge of his progress." [9]

Hewitt's duties became more complicated as the state's population swelled during the quarter century from 1875 to 1900. After his retirement as president of the American Public Health Association, he increased his interest in vital statistics and developed his laboratory.

[9] Hewitt, *Public Health a Public Duty: The Organization, Powers, and Relations of Local, State, and National Boards of Health* (Concord, New Hampshire, 1889).

Soon after arriving in Minnesota, he had suggested that the collecting and publishing of vital statistics be transferred from the assistant secretary of state, where it had been placed by a legislative act of 1871, to the secretary of the State Board of Health. His argument was logical: the assistant secretary of state was not a medical man; vital statistics depended upon medical knowledge; therefore, a trained physician should be placed in charge. The obvious candidate, of course, was the secretary of the board of health. Hewitt believed that local health officers should be made responsible for the collection of local birth and death records. He emphasized that birth certificates should be completed within five days and that death certificates should be returned within thirty-six hours. Local health officers were to submit monthly and annual reports to the state board, which would supply uniform blanks.[10] Not until March 8, 1887, however, did the legislature pass a vital statistics act which embodied most of Hewitt's recommendations.

Hewitt had his work cut out for him. Information concerning the births, illnesses, and deaths of Minnesotans had for years been incomplete and haphazard. Only in the larger cities — Minneapolis, St. Paul, and Duluth — did returns seem complete. In small communities and far-flung northern counties and townships, data all too frequently were garbled. C. F. Solberg, commissioner of statistics, complained in 1874 that "The Commissioner has been informed that the duty to give notice of births or deaths is very generally disregarded by parents and householders and not insisted upon by the local officers who defer the whole business of registration until the close of the year and then obtain their facts by making a house-to-house visitation." [11]

Incomplete as early statistics were, they did give a clew to health conditions, and they were of intense interest to the people. Urban newspapers frequently printed them with editorial comment. In 1888 Hewitt estimated Minnesota's population at 1,447,578. There were 38,149 births registered in 1886 and 29,211 in 1887. His report did not indicate the deaths in 1886, but he reported 13,262 deaths the following year, of which 7,093 were male and 6,049 were female. A comparative statement for the five years from 1882 to 1887 showed that in 1887 the percentage of deaths to population was .98. In 1893, after enormous labor, Hewitt brought together a composite picture of vital statistics covering the period from 1887 to 1891. He showed, in a series of graphs, that deaths from all causes in 1887 totaled 13,010 and in 1891 they num-

[10] State Board of Health, *Annual Reports*, 1874, p. 13.
[11] Commissioner of Statistics, *Annual Reports*, 1873, p. 4.

bered 14,714. The outstanding diseases were tuberculosis, pneumonia, typhoid fever, and diphtheria.[12]

Hewitt continued to pay special attention to the steady decline in the mortality from diphtheria, which he had been observing for nine years. "The use of antitoxine as a remedy for diphtheria," he wrote, "is increasing, and its success seems very encouraging. I am satisfied that its phophylactic use will prove of equal or greater importance than its curative influence, and respectfully urge the board to encourage observations in this direction, especially in the state institutions for children." [13]

As Hewitt obtained additional clerical help, he turned over more and more of the interpretation of vital statistics to assistants and devoted the time thus saved to his laboratory. Located in 1895 on the top floor of the Mechanics Arts Building on the university campus, the laboratory was Hewitt's pride and joy. A reporter who visited it said that "the atmosphere is pregnant with a mysterious odor, suggestive of witchcraft." The reporter found Hewitt in high humor, for he had just returned from Washington, D.C., where he had gathered new information about diphtheria. His caller asked him about the manufacture of antitoxin.

"We can't make anti-toxine like soapsuds," answered Hewitt. "That preparation takes months. Before we talk about it let us look into diphtheria." He explained, patiently and carefully, the technique for developing a pure culture of diphtheria bacillus. "I want people to know," continued Hewitt, after describing the diagnosis of diphtheria, "that I would like a couple of horses. If I can get one he'll be mine, not to drive, but for anti-toxine. Once we can get anti-toxine from a horse he becomes immensely valuable, for by a course of injections we can continue to get anti-toxine from him for two years. I will agree, if anyobdy gives me two horses, good sound horses, to begin to cultivate anti-toxine immediately and also to give the value of the horse in anti-toxine to poor children or any other charity the donor requests if I succeed in getting a proper preparation of anti-toxine. Is not that fair?"

The reporter agreed that it was and then asked Hewitt to tell him about the diagnosis of other diseases. He learned of sputum examinations for tuberculosis and also of Hewitt's labors in diagnosing diseases

[12]*Pioneer Press*, November 29, 1876, August 26, 1877, April 19, 1878, December 31, 1881, August 5, 1882, November 23, 1884, April 14, 1885; *Minneapolis Tribune*, August 5, 1879, December 30, 1886; State Board of Health, *Biennial Reports*, 1891-92, between pp. 34-35.

[13] State Board of Health, *Biennial Reports*, 1895-96, p. 10.

of cattle. Hewitt was anxious to receive animals that were suspected of being ill. "If the railroads and the local boards of health throughout the state," he said, "will comply with the suggestions of the state board which have been sent to them in the inspection and isolation of suspected animals and the disinfection of animals and things, these diseases can be easily crushed out. They have been brought into this state from adjoining states, and are now being spread from one place to another where precautions are not taken." [14]

The developing laboratory was concerned with diseases of animals as well as of men. Ever since Hewitt had become secretary, he had been forced to consider the relationship of the health of cows and hogs to human welfare. Glanders, lesions chiefly in the nose of horses, offered a special problem, as the disease was infectious and affected man. Local health officers frequently queried Hewitt concerning sheep scabies. A sheep farmer wrote angrily to Minnesota's attorney general, saying: "Now I am a resident tax payer of this town and I want a State Vetrinarian [sic] sent here to look into this matter and see what it is before it goes any farther at the Town's expense, and if the Chairman of the board has laid himself liable I want to see him have his just dues, for I think that there is a niger in the fence somewhere and I want him hunted out, and brought over the coals, and I think you are the man that can do it." The attorney general forwarded the complaint to Hewitt. In 1898 a St. Paul health officer quarantined more than two hundred sheep for scabies and then killed them all.[15]

Soon after Hewitt's appointment he was bombarded with questions about an epidemic referred to loosely as the "Canadian horse disease," or sometimes as the "epizooty," or even the "epizoozy." This was his initiation to a series of animal problems that continued for some twenty-five years. So troublesome did glanders become in 1884 that Hewitt twice contributed public announcements to the St. Paul press indicating the extent of the disease and urging stringent enforcement of quarantine laws. In September of that year Hewitt was instrumental in planning a detailed program for control of glanders, although he felt he could do little toward really allaying the disease without proper laboratory equipment. As is so frequently the case in public health problems, the public was indifferent. Dealers continued to traffic in diseased animals, even though the law provided that "Whoever knows or has reason to suspect the existence of any such disease (glanders, farcy,

[14] *Pioneer Press*, January 6, 1895.
[15] C. M. B. Livingston to H. W. Childs, November 24, 1893; memorandum by Myron H. Reynolds, February 17, 1898. Minnesota Department of Health, St. Paul.

etc.) among animals in his possession, or under his care, shall forthwith give notice thereof to the local board of health where such animals are kept, and for failure to do so shall be punished by a fine of not less than $50 nor exceeding $500, or imprisonment of not more than one year." When the laboratory finally was established, horse breeders began sending specimens to Hewitt for examination. The state board furnished free mallein for treatment, but even so, according to Hewitt in his last report as secretary, 507 horses were afflicted. He also stated, however, that the disease was diminishing.[16]

Eventually the laboratory aided cattlemen, but long before the primitive apparatus had been established on the university campus Hewitt had fought as best he could diseases of the mouth, tuberculosis, and blackleg. Of these, Hewitt recognized tuberculosis as the most significant. He spent tremendous energy attempting to control tuberculous cattle, not only because the death of cows was an economic loss to farmers, but also because of the danger of infected milk, butter, and cheese. The battle was a long one, and for many years it seemed that the state board was making little progress.

Veterinarians worked with the board of health, making post-mortem examinations and presenting findings. Investigators traveled the state, under Hewitt's supervision, to test suspected herds. An inspector found in a herd of thirty head of cattle nine cases of actinomycosis, a disease caused by the ray fungus affecting the jaws of cattle and swine. Health officers frequently wrote Hewitt asking how milk might be made pure. From Lanesboro, Dr. T. W. Hunt sent three questions that were typical of a large correspondence:

1. How can milk be made sterile of the tubercle bacilli?
2. Is the Pasteurization of milk a sure proof against the above germ? Or can the preparation termed "tuberculin" be used to better advantage? How & where could I best secure either or both of the above — "tuberculin," & Pasteur's apparatus?
3. I am desirous of learning the best method of sterilizing milk other than by that of boiling since sufficient boiling to destroy the tubercle bacillus renders the milk practically useless for table use.[17]

Time and again Hewitt urged the testing of herds. The results were forwarded to him for his recommendations. Frequently farm managers

---

[16] *St. Paul Daily Press*, October 24, 26, 1872; *Pioneer Press*, June 7, July 2, September 26, 1884, June 12, 1885; W. S. Webb to Hewitt, October 26, 1893, Minnesota Department of Health, St. Paul; State Board of Health, *Biennial Reports*, 1895–96, p. 11.

[17] *Pioneer Press*, December 19, 1889; letters to Hewitt from E. Mueller, May 17, 1894, and from T. W. Hunt, January 3, 1895, Minnesota Department of Health, St. Paul.

sent him rather informal accounts of what was going on. One of them wrote: "I attended a meeting today in Northcote of the Board of Supervisors of the town of Hampden to take under consideration the testing of all cows in the town for tuberculosis and they are greatly in earnest about it and want to investigate at once. I have assisted Mr. McFarlane in addressing for this evening on the subject and hope you will be able to send him about four bottles of tuberculine to make test and report to you. If you then think best to continue you can send more blanks and the necessary tuberculen [sic] and all shall be tested. I feel very solicitous about the stock on small farms in this community and am doing all I can to have an examination made."[18]

The extensive investigating work accomplished by the state board is indicated by the report of an agent working under the supervision of Dr. Franklin Staples of Winona. On June 26, 1895, the agent visited a farm located between Larnville and Pickwick, where he found in a herd of nineteen cattle animals suffering from actinomycosis. Proper treatment was commenced and the whole herd was quarantined. On June 27 he found one case at the city slaughterhouse at Winona. The place was immediately quarantined. On June 28 and 29 the investigator discovered on a farm near Stewartville nine cows afflicted with catarrh of the nasal chambers. He placed the entire herd of seventy-five head under quarantine and began treatment.[19]

During 1895 Hewitt used tuberculin for the diagnosis of tuberculosis in cattle, sending to the rural areas of Minnesota 3,185 doses. Of 2,975 animals tested, 6.27 per cent were condemned. "It seems advisable," he wrote, "that an examination of all herds of dairy cows furnishing milk for butter, cheese, or domestic consumption should be made. Tuberculin for such examination should be furnished by the state board of health, and used under the direction of the local boards. Condemned animals should be killed under inspection. The question of permitting carcasses lightly affected to be used for food will bear consideration. The mortality from tuberculosis in dairy herds costs the dairyman many times the amount incurred in carrying out the use of the tuberculin test."[20]

The laboratory, under the direction of Dr. Frank F. Wesbrook, gradually took over bacteriological animal work, paying particular attention to hog cholera and swine plague. Wesbrook, son of a former

[18] H. W. Donaldson to Hewitt, March 19, 1895, Minnesota Department of Health, St. Paul.
[19] *Pioneer Press,* July 2, 1895.
[20] State Board of Health, *Biennial Reports,* 1895–96, p. 11.

mayor of Winnipeg, Manitoba, had arrived in Minnesota in 1895, to accept an appointment as professor of bacteriology at the University of Minnesota Medical School and as director of the laboratory of the State Board of Health. He had been trained at the University of Manitoba and McGill University, and he had done graduate work at St. Bartholomew's Hospital in London and in the Rotunda Hospital in Dublin. Just before he came to Minnesota he had studied pathology at the University of Marburg, Germany, under the distinguished Karl Fraenkel. He was to remain in Minnesota until 1913, when he became president of the newly established University of British Columbia.

When Wesbrook took charge of the laboratory, the state board was reaching the end of an era. Hewitt's regime, although he did not realize it, was almost over. The public health service of Minnesota in 1895 consisted of the state board and approximately 1,780 local boards, of which 1,400 were in townships, 333 in villages, 40 in cities, and 3 in boroughs.[21] Hewitt had watched many of these boards develop, and he knew personally a majority of their health officers. He knew that forty-eight cities each had a board of health with a physician as health officer, but he also realized that in too many instances local health officials were not medically trained. This was particularly true in townships, where nurses as well as professional health officers were lacking.

The need for township nurses was especially serious. "Nurses trained to the care of infectious diseases are not to be had," wrote Hewitt, "and those of the average sort find better wages, accommodations and facilities in villages and cities, so that they are difficult to secure in townships even for greater wages than poor people can, or local boards are willing, to pay. . . . Common humanity and public safety demand that no time be lost in making the needful arrangements for providing a supply of competent women nurses, willing to serve in the care of infectious diseases in country districts, and arranging, in part at least, for their compensation."[22]

Hewitt had ambitious plans, now that the laboratory was under the competent supervision of Wesbrook, to strengthen rural health services and to continue his campaign against infectious diseases in both men and animals. He still maintained his vaccine station at Red Wing and he still took an active part in university affairs. Clerical help had relieved him of giving personal attention to the thousands

[21] State Board of Health, *Biennial Reports*, 1895–96, p. 5.
[22] State Board of Health, *Biennial Reports*, 1895–96, p. 8.

of letters that came to his office annually. He saw the State Board of Health as a helpful consulting agency always ready to supply local boards with advice and service. It was his earnest hope that more and more local health agencies would turn to the state board for the specialized assistance which only the state could furnish. He believed that many years were left to him to put into operation the policies he had been working for since 1872.

Unfortunately, he reckoned without giving proper regard to politics. Hewitt always had scrupulously avoided entangling himself in the snare of party ambitions. He had always believed that the state board must, of necessity, shun politics and be completely and totally nonpartisan. The health of the people was much too valuable to be involved in political scheming. For many years his feeling was justified. One governor after another reappointed him to the board. He asked no favors of them, and they apparently expected none from him. Nothing could have better satisfied Hewitt.

This was the situation until 1895, when David M. Clough became governor. Hewitt, if he followed his normal habit, probably paid as little attention to Clough's administration as he had to that of any other governor. Undoubtedly Hewitt was as brusque and straightforward in his dealings with the governor as he was with almost everyone else. It is certainly true that Tams Bixby, editor of the *Red Wing Republican* and private secretary to Governor Clough, asked Hewitt to contribute to the Republican campaign. "My husband declined," wrote Mrs. Hewitt years later, "stating that the State Board of Health had never mixed with politics and never would with his consent. Mr. Bixby then remarked that he had better change his mind as a matter of policy — and the matter was dropped between them." [23]

Perhaps Clough did not know and would not have approved, had he known, of Bixby's action. A close associate of Clough expressed the view that Bixby was "playing false" to Clough and said that the governor declared that Bixby was "trying to put him in bad with different men and organizations." Be that as it may, Clough failed to reappoint Hewitt. The doctor was sitting in his office on the afternoon of January 11, 1897, when the news was brought to him. Perhaps he had been expecting it, for he entered in his dairy that he had "long been prepared" for such an event.[24] Legend has it that within fifteen minutes

---

[23] Helen R. Hewitt to Folwell, September 19, 1927, Folwell Papers, box 52.
[24] L. G. Powers to Folwell, November 1, 1927, Folwell Papers, box 52; Hewitt Diary, March 7, 1897.

END OF AN ERA

after receiving the news Hewitt packed his few personal belongings, closed up his desk, and walked out. He never returned.

As might be expected, Hewitt's dismissal caused a furor. His old friend George E. Vincent called it a "brutal" proceeding. Newspapers in the Twin Cities and throughout the state tried vainly to explain the dismissal. The *St. Paul Globe* openly said that Dr. H. M. Bracken was a "candidate for the position of secretary and the salary attached thereto," and it was equally direct in charging that professional jealousy was responsible for Hewitt's nonreappointment. The *Pioneer Press* said editorially that it had been unable to discover any reasons for Hewitt's dismissal that would be satisfactory to the public. The activity and usefulness of Hewitt, the editorial continued, "is worth all the other members of the board put together. For twenty-five years he has been the state board of health. His ability and skill and zeal were so well recognized by the other members of the board that they have usually been content to support his suggestions and leave him to execute them. He has devoted himself to the work of the board for a quarter of a century with an absorbing and passionate devotion which has placed Minnesota among the first states of the Union in its freedom from epidemic or contagious diseases. They say he is arbitrary; but arbitrariness is one of the most valuable qualities of a good physician."[25]

At Mankato, the *Daily Review* said that "Gov. Clough has aroused the indignation not only of the old school physicians of the state but citizens generally familiar with and interested in the doings of the state board of health." The Ramsey County Medical Society passed a resolution requesting Clough to reinstate Hewitt, and eleven Mankato physicians urged their state senator to "use every lawful means in your power to have him retained, that the great cause of public health and honor of our state at home and abroad may be maintained." The desire to have Hewitt reappointed continued for many years. As late as 1901, he wrote: "Some friends (medical) are urging my reappointment on S. B. of Health. I think it useless & I could only serve as Ex officer if I were there. It is their belief that I would end the useless epidemic of Small Pox which prompts them I suppose. I could do it if given the position & power I had, Proof — my actual work for the last 15 years of my 25 years of successful service. I will go only if urged and promised support. Neither likely."[26]

[25] Vincent to Folwell, March 5, 1920, Folwell Papers, box 48; *Daily Globe* (St. Paul), January 15, 1897; undated clipping from the *Pioneer Press*.

[26] *Daily Review* (Mankato), January 12, 1897; *St. Paul Dispatch*, January 16, 1897; *Daily Globe* (St. Paul), January 18, 1897; Hewitt Diary, January 2, 1901.

Perhaps Hewitt never suspected, during those depressing days after his nonreappointment, that the real reason for his dismissal may have lain neither in his refusal to contribute campaign funds nor in the machinations of a professional rival. Some packers had been antagonistic because of what they considered to be Hewitt's too stringent crusade for wholesome meat. It is entirely possible that the University of Minnesota Medical School wanted him replaced by a man friendlier to its interests than Hewitt was. Dr. Perry Millard, dean of the school, long had been antagonistic to Hewitt, and he may have influenced the university to suggest to Governor Clough that it would look with favor upon a different secretary for the state board.

Hewitt sat down to write his final report with a heavy heart. "This, then, is my last report," he wrote. "I have helped and watched its development from the beginning to the present time. The 4th of next March the board will have completed its first quarter of a century, so that my service as secretary has been within two months of twenty-five years. The best of my life and effort have gone into this work. I have spared neither time, labor nor thought to make it what it ought to be. Such as it is, the record is made and closed." [27]

The morning after he was dismissed, Hewitt resumed private practice in Red Wing and saw his first patient. His services were not so much in demand as they had been when he took up public health work a quarter century earlier, but he said he found kind feelings directed toward him by those who had never previously employed him. Old patients returned to him.[28] He continued his habit of keeping meticulous case histories and he studied new medical texts and journals. He lectured frequently and began an intensive course of general reading. Yet it was many years before he could really reconcile himself to private practice. Meanwhile, the State Board of Health, which he had founded, was forging ahead under the supervision of a capable, but short-tempered, secretary.

[27] State Board of Health, *Biennial Reports*, 1895–96, p. 14.
[28] Hewitt Diary, March 7, 1897. Hewitt died at Summit, New Jersey, on July 7, 1910.

6

Years of Growth

THE FUROR caused by Hewitt's abrupt dismissal stirred the state long after his successor was appointed. For a short period rumor persisted that a veterinarian, Dr. Myron H. Reynolds, was to replace Hewitt as secretary. Reynolds had been appointed to the state board in 1897 to take charge of the rapidly increasing amount of animal work. He established his headquarters at the University of Minnesota Agricultural Experiment Station in St. Paul. Despite the fact that members of the state board felt that Reynolds was competent in his field, they were reluctant to make a veterinarian secretary.

The first meeting of the board after Hewitt's departure was held on January 12, 1897. No doubt vigorous discussion of possible successors took place, but no decision was then made. Wesbrook was elected secretary pro tem, and the board proceeded to routine business, including the re-election of Dr. Franklin Staples as president and the election of Dr. H. M. Bracken as vice-president. Dr. W. W. Mayo, familiar with the work of the bacteriological laboratory, moved the reappointment of Wesbrook at an annual salary of fifteen hundred dollars.[1]

When the board next met, on January 30, Bracken was elected secretary. Of the six ballots cast, five named Bracken and one was blank.[2] This choice was not unexpected, for intimates of Bracken's had long been aware that he was interested in becoming secretary. Yet there is no proof that he connived for Hewitt's dismissal in order to succeed him. A man of wide experience, Bracken perhaps was as well fitted for the arduous task of secretary as any member of the board. He came originally from the Keystone State, having been born in Noblestown, Pennsylvania, on February 27, 1854. Much of his boyhood was spent in Jersey, Ohio, where his father practiced medicine. He received an acad-

---
[1] State Board of Health, *Biennial Reports*, 1897–98, p. 51.
[2] State Board of Health, *Biennial Reports*, 1897–98, p. 53.

emy education, taught for a year at Boonton, New Jersey, and in 1874 entered the medical department of the University of Michigan. After another year of teaching, he became a student at the College of Physicians and Surgeons in New York.

Bracken was graduated in 1877 and almost immediately he sailed for Venezuela, where he became surgeon for a mining company. This type of practice irked him, and so he left for Edinburgh to do graduate work in Scotland's great clinics. In 1879 he passed the examination of the Royal College of Surgeons and then became physician in a boys' boarding school at Uppingham-by-the-Sea. In the fall he signed as ship's surgeon on the "Moselle," an untidy vessel which laboriously beat its way to ports in Central and South America and then on to the West Indies. For three years he bore with the "Moselle," and while he was with the ship he contracted both scarlet fever and malaria. He also served aboard the "Eider," touching at picturesque Barbadoes and Martinque, where he noted the "bare backs, bare shoulders, bare legs, bare feet" of "tall, supple, straight" natives, whom he described as one of the finest mixed races in the West Indies. He was impressed further by their dignity of carriage and easy elegance of motion. Finally he gave up the sea to practice for two years in New England. But in 1884 the wanderlust again seized him. This time he journeyed to Sonora, Mexico, to become a mining camp doctor. When the activities of the Apaches and of Geronimo forced mining activities to close down in 1885, Bracken returned to the United States for further postgraduate study in New York. The West lured him as it had Hewitt years earlier, and in December, 1885, he opened an office in Minneapolis. Two years later he was appointed professor of materia medica and therapeutics at the university, and in 1895 he was made a member of the State Board of Health.[3]

A man of vast energies and determination, Bracken set about an intensive program calculated to modernize the board's program. He realized as fully as Hewitt did that the local health officer was the keystone holding together the entire structure of the public health program. Bracken knew also that the primary functions of the state board were to consult with and advise local boards and to bring them specialized services. It was his belief that the more services the state board could

---

[3] "Henry Martyn Bracken, 1854–1938," in *Minnesota Medicine*, 21:811 (November, 1938); J. McKeen Cattell and Dean R. Brimhall, eds., *American Men of Science*, 77 (Garrison, New York, 1921); *Who's Who in America*, 11:325 (Chicago, [1921]); Bracken Papers, 3:30–45 ("Some Later Papers"). The Bracken Papers consist of five bound typescript volumes containing copies of Bracken's addresses and papers, as well as a history of the State Board of Health. They are in the possession of the Minnesota Historical Society.

YEARS OF GROWTH 79

build up, the greater would be the strength of the township health officer. Yet Bracken realized that he must not, as a state official, attempt to dictate overmuch to health officials in the field. Frequently, however, his extreme formality and sincere urge to help the cause led him to forget tact and caution. On those occasions — and they were many — he swung with a heavy fist. His official correspondence, in particular, was apt to ignore suavity and to be couched in blunt statements and heavy sarcasm, which alienated precisely those persons whom he wished to be his friends. Yet even Bracken's enemies admitted that, while they disliked him thoroughly, they considered him completely frank and honest.

Among Bracken's first chores was that of enlarging and staffing Wesbrook's laboratory. At the same time he put tremendous effort into energizing the veterinary department, of which Reynolds was the head. Wesbrook, with the assistance of Hewitt, had imported equipment from abroad and, when Bracken became secretary, was looking for competent assistants. His staff, he reported in March, 1897, consisted of himself as director, Dr. Louis B. Wilson as assistant bacteriologist, and Dr. Orianna McDaniel as temporary assistant. A janitor and two medical students kept the laboratory clean and did odd jobs. Clerical work was performed by W. P. Moorhead. For a short time Dr. Fritz Baumann, a graduate of Königsberg University in Germany and an experienced bacteriological chemist, voluntarily helped in the laboratory in exchange for what he could learn about pathogenic bacteria.[4]

Of all these assistants, Dr. McDaniel was to be associated with the state board the longest and for many years was to render distinguished service. She had been graduated in medicine from the University of Michigan in 1894. There she had been stimulated by the work of Dr. George Dock, professor of medicine, and there also the nineteen-year-old girl had been introduced to the fascinations of bacteriology. After graduation, the attractive Dr. McDaniel went to Minneapolis, where she interned at Northwestern Hospital. She visited wards filled with typhoid patients and she treated victims of the great Hinckley fire. She had determined to be a physician when she was only seven years old. Her second professional decision was made in Minneapolis, when she concluded that she would rather become a bacteriologist than engage in private practice. She therefore asked Wesbrook for an assistantship in pathology and bacteriology, which she received in the fall of 1895. Early the following year she began working in the laboratory of the

[4] State Board of Health, *Biennial Reports*, 1897–98, p. 123.

state board at fifteen dollars a month for half time. In April, 1896, she was appointed to the staff of the Minnesota Department of Health, remaining a vigorous member until her retirement in 1946. Although she did not know Hewitt well, she did become acquainted with Oscar C. Pierson. He had been a member of Hewitt's Episcopal choir in Red Wing. One day in 1888 after practice, Hewitt asked Pierson to help him temporarily. The short-term job became a permanent one lasting fifty-eight years. Pierson retired in the same year that McDaniel did.[5]

Well-trained and youthfully energetic, McDaniel plunged enthusiastically into her laboratory work. The big problem then was diphtheria, for the disease was widespread and not too much was known about it. Hewitt had examined throat cultures in 1894, but it remained for McDaniel to work up a pictorial classification of diphtheria bacilli. Both typical and atypical bacilli were described in an article written by her and some of her associates in 1898. A few years later Wesbrook added to knowledge of diphtheria in Minnesota in a paper read before the American Public Health Association at Havana, Cuba. "The experience of Minnesota," he said, "would seem to point decidedly to the conclusion that diphtheria infection is transmitted usually by almost direct exchange of the flora of the nose and throat." Then he concluded: "In institutional and school life the more independent the individual and the greater the facilities for individual isolation the greater the freedom from diphtheria infection and the easier is it to eradicate the disease."[6]

McDaniel played an important role in the work of the laboratory. "In the beginning we did things the hard way," she said. "In making a microscopic preparation of any culture, even though it would be destroyed immediately after examination, the smear was made on a coverslip, fixed by heat, stained and mounted in Canada balsam on a slide. Indeed it was a bit of a chore to prepare the mounts of from 50 to 100 cultures whether in the course of routine diphtheria examinations or in the study of diphtheria bacilli or other bacteria encountered. Incidentally the record says that frequently from 100 to 300 cultures of bacteria were under special study at one time." Not until 1903 or 1904 were "smears made on individual slides and directly examined

[5] Interview of the author with Dr. McDaniel, April 16, 1948. The Minnesota Department of Health is the operating force for the State Board of Health.
[6] McDaniel, paper read before the Society of American Bacteriologists, Minneapolis, May 11, 1948; F. F. Wesbrook, L. B. Wilson, O. McDaniel, and J. H. Adair, "A Preliminary Communication on Bacillus Diphtheriae and Its Variants in a School in Which Diphtheria Was Endemic," in the *British Medical Journal*, 1:1008–1011 (April 16, 1898); Wesbrook, *Diphtheria Infection in Minnesota*, 11 (reprinted from American Medical Association, *Journal*, 44:939–943 – March 25, 1905).

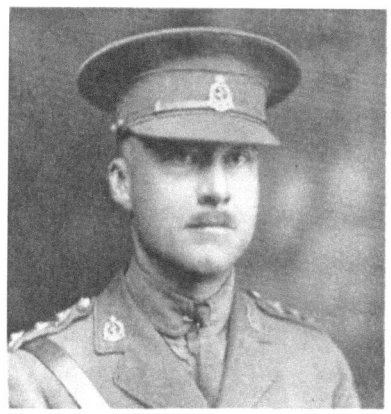
HIBBERT W. HILL

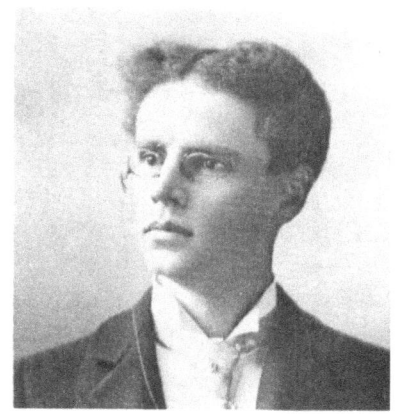
LOUIS B. WILSON

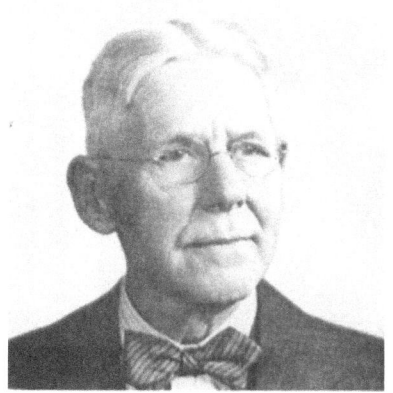
OSCAR C. PIERSON

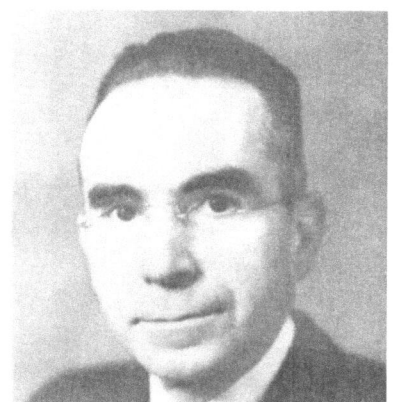
HAROLD A. WHITTAKER

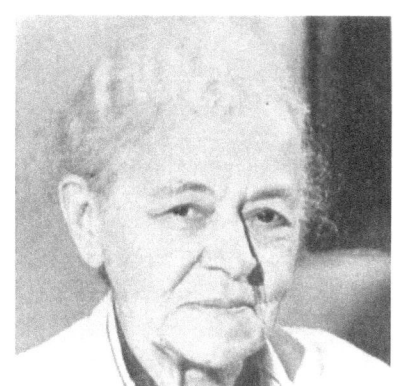
ORIANNA McDANIEL

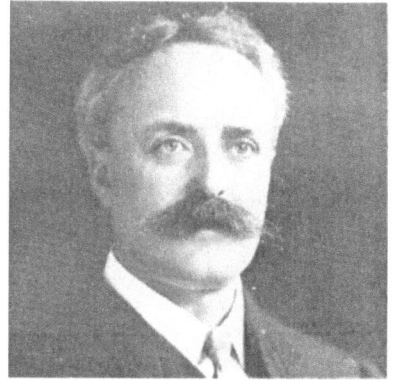
FRANK F. WESBROOK

Courtesy Dr. McDaniel, O. C. Pierson, and Minnesota Department of Health

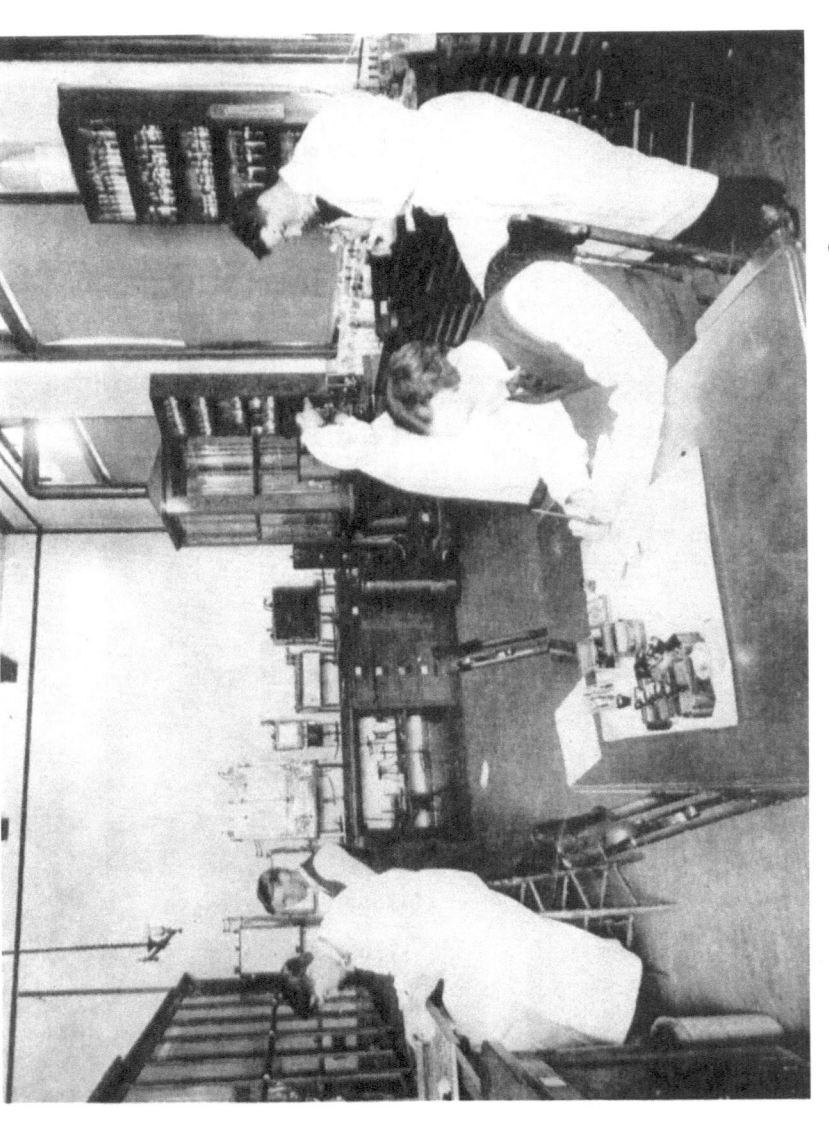

MINNESOTA DEPARTMENT OF HEALTH LABORATORY IN THE 1890s
A. W. Miller, Harry Charleston, Orianna McDaniel, W. P. Moorhead, L. B. Wilson
Courtesy Minnesota Department of Health

in oil without a coverglass and a few years later probably by 1906 the long slide suitable for receiving ten or more smears, so generally used now, was adopted."

"At first," continued McDaniel, "our diphtheria culture media, Loeffler serum modified by Dr. Wesbrook to contain 1.25% glycerine, was coagulated by dry heat in a homemade water-jacketed sloper and sterilized by the three-day fractional method. Soon after securing our first autoclave, an upright model, a method was worked out whereby coagulation and complete sterilization was accomplished at one process." [7]

The laboratory staff, during the early days when McDaniel was an assistant, did everything but mop, sweep, and dust. Soon there was one boy for general helpfulness, and then a half-time clerk-stenographer. "Before too long," recalled McDaniel, "the group grew and we were able to devote our time to the real work. But as new apparatus was received it had to be set up. Often it was extemporized in toto. Dr. Wesbrook was something of an expert in glass-blowing and we all did our best to emulate him." She remembered also when the Wyatt Johnston modification of the Widal test as an aid to the diagnosis of typhoid fever was begun in the laboratory in January, 1896. The outfit used by McDaniel and Wesbrook consisted of a small sheet of aluminum foil, an aluminum wire loop accompanied by a data card, and directions for collection. Dr. L. B. Wilson, McDaniel's colleague and the assistant bacteriologist, was as inventive as his chief. Wilson constructed a simple and convenient pipette device which permitted of easy sterilization and also insured accuracy of dilution. A few years previously he had also devised an apparatus for counting colonies in Petri-dishes, as the Petri plate was then called.

Bracken encouraged the laboratory to increase its services, so that by 1903 the Minnesota Department of Health proudly pointed to its work in diphtheria, typhoid fever, tuberculosis, rabies, water analysis, and routine investigations of meat and milk. Wesbrook, with Bracken's approval, divided the work of a state board of health laboratory into two classes:

1. Routine work whose aim should be to assist, when necessary, local health boards throughout the state in the exact determination of foci of known infectious diseases. This should include not only the examination of materials from human beings, but suspected water, milk, food and even domestic and other animals where the infection may be spread from them to man. The testing of new methods of bacteriological diagnosis; of the values of various commercial antitoxins and disinfectants; together with the investigation of other problems for which

[7] McDaniel, paper read before the Society of American Bacteriologists.

methods have been formulated, should constitute a part of the routine work of such laboratories.

2. Research work should be undertaken so that the etiology of obscure infectious diseases and their methods of transmission may be determined, new methods formulated and old ones adapted for the conditions which obtain in the particular locality; whilst in general all problems concerning which exact knowledge may benefit the state and protect its health should be studied.[8]

Wesbrook, fully aware of the increasing complexities of public health work, pointed out that routine laboratory tests — "tissues, tumors, pus, sputum, urine" — should not be made at state expense, but should be run in hospital laboratories and physicians' offices. State boards of health, he said, should only make investigations which are of especial use in the location and control of infectious disease. And Wesbrook, like Hewitt before him, felt the "necessity for the provision of special courses of instruction" for the training of health officers. "It is not too much to expect," he wrote, "that in a short time some special diploma, as indicating the possession of special qualifications for such a post as that of health officer, may be demanded." He urged that state universities, particularly if they were connected with state board of health laboratories, establish special courses and teach prospective health officers enough laboratory work "to insure successful collaboration of the state and local officers." He spoke, too, of a mutual stimulation as the result of the close relationship between the laboratory of the Minnesota Department of Health and the laboratories of the University of Minnesota.[9]

A few years later, when Wesbrook had had time to determine a little more fully the philosophy behind a health laboratory, he wrote: "In municipal health work, the laboratory is in close contact with the problems to be studied, but very frequently it is necessary for the laboratory men to leave the laboratory and to accompany executives, inspectors or others, so as to see and know the actual existing conditions and guide their work accordingly. In state or federal work, it is often imperative for the laboratory worker to visit the locality under investigation." He then continued, "It is impossible, in most instances, to render valuable service or to give intelligent advice based on shipped specimens and

---

[8] Wesbrook, *The Laboratory in Public Health Work*, 3 (Des Moines, 1904).
[9] Wesbrook, *The Laboratory in Public Health Work*, 5. An interesting elaboration of Wesbrook's thesis is the work accomplished on the etiology of Rocky Mountain spotted fever in 1902 by Dr. Louis B. Wilson, who was loaned to the Montana State Board of Health to investigate the disease. Wilson recognized the similarity of the causative organism to that which causes Texas fever in cattle and suggested that ticks were carriers of the disease.

meager data. Nor is it economical to spend days, weeks or months in working at problems which have been entirely obscured or at best rendered vastly more difficult by lack of foresight or of specific knowledge on the part of those for whom the investigations are to be made."[10]

While Wesbrook and McDaniel, with Bracken's encouragement, enlarged and intensified the activities of the laboratory, work also was increasing in the veterinary department. Supervision of infectious diseases of animals had been placed in the department in 1885 and was to continue until 1903, when, after violent discussion and much bitter feeling, a State Live Stock Sanitary Board was created by the legislature. Reynolds directed the veterinary department of the state board until August, 1900. He was succeeded by Dr. S. D. Brimhall in April, 1901, but later became director of the livestock board.[11]

Bracken opposed the creation of a livestock board, believing that the Minnesota Department of Health, through its many facilities and many contacts throughout the state, was better able to handle diseases common to both men and animals. He had taken pride not only in Reynolds' work, but also in the services that the health department offered to farmers and rural areas. In 1897 Minnesota had passed a law providing for the condemnation of cattle with tuberculosis. The tuberculin test was made by health officers acting under Bracken's orders. In addition, dairies were inspected and barns and milkhouses were examined. During a three-months period in 1902 inspectors reported to Bracken that, of 586 dairies visited, only 7 could be classed as excellent; 164 were called good, 186 fair, and 229 unsatisfactory.[12]

In addition to handling investigations of human diseases, the health department laboratory, aiding the veterinary department, attacked problems of tuberculosis in cattle, of hog cholera and swine plague; worked with trichinosis, a disease caused by the presence of trichinae larvae in insufficiently cooked pork; dealt with hemorrhagic septicemia in cattle; investigated cases of anthrax; and devoted much time to meningitis in horses, cattle, sheep, and swine. Sheep scab presented a major problem, as did "swamp fever" and glanders in horses. The laboratory was busy from morning until night. No problem was too big and none

[10] Wesbrook, *Co-Ordinated Specialism in Public Health Work*, 10 (reprinted from the *Journal of the American Medical Association*, 45:1835–1840 — December 16, 1905).
[11] State Board of Health, Veterinary Department, *Reports*, August 1, 1902–May 1, 1903, p. 8; [Bracken] to Franklin Staples, March 17, April 6, 9, 23, 1903, and Staples to Bracken, April 4, 22, 1902, Minnesota Department of Health, St. Paul.
[12] State Board of Health, Veterinary Department, *Reports*, 41. During this period the correspondence of the health department contains at least as many letters dealing with animal diseases as with human diseases.

was too small. The staff put as much energy into trying to determine whether or not a cat had diphtheria as it did into diagnosing rabies.[13]

Administering the department was no easy task, yet Bracken found time to make inspection trips and to deliver an astonishingly large number of speeches. He contributed articles to medical journals, including the *New York Medical Journal* and the *St. Paul Medical Journal,* and frequently participated in the meetings of out-of-state medical societies. He seldom missed an opportunity to forward the public health cause. Given to plain speech and not always cautious in what he said, Bracken nevertheless hammered home many a lesson that Minnesota needed.

A year before he became secretary, Bracken read a paper before the Minnesota Academy of Medicine in which he boldly challenged the prevailing practice of appointing inadequately trained men as health officers. "The appointment of health officers," he said, "should be made upon the basis of fitness, and should be free from all possible political taint. Do we find such men holding the positions of health officers? I am sorry to say that in many cases we do not. Representative medical men are rarely found holding responsible sanitary positions when the appointments are in the hands of politicians. . . . It is the man with a 'political pull' who secures the vote of the ordinary alderman. . . . Politicians think they are conferring a *favor* with their appointment, and that one or two short terms are quite sufficient for one man; that he should then yield his position to some other political pet. This is wrong. . . . It is the good of the *public*, and not of the individual, that should be considered in making an appointment, and the *public*, and not the individual, is the gainer." [14]

Close association with the work of Wesbrook and McDaniel led Bracken to have profound respect for the bacteriologist. "There ought to be bacteriologists in every city or town throughout the State," he once said, "in order that prompt examinations might be made when necessary." Bracken felt that work referred to a state bacteriologist often involved a considerable loss of time. In difficult cases, however, local bacteriologists could consult with the state bacteriologist, located at the health department. And, like Wesbrook and Hewitt, Bracken supported public health instruction in medical schools. He urged also a strong section on preventive medicine in the American Medical Association, pointing out, reasonably enough, that the American Public Health Association, the Conference of State and Provincial Boards of Health, the Conference of State Sanitary Executives, and the United

---

[13] State Board of Health, Veterinary Department, *Reports*, 189.
[14] Bracken Papers, 1:23.

States Marine Hospital services were not sufficient to cope satisfactorily with the prevention of disease.[15]

In May, 1901, Bracken outlined the demands of sanitary science to members of the Chicago Medical Society. His talk reflected admirably his program in Minnesota. Lucid, and lacking the rancor that Bracken sometimes interjected, the paper began quietly enough by stating that sanitary science rests upon both theoretical and practical knowledge. The laboratory provides theoretical data. Practical information, on the other hand, "is the natural outcome of the appreciation of reasonable rules and regulations shown by research and observation to be necessary for the comfort and well being of all." [16]

Then, carefully and in concrete language, Bracken discussed nuisances, emphasizing problems of tenement houses, of disposal of refuse, of sewerage systems, and of schools. He spoke, too, of the rise of tuberculosis and he talked of the ordinary methods of quarantine as "barbarous." He thought it unfair to tie up the well with the sick, and he advocated removing patients to isolation hospitals rather than permitting them to remain in the home. Finally, he said that physicians should take greater interest in public health.

Bracken understood as well as anyone the medical, social, and economic problems raised by tuberculosis. The disease in earlier years had brought countless sufferers to the state, thereby labeling Minnesota as a health resort, and it also had been the cause of a high percentage of deaths through successive decades. At least ten of Bracken's articles and addresses dealt with this problem directly and many others touched upon it indirectly. Given to short sentences when he was moved, Bracken told the Southern Minnesota Medical Association "Tuberculosis is recognized as a communicable disease, a preventable disease. If preventable, why not prevented? The only answer to this must be either because of ignorance or indifference. We can not now plead ignorance. We must, therefore, admit indifference." [17]

The public health program in dealing with tuberculosis, he continued, "is not to establish an unreasonable home quarantine of each case, but (1) to investigate every case in order to determine whether it is a source of danger in the home, and (2) to keep every closed case under observation in order to know at once if such a case changes to an open case. This work calls for a thorough health system for the entire state, with the visiting nurse as a part of the system." In Bracken's judgment,

[15] Bracken Papers, 1:36, 59.
[16] Bracken Papers, 1:72.
[17] Bracken Papers, 1:273.

control of tuberculosis or a reduction in the number of cases was not to be accomplished by expensive sanatoriums. Minnesota passed a state aid law for county sanatoriums in 1913, but Bracken felt that even this was not entirely satisfactory. "If county sanitoria," he argued, "are for the care of the patient only, and are to have no part in the control of the disease, then they are hospitals and should not be receiving state aid. The hospitalization of the sick is a very different problem from the special care of a group of patients as a part of the control of a disease. Patients who are able should pay their own hospital expenses. Patients who are poor and need hospital care should be provided for under the poor law." [18]

After summarizing the need for full-time, competent medical directors in county sanatoriums and showing how the department took quick and effective steps to prevent the use of unauthorized therapeutic agents in the treatment of tuberculosis, Bracken said that the tuberculosis situation in Minnesota, from a public health viewpoint, was most disappointing. "It was hoped," he concluded, "when the law of 1909 was passed that counties would become active in trying to care for their own tuberculosis, and this hope was still stronger when the law of 1913 providing state aid was passed, for it was the hope of health officials that the people would insist on protecting themselves from infection and that the counties would see the advantage of removing the burden of expense from the small municipality and the township, transferring such expense to the state. It remains to be seen what the future of this work is to be in Minnesota." [19]

Bracken's public life was so crowded with a number of things that it is practically impossible to record his wide range of interests and the innumerable topics upon which he wrote and talked. The papers he preserved — and they must be only a fraction of the whole — fill five fat volumes. These indicate his reactions to railway sanitary problems, including the protection of passengers; to preservation and transportation of dead bodies; to the needs of public health education in the United States; to reviews of legislation relative to sanitary problems; and to the history of his own department. In 1893 he published a text on materia medica, and many years later he prepared a typewritten history of the health department, which never was really completed and which was not published.[20]

[18] Bracken Papers, 1:276, 289, 291.   [19] Bracken Papers, 1:295.
[20] Bracken, *Outlines of Materia Medica* (Minneapolis, 1893); Bracken Papers, vol. 3, concerned primarily with railroad sanitation and the sanitary aspects of the care and transportation of dead bodies, and including also several historical sketches; vol. 4, "Fifty Years of Public Health Work in Minnesota, 1872–1922."

In the midst of a heavy speaking program and busy with plans for a reorganization of the board, Bracken fell ill with typhoid fever in May, 1910. During his convalescence he went abroad to study sanitary problems and to attend meetings of the third international congress on school hygiene at Paris. He also attended, as one of three American delegates, the third international congress on the physical education of the young at Brussels. Both conferences were held in August. Although not as vigorous as usual, Bracken not only took an active part in these meetings but also visited hospitals and schools in England, Scotland, and France.

"My first intention," he wrote after returning to the United States, "was to study public health methods in England and Scotland and I began this at Edinburgh. From Edinburgh I drifted down to Brighton, to the Royal Sanitary Institute. Then into the study of the tuberculosis problem; then into the study of hospitals for infectious diseases; then into the study of school inspection, open-air schools and school sanitation and finally into the study of the home conditions in and about Birmingham and Liverpool."[21]

This brief statement, unusually modest for Bracken, does not begin to cover his activities. He chatted with Edinburgh's chief veterinarian, learning to his surprise that the tuberculin test was not used in the inspection of dairy herds. He spent time at Sheffield, where he studied the city's milk supply and watched cows and hogs being led to slaughter. "Old Shambles" at Sheffield he compared with Minnesota slaughterhouses. "Altho old and considered disreputable by the city sanitary authorities, these places are ideal when compared with many of the slaughter houses thruout Minnesota. They are kept fairly clean and there was no disagreeable odor altho this visit was made during hot weather. The animals are badly housed in dark, close sheds for a day or two sometimes before killing. I saw live sheep standing huddled together against the wall in the same room where the butchers were killing and dressing sheep. This of course would not be permitted except for the present unsatisfactory condition of the old place. The cattle are killed with the poleax as at Paris and Edinburgh." He also visited the abattoirs and cattle markets of Paris. These he found in excellent condition. "Napoleon," he wrote in his notes, "in addition to being a great General, was apparently a leading sanitarian of his time." Bracken had learned that the emperor had insisted upon the establishment of abattoirs in 1810.[22]

[21] Bracken Papers, 5:164, "A Trip Abroad, 1910."
[22] Bracken Papers, 5:124, 135, 140.

At the Pasteur Hospital for Infectious Diseases, Bracken walked long, clean wards with nurses and staff physicians. He noticed a case of sleeping sickness, a case of cerebrospinal meningitis, a case of diphtheria, a case of measles, and two or three cases of scarlet fever all on one floor and under the care of one nurse. But he quickly learned that such an arrangement, because of the physical plan of the wards, did not make for spread of disease. Each ward had a central aisle, on each side of which were cubicles in pairs. Each cubicle was designed for one patient and was separated from the center aisle by a glass partition, so that a single nurse could care for a number of patients suffering from different diseases.

"It was stated to me," said Bracken, "that a special gown was provided in each cubicle for both nurse and attending physician but this I did not notice. It is my impression that the doctor may use a special gown for each cubicle but that the nurse goes from cubicle to cubicle without gowning, so long as she is taking care of ordinary cases, taking the precaution, however, to wash her hands thoroughly. The care of infectious diseases on the cubicle system is based on the idea that such diseases are carried rather by the nurses than by the air. The nurse is the chief point of danger and must therefore be above question as to her methods." [23]

Bracken returned to Minnesota with definite ideas gained from his trip. He strongly recommended the abandonment of the old type of isolation hospital with a ward for each disease, suggesting that the cubicle method he had observed in Paris might be cheaper and more efficient. But, he added, "the success of the cubicle method depends largely upon the loyalty and conscientiousness of the nurses and of the physician." [24]

At home again, Bracken plunged into routine work and also helped to work out details of a department reorganization which had been decided upon on July 12, 1910. The laboratory, under Wesbrook, was changed from a department to a division and was further divided into the main diagnostic laboratory, a chemical laboratory, and a Pasteur institute. A division of epidemiology was created with Dr. Hibbert W. Hill as director. It is said that Hill was the first man in the United States to bear the title of "epidemiologist." The reorganization also created a division of engineering, with Professor Frederic H. Bass of the University of Minnesota as director. Other members of the staff in 1910 included Orianna McDaniel as director of the Pasteur insti-

[23] Bracken Papers, 5:23.
[24] Bracken Papers, 5:41.

tute; Harold A. Whittaker as chemist and bacteriologist in charge of the chemical laboratory division; and Albert J. Chesley as a member of the epidemiological division.[25]

This staff was both competent and distinguished. Hill was a Canadian, who had had a wealth of public health experience. He had served as demonstrator bacteriologist and pathologist at Toronto, then had moved to Louisville to take part in filtration experiments, and from 1897 to 1898 had been chief of the Bureau of Sanitation of the Brooklyn watershed. Then he became director of the bacteriology laboratory of the Boston Board of Health and instructor in bacteriology at Harvard University. He came to Minnesota from Harvard in 1905 to assume two posts — assistant professor at the University of Minnesota and assistant director of the Minnesota State Board of Health. Bass also had had much practical experience. He was born at Hyde Park, Massachusetts, and was graduated from the Massachusetts Institute of Technology in 1901. Before he received his degree he had been employed by the Metropolitan Water Works of Massachusetts as assistant engineer. After graduation he became an instructor in engineering at the University of Minnesota, and in 1911 he was named professor of municipal and sanitary engineering. He had begun his duties with the Minnesota Department of Health in 1906. In 1910, the same year that Bracken made his European tour, Bass also went abroad to study "French, German and English municipal sanitation with special reference to water purification, sewage disposal and purification and refuse disposal." He returned saying that the United States had progressed more than European countries in the science of water purification, but that both England and Germany had made remarkable advances in the purification of sewage.[26]

Chesley, a member of the epidemiological division in 1910, was a native Minnesotan, having been born in Minneapolis on September 12, 1877. He received the degree of doctor of medicine from the University of Minnesota in 1907. His technical training had been interrupted by the Spanish-American War, when he enlisted in the Thirteenth Volunteer Minnesota Infantry, Company B, as a private. He was mustered out at San Francisco as a corporal on October 3, 1899. He became a member of the state health department in 1902.[27]

[25] Bracken Papers, 4:239.
[26] Cattell and Brimhall, eds., *American Men of Science*, 42, 316; State Board of Health, "Reports and Hearings," 1910–12, p. 366, Minnesota Department of Health, St. Paul.
[27] Franklin F. Holbrook, *Minnesota in the Spanish-American War and the Philippine Insurrection*, 239 (Minnesota War Records Commission, *Publication* 1 — St. Paul, 1923); *Who's Who in America*, 25:438 (Chicago, 1948).

Whittaker had been born in Wisconsin and had been trained at the University of Wisconsin. In 1906 he served as assistant chemist of the Ohio State Board of Health, and the following year he became chemist of the Minnesota Department of Health, where he remained for about a year. He then was attached to the United States Department of Agriculture as a scientific assistant. In 1909 he returned to the Minnesota health department as chief of the water and sewage laboratory and later became director of the division of sanitation. In 1946 he was made professor of public health engineering at the University of Minnesota.[28] The activities of Whittaker, Bass, Chesley, Hill, McDaniel, and Bracken not only centered in their offices, but also spread throughout Minnesota and extended to other states.

Hill, for example, visited Washington, Richmond, Columbus, and St. Louis in a three-months period and, in addition, made field trips to more than twenty Minnesota communities. His activities on these tours included the investigation of a drainage complaint, of an outbreak of dysentery, and of a minor smallpox epidemic. He also inspected a factory and made a diagnosis of scarlet fever. Chesley made twenty-five trips between December 28, 1910, and March 31, 1911, taking throat cultures of school children, offering advice, and talking on school problems in contagious diseases.[29]

The engineering division was equally busy with trips involving the sanitation of buildings, water supply problems, sewerage nuisances, and routine inspections. Bass worked in co-operation with the Minnesota Drainage Commission and the United States Geological Survey to secure a traverse of the shore of Mille Lacs Lake and also examined the East Grand Forks filter plant. Twenty-three Minnesota towns were inspected, with particular attention being paid to water supply and sewage disposal.[30]

In addition to purely routine matters, the department held hearings on a case arising from treatment at the Pasteur institute and on five slaughterhouse cases. Although Minnesota lacked a meat inspection law, the health department could initiate action against suspected slaughterhouses under the "Offensive Trades Act." Bracken reported that several of the abattoirs accepted the findings of the board and went out of business.[31]

Two rather unusual epidemics in 1910 brought unexpected prob-

[28] *Who's Who in America*, 25:2669.
[29] State Board of Health, "Reports and Hearings," 1910–12, pp. 314, 477.
[30] State Board of Health, "Reports and Hearings," 1910–12, p. 50.
[31] State Board of Health, "Reports and Hearings," 1910–12, pp. 71–95, 183–270; *Biennial Reports*, 1909–10, p. 171; Minnesota, *Revised Laws*, 1905, sec. 2143.

lems to the department and demanded the attention of practically every staff member. Hill wrote a special report covering an epidemic of anterior poliomyelitis, and later he investigated an outbreak of typhoid fever in Minneapolis. During the poliomyelitis epidemic he visited 27 different places, saw about 124 families in which the disease was suspected, investigated about 161 cases, recorded as polio 85 cases, rejected as not polio 58 cases, and failed, he said, to make a satisfactory diagnosis in 18 cases. Commenting upon the spread of polio, Hill wrote: "We may therefore assume that polio cases throw off the infective agent in great quantities and yet must admit that if so those associated with a case rarely receive the infection or, being infected, rarely prove susceptible — we do not know which." [32]

All the details of the typhoid epidemic were not clear, but Hill concluded that, of the 121 cases he saw, 88 were the result of infection from Minneapolis city water. He said that the reporting of typhoid cases in Minneapolis was "notoriously imperfect" and indicated that the methods of the Minneapolis Department of Health might be improved. Then he returned to a discussion of the city's water supply. "From the testimony of patients," he said, "many hotels in Minneapolis supply river water to their help and even to their patrons, and it is known that the Union Station at least supplies river water at two points for drinking. One hotel is said to have sent seven cases to the hospital. Many dry-goods stores rinse soda-water glasses in cold city water. In two or three instances persons who did not drink raw river water used it for their teeth, and in one case the patient, who did not drink river water, was very fond of lettuce well soaked in it." [33]

Wesbrook's laboratory, in which Bracken took much pride, was increasing the amount of work done almost every quarter. In a three-months period ending on March 31, 1910, the laboratory made 2,712 examinations of specimens received from 267 different localities. Diphtheria examinations averaged 37.5 daily, including Sundays. McDaniel's Pasteur institute also was busy, reporting that 21 persons had been treated during the quarter. Wesbrook's staff examined 22 different embalming fluids in order that Bracken might present the results, if he wished, to the Minnesota Funeral Directors' Association.[34]

These varied activities, however, did not exhaust the types of work performed by the department. Bracken also was interested in gathering vital statistics, feeling that, although it was important to collect such

[32] State Board of Health, "Reports and Hearings," 1910–12, p. 68.
[33] State Board of Health, "Reports and Hearings," 1910–12, pp. 120, 124; *Minneapolis Journal*, March 20, 1910.
[34] State Board of Health, "Reports and Hearings," 1910–12, pp. 125, 131, 135.

data, it was perhaps even more significant to interpret them. Early in 1911 he sent Oscar Pierson, whom Hewitt had brought to the department, to Washington, D.C., to receive instruction from the Bureau of the Census. Pierson also stopped in Harrisburg to see how Pennsylvania handled its vital statistics. He returned to Minnesota advocating a punchcard method of tabulating returns.[35]

A year later Pierson toured Minnesota to encourage registrars to make returns promptly and to see that the burial permit law was being enforced. "It was Dr. Bracken's desire," wrote Pierson, "that in addition to securing the delinquent reports I make the visit as educational as possible and in line with this I talked with as many officials, members of councils, newspaper editors, physicians, embalmers, etc., as possible, explaining the purpose and importance of the birth and death report. There is great need for public education on this matter. Almost all whom I talked with had but a vague idea of the value of these reports. 'A lot of red tape and expense for the purpose of giving the State Board of Health the reports to study statistics' being the general view taken." [36]

Although Bracken frequently irritated persons with his bluntness and all too often wrote letters that were almost completely lacking in tact, he did realize the value of keeping on friendly terms with the legislature. That he did not always succeed was admitted by many. Bracken was not a competent public relations man. Perhaps that is why in 1911 he asked Hill, a suave, friendly person, to prepare plans for winning the legislature to the support of the department.

Hill's program was a masterpiece, and it indicates how the state board operated: [37]

1. [Send] decision on bills, their wording, especially of titles, and distribution to clubs, societies, individuals for endorsement. Keep list of all clubs, societies and prominent individuals favorably disposed.

2. Careful selection and instruction of a group of legislative supporters for each bill.

3. Carefully arranged plans, understood by all supporters of bills, concerning the proposed course of each thru House and Senate.

4. Immediately on convening of the Legislature, early introduction, there posting of committee members in advance, brief hearings and prompt reporting-out, with an immediately following campaign of education amongst the House and Senate members, continuing that of the previous two years.

5. For educational purposes, prepare lists showing:
   (a) Daily calls for assistance received by the State Board of

[35] State Board of Health, "Reports and Hearings," 1910–12, p. 451.
[36] State Board of Health, "Reports and Hearings," 1910–12, p. 740.
[37] State Board of Health, "Reports and Hearings," 1910–12, p. 494.

Health, with reasons for same, and responses made, especially where aid is refused, with reasons therefor.

(b) Summaries of investigations made, with results, and cost to State Board of Health of the same, showing cash expended in traveling; in investigating; in resulting office or laboratory work.

(c) Actual records of the cost of infectious diseases to families thruout the state — by means of printed forms sent out to heads of families.

6. Secure written endorsement from prominent lay bodies of all descriptions.

7. In the case of permissive bills, secure representatives from districts, counties or municipalities to which such permission would apply, showing demand for such legislation.

8. By lectures, tuberculosis exhibits, writings and newspaper articles, keep the general public informed of State Board of Health activities, especially giving results of work done.

9. Secure from County Superintendents records of schools closed on account of infectious diseases, showing the time lost, the number of pupils and teachers involved, and the extent of the direct financial loss.

10. Avoid asking for the creation of new agencies, but rather for the extension of existing agencies.

There was real reason, of course, why both Bracken and Hill should take special pains to outline a regular campaign of political action. The legislature of 1911 had not been particularly friendly to bills in which the state board was interested. A bill to prohibit the use of unsanitary school buildings had ended on general orders in the House, and had been overwhelmingly defeated, after acrimonious debate, in the Senate. A bill to create the full-time position of medical school inspector and health officer combined had failed to secure a majority in the House. Hill campaigned hard for a bill to provide for district public health inspectors, even accompanying Senator Joseph M. Hackney to a meeting of the finance committee. Hill then told what happened: "On bringing up the bill before the Committee, Senator [Frank] Clague denied having stated that he would allow four men [*inspectors*], and expressed hearty disapproval of the whole plan. Senator [Charles S.] Marden said in the committee it was all d—— foolishness, and the bill was indefinitely postponed." [38]

Even with Hill's tactful assistance, politics became an increasing vexation to Bracken. "The board," he once wrote, "was handicapped in matters pertaining to politics. Politics made queer bed fellows." He then pointed out that he lived in Minneapolis and that the "Minnea-

[38] State Board of Health, "Reports and Hearings," 1910–12, p. 491; Hill to W. C. Chambers, June 21, 1911, Minnesota Department of Health, St. Paul. The bills were H. F. 287 and S. F. 235; H. F. 294 and S. F. 366; and H. F. 771 and S. F. 562.

politans in state politics were deeply interested in securing appropriations for the University. They could not take on the additional burden of trying to secure favorable legislation for the state board of health." He also indicated, in his blunt, forthright manner, that St. Paul was the home of Dr. H. L. Taylor, a physician in charge of the state antituberculosis movement. St. Paul legislators, therefore, were more likely to support bills encouraged by Taylor than to give their assistance to bills approved by Bracken and Hill. Taylor's interests, commented Bracken bitingly, "were in the *care of the tuberculous*, while the secretary of this board, supported by the board, was in favor of both the *control of the disease* and in the *care of the patient*." And Bracken said with perfect candor that the antagonism between himself and Taylor interfered with support for public health from St. Paul state politicians.[39]

But that was not all. Two other factors impeded Bracken's program for political support. In the first place, since 1898 he had been involved in a feud with a county attorney whom he said had refused to prosecute patients who broke quarantine. Then the attorney was elected a state senator. It seems that one of his consistent policies thereafter was to oppose legislation endorsed by Bracken. The other factor was Bracken's inability to get along with politicians, which he readily admitted. He said he was not a born lobbyist, he despised political methods, and he was tactless. Dr. W. J. Mayo once told him that he was the most tactless man he ever knew and that he thought Bracken was rather proud of the fact. "This latter was not the case," said Bracken, writing in the third person. "However, when he went into office in 1897, he knew that some people would damn him if he did his duty; others would damn him if he did not do his duty. He determined to do what he considered his duty and not care a damn what people said. In this he was tactless." [40]

Regardless of the reasons for friction between Bracken and the legislature, the results were detrimental to the board. Appropriations were trimmed, the secretary's salary was cut, and dissensions developed within the health department. Wesbrook in 1910 asked for "complete autonomy" for his laboratory, offering his resignation as an alternative. Bracken said that Wesbrook's proposal meant "a willingness to do the work *for* the board but not under the board." Perhaps Bracken felt also that Wesbrook wanted to turn the laboratory over completely to the University of Minnesota. Certainly Wesbrook looked with favor upon

[39] Bracken Papers, 4:269.
[40] Bracken Papers, 4:270.

YEARS OF GROWTH 95

a university laboratory, and he may have felt that the university was in a better position to render state-wide laboratory service than was the health department.[41] When the board did not accept his proposal, Wesbrook resigned on December 14, 1910, with the stipulation that he would continue to serve until January 1, 1911. Dr. R. J. Mullin succeeded him.

Within the next few years other staff changes occurred. Dr. F. L. Watkins, who had been helping with vital statistics, resigned in 1912 to become deputy registrar of Mississippi. Hill also left in 1912 to become director of the Institute of Public Health at London, Ontario. Chesley succeeded Hill as director of the division of epidemiology. But Bracken's difficulties were not yet over. In December, 1912, he was dropped from membership on the board because he was also an employee of the board. To meet this situation the board gave Bracken all the privileges of a board member except that of voting. Then to add to his embarrassment, his appropriations were cut from $84,000 in 1913 to $73,500 in 1914. "Minnesota," said Bracken, "which has been in the foreground of public health for many years, is apparently losing ground due to lack of interest on the part of the legislature." The same year, Dr. Carroll Fox, surgeon of the United States Public Health Service, surveyed public health administration in Minnesota, and he later reported that "it is probably the most progressive that we have in the United States." [42]

No sooner had Bracken reorganized his staff on what he hoped was a harmonious basis than another problem rose to plague him. This was the Efficiency and Economy Commission, which had been appointed by Governor Adolph O. Eberhart for the purpose of reducing state expenditures and increasing the efficiency of state government. Charles P. Craig of Duluth was chairman. The commission's work excited the state and drew both applause and disapproval from newspapers. No editor, however, was more sensitive than was Bracken, who believed that Craig's reorganization plan would strip the board of its independence and subordinate it to lay control and to political influence.

Indeed, Bracken had cause to be fearful. The commission's report, transmitted in November, 1914, actually recommended that both the

[41] Bracken Papers, 4:266; State Board of Health, "Reports and Hearings," 1910–12, pp. 111–115; Wesbrook to E. L. Touhy, March 29, 1910, State Department of Health, Minneapolis.
[42] Bracken Papers, 4:301–303; Carrol Fox, *Public Health Administration in Minnesota* (*Reprint* 223 from *Public Health Reports*, October 2, 1914 — Washington, D.C., 1914).

board and the office of secretary be abolished and that control of public health be placed under a department of public welfare. Fortunately, although hearings were long and bitter, the commission's recommendations were not enacted into law. The State Board of Health was able to maintain its independent status.

In 1915 Bracken was forced to tell Bass that the board no longer could afford to employ him. The services of two other employees also were terminated. Thinking that a change of secretaries might reconcile the board and the legislature and might relieve departmental discontent, Bracken, "thoroughly disgusted with the treatment given the board by the legislature," suggested to Chesley that he become secretary. When Chesley refused, Bracken on July 13, 1915, presented his resignation, but the board refused to accept it.[43]

Encouraged somewhat, Bracken reorganized the department with Pierson as assistant secretary, McDaniel as director of the Pasteur institute, Chesley as director of the division of preventable diseases, Whittaker as director of sanitation, and Mrs. O. C. Pierson as director of the division of vital statistics. From this reorganization of August 1, 1915, the work of the board, said Bracken, "moved very smoothly." Yet the respite was not long.[44]

Governor J. A. A. Burnquist, in his inaugural message of 1917, spoke favorably of public health work, saying that in spite of the low appropriation for the purpose, Minnesota ranked fourth among the states. The governor added, however, that "it is impossible for our health department, with such small amount as is now given it, to make as rapid progress as it could if more funds were made available for the advancement of public health. If necessary, less money should be appropriated to other departments in order that more money might be used for the purpose of preventing the spread of disease through the enforcement of proper health regulations and the necessary propagation of health education."[45]

Bracken thoroughly approved these sentiments, but he violently disliked Burnquist's method of gathering public health data. According to Bracken, Burnquist asked Dr. Ignatius J. Murphy, executive secretary of the Minnesota Public Health Association, for information. Bracken thought the governor should have approached him directly, especially as Murphy got the material from Bracken and then sent it on to the governor.[46] Bracken also felt that Burnquist was unfriendly

[43] Bracken Papers, 4:340.
[44] Bracken Papers, 4:341.
[45] Burnquist, *Inaugural Message*, 7 (St. Paul, 1917).
[46] Bracken Papers, 4:367.

to him and that he wished to abolish the state board as it was then organized.

There probably was some truth to this suspicion, for Governor Burnquist did advocate the creation of a commission of public health, a move supported by members of the Minnesota Public Health Association. Briefly, the plan proposed by the governor and the association was as follows: [47]

1. The State Board of Health should be reorganized and made to consist of five instead of nine members.

2. The State Board of Health should be granted broad, general powers, instead of specifying in detail in the law the limits of its duties and activities.

3. The Board of Health should be empowered to appoint a Commissioner of Public Health.

4. The present Advisory Commission should be discontinued and its powers and duties transferred to a new division of the State Board of Health, to be headed by a man especially trained in tuberculosis work.

5. Industrial Hygiene should be transferred from the Department of Labor to the State Board of Health.

6. All existing state financed activities relating to public health should be organized under the State Board of Health.

7. Larger appropriations for the State's public health service should be granted.

The bill before the legislature, however, altered the governor's proposal, the most drastic change being that the governor, not the board of health, should appoint the health commissioner. This Bracken opposed violently, and, much to his delight, the bill died in the Senate after a stormy session. But years of fighting had left their scar, and Bracken once more felt that he should retire. He made an effort to secure a commission in the British Army, but he was then sixty-three years old and was rejected. The sight of members of his staff leaving for military duty or for Red Cross work in World War I depressed Bracken even more. He found little satisfaction in his duties and said he was "thoroughly tired of the disagreeable interference with his work." [48] He found it difficult to work harmoniously with Dr. Charles E. Smith, Jr., who had been appointed assistant secretary in 1917, and he said that it was only the loss of staff members to war service and epidemics of anterior poliomyelitis and influenza which prevented him from resigning in 1918.

[47] Burnquist, *Inaugural Message*, 8; form letter sent out by Dr. W. A. Jones to Minnesota physicians, February 19, 1917, Minnesota Department of Health, Minneapolis.
[48] *Senate Journal*, 1917, pp. 548–550; Bracken Papers, 4:369.

Bracken's resignation was precipitated, but not caused, by criticism from Hill, who had returned from Canada in 1918 to become executive secretary of the Minnesota Public Health Association. Early in April, 1919, Bracken said, he received word indirectly from Governor Burnquist that unless he resigned, the governor would replace him.[49] For almost four months Bracken pondered the problem. Finally, on July 8, 1919, the board accepted his resignation to take effect on September first. At that time Bracken became supervisor of District Number 10 of the United States Public Health Service. His duty was to aid beneficiaries of the War Risk Insurance program.

When Bracken closed his desk, he had been secretary of the State Department of Health for twenty-three years. Every activity of the department had grown under his administration and several new divisions had been created, among them the divisions of tuberculosis, venereal diseases, and child conservation. Although reorganizations had been attended with internal bickering and dispute, the over-all result was increased efficiency. Bracken also had co-operated well with national health organizations and had, in most cases, given sound advice to local health authorities. He shared the view of a colleague who, speaking of the relationship of the private physician to the department, said: "The physicians here are all good fellows and mean to do what is right but they are damnably lax and careless, they rarely report to me on the blanks provided by the S. B. of H. and prefer to yell their diagnoses to me across the street, leaving it to me to make out the reports."[50] But Bracken kept continually at the careless doctor, so that year by year his returns improved both in quality and quantity. To offset these contributions, the Bracken administration was marred by loss of distinguished personnel and by failure to win and keep legislative support.

[49] Bracken Papers, 4:416, 417; *Pioneer Press*, April 12, 1919. Bracken indicates that Hill also criticized him in the *Pioneer Press* during March, 1919, and in the *Journal* of the Minnesota Public Health Association, April 5, 1919. A careful check of these two publications reveals no such attacks for the period indicated.

[50] Tuohy to Wesbrook, March 25, 1910; Wesbrook to Tuohy, March 28, November 2, 1910; Alexander Barclay to T. R. Martin, October 7, 1914. Minnesota Department of Health, Minneapolis.

7

The Fight for Pure Water

MINNESOTA is a land of flowing streams and placid lakes. This surface water quenched the pioneer's thirst when the state was crisscrossed by emigrant caravans and when its population was small and scattered. But it was inconvenient for the settler, once he had chosen his homestead, to carry a sloshing pail from river to kitchen. Usually he wanted a nearer source of supply, and so he shoveled out a hole in the ground, erected a crude windlass from which hung a bucket, and called the result a well. These primitive wells, popular in both country and town, tapped underground water that, generally speaking, flowed over rock. Only in the southeast corner of the state is there a sinkhole area, where the limestone lies in vertical and horizontal channels and where openings in the covering loam or drift connect directly with the underlying rock.[1] Minnesotans, then as now, could almost be assured of a pure water supply no matter where they located a well, if only they would construct their well properly and prevent outside contamination from seeping in.

In the early days, when growing communities took their raw water supply from such rivers as the Mississippi and the St. Croix, there was little danger, because then municipal sewage was not disposed of into streams and because no smoke-belching industries nor modern canneries and creameries clouded rivers with murky waste. Yet almost from the very first both rural and urban residents became ill as the result of drinking impure water. By the time the State Board of Health was created, typhoid fever, a water-borne disease, annually was taking a large toll of lives. Newspapers almost constantly reported cases, and editors lugubriously commented upon the spread of the disease. A policeman in St. Paul lost three children in one day, and a Norwegian

[1] S. P. Kingston, "Contamination of Water Supplies in Limestone Foundation," in American Water Works Association, *Journal*, 35:1450–1456 (November, 1943).

family living on Highland Prairie had nine children sick with typhoid at one time. The Cataract House, a Minneapolis hotel, was supplying patrons, from a well sunk in boggy ground, with water that was a "stench in the nostrils" and that caused the death of several roomers. Hewitt, after inspecting the state prison at Stillwater, said that prisoners drew water from a well into which poured surface drainage. Nineteen cases of typhoid fever were the result, although in the 1870s the disease was not believed to be water-borne.[2]

The prevailing opinion, in Minnesota and elsewhere, was that typhoid fever was of miasmatic origin, caused from the decomposition of animal and vegetable substances, from foul drains or leaky sewers, from neglected outhouses and cellars, from the breaking up of new soil, or from the disturbance of sluggish streams or ponds. Although Dr. D. W. Hand, president of the state board in 1873, commented upon the infectious character of the stools of typhoid fever patients, he did not believe the disease was contagious.[3] He had no suspicion, of course, that the disease could be spread not only by human carriers, but also by flies, and that it was milk-borne as well at water-borne. Local health officers and private physicians shared this ignorance.

In 1880, however, the situation changed, for in that year Karl Joseph Eberth described the typhoid bacillus. Nine years later the idea that typhoid was water-borne was prevalent in Minnesota, but it was further held that human or animal excrement must first pollute the water supply. The germ theory took hold slowly, some medical men refusing to accept it until public health officials demonstrated its validity beyond a shadow of a doubt. "Without entering into the discussion of the germ theory at all," said Dr. J. C. Rosser, chairman of the committee on epidemics and hygiene of the Minnesota State Medical Society, "I shall answer your first question, that I do not believe the germ theory sufficient to explain all the phenomena in the so-called zymotic diseases; neither is there evidence enough produced, to my mind, to prove the existence of a specific bacterium for each of the infectious diseases; neither do I believe bacteria or any of the other little bugs to be the cause of disease, but rather the result of the same — that is, diseases of a certain kind are favorable for the development of bacteria." Regardless of Rosser's opinion, the state health department not only held to the germ theory, but also believed that typhoid was carried in contami-

[2] *St. Paul Daily Press*, June 12, 25, September 12, October 11, 29, 1872, September 30, 1874; *Duluth Daily Tribune*, January 4, 1873; *Minneapolis Tribune*, June 20, 22, 1875; State Board of Health, *Annual Reports*, 1873, p. 86.
[3] State Board of Health, *Annual Reports*, 1874, pp. 64, 67.

nated water. The typhoid epidemic of September, 1881, in Minneapolis seemed to prove that. Eight years later, Hewitt said bluntly that a "foul water supply" was one of the commonest methods of propagating typhoid fever.[4]

Illustrations showing the relation of impure water to disease were numerous. At a conference of state and local boards of health in 1885, Dr. Charles Berry of New Ulm told of a family having three or four cases of typhoid fever. Berry made several visits, but he could find no local cause for the disease and finally decided the water must be at fault, although it looked and tasted pure. Shortly afterwards an abandoned privy vault was found near the well. Dr. C. F. Warner of Mankato reported at the same conference that there was more sickness in the portions of the town using shallow wells than in the low-lying districts, where sickness naturally would be expected. A St. Paul physician said that complaints of poor water were numerous, and in every instance analysis revealed contamination by cesspools and vaults.

When Hewitt rose to speak, the delegates listened respectfully. Many of them knew that for years the laboratory of the state board had made analyses of suspected water. Hewitt had reported in 1879 that the "samples examined came from various towns and cities of the State, and some of them were found to be so bad . . . as to have been directly instrumental in causing typhoid and other fevers in the families which used them. In this way much assistance has been afforded health officers and physicians in finding and destroying causes of disease." As early as 1876 the state board listed water supplies as one of its major projects, and in that year a warning was issued for citizens to clean roofs and water pipes to prevent pollution before water reached cisterns. Hewitt told the delegates that it was the duty of health officers to make more water analyses than was the practice. He suggested that surface waters be kept from running into wells by erecting tight metal curbs around wells and by digging wells deeper. He thought all wells should be condemned until proved safe, and he spoke of the serious contamination of river water by night soil (sewage), and garbage.[5]

Although several Minnesota cities located on rivers took their water from streams, St. Paul early began drawing its water supply from lakes, particularly Lake Phalen. Yet drawing water from lakes presented difficulties. In 1873 summer grasses, weeds, and slimy accumulations

[4] *Public Health in Minnesota*, 1:21 (May, 1885); 5:71 (September, 1889); Minnesota State Medical Society, *Transactions*, 1883, p. 209; State Board of Health, *Biennial Reports*, 1881–82, p. 14.

[5] *Pioneer Press*, April 16, 1876, December 31, 1879, January 29, 1885; *Pioneer-Press and Tribune*, May 5, 1876.

clogged the strainer near Lake Phalen, and shut off the water supply. Water drawn from White Bear Lake was criticized merely because it looked injurious, but it had at least one stout defender, who argued thus: "Water drawn from the swamps and bogs near White Bear Lake flows into and over the surface of six lakes before it reaches the inlet pipe of the Water Company — is spread out over the surface of thousands of acres of water, reaching the direct feeding works of the company some ten days after leaving its swampy beds, the malarious taints ... in the meantime having vanished into the air."[6]

Other objections were made to water drawn from lakes. Fastidious citizens were averse to drinking water in which people had bathed, and others were annoyed when a live snake was drawn from a water hydrant. Nor was that all. It was customary in the 1870s for water merchants to cart drinking water and retail it to families living at a distance from regular waterworks or springs. When a vigilant citizen discovered that one purveyor was labeling his merchandise "Lake Phalen Water" and drawing it from slaughterhouse-contaminated Phalen Creek, a terrific howl went up. St. Paulites wondered if water kept in public drinking barrels was pure and later speculated as to whether a drinking fountain for "thirsty horses, dogs, and men" was safe to use. Even the public supply near the Park Place Hotel was suspect. Health seekers attributed its reddish color to the presence of beneficial iron, and skeptics maintained that the discoloration resulted from unsanitary vegetable matter.[7]

Discussion became so vigorous that Dr. Brewer Mattocks, St. Paul health officer, in 1878 tried to ease public feeling with a long explanation of what constituted pure drinking water. He pointed out that chemically pure water was unnecessary to maintain health, but that it was essential that water be free from harmful animal and vegetable matter. "A healthy man," Mattocks continued, "may drink impure water year in and year out, without positive detriment to health, but the time will sooner or later come when the system is run down and debilitated; and then impure water often is the turning-point of disease." He suggested a simple method of testing water: place a glass container of well water, Phalen water, or cistern water next to a container of filtered water. If after three days the unfiltered sample remains clear, it is not seriously impregnated with decaying matter. Mattocks recommended filtering impure water through a large flower pot filled with

[6] *St. Paul Daily Press*, July 8, September 3, 1873.
[7] *St. Paul Daily Press*, June 18, August 7, 1874; *Evening Dispatch* (St. Paul), May 27, 1874; *Pioneer-Press and Tribune*, May 16, 1876; *Pioneer-Press*, March 10, 1875.

washed sand and coarse gravel, with a layer or two of pounded charcoal added. He thought water from Lake Phalen was more healthful than well water.[8]

A rapidly growing population and an increasing number of industries forced St. Paul to consider exactly what type of water management it wanted. Before 1875 opinion was split, one group holding that a private water company would give better service and another believing in municipal ownership and control. In 1875, however, advocates of a city owned and operated waterworks prevailed. Opponents of this plan argued that it would not pay unless all parties on different lines became patrons; that it would require arbitrary, if not despotic rules, and hence would be difficult to uphold in court; and that it would require an outlay of money necessitating loans that the people were not yet ready to meet.[9]

By 1881 it was clearly evident that no private enterprise could meet the water needs of St. Paul. Not even the building of an inexpensive embankment at the outlet of Lake Phalen, which would, it was thought in 1876, increase the city's water supply, could solve the problem.[10] Champions of a municipal waterworks pointed out that, when the private company was established in 1868, provision had been made for its eventual purchase by the city. With this in mind, a commission, comprising the committee on legislation of the St. Paul City Council, a committee of the Chamber of Commerce, and members of the state legislature from Ramsey County, went to work.

A bill was introduced into the legislature and was approved on February 10, 1881. It provided, in brief, for the purchase of the property, rights, and franchises of the St. Paul Water Company by the city for a fair sum. Management of the municipal company would consist of four water commissioners to be selected by judges of the district court. The engineer, surveyors, agents, and other employees would be hired by a board with the mayor of St. Paul as an ex-officio member. One of the first duties of the board would be to extend the works and to tap sources of supply other than Lake Phalen, "after which the system will be enlarged and extended on a basis equal to the demands of a city that is growing with extraordinary rapidity, and whose wants in the matter of water can only be supplied by the people themselves in their corporate capacity." [11]

[8] *Pioneer Press*, May 12, 1878.
[9] *St. Paul Daily Press*, January 27, 1875.
[10] *Pioneer Press*, November 14, 1876.
[11] *Pioneer Press*, January 23, February 8, 1881; St. Paul Common Council, *Proceedings*, 1882, pp. 54–68; Minnesota, *General Laws*, 1881, p. 753.

In August, 1882, the deal was consummated, and St. Paul, for the first time in its history, controlled its water supply and its distributing system. Extension went ahead rapidly, until it no longer was proper to speak of the city receiving its water from Lake Phalen, for that lake supplied only the section known as Bronson's Addition. By 1883 most of St. Paul was being supplied with water from Lake Vadnais and the Vadnais chain. The board also considered the possibility of expanding water sources to include some, if not all, of the lakes lying north and northeast of St. Paul and varying in size from large ponds to the broad waters of White Bear, Bald Eagle, and Forest lakes. This supply, from an area lying about two hundred feet higher than the Mississippi River, was believed to offer purer water from a practically inexhaustible source. A high service reservoir was also planned to supply St. Anthony Hill, which could not be serviced by a low-pressure plant.[12]

Both health officers and private physicians enthusiastically endorsed a municipality-owned waterworks and the water which was drawn from Minnesota lakes. "Every family in town should have this water in their homes," commented a doctor, "then flush the sewers, and have good ventilation, and doctors will soon cease practising." This was good advice, but many St. Paul residents still preferred, for one reason or another, to draw drinking water from shallow wells that were in constant danger of contamination from seepage from creeks, cesspools, and water closets. Dr. Talbot Jones reported in 1885 that specimens of well water taken from almost every section of the city showed impurity in the vast majority of instances. And in 1884 local newspapers had said that well water showed evidence of contamination with cesspool matter. Dr. D. W. Hand, president of the State Board of Health, endorsed these analyses and warned St. Paul that well water was an influential factor in the spread of disease.[13]

Many factors stood in the way of residents abolishing wells and subscribing to city water service. In the first place, the extension of mains was slow, for the new city-owned company could not begin to pipe water wherever it was needed. In the second place, water rates were high for families living in poor districts, such as Swede Hollow. In the third place, the cost of home plumbing was beyond the reach of many middle-class families. Finally, as St. Paul's health officer pointed out, there was a surprising amount of skepticism concerning the defects of wells.[14]

[12] *Pioneer Press*, June 1, 1884, December 18, 1887.
[13] *Pioneer Press*, October 12, December 11, 1884, March 23, 1885; St. Paul City Officers, *Annual Reports*, 1885, p. 276.
[14] *Pioneer Press*, March 23, June 24, 1885.

Gradually, however, the combined efforts of state and local health officers and almost constant newspaper warnings took effect. The process was slow, as is all social development, but it was also persistent. Residents of the Sixth Ward and Dayton's Bluff protested vigorously against stagnant pools of water, claiming that these pools produced the contagious diseases that were afflicting them. Children in the Van Buren School were said to have taken sick as the result of drinking polluted water. Irate citizens even complained when a movement was inaugurated to establish a public park on the shores of Lake Phalen, maintaining that a recreation center would contaminate the water. Objection also was made when St. Paul planned to cut ice from the Mississippi River, and an ordinance prohibiting the taking of ice anywhere below the Falls of St. Anthony was passed. The state health department was quoted as saying it had "ascertained that the filth and sewage of Minneapolis emptying into the river rendered the ice impure, and liable to affect the health of the people using it." [15]

This increasing public interest in pure water no doubt prompted city fathers to redouble their efforts to extend mains and stimulated health officers to sing the praises of water drawn from city pipes. Hewitt lent his aid to St. Paul in 1889 by saying he was surprised at the purity of its water. The St. Paul Department of Health, pleased with this praise, nevertheless realized that not all its water was safe. It continued the fight by pointing out that, of the patients involved in the sixty-four cases of contagious diseases reported in May, 1890, thirty-six had used lake water, twenty-two, well water, and six, cistern water. Of these, only nineteen had sewer connections in their homes.[16]

Indeed, an attempt was made to show that St. Paul was a healthier city than Minneapolis to live in because its water was purer. A physician argued this way: "I know no measure which is so thoroughly reliable in case both cities have the same environment. For instance, in the case of St. Paul and Minneapolis, the two cities have almost identi-

[15] *Pioneer Press*, June 15, 1885, May 25, November 25, 1886; *Minneapolis Tribune*, July 24, 1887; *Amendments to the St. Paul City Charter and Laws Relating to the City Government and Ordinances of the City Council*, 254 (St. Paul, 1887). For Hewitt's analysis of water, see St. Paul Water Commissioner, *Annual Reports*, 1886, p. 33. For many years the Minnesota Department of Health concerned itself with investigating the bodies of water from which ice supplies were obtained, but in 1915, in line with the conclusions of the United States Public Health Service, this practice was discontinued. "Studies of ice formations have shown that even where the ice is collected from waters so polluted as to be absolutely unsafe for drinking purposes, the ice itself seldom shows any evidence of pollution." Bracken to Charles F. Lewis, October 7, 1915, Minnesota Department of Health, St. Paul; State Board of Health, *The Natural Purification of Water by Freezing* (February, 1917).

[16] *Pioneer Press*, November 20, 1889, June 5, 1890.

cal conditions in regard to climate, atmosphere, etc. The only difference is in the water supply, and it is generally conceded that Minneapolis has not as good a supply as St. Paul. This would tend to make the Minneapolis death rate a trifle higher. At present Minneapolis is supplied with river water, but if the quality were as good as that furnished St. Paul the death rate ought to be about the same in both cities, for each has about the same amount of sewers, and they are equally well drained. In zymotic diseases Minneapolis generally runs higher in death rates than does St. Paul. In 1888, for instance, Minneapolis had 160 deaths from typhoid fever, against 142 in St. Paul, while cases of diphtheria were as 148 to 111 and of diarrhoeal diseases 267 to 227. St. Paul is unusually healthful, and there are few, if any, cities in the country that can show as good a record. Minneapolis while existing under almost the same conditions, cannot show any better record, and it is doubtful if she can show one quite as good." [17]

Despite such boasting, St. Paul was not without its tribulations. Housewives complained that water had "masses" of minute vegetation in it and that its color was darkish. This was generally attributed to flushing the mains and was considered harmless, although subscribers were told they might filter or boil their water if they were fearful. Hewitt, receiving almost half a gallon daily for analysis, found nothing deleterious in it and suggested that the trouble might be due only to microscopic fungi lodged in smaller mains and service pipes.[18]

Modern technological engineering was to solve these problems with the addition of reservoirs and improvements in purification. Artesian wells also assured cleaner water at a time when the entire city could not be supplied from regular mains. In 1888 a sixteen-million-gallon open reservoir was completed at the head of Dale Street, which served the high areas of the city until its abandonment in 1918. By July, 1896, the system was extended to tap the water of Otter Lake, north of Pleasant Lake, and work was begun on the construction of a forty-two-inch wooden conduit north to the Centerville lakes system and the construction of a pumping station and twenty-eight artesian wells along the shore of Centerville Lake. Additional artesian wells were sunk in 1910, an exceptionally dry year, but little more was accomplished until 1925, when it was found necessary to use Mississippi River water to supplement Lake Vadnais sources. A modern electric pumping station was constructed on the east bank of the Mississippi River north of Minneapolis.

[17] *Pioneer Press*, September 24, 1890.
[18] *Pioneer Press*, June 30, 1893, July 26, 1895.

THE FIGHT FOR PURE WATER

Three years later a Highland Park water tower went up to supplement the capacities of an eighteen-million-gallon reservoir on South Snelling Avenue and a sixteen-million-gallon low service reservoir. By then wells were almost a thing of the past, and St. Paul possessed a filtration and purification plant that would have been the envy of both Hewitt and Bracken. In 1920 the St. Paul Water Department had added a chemist and a bacteriologist to its staff, so that the people "may have confidence and shall need have no fear as to the purity and healthfulness of the water furnished them."[19]

Minneapolis also waged a fight for pure water. Like St. Paul, Minneapolis was ridden with typhoid fever resulting from the use of contaminated water drawn from private and public wells. But for Minneapolis the great water source was the Mississippi, from whose depths raw water was sucked and distributed to thousands of defenseless families. The pipes through which this water ran leaked to permit entry of ground water, rats chewed holes in them, and poor connections and joints invited seepage. In winter, water mains in the heart of Minneapolis were frozen solid for weeks.[20]

Many resented water superintendents whom they considered incompetent, and others were suspicious of the quality of water itself. "It is well for our Minneapolis people to take all necessary precautions to secure themselves with pure water," commented a St. Paul editor in 1876, "but it is not well for them to grope blindly in this or any other matter involving the health of 24,000 people and no inconsiderable fraction of their wealth. If the water of the Mississippi . . . is either impure or unhealthy, the city will be justified in taking steps at whatever cost to remedy the situation."[21]

Not only was the Mississippi contaminated by sewage from Bassetts Creek and from towns to the north, but it also was fouled by the dead bodies of horses and other animals, which were caught and held by floating timbers. An observer in 1876 counted twenty-seven bloated carcasses of horses, cattle, hogs, sheep, and deer directly above the pipes leading to the waterworks. Yet, even with such dramatic evidence, some individuals held that raw Mississippi water was less contaminated than water drawn from city wells. Regardless of differences in opinion, it

[19] St. Paul City Engineer, *Annual Reports*, 1894, p. 835; St. Paul Board of Water Commissioners, *Annual Reports*, 1920, p. 9; St. Paul Water Department, *Romance of the Water Department*, 4 (St. Paul, 1934). See the map facing page 5 and the diagram showing the course of water during the process of purification, facing page 6.
[20] *Minneapolis Tribune*, March 24, 1875.
[21] *Pioneer-Press and Tribune*, September 2, 1876.

was thought desirable not only to investigate thoroughly the defects of the Minneapolis water supply, but also to see whether or not it might be possible to pull water from lakes as St. Paul was doing. Cedar Lake, Lake of the Isles, and Lakes Calhoun and Harriet were all suggested as possible sources.[22]

In 1877 Mayor A. A. Ames invited the city engineer and Professor Stephen F. Peckham of the University of Minnesota to study water supply in detail and to report to the city council. Peckham, after exhaustive water analyses, concluded that river water above Minneapolis was suitable for domestic use; that local contamination from city sewage, especially from Bassetts Creek, was sufficient to cause apprehension of disease; and that local contamination would become increasingly dangerous, because of an essential change in sewerage plans that would send municipal sewage directly into the river at a point which would make the Mississippi totally unfit for use as a source of water supply.

T. L. Rosser, the city engineer, was not so disturbed as was Peckham, saying that no city was more fortunately located in regard to water supply than was Minneapolis, where the Mississippi and near-by lakes offered purity on all sides. "Most of the citizens of our city," continued Rosser, "are possessed with the conviction that the water of the Mississippi river in the vicinity of the pump house is unwholesome, and saturated with latent disease. Whether this is due to a blind prejudice, or the results of scientific demonstrations, I will not assume the province of deciding. Neither will I assume the function of a sanitary engineer and attempt to measure the germs of disease and death which are constantly being carried by our cesspools through a sandy soil into our wells without being purified. Nor will I attempt to measure the amount of filth which pollutes and befouls the river near the pump house. These are questions for the Health Commissioner and the death rate to answer, and so far as I am informed, the facts in the case are not of an alarming character at the present time."[23]

Rosser got little support from the Minneapolis health officer, G. F. Townsend, who endorsed Peckham's report with enthusiasm and added some findings of his own. Peckham argued the "imperative necessity of taking the supply of water for the city from some point in the river above the city limits, where the pure river water will be free from the contamination of the city sewerage." The fact that even a small amount of contamination might be present in river water was

---

[22] *Pioneer-Press and Tribune*, June 3, 26, July 23, August 31, September 5, 1876.
[23] *Pioneer Press*, March 17, 1877; Minneapolis City Council, *Proceedings*, April, 1876–April, 1877, p. 192.

THE FIGHT FOR PURE WATER 109

sufficient to convince Townsend that water should be taken from the very best spot on the river. In his annual report he urged early action to insure a purer supply.[24]

Despite much favorable endorsement, little was done to move the Minneapolis water intake farther upstream. The delay was due not only to a sluggish attitude on the part of the city council, but also to the fact that the council wished to alter the sewerage system at the same time that it changed the source of water supply. While bickering went on as to where both water and sewerage system should be located, a new health officer, Dr. A. H. Salisbury, spoke out plainly. He said that fifty years earlier Minneapolis had been one of the healthiest cities on the globe, but that now it had a higher death rate than many communities less favorably located. He listed the outstanding diseases as scarlet fever, diphtheria, typhoid fever, and diarrheal diseases, and he deplored the fact that children should die at the rate of forty or fifty a month. Then he continued graphically: "But when the water they drink is first filtered through stable refuse and privy-vaults; when the air they breathe comes from cess-pools and sewers; when their food is drawn from diseased slop-fed cows, this infant mortality is not so surprising. . . . Let us, then, no longer drink the filth drained from ten thousand cesspools and flavored with the putrid carcasses of dead animals, but unite in demanding, pure, wholesome, healthful water." In his official reports he spoke of the paramount importance of safe water for culinary and drinking purposes, agreeing with the city engineer that disastrous results were the natural outcome of the cesspool system.[25]

But Salisbury was not content merely to describe unsanitary conditions in the press and to nag at the Minneapolis city fathers. He called in Hewitt, asking him not only to analyze water but also to make public addresses. Hewitt spoke at Harrison Hall on "The Water Supply of Minneapolis." If Salisbury thought that lectures by Hewitt would promptly result in better drinking water for the citizens of Minneapolis, he was disappointed.[26]

Nothing was accomplished until 1883, when another special committee was appointed by the city council to investigate the same old water problem. Undoubtedly Mayor Ames, himself a physician, had stimulated this action in his inaugural address a year earlier. Professor James

[24] *Pioneer Press*, March 18, 1877; Minneapolis City Council, *Proceedings*, 1876–77, p. 192, appendix, 54.
[25] *Pioneer Press*, April 20, 1878, November 1, 1879; *Tribune*, July 28, 1879; Minneapolis City Council, *Proceedings*, April 9, 1878, April 8, 1879, appendix, 102, 110.
[26] *Tribune*, December 23, 1879; *Pioneer Press*, January 11, 1881.

A. Dodge was asked — as Peckham had been a few years earlier — to take water samples and to recommend a safe intake location. He concluded that water should be drawn from the channel of the river above Minneapolis. In 1885 Dodge again submitted a report, this time a detailed analysis of water samples drawn from six different areas. He drew attention to the fact that an analysis of water was not always sufficient to warrant positive conclusions, saying that it was equally necessary to study the environment through which the water ran or from which it came. He favored a system of home filtration instead of a city owned and operated filtration system.[27]

Although action was stimulated by public sentiment, by Dodge's report, and by the fact that typhoid fever in Minneapolis in 1883 had caused more deaths than any other one disease, it was not as far reaching as friends of pure water had hoped it would be. The water board, meeting behind closed doors, apparently considered abandoning the Mississippi and substituting water drawn from artesian wells. Hewitt, hearing of this, argued that, despite popular notion, not all spring water was pure. Another physician pointed out that even artesian wells were open to contamination, and he estimated that Minneapolis contained over fifty thousand cesspools and privy vaults that could not fail to seep into even deep wells.[28]

The board also considered the installation of a filtering plant, an idea which Dodge pushed vigorously. Speaking on filtration before the Minnesota Academy of Natural Sciences, Dodge carefully and tactfully explained that, while the water supply of Minneapolis was no worse than that of many other cities, there was need for improvement. He thought filtration was the answer, and he described varieties of filters in common use. Certainly Dodge did not hold that the sinking of artesian wells was the answer to the Minneapolis water problem. He probably looked askance at the magnificent Bryn Mawr well, where the water spurted some six feet above the ground, and no doubt he was dubious, too, of the well in Central Park. Dodge's skepticism was justified, for in 1890 a health department analysis of samples showed forty wells giving water inferior to that drawn directly from the Mississippi.[29]

[27] Minneapolis City Council, *Proceedings*, April 11, 1882–April 10, 1883, p. 6; *Tribune*, March 7, 1883; *Pioneer Press*, January 3, 1885.
[28] Minneapolis City Council, *Proceedings*, 1882–83, appendix, 141; *Pioneer Press*, August 2, November 4, 1885, June 8, 1887. Gradually, through the years, many of the downtown hotels, department stores, and office buildings drilled their own artesian wells. Because of the labyrinth of sewers tunneled through the underlying rock, contamination of these wells was an ever-present danger. A. J. Chesley to H. P. Howard, March 4, 1926, Minnesota Department of Health, St. Paul.
[29] *Pioneer Press*, April 4, 1888, May 7, 1890.

THE FIGHT FOR PURE WATER

Hewitt, too, was suspicious of well water. He declared openly that the only logical source for Minneapolis water was the Mississippi River, and he, like Dodge, championed filtration of water for domestic use. Hewitt recommended a natural earth filter. The Minneapolis City Council, wearied by years of debate and frightened by the prevalence of water-borne diseases, resolved to float a bond issue of $500,000 for the construction of a reservoir and the establishment of a filter system. The date of this action was August 3, 1894, and the event was the first great decisive forward step taken in many years.[30]

Saying that the citizens of Minneapolis were entitled to get drinking water that was above suspicion, F. W. Cappelen, the city engineer, listed the benefits which a filtration plant would confer:

First — All odor, color and impurities in suspension shall be removed.

Second — The free ammonia shall not exceed 0.05 in one million parts.

Third — The albuminoid ammonia shall not exceed 0.1 per million parts.

Fourth — No measurable amount of the coagulant or other purifying agent used shall be left in the filtered water.

Fifth — The microbes in the filtered water shall not exceed 100 colonies per cubic centimeter.[31]

Work on two reservoirs at Columbia Heights was begun and completed in 1896, but the filtration plant did not materialize. The city engineer placed the blame squarely on the waterworks committee of the city council, saying that the committee did not hurry a filtration plant along. Hewitt found *coli communis* in the water, and he, too, did his best to push action. A year later the plans for a filtration plant again were postponed, this time because the committee wished to wait to see the results of filtration at Louisville, Kentucky. Meanwhile, so many frogs were jumping into reservoirs and squirming through mains to plug outlets of fire hydrants, taps, and sprinkling systems that wire screens three feet high were erected to keep out the jumping hordes. City fathers were plagued also by typhoid cases, by threats of insurance companies to raise rates unless a more adequate supply of water was assured, and by a growing popular demand for filtration.[32]

Something, it was clearly apparent, had to be done. City engineers presented a fairly complete picture of the situation in 1900. Water problems were vastly different then from those of 1867, when the

[30] *Pioneer Press*, August 4, November 14, 1894; Minneapolis City Council, *Proceedings*, 1894–95, pp. 471.
[31] Minneapolis City Council, *Proceedings*, 1894–95, p. 466.
[32] Minneapolis City Officers, *Annual Reports*, 1895, p. 157; 1896, p. 140; 1899, p. 174.

THE PEOPLE'S HEALTH

Minneapolis waterworks was authorized by the city council as an auxiliary to the fire department. A small rotary pump, installed in the Holly Sawmill, brought the first pumped water into Minneapolis. Not until 1872 was a vertical double-acting piston pump located at the foot of Fifth Avenue South and the Mississippi River. Five additional pumps were installed in 1884, making a total pumping capacity of thirty-three million gallons per day. Other pumping stations were placed in operation in 1885 and 1888, the last located at Camden, three miles north of the center of Minneapolis business.[33]

The 1900 proposal called for the construction of basins, new pipe lines, and additional pumps to carry water from the Mississippi to a settling basin close to the shore. Water piped from the sedimentation basin would, it was believed, be somewhat clarified before reaching the pumps and thus would be ready to pass through filters. Engineers thought that increased filtration would become necessary as upriver towns swelled in population and their sewage became more objectionable. "If the water is properly sedimented before it is pumped," said Minneapolis engineers, "filtration will not be so much a necessity for several years to come and pump injuries on account of grit will be reduced one-half. Sedimentation is not expected to remove all the bacteria but, when properly conducted, will remove a considerable part of them from the water."[34]

In 1901 and again in 1902 superintendents of waterworks and engineers still were debating the merits of a filtration plant, and citizens were growing weary of so much talk and so little action. Finally, on February 18, 1910, the city council authorized the establishment of a sterilizing plant which would treat water with hypochlorite of lime, and recommended that one basin should be covered and used as storage for clear water as part of a filtration plant. It was at first believed that water could be purified by the so-called Johnson system, a procedure by which ozone produced by an electric current passing through the water was supposed to decontaminate it. This, however, was found to be too costly.[35]

The introduction of hypochlorite into Minneapolis water was, of course, an outstanding sanitary step and a relatively new procedure. The original experimental work had been done in Chicago only a few years

[33] *The Water Works of the City of Minneapolis. . . . A Brief Historical Sketch and a Description of the Present Water Works*, 3–5 (Minneapolis, 1919).
[34] Minneapolis City Officers, *Annual Reports*, 1900, p. 160.
[35] Minneapolis City Officers, *Annual Reports*, 1901, p. 303; 1902, p. 281; 1910, p. 24g; Minneapolis City Council, *Proceedings*, 1910, p. 129.

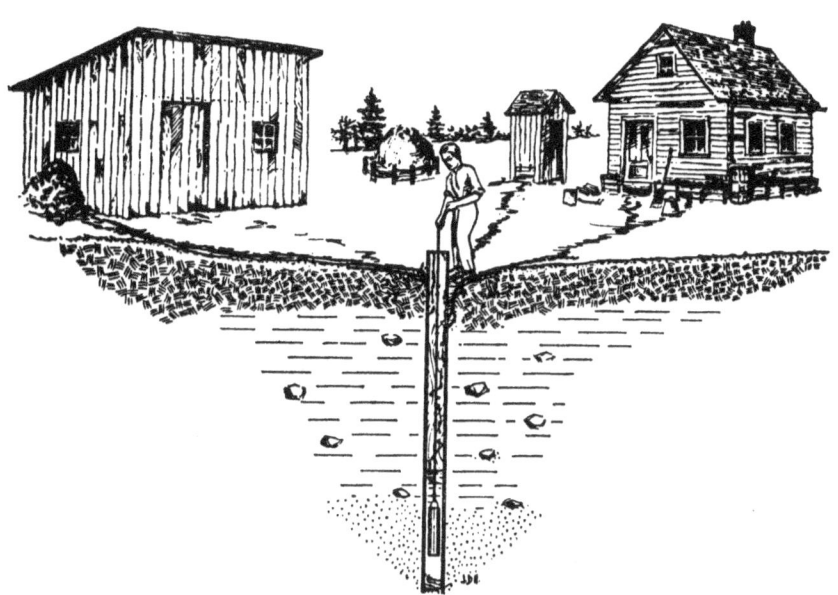

HOW POLLUTION MAY ENTER A POORLY CONSTRUCTED WELL
From State Board of Health, Farm Water Supplies, 1915

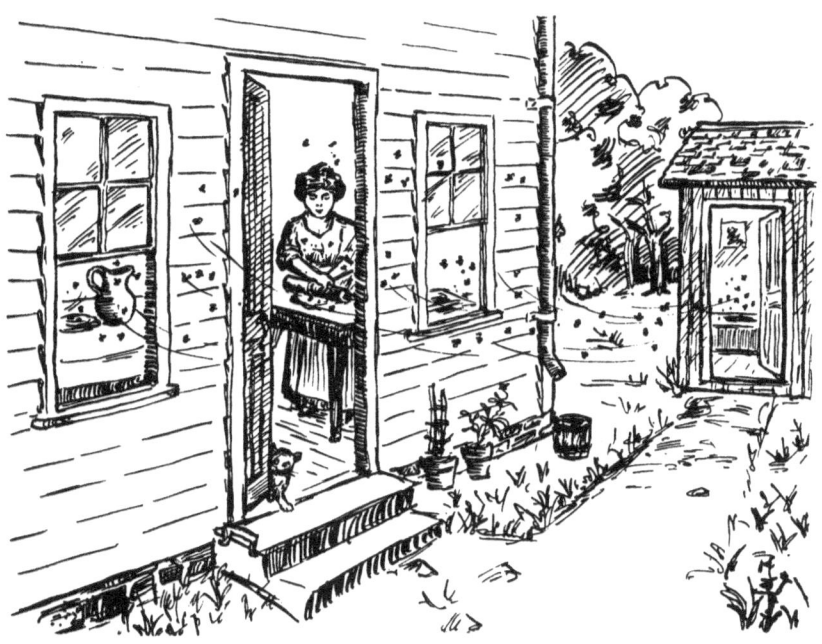

HOW FLIES MAY SPREAD DISEASE
From the author's collection

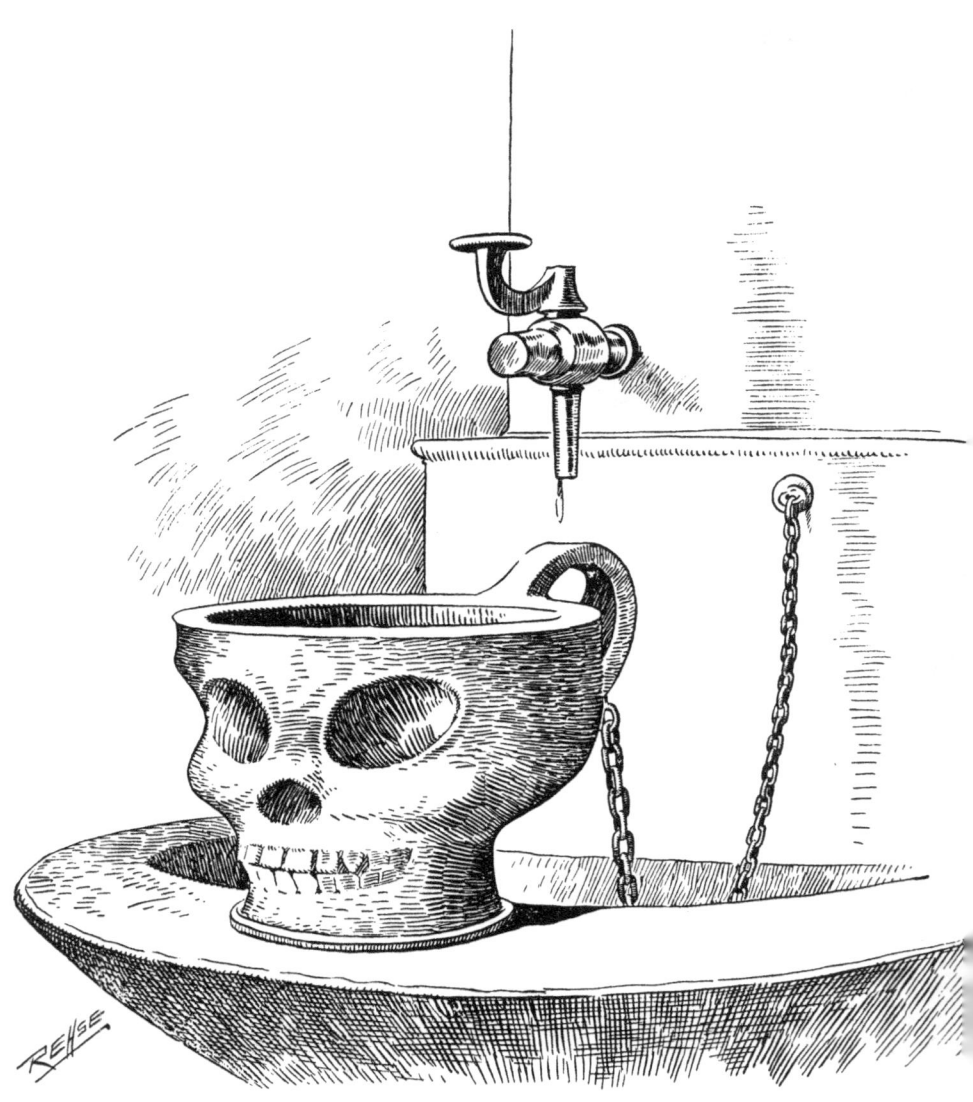

The Public Drinking Cup

A State Board of Health Circular
From the author's collection

THE FIGHT FOR PURE WATER   113

earlier. Chlorination of water, if done properly, would make it absolutely safe for drinking purposes and thus would free mankind from its age-old fear of typhoid epidemics and other water-borne diseases. The state health department, recognizing the significance of this new water treatment, had a homemade, portable hypochlorite plant for emergency use in typhoid and dysentery epidemics throughout the state. A dramatic demonstration by the department took place at Hibbing in May, 1910, when an outbreak of dysentery "stopped as soon as the hypochlorite treatment commenced, and . . . at no time since has the water, in any of the samples taken, shown the presence of pathogenic bacteria." In 1910 not only Minneapolis, but also Hibbing, East Grand Forks, Breckenridge, Brainerd, and Baudette were chlorinating water. St. Paul was using chlorine by 1919 and was sending two samples weekly for analysis by the state health department.[36]

St. Paul and Minneapolis were not alone in their campaign to secure pure water. Scores of smaller communities, under the urging of local health officers, patiently and persistently labored to prevent contamination of wells and cisterns and to find a method to make river water safe. The decades following 1870 saw towns and villages reach their goal — objectives not always achieved in whole, but usually in part. The Minnesota water picture in 1900 was far better than it had been thirty years earlier, but even so it was far from perfect.

In 1873 the people of Mankato were discussing a plan, later adopted, by which their "progressive and wide awake city" would draw water from a lake on Shaubut's Hill. At Winona the city council authorized the construction of waterworks in 1874 and found considerable popular support of the plan. Perhaps the proposal was stimulated by an unusually dry and hot summer. The failure of the Stillwater waterworks in 1877, resulting in clogging of pipes and the shutting off of two principal fountains, forced citizens to carry their water from springs, streams, watering troughs, and abandoned wells and lent emphasis to a movement already under way for the development of a more modern water supply. [37] Stillwater installed the first filter in Minnesota in 1881, and Brainerd put in use Minnesota's first mechanical filter four years later.

A newspaper reporter, in the early summer of 1872, commented upon the source of city water in Duluth and described his sickening reactions. "The bottom of the lake," he wrote, "is completely covered with

[36] State Board of Health, *Biennial Reports*, 1909–10, p. 271; St. Paul Board of Water Commissioners, *Annual Reports*, 1919, p. 11.
[37] *St. Paul Daily Press*, March 15, 1873, July 29, 1874; *St. Paul Pioneer*, May 13, 1874; *Pioneer Press*, January 17, May 31, 1877.

decayed fish entrails and other offals; while the surface, in calm weather, is thickly coated over with a slimy, greasy substance resembling dishwater. Indeed the same state of affairs would apply to a greater or less extent, to the whole distance along the shore, from the railroad to the citizens' dock; and, knowing as we do, that the water which *nine-tenths* of our people drink is taken *from between these two points*, it must be a 'strong' stomach, surely, that will receive it unhesitatingly." Then he added, a bit pathetically: "It is conceded that no better drinking water is found upon the globe than this of Lake Superior; and it is really a shame that we cannot have it in its purity, when only a little city legislation would effectually remedy the gross evil." Duluth wells were described as "smelly" and "sickening," even though residents sought to purify them with lime.[38] These conditions gradually were eradicated as Duluth improved its water supply and constructed modern waterworks. In 1912 Duluth began chlorination.

St. Cloud, a thriving community on the banks of the Mississippi, completed its waterworks in 1888, erecting a large crib near the middle of the river and constructing a twenty-nine-thousand-gallon cistern. Divided into two parts, the cistern was so constructed that all water was forced through a sponge filter. By 1910 St. Cloud had made additional improvements, and other Minnesota towns had vastly altered primitive waterworks to conform to more sanitary standards.[39]

Generally speaking, progress toward purification of water was easier in urban centers than in rural areas. Cities were forced by public opinion and by recurrent epidemics to provide protection for residents. People demanded a water supply both adequate and pure. They wanted an abundance of water for the use of their fire departments and they wanted uncontaminated water for drinking. Then, too, municipalities could find ways to finance waterworks. But in country areas, where most of the people lived on farms and where villages were small and impoverished, progress was slow and, in many instances, disheartening. In these rural districts the well continued to be the chief water source.

It was difficult, indeed, for the state health department to convince individualistic farmers that wells could be dangerous. The water looked clear and sparkling, and so it must be good. The farmer frequently argued that his father and his grandfather had dipped the bucket into the old well and had got along all right. This was a difficult argu-

[38] *Duluth Daily Tribune*, June 5, 12, 1872.
[39] *Pioneer Press*, December 21, 1888. For a description of the water supply in fifty Minnesota communities in 1910, see State Board of Health, *Biennial Reports*, 1909–10, pp. 248–256.

ment for health authorities to meet, and it was even more difficult to explain the relationship between the moss-covered well near the manure pile and the moss-covered gravestones in the family cemetery. Yet, difficult as the task was, the state department undertook it, with the assistance of county health officers.

The first great survey of rural water supplies was undertaken in 1877. Hewitt and Professor N. H. Winchell, state geologist and professor of chemistry at the University of Minnesota, took the Northern Pacific Railroad en route to the Red River Valley. Professor Peckham accompanied the party. Among the localities visited were Campbell, Breckenridge, and Moorhead, and samples were drawn from the waters of the Bois des Sioux, Otter Tail, and Red rivers. Two types of wells were found, a shallow pit which penetrated only the lacustrine clay and a deep-shaft well which penetrated the drift clay. Winchell thought that, as a rule, water from these shallow wells was free from alkaline qualities and was safe for domestic use. Deep-well water, he said, was always alkaline, cool, clear, and sparkling.

The party found scores of stagnant wells whose waters were turbid and on whose surface floated small globules of colored and oily film. This was said to be due to housing made from pine timber. Deep wells sometimes showed the formation of organic salts and the liberation of free sulphureted hydrogen, so that sometimes a real "sulphur" water resulted. Several recommendations were made, including the lining of wells with cement, the avoidance of zinc pipes, the use of properly constructed cisterns in preference to the average well, and the boiling or filtering of well water to remove organic impurities.[40]

In 1878 Hewitt, encouraged by the results of the Red River Valley investigation, began a systematic survey of the domestic water supply of the state. His report was ready in 1880, after he had examined some two hundred samples taken from Minnesota's lakes, rivers, springs, wells, and cisterns and from melted snow. These were tested for physical characteristics, including color, turbidity, sediment, luster, taste, and smell. Both qualitative and quantitative chemical analyses were also made. Hewitt found, as might be expected, that common causes of contamination included cesspools, outhouses, and manure heaps. Many of his samples were of water utterly unfit to drink.[41]

Hewitt was so impressed by the prevalence of contamination in both

[40] *Pioneer Press*, June 22, September 18, 1877, February 28, 1878; State Board of Health, *Annual Reports*, 1878, pp. 57–64.
[41] State Board of Health, *Biennial Reports*, 1879–80, pp. 129–141; *Pioneer Press*, November 12, 1880.

urban and rural waters that in 1883 he drew up for presentation to the legislature a bill to prohibit the discharge of excrements, sewage, and other polluting matter into any pond or river. The bill also provided for general supervision by the State Board of Health of all rivers, streams, and ponds used as sources of water supply by any town or city. In addition to this bill, which, however, was not enacted into law, Hewitt fathered a rather definite water campaign. When occasion arose, he spoke to farm groups, hammering home the lesson that air and water are the vehicles for the transmission of disease. At Faribault he told a meeting of citizens and farmers that "more danger is lurking in polluted well water than can easily be imagined. A well as ordinarily used drains a strip of land, having for its center the center of the well. . . . Do away with vaults, cess pools and other nuisances and the health of your city and state will remain unexcelled." [42]

This eternal vigilance and constant harping against impure water paid off. Hewitt was gratified when Governor William R. Merriam spoke of the valuable accomplishments of the state board in making water investigations, but he was more pleased by countless letters of inquiry that began pouring into his office. Many of these notes described or complained of unsanitary wells and others were requests for water analyses. A Lutheran pastor, for example, complained that his well was located only twelve feet from his stable. His predecessor had lost three children and he had lost one. The minister thought "a strong remonstrance based on the analysis" would cause his parishioners to give him a new well. "I am not satisfied with my well water," wrote a Centerville resident. "How much will it cost me to get it analyzed to find out if it is fit for human use?" [43]

No doubt Hewitt smiled at complaints couched in miserable English, such as this one from a resident of Sunrise City: "five miles west of here in the town of North Branch, there are two Starch Factoryes the refuse from them run into the Sunrise River, this river runs through the Sunrise Village the smell of this is unendurable. the Water is so pregnant Cattle will not drink it." [44] The humorous complaint was referred to Dr. Thomas Zeien of North Branch for investigation.

Requests for water analyses became so numerous after Bracken became secretary that the health department, in self-defense, considered

[42] *Pioneer Press*, February 7, 20, 1883, October 3, 1888.
[43] Merriam, *Inaugural Address*, 23 (St. Paul, 1889); Edward S. Frost to Hewitt, January 10, 1893, J. W. Holinquist to Hewitt, April 19, 1894, Minnesota Department of Health, St. Paul.
[44] E. E. Chase to Hewitt, February, 1896, Minnesota Department of Health, St. Paul.

THE FIGHT FOR PURE WATER 117

the distribution of a printed circular telling what people might expect in the way of assistance. For some years Bracken held to the older policy of answering each individual request, but he finally was forced to prepare printed form replies. In addition, the department issued or reprinted digests of water regulations, distributed pamphlets pertaining to water supply on the farm, published for free distribution results of water investigations and of typhoid pollution of wells, and prepared plans and sketches for a portable hypochlorite treatment plant. Even these aids did not satisfy public demand. Year by year requests for information about how to dig a well and where to locate it poured in. Innumerable citizens telephoned the health department to request water analyses and investigations or to ask about safeguarding springs and cisterns. To answer these requests today, the department distributes a set of fifteen pamphlets that explain in detail most questions pertaining to private water supply sanitation. The effectiveness of this manual may be judged by the fact that not only other states but also foreign nations have requested it in large quantities.[45]

This procedure of sending manuals to private citizens differs widely from earlier activities, when the department itself was able to analyze water samples from all sources. Today water samples from private supplies are not accepted for analysis, because a single sample can reveal only the quality of the water as it was at the time it was drawn and because such an analysis may be misleading. The department feels that only an environmental survey in conjunction with water analyses can insure a complete and trustworthy report.

Progress toward a clean water supply did not suddenly and dramatically wipe out water-borne diseases, but, as the public learned more about the proper construction and location of wells and cisterns and as water superintendents experimented with chlorination, the number of typhoid cases dropped. Outstanding exceptions were several severe typhoid epidemics.

Until 1910, when water chlorination was first tried in Minnesota, the state, as has been indicated, constantly was fighting typhoid fever.

[45] H. C. Carel to Bracken, March 3, 1902, Bracken to Carel, March 10, 1902, Minnesota Department of Health, St. Paul; Rome G. Brown, *A Summary of the Law Relating to Pollution of Water of Lakes and Streams* (Minneapolis, 1900); Karl F. Kellerman and Harold A. Whittaker, *Farm Water Supplies of Minnesota* (Washington, D.C., 1909); State Board of Health, *Farm Water Supplies* (St. Paul, 1915); F. F. Wesbrook and R. B. Dole, *Water Investigations in Minnesota* (reprinted from *Northwestern Lancet*, 25:81–85 – March 1, 1905); H. W. Hill, *Typhoid Pollution of Wells* (reprinted from Illinois Water Supply Association, *Proceedings* – February, 1911); H. A. Whittaker, *Hypochlorite Treatment of Water Supplies* (*Reprint 261* from *Public Health Reports*, February 26, 1915 – Washington, D.C., 1915); Minnesota Department of Health, *Manual of Water Supply Sanitation* (1941–47).

Minneapolis, for example, reported between 450 and 600 cases in September, 1881. Deaths were about one in ten. An outbreak, reported to be of epidemic size, occurred in Minneapolis in 1893, and Hewitt wrote that other cities continually were complaining of infection. The following year a local health officer said that typhoid was rampant in Grand Forks. During the Spanish-American War an outbreak among troops stationed at Camp Ramsey caused great consternation and filled St. Paul hospitals with patients. To list all communities, summer resorts, and railroad, mining, and lumber camps that reported typhoid between 1890 and 1910 would be useless. Chesley was certainly correct when he wrote in 1912: "In Minnesota we have an enormous amount of typhoid fever." [46]

Local and state health officials developed through the years a multiple-point campaign designed to reduce the number of cases. They knew that typhoid could be transmitted by flies and human carriers and could be borne in water, food, and milk. Therefore they determined to try to locate and control human carriers, to wage war against the fly, to distribute literature explaining the causes and methods of prevention of typhoid, to print approved methods to be followed in a typhoid outbreak, and to make available to the public reports of researchers and committees. Attempts were made also to improve sewerage systems, to oversee waterworks, and to safeguard milk supplies. [47]

To fortify this program, local health officers were encouraged by Bracken in 1911 to try "vaccination" as part of a preventive program against typhoid. A consistent effort to introduce vaccination into state institutions met with varying success. Superintendents in general en-

[46] *Tribune*, October 13, 1881; *Pioneer Press*, September 17, August 11, 16, 19, 23, 25, 26, 28, 1898; Hewitt to F. A. Dodge, October 18, 1893, A. A. Miller to Hewitt, January 31, 1894, C. E. Dampier to Hewitt, February 3, 1894, Chesley to R. B. Watrous, March 28, 1918, Minnesota Department of Health, St. Paul.

[47] H. W. Hill, *The Care and Control of Typhoid Carriers* (reprinted from *St. Paul Medical Journal*, 18:46–48 – February, 1916); A. J. Chesley, H. A. Burns, W. P. Greene, and E. M. Wade, *Three Years' Experience in the Search for Typhoid Carriers in Minnesota* (reprinted from *Journal of the American Medical Association*, 68:1882–1885 – June 23, 1917); "Important Facts about the Fly," in *Minnesota Health Journal*, 1:3–5 (May, 1917); L. L. Lumsden, *Typhoid Fever: Its Causation and Prevention* (United States Public Health Service, *Bulletin* 6 – Washington, D.C., 1917); T. J. Malone, *Protection Against Typhoid Fever* (reprinted by the State Board of Health from the *Tribune*, November 16, 1913); H. W. Hill, *The Detailed Procedures to be Followed in an Epidemiological Determination of the Origin of a Typhoid Outbreak* (reprinted from Illinois Water Supply Association, *Proceedings*, March, 1912); H. W. Hill, *Report of Committee on Typhoid Fever* (reprinted from *American Journal of Public Hygiene*, 20:50–53 – February, 1910); A. J. Chesley, *Typhoid Fever* (reprinted from *Minnesota Medicine*, 2:146–148 – April, 1919); W. P. Greene, *Endemic or Residual Typhoid Fever in Minnesota* (reprinted from *Journal-Lancet*, 40:248–251 – May 1, 1920).

THE FIGHT FOR PURE WATER

dorsed it, although not without reservations. Bracken thoroughly approved the use of typhoid vaccines, saying that he "would rather advise a man who had not had typhoid and who is knocking about a good deal to be vaccinated." The board furnished this prophylactic treatment free to any physician in the state, but Bracken made it clear that free distribution did not mean "free medical service in the administration of the prophylactic." [48]

Despite all the best efforts of health officials, typhoid epidemics flared up periodically. The first great twentieth-century epidemic — one that still is remembered for its enormity — occurred at Mankato in 1908. The last large and serious outbreak took place in Minneapolis in 1935. Between these two, at least four others varying in severity developed. Of the six, several were caused by contaminated water supplies, one by carelessness in failing to inject a sufficient quantity of chlorine into the water, another by infected cheese, and still another by a human carrier.

The Mankato epidemic, which began in June and first manifested itself as a widespread diarrhea, was the result of sewage entering the water supply. The initial diarrhea involved from four thousand to six thousand adults and children of both sexes and all ages — fully half of the drinkers of city water, it was estimated. "The origin of the outbreak," wrote Hill, who was sent to Mankato, "is doubtless due to the extremely heavy rains, washing the streets, yards, closets and cesspools of the high part of the city, behind the 3rd St. well, down and into the well-pit — perhaps also to sanitary sewer overflows reaching the well-pit of the 2nd St. well or even backing into the well-pits directly through the overflow pipes in the well-pits, although this possibility is denied by the City Engineer and by the waterworks engineer." By early July typical typhoid cases were showing up, and by the afternoon of July 18 about a hundred cases had been reported. "My own observations showed that new cases were developing every hour," said Hill. On July 26 some 260 typhoid cases had been reported, 7 deaths had occurred, and 3 deaths were imminent. Hill concluded that possibly cases should begin to diminish, not only because the period of incubation should be about over, but also because citizens were boiling water to protect themselves. This, in general, was the situation, but additional cases were reported during early August. Hill continued his investi-

[48] G. O. Welch to Bracken, December 8, 1911; A. C. Rogers to Bracken, December 11, 1911; Bracken to Arthur J. Gillette, July 26, 1913; form notice sent to secretaries of the councils of towns and cities, 1913. Minnesota Department of Health, St. Paul.

gations throughout that month and into September. Bacteriological samples from the Mankato water supply were reported upon in October. The total number of cases reported was 1,022 and the total number of deaths was 70.[49]

Early in 1909 typhoid fever in epidemic proportions was reported at Breckenridge, on the line between Minnesota and North Dakota at the junction of the Bois des Sioux and Otter Tail rivers. The town had a population of between a thousand and eighteen hundred persons. It had presented a health problem since 1906, when the state department had investigated the prevalence of typhoid, and Hill had determined that the Otter Tail River was contaminated. Indeed, Hill felt that Breckenridge health officers had not taken "any adequate steps for its typhoid suppression so far or even notification to us in time to prevent its present extreme development." In addition to being annoyed with the lax tactics of the health officers, Hill had little respect for Breckenridge's physicians; one of them, he said, owned a drugstore and advertised patent medicines, and the other was a "white-bearded old German who has been there a long time and seems never to have passed any examination for his license."[50]

Despite Hill's recommendations in 1906, little had been done to safeguard Breckenridge's drinking water. Hill was not surprised, therefore, when typhoid again broke out three years later. Once again he repeated his advice that Breckenridge substitute deep water for the Otter Tail River water then in use. This time he got action, for Breckenridge had become a city and was able to issue bonds for the construction of public utilities, including waterworks. In 1910 a filtration plant was installed and the use of hypochlorite was begun. Said the engineer: "There has been no typhoid fever in Breckenridge since we began the sedimentation and filtration process in August, which is a remarkable record for Breckenridge." But the troubles of Breckenridge were not yet over. Tests by the Minnesota health department showed that the average bacterial count in water that had gone through the waterworks was much higher than it should be and that *Bacillus coli* was "con-

[49] H. M. Bracken, F. H. Bass, F. F. Wesbrook, H. A. Whittaker, and H. W. Hill, *The Mankato Typhoid Fever Epidemic of 1908*, 439 (reprinted from *The Journal of Infectious Diseases*, 9:410–474 — November, 1911); H. W. Hill, "Mankato-Report on Diarrhea Outbreak: [Notes of a] Trip, June 29, 1908," "Report of Typhoid Investigation at Mankato, July 17–19, 1908," and "Report of Progress on Typhoid Investigation at Mankato, July 24–27, 1908 (typescripts), Minnesota Department of Health, Minneapolis; Hill to Bracken, August 10, 12, 20, September 10, October 13, 1908, Minnesota Department of Health, Minneapolis.

[50] Hill to E. W. Gag, March 8, 1906; H. W. Hill, "Breckenridge, Minn. — Typhoid Fever Outbreak Investigated Mar. 14–15–06" (typescript). Minnesota Department of Health, Minneapolis.

THE FIGHT FOR PURE WATER

stantly found present in the effluents of both filters, indicating an unsafe water for public use." This difficulty eventually was overcome, and no longer did Breckenridge citizens see displayed in public places the poster headed: "Typhoid fever is epidemic in Breckenridge." [51]

In general, deaths from typhoid fever in Minnesota decreased from 1905 to 1906 but increased steadily thereafter to 1910. In that year Minneapolis had an epidemic which sent deaths skyrocketing to an all-time high since 1900. During the Minneapolis epidemic Hill investigated fifteen cases in the University Hospital and about thirty cases in the Minneapolis General Hospital. The cause, in almost every instance, was contaminated Mississippi River water.[52]

Contaminated water was again the villain in 1914, when typhoid epidemics occurred at New Ulm and Benson. Forty-eight cases were reported at New Ulm and in the adjacent countryside. Epidemiologists said definitely that contaminated city water caused the disease and concluded that "this outbreak again demonstrates the apathy which frequently exists wherever local action is needed to protect the public from disease. In this case the authorities had been previously informed that the water supply was seriously polluted. It only remained for a 'carrier' of typhoid bacilli to take part in such pollution and an outbreak of typhoid fever was inevitable." From July 25 until December 27, 1914, one hundred and eighteen typhoid cases and four fatalities were reported in Benson. Investigation showed that the disease was water-borne and that it was due to deficient waterworks.[53]

Two other epidemics are interesting, not because of the number of cases involved, but because of their rather unusual sources. One hundred and six students and employees of the University of Minnesota fell ill after dining at the men's union cafeteria on the campus. The state health department began its investigations on March 25, 1921, and finally concluded that the paratyphoid fever was occasioned by pasteurized milk, "sold in bulk . . . the probability being that the milk was infected after delivery to the cafeteria." In this instance it was impossible to fix on any one individual as the carrier. Four years later

[51] H. W. Hill, "Report on Typhoid Investigation at Breckenridge, Feb. 2–6" (typescript); Edward P. Burch to Wesbrook, December 15, 1910; State Board of Health, "Report of the Laboratory Division . . . on Water Investigation at Breckenridge, Minn., May 31 and June 1, 1911" (typescript); Breckenridge Board of Health, Typhoid Fever Poster, March 12, 1906. Minnesota Department of Health, Minneapolis.

[52] State Board of Health, "Reports and Hearings," 1910–12, p. 117.

[53] State Board of Health, *Reports on Epidemics of Typhoid Fever at New Ulm, Minn., in 1914* [and] *Benson, Minn., in 1914*, pp. 86, 102 (reprinted from State Board of Health, *Biennial Reports*, 1914–15, pp. 77–102).

an epidemic of twenty-nine cases of typhoid fever was reported from four Minnesota counties, and epidemiological investigation showed the source of infection to be cheese manufactured in a co-operative factory.[54]

Among the last typhoid epidemics in Minnesota was one that began in May, 1935, as the result of insufficient chlorination of the Minneapolis water. The year started with no more cases than there had been in preceding periods. Until May only three cases had been reported; but, beginning early that month and continuing until August 10, new cases developed rapidly. Although the disease spread to residents of Robbinsdale and St. Louis Park, it never assumed the proportions it might have, because of prompt investigation and recommendations made jointly by the Minneapolis health department and the state board. Fortunately, illnesses were mild and the death rate was low. A total of 175 cases and 6 deaths were reported. The most exhaustive epidemiological and engineering researches pried into every possible source of contamination, including the Columbia Heights waterworks and the Fridley purification plant. The water distribution system of Minneapolis was examined thoroughly and notice was taken of miscellaneous sanitary defects. Case histories were studied clinically and epidemiologically, special care being taken to investigate the sources of food eaten by patients. Milk, cream, butter, cheese, salad dressings, green vegetables, and even Eskimo Pies and Chilly Charlies — all were examined and given a clean bill of health. Typhoid bacilli were not present in any of them.

Finally, after long weeks of weary labor, it was reported officially that "post-chlorination had been discontinued at the Fridley plant on March 23 and was resumed on May 6; that the amount of residual chlorine present in the treated water as it entered the distribution system fell to the low level of 0.1 part per million on April 9 and with few exceptions remained at or below this level — falling April 30 to 0.03 part per million — until June 22; that the residual chlorine remained below 0.3 part per million until July 9 and was raised to 0.5 part per million a few days later. . . . In other words, if the period of incubation of typhoid fever and the conditions of flow of the water in the distribution system be taken into consideration, it appears that this sharply defined epidemic, May 4 to Aug. 10, coincided with the period

---

[54] E. M. Wade and O. McDaniel, *Report of an Epidemic of Paratyphoid Fever in Patrons of a Cafeteria* (reprinted from American Medical Association, *Journal*, 83:1416–1420 — November 1, 1924); E. M. Wade and Lewis Shere, *Longevity of Typhoid Bacilli in Cheddar Cheese* (reprinted from *American Journal of Public Health*, 18:12 — December, 1928).

THE FIGHT FOR PURE WATER 123

of low residual chlorine in the water supply, April 9 to July 9–13." Many laymen, perhaps correctly, interpreted this to mean that, for some reason or other, the amount of chlorine introduced into Minneapolis water was insufficient to kill harmful bacteria, and they felt that the lives of six persons might have been saved if the chlorine content of drinking water had been maintained at a safety level. Certainly chlorination, costing only from two to four cents per capita per year, is one of the cheapest forms of health insurance a municipality can invest in.[55]

There have been times, of course, in the history of the state when bizarre incidents have threatened water purity and caused consternation among sanitarians. One of these occurred in Duluth in December, 1920. A bacteriologist, at the request of a local newspaper, induced the attendant in charge of the chlorination plant to turn off the chlorine with which all city water was treated in order for him to take samples of raw water for bacteriological examination. Apparently some twenty-five thousand gallons of raw water entered the Duluth distribution system during a thirty-five-minute period, so that potentially the health of the citizens was endangered. Only a year earlier the sanitary aspect of Duluth water had been declared unsatisfactory. Consequently, when the newspapers reported the city water unfit to drink, public uproar was tremendous. The situation, of course, was not as critical as it was first thought to be, but it dramatically pointed up the need for purer water than Duluth was receiving. Subsequent investigations by the state health department showed continual improvement.[56]

After the unfortunate Minneapolis typhoid epidemic of 1935, the number of both cases and deaths fell off rapidly, although in 1939 and 1940 there was an outbreak at Harmony.[57] By 1948 the disease was such a rarity in Minnesota that a younger generation of physicians sel-

[55] Frank R. Shaw to Whittaker, February 14, 1936, Minnesota Department of Health, Minneapolis; Minnesota Department of Health, *Report of Investigations of the Typhoid Fever Epidemic, Minneapolis, 1935,* 9, 95; interview of the author with O. E. Brownell, June 21, 1948.
[56] *News Tribune* (Duluth), December 19, 1920; *Duluth Herald,* December 22, 1920; Chesley to Warren E. Greene, December 23, 1920, January 8, 1921, Greene to Chesley, December 29, 1920, Minnesota Department of Health, Minneapolis; State Board of Health, "Report on the Water Supply of Duluth, February 18, 1919," "Report of Water Supply of Duluth," March 22, 1922, and "Investigation of Duluth Water Supply," December 30, 1929 (typescripts), Minnesota Department of Health, Minneapolis; Duluth Health Department and Works Progress Administration, "Sanitary Survey of Duluth," September, 1949 (typescript), Minnesota Department of Health, Minneapolis.
[57] Kingston, in American Water Works Association, *Journal,* 35:1450–1453 (November, 1943); F. M. Feldman to McDaniel, September 20, 1939, and Chesley to the Harmony Village Council, September 18, 1940, Minnesota Department of Health, Minneapolis.

dom, if ever, saw a case. No longer need modern parents, like pioneers of old, count with almost mathematical certainty on losing at least one child to typhoid. The subjugation of this disease is one of the most dramatic victories won by public health authorities. Yet even today eternal vigilance is the price of victory.

When a child or his mother places a cup under the faucet and drinks, the safety of the water is assured by a long chain of strict supervision. Whether the family travels in railroad coach or aboard a mighty liner of the skyways, it knows drinking water has been rigorously inspected and approved by the Minnesota Department of Health. This safeguard is the result of a quarantine regulation passed by the United States Treasury Department in 1913, which required railroads to obtain approval from a state or local board of health of all water supplies placed on trains engaged in interstate traffic.[58] By 1940 investigations covered the method of handling water from the point of discharge to the tanks in the coaches and included the examination of containers, hoses, and ice pails.[59] Let one link in this chain of control from source to consumer weaken or break, and deadly typhoid may appear.

To be constantly alert to potential danger demands a high degree of supervision. That is why Minneapolis drinking water is tested at the waterworks once every eight hours and why St. Cloud runs a routine test every hour. And that is why the Minnesota Department of Health, as one of its obligations to every citizen, approves plans for the remodeling of old waterworks and the construction of new ones. The department also inspects the water supply of rural schools, state institutions, scout camps, and resorts. During flood periods sanitary engineers hasten to inundated areas to attempt to prevent contamination of both private and public water supplies. Health officials took an emergency chlorinator to Virginia in 1947, when a heavy rain flooded the source of water supply and exposed citizens to water into which surface drainage poured.[60] Engineers, blueprints in hand, check plumbing in uncompleted public buildings to make sure that no sewage can contaminate drinking water. Indeed, Minnesota led the way in prohibiting deadly "cross-connections," which make possible the contamination of pure water with sewage.

[58] R. H. Mullin, H. A. Whittaker, and B. M. Mohler, *Railroad Water Supplies in Minnesota* (*Reprint* 191 from *Public Health Reports*, May 15, 1914 — Washington, D.C., 1914); State Board of Health, Division of Sanitation, "Quarterly Reports," December 31, 1916, p. 8. On January 1, 1947, the division became the "Section of Environmental Sanitation."
[59] Division of Sanitation, "Quarterly Reports," June 30, 1940, p. 1.
[60] Report of the Division of Municipal Water Supply and Plumbing, in Section of Sanitation, "Quarterly Reports," September 30, 1947.

8

With Pump and Pipe

A CITY resident in 1872 needed a strong body and an iron will. He lived in the midst of filth and at a time when disposal of sewage was a personal problem and not a municipal responsibility. The citizen of Minneapolis, St. Paul, or any of the smaller towns depended upon a sturdy constitution to breathe successfully the pestilential air from reeking yards, alleys, and privy vaults, to drink water polluted by sewage carelessly and promiscuously dumped, and to leap over filthy mudholes in poorly drained streets. He needed an iron will either to close his mind to existing evils or to lead him to agitate, in the face of general indifference, for sanitary reforms.

As early as 1857 disgruntled residents had complained bitterly of the St. Paul approaches to the lower Mississippi levee. There, street gradings had dug out holes, creating ponds, ditches, and canals filled with green, slimy, stagnant water. Under a sultry July sun these cesspools emitted stifling stenches and caused inhabitants of near-by dirty shanties to fear for their health. "The malignant Typhus will not only be there, but a dozen other fatal diseases, to depopulate the neighborhood," warned a reporter after visiting the levee district. "Under any other climate than that of Minnesota, it would have been so before now. But even here where men can expose health, and risk life with greater impunity than anywhere else, almost, so certain a penalty cannot be much longer avoided."[1]

Nearly a decade later people were encouraged to dump their refuse in the Mississippi rather than let it rot on the bare ground. Police, acting under local health regulations, did what they could, but it was difficult to enforce sanitary codes when the city made no provision for gathering and disposing of refuse nor for plants designed to treat sew-

[1] *Daily Minnesotan* (St. Paul), May 21, 1857.

age. A St. Paul offender received an official reminder that he had been throwing "slops in the wrong place, which was against the peace and dignity of the State of Minnesota." The courts dismissed a hotelkeeper only after he promised to remove filth near his building. But the few who were apprehended and forced to clean up were only a fraction of the total number of offenders.[2]

Health officers did their best, and occasionally they received praise when nuisances were abated. Their early attempts at civic sanitation were crude indeed, in the light of what was to come, but local health officers, attempting to drain pestilential ponds, clean filth from vacant lots, and plug a stinking hole under the steps of the St. Paul Post Office, could not foresee the day when municipal street departments, garbage collectors, and sewage disposal plants would give St. Paul the reputation of being a clean city. These early sanitarians, however, were constantly rebuked for not accomplishing more. Private citizens erected signs over rubbish piles, which they themselves had heaped there, asking that they be removed. When St. Paulites appealed to the health or public works boards or the city council for someone to fill in a stagnant pool on an unfilled lot, they forgot that they were largely responsible for its existence.[3]

The stench from a toilet, with neither air vent nor sewer connection, at the Milwaukee and St. Paul Depot caused protests, but St. Paul residents were not ready to endorse plans for a city-wide sewerage system which would stop individual nuisances at one fell swoop. There was a crying need for sewers in all Minnesota cities in 1872. Water backed up from drains into basements of private residences. Most river cities dumped sewage directly into the streams with only the most casual consideration of resulting pollution. A tremendous deposit of filth was discovered at the base of Minnesota Point in Lake Superior, whence Duluth drew its water supply.[4]

The dumping of sewage into rivers was further complicated by street-sprinkling systems. During hot summer months innumerable cities drew river water into tanks and then allayed dust with it. The result, of course, was obvious: sewage-filled water was brought back into towns and, it was believed, scattered about to the detriment of health. Stillwater practiced this system, but St. Anthony Falls, whether for convenience or sanitation, drew its sprinkling water from a spring.[5]

[2] *St. Paul Pioneer*, April 19, 1866; *St. Paul Daily Press*, May 3, July 3, 1872.
[3] *St. Paul Daily Press*, April 12, June 28, July 30, 1872.
[4] *St. Paul Daily Press*, October 8, 1872; *Duluth Daily Tribune*, June 5, 1872.
[5] *Stillwater Gazette*, April 30, 1872; *Weekly Democrat* (St. Anthony), June 1, 1871.

Other progressive cities adopted the latter plan, including Minneapolis and Duluth.

These were a few of the baffling problems facing early local health officers. The St. Paul Board of Health had been established in 1854, and a committee on health was active before that. Minneapolis had secured its first health officer in 1867, an event which caused the *Minneapolis Chronicle* to say wistfully: "We hope now that we have a health officer, and a good one, that this city will be put in a suitable condition to receive any visitation that may reach us." By 1872, when Hewitt became secretary of the state board, many communities had health officers. It was Hewitt's idea that local health boards should be "permanent and independent, constantly looking after sewerage, water supply and nuisances" and that their duty was to "prevent disease, not to wait for its appearance." If local boards refused to act, Hewitt maintained with considerable vigor, the state board should have the right to go anywhere and to establish quarantines.[6]

Among the first problems confronting Hewitt and the local boards was that of the systematic removal and disposal of sewage and general surface water by sewers. He knew only too well that "the sewage of city sewers is composed of human excrement, urine, water from kitchens, vegetable, animal and other refuse, drainage from stables and cow houses; also from slaughter houses, etc. That is, this sewage is a hotbed in which disease germs can freely and easily germinate and spread if once introduced." It was his job to help devise a system whereby sewage could be collected systematically and disposed of scientifically and in a sanitary manner.[7]

In 1885, at the time of the greatest concern about sewage in the Twin Cities, one of the nation's most noted engineers concisely stated the cardinal principles upon which the sanitation of towns should be based: "Excreted filth, domestic refuse and dangerous waste products of manufactures completely removed beyond inhabited districts and properly disposed of before a putrefactive change takes place. Objectionable matters to be so removed as to not render foul the conveying apparatus, channels or rivers used. No system of sewerage is complete until all nuisances from sewage are prevented. Scavenging should be complete. Storm water should be conveyed without damage or inconvenience. The underground water level should be permanently lowered by means of subsoil drainage to suitable depth below all habitations.

[6] *Daily Minnesota Pioneer*, May 29, 1854; *Minneapolis Chronicle*, May 2, 1867; *Pioneer Press* (St. Paul), February 18, 1881.
[7] *Pioneer Press*, March 8, 1885.

Effective sanitary laws and inspection should be enforced." The privy vault and the cesspool were condemned and the pail system was described as offensive.[8]

For many years St. Paul was without a sewerage system. A reporter in 1872 listed specific shortcomings in city sanitation and made seven recommendations which he felt would improve the frightful conditions. He said that many fevers were attributable to the faulty system of sewerage, which was little more than a helter-skelter of ditching and small tunnels. He found sewers with outlets into the Mississippi above the high-water mark and observed innumerable pools of stagnant water. Piles of garbage and filth in back yards indicated that property owners were either too niggardly or too disinterested to preserve their health, or both. Finally, the roving reporter called on the council to sponsor thorough cleaning of premises immediately after frost disappears; to provide thorough surface drainage; to give the board of health full power and sufficient means to carry out expedient sanitary regulations; to see that street commissioners do not "botch the job"; to empty stagnant pools; to adopt mechanically or scientifically good sewerage systems; and to begin by setting a good example at home.[9]

Some of these suggestions were not new, for they had been made by Captain James Starkey in a pamphlet on sewerage and street grades published in 1857. In 1869 the council had rejected a sewerage plan prepared by J. S. Sewall, but the following year a special council committee approved a modified version of Sewall's proposal. Subsequent opposition, however, prevented active steps to put this scheme into operation. In March, 1872, the council again considered proposals for a sewerage system. The city surveyor was ordered to prepare a plan of main and lateral sewers. On May 23, 1872, Starkey reported the following recommendations for sewers: The main sewers should run parallel to the Mississippi; sewer districts should be established for stated purposes; outlets should be made as far below thickly settled districts as possible; brick sewers should be egg-shaped; small sewers and house drains should be constructed of glazed stoneware pipe with curves and branches; all connections should have curves; and construction details should be referred to a public works board or similar authority.[10]

[8] Samuel M. Gray, *A Proposed Plan for a Sewerage System and for the Disposal of the Sewage of the City of Providence* (Providence, 1884), quoted in the *Pioneer Press*, March 8, 1885.
[9] *St. Paul Daily Press*, March 28, 1873.
[10] Starkey, *Suggestions Relative to the Sewerage and Street Grades of St. Paul* (St. Paul, [1857]); St. Paul Common Council, *Proceedings*, April 11, 1871, p. 61; April 9, 1872, p. 222; April 9, 1872, to January 6, 1874, p. 43. The early development of the St. Paul sewer system is summarized in the *Pioneer Press*, October 4, 1885.

Starkey was elected superintendent of sewers in April, 1873, and he immediately prepared a sewer ordinance. He remained in full charge of St. Paul's sewerage system until 1875, when his office was merged with that of the city engineer. His problems were staggering, for the hit-and-miss system of locating sewers had had some strange results. For example, the Capitol's sewer had been laid up hill, and the placement of pipes beneath the City Hall resulted in such a stench that the seat of city government was compared with the Black Hole of Calcutta. In other parts of the city sewers were caving away at important intersections and were either losing their linings or draining into the open. Complaints of sewer gas were numerous. Carelessly or dishonestly constructed sewers were called "underground sinks of poisonous filth and nurseries of disease and death." [11]

If Starkey found sewers improperly constructed, he also knew that they were improperly cleaned and flushed. Until about 1885 St. Anthony Hill residents had no water supply to cleanse sewer pipes. Another large area of contamination lay near the stockyards, where sewers were needed desperately to carry away waste from slaughtering houses and rendering establishments. The city health department stated that unless the stockyards were furnished with sewer pipes, the health of the district would be in peril. Without sewers, refuse drained into cesspools which filled rapidly with water impregnated with animal matter. The bulk of stockyard waste was carted off to low-lying districts where it was dumped and buried, but when this rotted it, too, was carried in fluid form into deep pools.[12]

Dr. Talbot Jones, St. Paul health officer, saw a clear relationship between these primitive sewerage conditions and the large number of illnesses reported to him. "Out of the 50 cases of scarlet fever and diphtheria, 48 resulted where there was no sewer drainage, and only two where there was," he said in 1886. The city board of health once officially condemned St. Paul's attitude, which permitted cesspools and filth to remain undisturbed. Time and again newspapers exposed menaces and urged that householders connect their plumbing with street sewers. Local health officers reported that they, too, had used every exertion short of prosecution to induce citizens to connect their houses with sewers. Finally, by 1890, a city health ordinance made it the duty of every householder to connect his building with a sewer, if the house

[11] *St. Paul Daily Press*, January 21, February 7, September 9, November 6, 1874, January 26, 1875; *Pioneer-Press*, April 28, 1875.
[12] *Pioneer Press*, January 13, 1884, March 8, 1885; St. Paul City Officers, *Annual Reports*, 1885, pp. 234, 278.

stood on a sewer line. Failure to comply subjected an offender to a fine of from twenty-five to one hundred dollars, which became a lien upon the real estate and could be repeated until the owner complied with the ordinance.[13]

Although the *Pioneer Press* reported in 1890 that the city had about fifty more miles of sewers than any other community of comparable size, those boastful figures did not reveal the full story. It was estimated that about one-half of St. Paul homes had faulty sewer connections and that far too many residents still considered the private cesspool and vault to be far superior to the public sewers. The only answer was to prove by education and by scientific sewer construction that a city could do a better job of waste disposal than could the average resident.[14]

Before modern construction could begin, a survey of all existing pipes and connections had to be made. This was a stupendous undertaking, for it not only involved an inventory of both private and public sewers, but it also meant that weeks of time had to be spent in attempting to locate long-forgotten and hidden drains. It also meant hours of discussion concerning the respective merits of concrete versus vitrified pipes. Sewer sizes were hotly debated, one school holding that pipes should be relatively small and the other believing that they should be large enough to admit a workman, who then could examine, repair, and clean them. City engineers argued, too, that the larger the pipe, the larger the amount of water to be pushed through for flushing. Bickering over all these points continued for years. An Eastern advocate of vitrified pipe, for example, argued the positive evils of iron, but a St. Paul inspector not only ordered the use of extra heavy iron piping, but also favored iron joints.[15]

Another construction problem was brought to light in 1890. Critics claimed that St. Paul was building sewers from soft brick, a technique that resulted in leakage and the gradual breakdown of sewers. Other residents complained that construction engineers tore up streets and marred the beauty spots of the city when visitors were arriving for the State Fair. Yet visitors expressed surprise at paths which wound "among barns and cesspools and along piles of filth and rubbish" breeding stench and contagion. St. Paulites frequently thought their taxes were

[13] *Minneapolis Tribune*, July 3, 1886; *Pioneer Press*, March 26, 1881, November 19, 1888, November 12, 1890.
[14] *Pioneer Press*, November 14, 16, 1890.
[15] *St. Paul Daily Press*, March 15, 1873, January 16, 1875; *Pioneer-Press*, August 26, 1875, April 12, August 28, 1885; St. Paul City Officers, *Annual Reports*, 1885, p. 243.

too high, and blamed them on sewer assessments. In 1893 property owners vigorously fought an assessment for draining vacant lots. Indeed, draining contracts, let through the efforts of the St. Paul Department of Health, caused more trouble to the Board of Public Works than any others.[16]

Public apathy, and even antagonism, was complicated by the attitude of institutions and of individuals intent upon following age-old procedure. Macalester College, for example, ignored complaints of the health department until threat of arrest finally forced the administration to alter locations of toilets and to provide a cesspool for college sewage.[17] Citizens objected to a plan of the health department for the disposal of night soil. There were several ways to rid St. Paul of this human excrement collected at night. One was to dump it directly into the Mississippi, but that, of course, was a source of contamination. Another was to carry it on barges down the river to a point about a mile beyond the city limits and dump it there. A third was to let scavengers carry it away for burial. A newer plan was to collect it and then burn it in a crematorium. The fifth method involved chemical conversion of portions of the waste into fertilizer.

All these disposal systems were debated actively. When the Waring system was developed and successfully introduced in Memphis, where sewer construction was of vital concern to inhabitants besieged by yellow fever, it, too, had its champions. This system involved the laying of two small sewer pipes underground, one to drain off surface water and the other to carry sewage. Both pipes were laid in one ditch about four feet under the surface. The advantages claimed for St. Paul were greater sanitary protection, simplicity of design, low cost, and the belief that there could be no escape of gas.[18]

Another popular plan, competing with the Waring system, was the New Orleans method, which involved no underground drainage, but made use of cesspools and dry earth closets. These were emptied by odorless excavators and their contents were dumped into a deep section of the river. After debating the merits of the Waring system and the New Orleans plan, St. Paul authorities made arrangements to adopt a modification of the latter. An ordinance regulating the location of cesspools in relation to dwellings and wells was passed on October 16, 1883, and approved the next day. Once again health officers found citizens careless and even contemptuous in their observance of the ordi-

[16] *Pioneer Press*, June 19, 1875, September 24, 1890; *Tribune*, August 6, 1879; St. Paul City Officers, *Annual Reports*, 1893, p. 835.
[17] *Pioneer Press*, December 6, 1888.
[18] *Pioneer Press*, January 18, 1881.

nance. Yet attempts were made to enforce this law vigorously. Erring residents were first to be given a twenty-four-hour warning and then, if they failed to comply, were to be arrested.[19]

The modified New Orleans plan also broke down when scavengers were licensed. These collectors of night soil cut rates, fought among themselves, and generally reaped huge profits without performing adequately the service for which they were paid. Not even the carefully worded ordinance of October 16, which prescribed the method of collection, could force scavengers to perform their work in a sanitary manner. St. Paul found also that the New Orleans system was deficient because it did not make adequate provision for the final disposal of night soil. St. Paul would not do what New Orleans did. Therefore, a modified European program was proposed by which chemicals were to be added to night soil, so that this refuse could be turned into fertilizer and sold to gardeners and farmers.[20]

While the merits of such varied plans were being debated and until a modified New Orleans plan could really be made effective, St. Paul provided for the removal of night soil in air-tight and water-tight wagons, which were inspected by the health department. Night soil was collected under contract and dumped at designated locations. A St. Paul health officer declared this procedure to be one of the best in the nation. Yet it was not without its drawbacks. A disposal problem arose during the summer of 1885 when an injunction was served upon the Odorless Excavating Company "to prevent its dumping night soil into the river." The company refused, "on account of the distance, to comply with the request of the city council to dump at the eastern limits of the City." The situation was critical, for no collections had been made for several days. Before the company and the city could come to an agreement, several solutions were proposed. St. Paul toyed with the idea, for example, of constructing dumping wharves jutting out about a hundred feet into the Mississippi. There, it was thought, the current would be strong enough to carry night soil directly downstream, so that it would not fan out and be deposited in shallow water and along the banks.[21]

---

[19] *Pioneer Press*, November 18, 1884; St. Paul Common Council, *Proceedings*, 1883, p. 403. Ordinance 355, section 93, reads in part: ". . . no water closet, privy vault or cesspool shall be so constructed within twenty feet of any house, residence or building without a permit from the owner or agent of said house, residence or building." This ordinance comprised a complete rewriting and revision of St. Paul's health and sanitary regulations and a reorganization of its health board. *Pioneer Press*, October 28, 1883.
[20] *Pioneer Press*, January 25, 1885.
[21] *Pioneer Press*, April 12, June 5, 1885; *Tribune*, June 5, 1885.

What actually happened, of course, was that St. Paul operated a number of disposal schemes simultaneously. None of them solved the problem, for one was always breaking down. The problem was complicated also by the fact that St. Paul was growing so fast in 1886 that a sewer system could not keep up with the growth of population and it was necessary to utilize scavengers to supplement the more permanent sanitary system. It was estimated that not one-fifth of excreta deposited in privy vaults was removed by night-soil men. The remainder polluted the air, stimulated disease, and lowered living standards. This was true in fashionable districts as well as in shantytown. Under the front walk of the imposing Capitol itself great cesspools emanated putrefactive odors.[22]

So many areas of town were in need of proper drain and sewer pipes that Talbot Jones, the health officer, whose duty it was to recommend districts for the installation of sewerage tunnels, found it difficult to establish priorities. He had to choose between a low swampy section and a rather thickly populated and most unhealthful area. "It is almost impossible to keep water out of the cellars of dwelling houses," Jones reported. "Cisterns cannot be made, and as for the well water, which is almost wholly relied upon for drinking purposes, it has been analyzed time and again, and in the great majority of instances has been found to contain sufficient organic impurities to condemn it for drinking. These various conditions combine to produce much sickness which an efficient system of sewers would, in a large measure, tend to remove. The construction of this system of sewers is also strongly recommended by the city engineer in his annual report to the board of public works." [23]

Progress was infuriatingly slow. As health and other public officials struggled to improve sanitation, citizens doggedly balked plans for improvement, resurrected old arguments, and thought up new ones. It was said that a sewer connection between street and house cost a hundred dollars and that was too much; it was argued that houses were built so poorly that inside plumbing froze during winter months; and it was stated that a city-wide sewerage system would deprive farmers of valuable fertilizer. Estimates of the number of houses on sewer lines that did not have connections ran from six thousand to eleven thousand. Scavengers still "reaped a rich harvest" from their labors, and health officials continued to harp about a system they believed to be outdated and detrimental. In 1911 about forty per cent of St. Paul's population

[22] *Pioneer Press*, July 17, 1886; *Tribune*, July 27, 1886.
[23] *Pioneer Press*, April 7, 1886; St. Paul City Officers, *Annual Reports*, 1885, p. 233.

was without sewer service. Actually St. Paul was better than other, smaller cities in this respect. Stillwater, Brainerd, Crookston, St. Peter, Winona, and Fergus Falls — to mention only a few — ranged from sixty-six and two-thirds to seventy-five per cent without such service.[24]

The twentieth century, with its tremendous new engineering knowledge and new concepts of municipal sanitation, brought modern, scientific sewage disposal to St. Paul. Laboratories tested and made reports on different types of pipes; research institutes attacked city sanitation as an over-all plan rather than in the haphazard manner of the past; and an increasing knowledge of public health finally led a sluggish public to endorse inside home plumbing and to consider the chamber pot and the privy relics of a bygone age. The very term "night soil" was to disappear from the people's vocabulary. No longer did the St. Paul Street Department and the Board of Public Works annually inventory horses, harness, wagons, and sleds. Tools had changed too. The pick and shovel, time-honored equipment of the sewer digger, were replaced by mechanical monsters that could dig a ditch, lay a pipe, and cover it over almost in one operation.

The Mississippi, for decades a dumping ground for sewage, was now regarded with new respect by the people. They considered it an asset rather than a convenience. The great river no longer was to be a breeding place of disease, but was to become an aesthetic highway, given over to fishing, swimming, and boating. One of the major factors in this accomplishment was St. Paul's construction of a modern sewage treatment and disposal plant. But this innovation was completed only after the state health department had condemned the increasing pollution of the Mississippi and when both St. Paul and Minneapolis had been persuaded to fight contamination on a co-operative basis.

Minneapolis, like St. Paul, had had a long history of fumbling with the problem of sewage disposal. It, too, had begun as a town without sewers and with piles of slops and garbage tossed carelessly on streets. Minneapolis residents opposed the construction of sewers and seemed not to care that the sewerage of the City Hall was "exceedingly defective, and people engaged on the upper floors are in constant peril from typhoid fever or other deadly diseases." Poisonous gases were said to fill public buildings to a sickening degree. Lower Washington Avenue, the mecca of lumberjacks on a spree, was heaped with accumulated

[24] *Pioneer Press*, April 22, 1893, March 9, 1897; Caroline B. Crane, *Report on a Campaign to Awaken Public Interest in Sanitary and Sociologic Problems in the State of Minnesota*, 46 (St. Paul, 1911).

filth, and a reporter noted that the street facing the jail was "adorned" on both sides with "immense piles of manure, privies, old barrels, boxes, and refuse of back yards generally." Sidewalks were lacking, and the citizen had to pick his way gingerly, hoping against hope that his shoes and clothes would not be ruined. After heavy rains thoroughfares were ankle-deep in water and floating garbage. "Isn't it about time," queried an annoyed resident, "that the planking was lifted from these gutters, and the underlying accumulations of filth and rubbish removed?" North Minneapolis was almost literally a pest district, honeycombed with sink holes, pockets, and marshes and with no natural outlet for drainage. Persons moving in to the rapidly growing vicinity of Hoag Lake lived on the edge of a marsh and breathed obnoxious odors.[25]

No one recognized the evil situation better than did Hewitt. In 1882 he met with Minneapolis health officers to discuss existing conditions and to talk over proposals necessary to assure the city's health. Seven years later he wrote emphatically: "I sincerely hope they [*Minneapolis*] won't go back to the position of St. Paul, but keep under the state law and get at the work in a business like way." He recommended a house-to-house survey to ascertain the actual sanitary condition of the city, the actual methods used in the disposal of sewage, night soil, and garbage, and the actual state of water supply and ventilation in public and private buildings. So significant were the sanitary needs of Minneapolis that ministers preached on the subject and countless newspaper editorials deplored existing conditions.

"The building of sewers is a sanitary reform only so far as it goes," commented the *Pioneer Press* in speaking of Minneapolis. "People may use the sewers, and a great many people will undoubtedly use them when they become available, or as the filling up of cesspools and privy vaults may compel them to seek some other method of disposing of sewage. But while a property owner may be compelled to pay his proportionate tax for the construction of a sewer, there is no law to compel him to use it when it is once constructed; neither is there any power to compel him to abandon the primitive methods of disposing of his filth now in force throughout a large part of the city. The very nature of the soil on which the city is built is a temptation to that large class of people who weigh temporary expenditure with more jealous attention than the ultimate welfare of the community. . . . The connection

[25] *Pioneer-Press and Tribune*, May 21, August 20, 1876; *Pioneer Press*, June 1, July 31, 1877, October 30, 1880, July 1, 1883; *Tribune*, May 28, 1878.

[between sewer and house] should be made obligatory within a reasonable time after the sewer is made available, and the abandonment of the old methods of disposing of filth compelled."[26]

Not only did the City of Minneapolis empty its sewage into the Mississippi, but so also did slaughterhouses and the University of Minnesota. As late as 1910 Bracken complained officially of the university's dumping untreated waste materials into the river. Years earlier the mayor of Minneapolis had suggested the construction of a deep cesspool, lying well below layers of clay and gravel, to catch and hold the city's sewage. Plans were made, too, for the hauling away and burying of night soil.[27] As a matter of fact, several disposal systems were operating simultaneously. All through the 1880s and 1890s Minneapolis was extending its municipal sewerage system, and each decade showed more homes and businesses making connections. But, at the same time, hundreds of homes continued to use the privy or to contract with scavengers to haul away night soil. Minneapolis itself utilized scavengers when occasion demanded. It is safe to say that, no matter what the plan of collection, the bulk of night soil, contents of vaults, and garbage eventually found its way into the Mississippi. Not even Hewitt's recommendations for Minneapolis, made following his trip to Europe in 1890, when he studied sewerage systems of London and Paris, affected the general picture.

In 1891 the Minneapolis City Council approved a night-soil dump, but the city's rejoicing was short-lived. Residents in the vicinity of the projected disposal area objected so vigorously that the plan was abandoned. "In the meantime, the mercury moves up a notch in the thermometer every day," said a newspaper, "and the garbage situation grows more alarming."[28] This situation, in general, was to continue until after World War I, when the labors of the Metropolitan Drainage Commission were to alter radically sewage disposal in both Minneapolis and St. Paul.

Small urban areas watched with intense interest the way St. Paul and Minneapolis handled their sewerage problems in the thirty years from 1870 to the turn of the century. Perhaps they resented a description of Minnesota's outlying areas: "Dreary, treeless, muddy or dusty, desolate, disordered and disreputable appearing villages, and country places out at elbows, are in many parts of Minnesota and adjoining States the

---

[26] *Tribune*, December 24, 1882; *Pioneer Press*, November 24, 1884, May 21, 1888; Hewitt to Folwell, February 8, 1889, Folwell Papers, box 34.
[27] Bracken to Richard Olding Beard, October 31, 1910, Minnesota Department of Health, St. Paul; *Pioneer Press*, June 25, 1886.
[28] *Pioneer Press*, May 28, June 12, 1891.

rule, not the exception. . . . In many of our new railroad towns . . . the first thing that offends the eye of a visitor is a disorderly mass of agricultural machinery heaped around the station and in front of stores of dealers. . . . Then his attention is arrested by the fact that the village cows and hogs are allowed to have their own way among the unsightly salt barrels and dilapidated dry goods boxes that disfigure the public squares; and he turns away . . . disgusted by the miscellaneous display of empty fruit cans and kitchen debris that litter even the purlieus of the village hotel." [29]

When Hewitt, in 1881, advocated the establishment of voluntary sanitary associations, modeled after those of Scotland, he knew the Minnesota need for such groups. "Nothing more pitiable can be imagined than the condition of a thinly settled township or a small village in the presence of epidemic disease other than smallpox," he said. "The suffering, hardship, and premature death which has occurred simply because people did not know what to do, and local authorities were alike or indifferent, cannot be estimated." [30]

To attempt to control sewage disposal in small towns and cities, the state health board in 1885 instructed Hewitt to suggest that sanitary inspectors survey their communities to discover the location and character of all vaults or other receptacles of human excreta and to determine the relations of these to the water and air supply of each house. The board declared the privy to be a great danger to health, and it ordered local boards to clean and fill up all privies that were not watertight and to substitute for them a cheap, above-ground construction. A closed-tub system for the removal of night soil and garbage was recommended, as was the organization of a scavenger force under the direction of the health officer. Burial in trenches was recommended.[31]

Year after year Hewitt advocated the earth closet as a substitute for the ancient privy, and people gradually became aware of the necessity for sanitary privies and wrote him for advice on how to build them. "If you have any circulars or information in regard to the construction of tight movable privy vaults suitable for small villages, or any system for the solution of the Back House problem where sewers are out of the question, please send us some," wrote a physician from Morgan. A rural resident also requested instructions on how to build an earth closet, which "you speck [sic] so hily [sic] of." So many similar requests arrived that Hewitt published an article on the earth closet in *Public*

[29] *Pioneer Press*, October 17, 1880.
[30] *Pioneer Press*, February 17, 1881.
[31] *Pioneer Press*, April 10, 1885.

Health in Minnesota. Written so that the average layman could understand it, the article carried detailed plans and drawings.[32]

The dry-earth closet championed by Hewitt, when properly constructed and used, was far superior to the urban privy common in St. Paul, Minneapolis, and Duluth. By 1889 smaller cities, including Faribault, Northfield, and Winona, had waged fairly successful war against the "hole-in-the-ground" privy and were substituting the dry-earth closet.[33] It was a simple affair consisting of a box saturated with petroleum paint. Excreta was deposited in this box and immediately covered with dry earth from a barrel which stood inside the outhouse. When full, the box was hauled away and its contents were buried. Hewitt maintained that this process resulted in the return of dead and offensive matter in an odorless and cleanly fashion to the ground.

Health officers were quick to see the advantages of the dry-earth closet over the hole-in-the-ground privy common in Hewitt's day. Most privies were seldom cleaned, some not for two or three years. All too frequently a filled privy hole was covered superficially with a sprinkling of earth and another pit was dug at a new location. With this continuing process, it was thought that a man's back yard was pitted with pools of contamination within a decade or so. But for some unaccountable reason, private citizens were not so quick to realize the advantages of the dry-earth closet as were health officers. Innumerable complaints from harassed local health officials told of the difficulties they had in persuading residents in their communities to substitute the newer type closet for the old-fashioned privy.[34]

Sometimes, as in Austin in 1898, a health officer took matters into his own hands and reported his activities as follows: "I personally superintended the filling and closing of the well, and ordered my men to load up privy buildings and haul them out of town, and fill up vaults with fresh earth, this met with such opposition from the business men who — to avoid expense would not connect with the sewer — that my orders had to be carried out in the night and one morning the above gentlemen missed their $25.00 buildings and found in their stead a beautiful clean spot of fresh earth — which is no doubt greatful [sic] to the aristocratic noses of would be dictators who are forced to live in

---

[32] J. L. Adams to Hewitt, May 1, 1894, and John Gallagher to Hewitt, May 8, 1894, Minnesota Department of Health, St. Paul; *Public Health in Minnesota*, 10: 10–12 (March–April, 1894).
[33] *Public Health in Minnesota*, 5:48 (July, 1889).
[34] J. A. Regner to Hewitt, May 30, 1894; J. W. Scott to Hewitt, June 30, 1894; Jacob W. B. Wellcome, Jr., to Bracken, June 12, 1902. Minnesota Department of Health, St. Paul.

that neighborhood." Now and again an aroused and irate citizen complained directly to the Minnesota Department of Health that local health officers were lax in enforcing ordinances against deep-pit privies. One such complaint came from Worthington: "Privy vaults are built which are water tight and deep enough to drown a person and are untouched for a decade — until the floor decays and goes down, as one did with me last Nov., nearly costing me my life."[35]

Bracken, although as interested in sanitary sewage disposal as was Hewitt, was not so patient nor so gentle in answering letters requesting information about sanitary outhouses. "I can give you no plans for the construction of vaults as asked for by you," he wrote to a Hanska physician in 1902. "I can only state that the only satisfactory vault should be water tight, that is constructed of brick or stone with cement or with lumber so closely joined as to make it water tight. Provision should be made for cleaning out such a vault. I may suggest that in some cases it is well to use a dry earth closet rather than a vault. You can find plans for such closets in various works on sanitation. The enclosed circular may be of some service to you, although it is not up to date in the general plan outlined."[36]

In 1916 the state health department issued exactly the type of bulletin which Bracken told the Hanska physician was not available. A simply worded introduction told the reader that before it was discovered that diseases were transmitted by improperly caring for human excreta, privies were used only for the purpose of privacy and protection. It went on to explain that now a major function of the privy was to provide a *safe* receptacle for the deposit of human excreta. The bulletin explained why this safety factor was important. Diseases most commonly transmitted by improper disposal of waste are typhoid fever and dysentery. The route of infection, said the bulletin, is well known: animals may have access to the privy and humans may touch the animal; then the human puts his fingers in his mouth or neglects to wash before eating and thus transfers minute particles of excreta. Flies also may carry disease from privy to table and then to man. In order to obtain and maintain a sanitary privy, continued the bulletin, three important points must be given consideration — location, construction, operation. Location must not endanger water supply; construction must prevent contact of excreta with persons, animals, and insects;

[35] W. H. McKenna to Bracken, August 18, 1898; Mrs. Hammond to Hewitt, March 4, 1895. Minnesota Department of Health, St. Paul.

[36] Bracken to Douglas Wood, March 17, 1902, Minnesota Department of Health, St. Paul.

and operation must demand keeping the privy clean and in good repair. Several revisions of this manual were published, each incorporating new ideas.[37]

The suggestion was made that model privies be demonstrated in towns needing sanitary instruction. These should be flyproof, well ventilated, and provided with toilet-paper holders and circulars explaining the fly menace. In addition, a card stressing the importance of washing hands was to be posted. Plans were made and designs drawn for concrete bases for privies in the hope that cement would keep out flies more effectively than other materials.[38] The best method of removal of excreta, however, according to the state board, was the water-carriage system, for it was easy to clean and keep clean, was convenient to use, was free from flies, was no danger to the housewife who cleaned it, and it promoted frequent use and better health. Such a system, although ideal, had obvious disadvantages. In the first place, it was costly to the citizen, for it demanded toilet fixtures, a house drainage system, main drains or sewers, and a disposal or purification plant. Moreover, a water-carriage system for a cold climate such as that of Minnesota requires that pipes be laid deep enough under ground to prevent freezing. That, too, is expensive. In the second place, this type of system is planned to drain into an underground disposal plant, which is really a cesspool. The average cesspool leaks notoriously, and "it is extremely difficult to predict just what direction the underground flow from a cesspool may take." It is possible, of course, for contaminated matter to seep into wells or cisterns.[39]

The Iron Range, beginning to show promise in the 1880s when other sections of Minnesota had already passed through a pioneer period, used four kinds of privies, ranging all the way from primitive makeshifts to the pit type. A refined water-carriage system was much too advanced to be generally used there until long after 1900. The most desirable type in flourishing mining towns and busy camps was the pit privy, because it could be made fly-tight by banking earth around the base, because it was simple to construct, and because it did not require handling excreta. On the other hand, this style of privy could discharge its contents by seepage into the soil and it might pollute wells used as sources of water for domestic use. The state health department, after a survey, said that practically all "the people living on the locations of

[37] State Board of Health, *The Sanitary Privy*, May, 1916; 1940.
[38] Chesley to Bracken, June 17, 1912; Bracken to Bass, July 19, 1912. Minnesota Department of Health, St. Paul.
[39] State Board of Health, *Sewage Disposal in Unsewered Districts*, 3, 9 (Minneapolis, [1916]).

the Oliver Iron Mining Company are provided with water from protected sources which is in no danger of contamination from privies [and] there is no real reason why the pit type of privy cannot be used on the locations where safe water supplies are available." [40]

Whenever possible, however, private citizens and industrial concerns were urged to install a sewage disposal plant that included a settling, or septic, tank, where bacterial action prepares, but does not purify, sewage for disposal in the soil; a dosing tank, where overflow from the settling tank will pass and where the action of an automatic siphon will cause liquid to flow intermittently; and a set of tile pipes laid in dry, porous soil for wide distribution of the waste. Such a plan, as is obvious, was recommended only for localities which had no municipal sewerage systems. Later, traps or water seals to prevent offensive gases from entering residences were approved, and grease traps to be placed on outlets from kitchen sinks were recommended. Special warnings were issued concerning the type of pit to be used for receiving sewage from a domestic disposal plant. Regulation 226 of the Minnesota State Board of Health says: "No well, abandoned well or sink hole shall be used as a receptacle for sewage, industrial waste or other wastes. Cesspools, soil absorption systems, shafts or similar structures, excavations or natural earth formations used for the disposal of sewage, industrial wastes or other wastes shall be located and operated so as not to jeopardize the safety of underground water supplies or otherwise render them unsuitable for domestic use." [41]

Drainage was a perennial problem for both private plants and municipal sewerage plants. The individual usually, with intelligence and by co-operation with local and state health authorities, could solve his problem with relative ease. In small towns and cities where there was local prejudice, political influence, or sheer ignorance, however, the situation was apt to be complicated. Rochester, for example, was built on sloping ground which ran toward running streams. This was almost ideal for drainage. Yet in 1884 the city was drained by only two short underground pipes. There were no sewers. "In the rear of almost every house in the city may be found during the winter season frozen masses of ever-increasing accumulations of kitchen debris," affirmed a St. Paul reporter, who had been sent to Rochester to investigate an outbreak of diphtheria. "These accumulations are, of course, innocuous as long as

[40] State Board of Health, *Report on Sewage, Excreta, and Garbage Disposal at Certain Locations of the Oliver Iron Mining Company on the Minnesota Iron Range*, June 22–27, 1915, p. 65.
[41] Minnesota Department of Health, *Small Water Supplies and Sewerage Systems*, 1940, p. 38.

they remain frozen. But in the spring when the refuse matter melts, part of it passes away in noxious gases, and the remainder putrefies where it lies, penetrating the soil below more deeply with each successive season, besides continually poisoning the air at the surface."

The reporter, stepping out of his role as newspaperman and into that of sanitary engineer, suggested that Rochester hire a competent engineer and plan for a complete system of sewers. If this were done, the city would be thoroughly drained within a few years and taxes would not be appreciably higher. "And," he added, "there will be no excuse for such plague spots as the present diphtheria center, where all the slops are thrown out beside the well, and where the waste-pipe from the common sink discharges directly below the floor with no drain to carry away even what the super-saturated soil refuses to absorb."

Irate Rochester citizens denied this appraisal of their city, maintaining that the town had a good health record, that the diphtheria cases were largely in one house, and that filth accumulations in streets, alleys, and back yards were carefully looked after and removed by an efficient board of health. "Sewers," said a Rochester defender, "in a large city are an absolute necessity, and at no distant future will have to be adopted in this city; but for the present, I believe there is no cause for alarm." [42]

Rochester need not have been too sensitive, for criticisms directed against it could have been duplicated many times over throughout the state. New Brighton, center of slaughterhouse and packing activities, was dumping offal into Mud Lake and discharging it into sand pits. Fairfax wanted to drain a swamp but did not know how to proceed. Citizens of Shakopee were up in arms because no sewerage system existed there and night soil was being dumped in the river close to the mill. A Willmar resident described a stagnant pool close to town into which sewers with water closet connections emptied. At Sleepy Eye a cesspool stood in front of a Catholic church and school and emitted an "unbearable" stench during warm weather.[43]

Bracken, late in 1897, made a special trip to New Ulm to discuss the establishment of a city hospital for infectious diseases, to urge the construction of a public abattoir, and to give advice on water supply and sewerage. His trip was the result of complaints similar to those received from other Minnesota towns. When he returned to St. Paul he

[42] *Pioneer Press*, January 11, 19, 1884.
[43] Letters to Hewitt from A. A. Stoddard, June 25, 1892, from C. T. Buchanan, July 22, 1893, and from E. S. Frost, April 11, 1896; Jacob W. B. Wellcome, Sr., to Bracken, May 10, 1897. Minnesota Department of Health, St. Paul.

wrote a long letter advocating the installation of a sewerage system; such a system, he said, in the long run was a matter of economy. He warned New Ulm not to plan to empty its waste into the river, "first, because the river is too small to serve as a carrier for sewage (undoubtedly a nuisance would be created) and second, because there is a law against the pollution of streams." A year later, when New Ulm was about to install a sewer system, Bracken congratulated the community. "You certainly need one," he wrote. "Some of the vaults that I saw on a recent visit to New Ulm were in a condition that no city should tolerate. They pointed very plainly to the need of sewers, especially through the business part of the city." After sewers were installed, Bracken again visited New Ulm. "What is the use of having a sewer and not using it?" he wrote on his return. "Your city should pass an ordinance requiring all blocks, saloons, hotels, butcher shops, laundrys [sic] etc., to make sewer connections within a reasonable time; say within six months. You should not allow any new cesspools or vaults to be constructed within the sewer area; nor should old ones be allowed use longer than six months after sewer construction has been completed along the property where they are located."[44]

No matter how hard Bracken and the department worked to discourage use of antiquated privies and vaults and to encourage the installation of modern sewerage systems, it seemed as if little progress was being made. Bracken was forced to tell the director of a New Jersey state hospital that Minnesota state institutions had practically no systems of sewage disposal, and he was tremendously concerned over the continuing pollution of streams with sewage from villages and cities throughout the state. He pointed out frequently that raw sewage must not be emptied into lakes and tried, sometimes vainly, to explain the difference between *raw* and *treated* sewage to town officers.[45]

Yet the situation certainly was not completely disheartening in the first decade of the twentieth century. Brainerd was planning a sewerage system, filter beds were considered for the University of Minnesota experiment station at St. Anthony Park, and the university's Board of Regents had been approached with a plan for the establishment of a small sewage disposal plant for experimental purposes on the campus. Indeed, the number of towns constructing municipal sanitary sewer

[44] Bracken to O. C. Strickler, November 16, 1897, July 5, 1899, and to the president of the New Ulm City Council, June 20, 1898, Minnesota Department of Health, St. Paul.
[45] Bracken to B. D. Evans, February 10, 1902, and to C. I. Oliver, September 3, 1903; State Board of Health to Persons Interested in Sanitary Matters, July 10, 1903. Minnesota Department of Health, St. Paul.

systems had increased rapidly since 1872, when both St. Paul and Minneapolis started construction. During the next decade three communities — Fergus Falls (about 1882), Duluth (1883), and Redwood Falls (1887) — began building sewer systems. The 1890s saw eight towns begin construction of municipal sanitary sewer systems. The first three were Austin (1892), Winona (1892), and Ada (1895), and they were followed by Moorhead, New Ulm, Benson, St. James, and Wells. The boom really began after the turn of the century, with at least twenty-eight cities falling into line. Eveleth and Hibbing began construction in 1900, Ely and Sauk City in 1901, and Hutchinson, Rushford, and Slayton the next year. The first three cities to construct sewage treatment plants were Hallock (1904), Baudette (1909), and Canby (1910).[46]

The most extensive and perhaps the most dramatic sewage treatment project involved the Twin Cities and was initiated on July 31, 1923, when Chesley, acting under instruction of the State Board of Health, called the attention of the two city councils to the polluted condition of the Mississippi. Again on July 28, 1925, Chesley referred to the insanitary state of the river and urged that early action be taken to avoid more serious difficulties. He offered the co-operation of the board. City councils of both cities then appointed a joint committee, which advised that the United States Public Health Service be requested to make a survey of the Mississippi adjacent to the Twin Cities. Local and state agencies enthusiastically endorsed the project. An interim committee was appointed in the legislative session of 1925, the Izaak Walton League became interested, the Engineers' Society of St. Paul and the Engineering Club of Minneapolis held special meetings, and, finally, a Metropolitan District Planning Association was formed. On April 14, 1927, the legislature created the Metropolitan Drainage Commission, with powers "to study the subject of sewage disposal and treatment, to make surveys and collect data relating to the methods which might be used in disposing of such sewage or of treating the same so as to protect such water course from pollution, as well as any other water courses or bodies of water lying within the drainage area of which such cities are a part." Members of the commission were C. F. Keyes of Minneapolis, chairman; Oscar Claussen of St. Paul, vice-chairman; and Russell H.

[46] John J. Flather to Bracken, September 21, 1903, Bracken to W. M. Hays, April 16, 1902, and to F. S. Jones, August 25, 1904, Minnesota Department of Health, St. Paul. The data on the municipal sewer systems constructed between 1872 and 1910 were compiled from Minnesota Department of Health, *Municipalities Having Sewer Systems with Sewage Treatment Plants, January 1, 1947.*

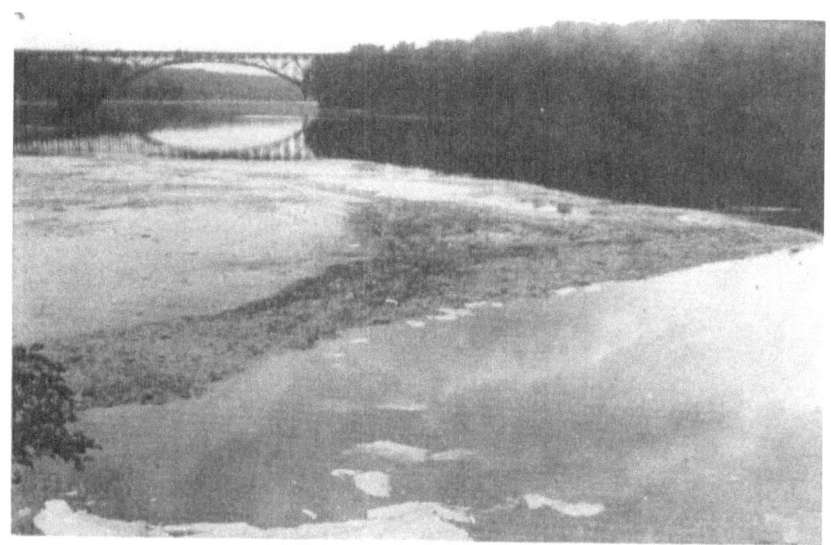

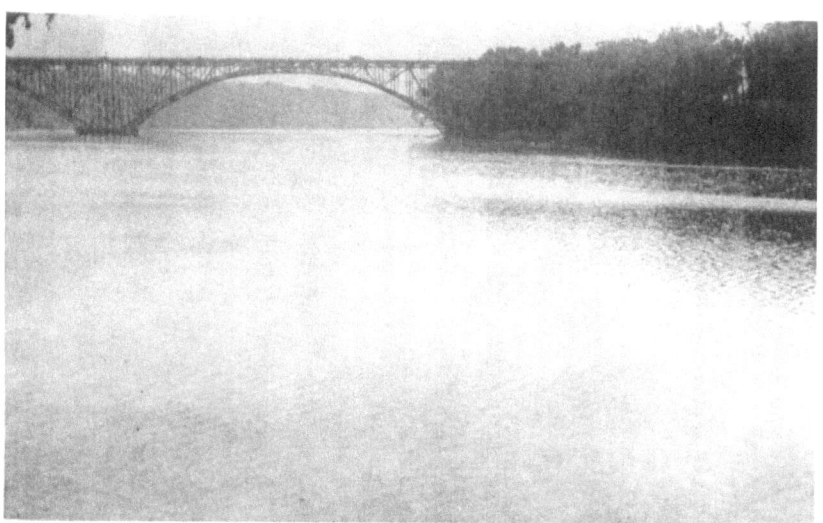

MISSISSIPPI RIVER BEFORE AND AFTER CONSTRUCTION OF THE
TWIN CITIES SEWAGE TREATMENT PLANT
Courtesy Minneapolis-St. Paul Sanitary District

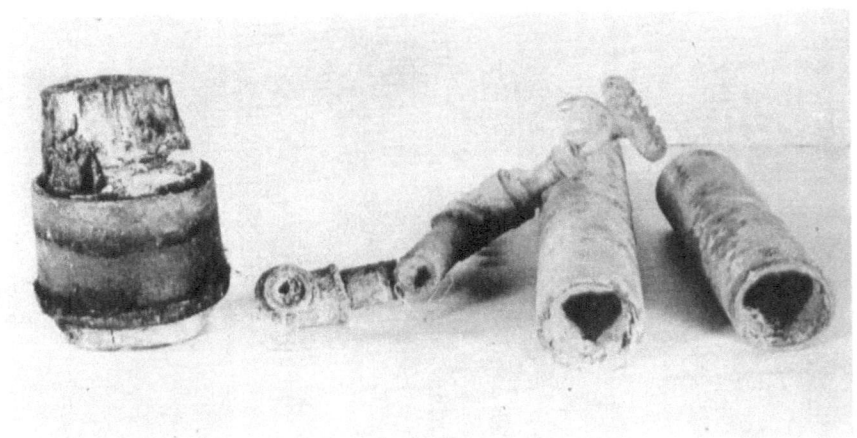

OLD TYPE WATER PIPES

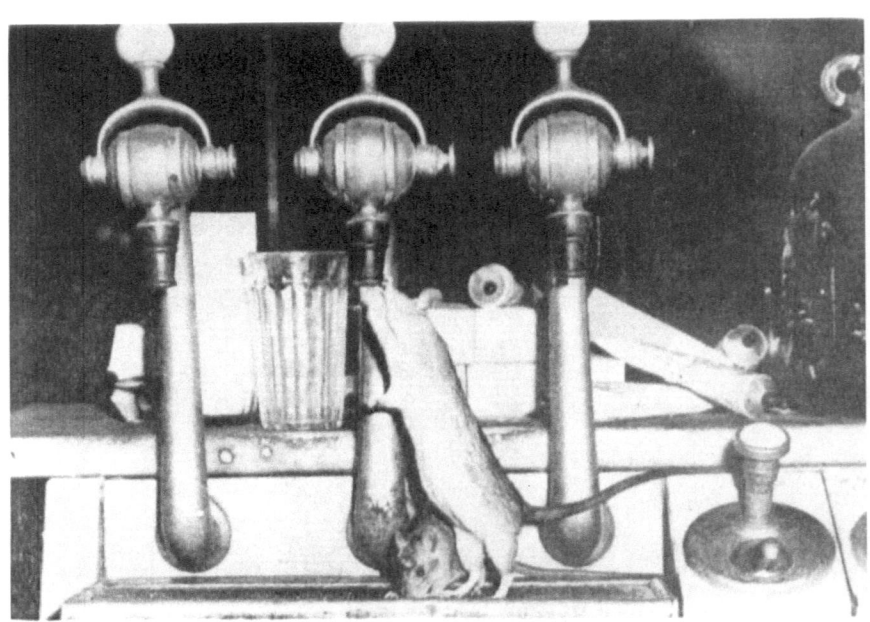

RATS ARE A MENACE TO HEALTH
Courtesy Minnesota Department of Health

Bennett of Minneapolis and George M. Shepard of St. Paul. C. D. Tearse of Winona was directly appointed by Governor Theodore Christianson.[47]

Progress was necessarily slow, for preliminary work involved tremendous labor in office, laboratory, and field. The division of sanitation of the Minnesota Department of Health made bacteriological examinations of sewage samples. The department also aided the investigation undertaken by the United States Public Health Service, assembling biological, physical, bacteriological, and chemical information. On December 1, 1927, the commission requested the Minnesota State Board of Health to express an opinion on (1) the public health aspect of the problem, (2) the classification of various sections of the river under consideration, and (3) the economic value of preserving fish life in that portion of the Mississippi which was or might be affected by the discharge of sewage from the Twin City area.

The board found that a "condition of public nuisance exists, except during periods of relatively high water, in the section of the river from the head of the pool above the Twin City Lock and Dam in Minneapolis to the influx of the St. Croix River at Prescott. This condition is evidenced by odors, floating and suspended material, sludge deposits, and by the ebullition of gas." From Prescott to the head of Lake Pepin, water was unfit for either drinking or swimming, and the waters of Lake Pepin itself did not comply with the standards set by health authorities for bathing purposes. It was the opinion of the Minnesota and Wisconsin health boards and the Minnesota commissioner of game and fish that the pollution of the Mississippi should be so restricted that the public health hazard would be reduced to a minimum and the health of livestock would not be endangered. Fish life, at least below the mouth of the St. Croix, should not be jeopardized.[48]

Between 1927 and 1933 the Metropolitan Drainage Commission supervised a tremendous amount of work, including preliminary surveys, analyses of population trends, and the gathering of data concerning sewage and sewage treatment. Its reports were published in five volumes. During the six years of its existence the commission held seventy-eight meetings and spent $246,297.50. On April 19, 1933, the work of the commission was terminated when a legislative act providing for a Minneapolis–St. Paul Sanitary District was passed. Briefly, this act im-

[47] Minneapolis and St. Paul Metropolitan Drainage Commission, *Annual Reports*, 1927, pp. 1, 9; Interim Committee, *Reports*, 1927.

[48] Minneapolis and St. Paul Metropolitan Drainage Commission, *Annual Reports*, 1928, pp. 4–6.

posed upon the State Board of Health the duty of making certain investigations and carrying out certain legal proceedings preliminary to the establishment of the sanitary districts of two or more cities of the first class. On July 3, 1933, the board issued an order declaring Minneapolis and St. Paul to be a single sanitary district.[49] Critics who delight in pointing out the fierce rivalry and lack of co-operation between the two cities usually neglect to mention the Minneapolis–St. Paul Sanitary District, one of the finest examples of municipal co-operation in the United States.

The year 1934 saw this co-operative venture begin to take tangible form. The Federal Emergency Administration of Public Works allocated eighteen million dollars for the project and the district borrowed additional substantial sums from the cities of Minneapolis and St. Paul. Harold Ickes approved the appointment of a three-man board of engineers composed of Brigadier General C. W. Kutz of Washington, D.C., chairman, Professor Frederic Bass of the University of Minnesota, and William N. Carey, state engineer from Minnesota, for the Public Works Administration. The Chicago firm of Consoer, Townsend, Older, and Quinlan was engaged as consulting engineers, and the first contracts were let to the Middle Roads Company of Flint, Michigan, for the construction of a tunnel section, and to the Feyen Construction Company of St. Paul for another tunnel job. Workmen were employed in the ratio of two from Minneapolis for every one from St. Paul, as the former city was paying approximately two-thirds of the cost of the project and the latter approximately one-third.[50]

In October the engineering board recommended that chemical treatment of sewage be adopted for the project, and plans were made for the installation of a plant for this purpose at an estimated cost of $3,376,000. It was to be located at Pigs Eye Lake in St. Paul, an old landmark and one well known to the earliest pioneers. Meanwhile, citizens who for years had complained of sewage conditions watched proceedings with unusual interest. The state health department continued its investigations of the pollution of waterways, submitting a long series of reports that were to continue after the district treatment plan was completed. Arrangements also had to be made to consider the disposal of waste from the Veterans' Hospital at Fort Snelling and to keep constantly in mind the pollution not only of the St. Croix but also of smaller bodies of water. Another pollution problem was waste from

[49] *Minneapolis Star*, July 8, 15, 1933; *St. Paul Dispatch*, July 8, 15, 1933.
[50] Minneapolis–St. Paul Sanitary District, *Annual Reports*, 1934, p. 3.

canning factories, which in eighteen years had increased their output from an equivalent of 12,000,000 cans to over 142,000,000 in 1937. The waste from a single plant, said health authorities, had an affect upon the oxygen resources of a stream equivalent to the sewage from a city with a population of forty thousand.[51]

With the state health board constantly advising, work on the huge disposal plant moved ahead with extreme rapidity, considering the intricate engineering problems involved and the tremendous amount of labor necessitated by the removal of 650,000 cubic yards of earth and the pouring of 170,000 cubic yards of concrete. More than 30,000,000 pounds of reinforcing and structural steel went into the project. The plant was designed to handle an average sewage flow of 134,000,000 gallons a day and to remove a total of 150,000 pounds of sewage solids daily, with provision made to increase this to 650,000 pounds.[52]

When the plant was dedicated on May 16, 1938, Minnesota's largest cities, including Duluth, could say that pollution had been reduced and that great progress had been made toward safeguarding the public health. Pipe and pump finally had conquered and made obsolete the deep-hole privy which had been a factor, in conjunction with the fly, in spreading so much disease and causing so many deaths.

[51] Community Alliance of South St. Paul, *Sewage Conditions in the Metropolitan Drainage District* ([South St. Paul?]), 1930); Minnesota Department of Health, "Resumé of Stream and Lake Surveys and Investigations Undertaken in Cooperation with the Department of Conservation, Sept. 1927 to March, 1934," "Report of Special Investigation of the Pollution of the Mississippi River, May and June 1933," "Preliminary Report on the Pollution of the Minnesota River from Mankato to the Junction with the Mississippi River at Mendota, March–April, 1934," "Status of Pollution Abatement Activities along the Mississippi River in Minnesota between Minneapolis and La Crosse, July, 1935," "Memorandum of Pollution of the Mississippi River above the Minneapolis Water Supply Intakes," March 3, 1936, "Stream and Lake Pollution," April–June, 1936, and "Policy on Pollution of the Upper Mississippi River (above St. Anthony Falls) and Tributary Streams," September 16, 1942 (typescripts), Minnesota Department of Health, Minneapolis; Chesley to the chief medical officer, U.S. Veterans' Hospital, December 29, 1934, and to E. V. Willard, May 17, 1935, Minnesota Department of Health, Minneapolis; Division of Sanitation, "Quarterly Reports," March 31, 1934, p. 7, June 30, 1938, p. 2. For a study of the cannery waste disposal problem in Minnesota, Wisconsin, Illinois, Indiana, Iowa, and Missouri, see L. F. Warrick, T. F. Wisniewski, and N. H. Sanborn, *Cannery Waste Disposal Lagoons* (April, 1945).

[52] Minneapolis–St. Paul Sanitary District, *Intercepting Sewers and Sewage Treatment Plant* ([St. Paul?], 1938).

9

Toward Better Food and Drink

THE CENTENNIAL year is now fairly ushered in, and it is a year destined, we trust, to be the proudest in the American calendar," commented the *St. Paul Pioneer-Press* in 1876, when the nation was rejoicing in Philadelphia at the end of a hundred years of progress. The St. Paul editor thought there were many ways of celebrating, and he suggested, among others, that 1876 was a good year "for grocery-keepers to stop sanding their sugar."[1] This advice, although offered waggishly, carried a barb. For decades the American consumer had been hoodwinked and imposed upon by unscrupulous retailers and commission merchants, who not only sanded sugar but also ground beans into coffee, sold soda crackers that the store cat had nested in, and cut steaks from beef butchered under filthy conditions. The general store, located in towns and at hundreds of Minnesota crossroads, was apt to keep its milk in dirty containers, to retail butter dotted with flyspecks, and to dispense a variety of adulterated flavorings and syrups. A customer literally took his life in his hands when he purchased half a pound of headcheese or asked the baker for a loaf of bread. The cheese might have been made from diseased pork, and the loaf could have contained cockroaches.

No wonder that scores of Minnesotans became ill after drinking milk, eating pork, or using impure baking powder. The adulteration of food and drink, said an editor sadly, had become almost as general as the use of them. Rochester was tremendously excited in 1880, when Dr. W. W. Mayo reported upon the impurity of sugars and syrups which he had purchased and analyzed. His action was called the opening of a "war on adulteration, which can only benefit the public." The St. Paul Chamber of Commerce interested itself in the problem

[1] *Pioneer-Press*, January 2, 1876.

of unclean foods and adulterated drugs, and in 1883 dairymen were urging national legislation to prevent the adulteration of butter, cheese, and milk. They were fearful that unless drastic action was taken the entire dairy business would fall into disrepute. The Minnesota dairy industry was well acquainted with what was happening in New York. Public health experts, after gathering samples throughout that state, reported that purity was the exception rather than the rule. They continued: "Butter, milk, lard, baking powder, sugar, tea, coffee, and a multitude of other commodities were found to be mingled with foreign substances to an extent that not only defrauds the purchaser, but puts him, in many instances, in imminent danger of sacrificing his health to the cupidity of unscrupulous dealers." [2]

This moral indignation, bubbling in the white heat of an aroused public opinion, was not new in Minnesota. As early as 1855 St. Paul had passed an ordinance requiring the inspection of flour and the gauging of all liquors sold in the market, and after the Civil War the movement for pure foods and drugs gained impetus. Yet there was a great gap between law and practice in the early days when public health was in its infancy and when health officers had to fight against apathy of city fathers, and against public indifference too. Fortunately local health officers were encouraged by Hewitt to insist that laws to control unsanitary food be passed. The state health department almost from its beginning took an active interest in safeguarding the public from diseased foods and unclean milk, butter, and cheese. It urged cleanliness, inspected dairy cattle and farms, stood behind local health officers, drew up model acts designed to prohibit adulteration, and, after many years, finally succeeded in establishing a restaurant and food inspection program that was independent of politics. In 1879 Hewitt said that the state board stood ready to help individuals and communities investigate suspected food.[3]

Perhaps the most dramatic problems tackled by the board, in conjunction with local officials, concerned meat and milk. Americans always have been great meat eaters, and the men and women of the North Star State were no exception. Long before 1884, when it was estimated that at least seventy-five thousand head of cattle had passed through St. Paul bound for Eastern markets and when it was pre-

[2] *Pioneer Press*, February 3, 1879, November 20, 1880, January 25, 1881, February 18, 1883.
[3] *Daily Pioneer* (St. Paul), September 7, 1855; *Pioneer Press*, March 1, 1879; State Board of Health, *Biennial Reports*, 1883–84, p. 11; *Public Health in Minnesota*, 7:72 (January, 1892).

dicted that both St. Paul and Minneapolis would become important stock centers, private slaughterhouses and individual butchers were killing and dressing a tremendous number of hogs and beeves. St. Paul and Minneapolis as well as other Minnesota cities faced the problem of how to make certain that meats would be prepared in a sanitary manner and be free from disease. This was a difficult task. Some butchers did try to make their establishments neat and odorless, but, said an observer in St. Paul in 1873, there "are strong reasons to believe that the butchers of the city do not obey all the ordinances regulating the health and cleanliness of the city."[4]

F. R. Potts, St. Paul health officer, was kept busy inspecting butcher shops in 1873. He recommended that all slaughterhouses be removed outside the city limits, but his advice was not taken. As a result Phalen Creek was polluted with offal. Two years later another health inspector said a butcher was selling beef that was "black as a hat." Yet it was most difficult in those early days for an inspector to bring a butcher into court and get a conviction. When, for example, Gottlieb Houck was hailed into court on a charge of selling diseased meat, he pleaded that he did not do it deliberately and that he had refunded the purchase price when the customer complained. The court discontinued the case after a payment of costs amounting to two dollars. Meanwhile, one case of "meat poisoning" after another was being reported. Complicating an already confused situation were peddlers who had no shops and sold meat from pushcarts. It was almost impossible for authorities to find these meat bootleggers, for they disappeared quickly into alleys and down tenement streets if they thought an inspector was after them. They held no licenses, and their meats were said to be cut from diseased animals and to be "entirely" bad.[5] Minneapolis butchers complained that there were "rogues in all trades" and suggested that the 130 city butcher shops be licensed by the city. A regular butcher would pay $100 annually, and a pushcart butcher would be charged $250. Proceeds from license fees would be used to pay the salary of a full-time city meat inspector.

St. Paul attacked the problem by sending its health officer, Dr. Henry F. Hoyt, to Kansas City, St. Louis, and Chicago to study how those municipalities protected the health of citizens and assured a supply of wholesome meat. Hoyt returned with a plan for rigorous

[4] *Pioneer Press*, October 12, 1884; *St. Paul Daily Press*, December 7, 1872, July 16, 1873.
[5] *St. Paul Daily Press*, July 15, 1873; *Pioneer-Press*, November 24, 1875, April 25, 1881, January 7, June 14, 1882, January 11, April 12, 1884.

inspection, beginning at the stockyards and continuing through the slaughterhouse and the butcher shop. The St. Paul health board approved this arrangement, and it was started within a few days. Before two weeks had elapsed the system was working so well that it was rumored that purveyors of diseased meat were ignoring St. Paul entirely and disposing of it in Minneapolis. This rumor was quickly denied by Mill City officials, who maintained that the beef was sent to Minneapolis rendering establishments and not to butcher shops. By November, 1884, Hoyt was able to order thorough inspection of slaughterhouses and meat shops once a week. By the end of the month, before Hoyt's system had run more than a few weeks, the reaction set in. Butchers who had been eager for a strict inspection system and had endorsed Hoyt's program now claimed that he was too strict, that he was injuring the reputation of the better butchers, that he was appointing incompetent inspectors. The bewildered Hoyt said he did not know what St. Paul butchers wanted, but added that he was certain of one fact: "He has been appointed to inspect the meats sold in St. Paul, and the public look to him to protect their interests, as far as lies in his power. This he proposes to do, regardless of the harpings of anybody or any class of men." Regardless of the merits of the criticism against Hoyt and his inspectors, this much must be said: they were giving St. Paul its first real protection against spoiled meat. Of a total of 520 cattle inspected at the Minnesota Transfer, only 12 were found to be unfit for use. And out of a total of 3,974 cattle, sheep, and hogs inspected, only 612 were condemned and sent to a fertilizing company.[6]

Minneapolis watched Hoyt's work critically and early in 1885 decided to adopt a similar, but not identical, program. The council committee on health and hospitals on February 16 heard evidence that farmers were bringing spoiled meat into town and recommended the appointment of a city meat inspector. In March an ordinance was passed which created the office of inspector of meats and defined his duties. Another ordinance regulated the sale of meats and other foods and prohibited the sale of all unwholesome or impure articles used for food. Violators were subject to a fine of not more than fifty dollars or imprisonment in the city workhouse or county jail for a period not exceeding ninety days. With inspectors in both cities, control was easier, and it became increasingly difficult, although not impossible, for butchers to sell meat that threatened public health.

[6] *Pioneer Press*, October 18, 26, 31, November 18, 24, December 11, 1884.

More than a thousand pounds of chicken were condemned in one market on one afternoon. A butcher selling beef from a cow that had died from consumption was arrested and fined ten dollars. Incidents like these were numerous, and they served to deter packers and retailers who might otherwise be lured into temptation.[7]

Mayor George A. Pillsbury praised the work of John T. Lee, Minneapolis' first meat inspector, and said that the office was a most important one. The mayor was gratified that in a few weeks Lee had condemned 18,761 pounds of fresh pork and 1,100 pounds of salt pork. The inspector also condemned almost 6,000 pounds of hams and shoulders, and refused to approve nearly 4,000 pounds of fresh beef. Quantities of sausage, mutton, venison, and poultry also were condemned. "It is not too much to say," concluded Pillsbury, "that the condemnation of the above alarming quantities of unwholesome provision has promoted the general health of the city." So zealous was another inspector that in July, 1887, he condemned more than 30,000 pounds, causing the *Minneapolis Tribune* to comment, "Meat Inspector Mea, if he keeps up the present racket, will reduce Minneapolis to a vegetarian diet."[8]

Meat inspectors knew what they were doing. They realized more than the public ever could the unsanitary conditions of packing houses and the slovenly manner in which the corner butcher prepared and packaged meats. On July 4, 1886, at least forty persons at Hutchinson were poisoned as the result of eating locally made spiced beef. The Hutchinson Board of Health condemned about a ton of meat, but not before several consumers had died. Duluth reported cases of food poisoning, as did smaller communities, including Winona and Rochester. Most areas approved city ordinances that provided for meat inspection. In 1889, however, the St. Louis County district court held a meat-inspection law to be unconstitutional. The court said that such a law not only interfered with interstate commerce, but even went too far as a police regulation. This decision, handed down in Duluth, annoyed St. Paul stock dealers, who supported vigorously the principle that meat must be inspected to protect both retailer and consumer.[9]

Hewitt, of course, believed thoroughly in this type of legislation

[7] *Pioneer Press*, February 17, March 26, June 2, 1885; *Daily Globe* (St. Paul), June 13, 1886; St. Paul City Officers, *Reports*, 1885, pp. 278–280, 294; State Board of Health, *Biennial Reports*, 1886–88, pp. 21–23.
[8] *Pioneer Press*, April 14, 1886; *Minneapolis Tribune*, July 2, 1887; Minneapolis City Officers, *Reports*, 1889, p. 437.
[9] *Pioneer Press*, July 27, August 15, 1886.

TOWARD BETTER FOOD AND DRINK 153

and, on one occasion, prepared an elaborate outline explaining why animals should be inspected before slaughter. He argued that examination of animals before killing would prevent the slaughter of well animals which were not fit for food because of age, injury, or fatigue. It would also prevent the slaying of sick and diseased cattle. Slaughtering, he said, is a sanitary matter. He recommended the appointment of additional inspectors to work in specific localities throughout the state. They would oversee the method of slaughter and supervise the care of the carcass until it was sold or cured. An act, modeled on Hewitt's notes, was approved on April 16, 1889.[10]

In many instances the state department recommended or approved inspectors for towns or specific packing plants. This presented complications, for it involved the vexing problem of personnel and was apt to lead to political entanglement, which the department was most anxious to avoid. The extreme care with which the department approached the problem is indicated in Bracken's discussion of municipal meat inspection. He pointed out in 1898 that no definite policy had been agreed upon. Then he continued: "It certainly is a fact that is quite generally recognized that there should be careful inspection, both ante and post mortem. In connection with the inspection of dairy cattle, as carried on by the city board of health of Minneapolis, it seems advisable that an authorized inspector from our board should keep such cattle as are condemned by the tuberculin test under observation until they are finally disposed of. I understand that it would be quite agreeable to the Minneapolis board of health that we should give such authority to their meat inspector." His caution becomes increasingly apparent: "I would, therefore, recommend that Charles Tilbury be given authority to act as meat inspector for the state board of health; this, without financial obligation on the part of the board, and with power of cancellation at any time, at the discretion of the secretary and executive officer of the state board, by properly rendering notice to that effect to the commissioner of health of Minneapolis." [11]

The Bracken administration, determined to keep the most careful watch over the meat supply of the Twin Cities, met periodically with health officials from both St. Paul and Minneapolis. A result of these conferences was an agreement that each city must establish a public abattoir if the state department was to see that meat was properly

[10] Minnesota, *Laws*, 1889, p. 52; typewritten notes in the Hewitt collection, Minnesota Department of Health, St. Paul.
[11] State Board of Health, *Biennial Reports*, 1897–98, pp. 67, 98.

inspected. It was also determined that cattle reacting to the tuberculin test should be permanently branded with a hot iron upon the left hip. Bracken offered to furnish uniform branding irons. A third point was a recommendation that the federal regulations covering the inspection of tuberculous cattle to be slaughtered would be followed. The Minnesota health board would supervise the killing.[12]

There was real reason, of course, why Bracken was concerned about the state's meat supply. In June, 1898, he had sent a most complicated questionnaire to health officers of 228 cities. Among the questions asked were: Is the meat consumed as food subject to inspection? What is the character of beef furnished? To the first inquiry, 210 returns were made. They revealed that only 20 communities were inspecting meat, among them Aitkin, Brainerd, Duluth, Hinckley, Eagle Bend, and Winona. The second query brought 170 returns; 96 communities said the quality was good, 56 fair, 11 tough, and 1 old. Bracken also asked about the condition of local slaughterhouses. Returns indicated that most of them were maintained in good condition.[13]

Despite all this, the board received innumerable complaints. One health officer said that a local slaughterhouse was "a terror to civilization truly, a pile of offal near the house made it a daring thing to go near, and the flies attacked anyone approaching so fiercely that it seemed too bad to overcome them. The house has a hog pen around three sides, scattered about with offal, and 4 hogs kept there. No water is used evidently, about the place." A later observer, speaking of slaughterhouses in country towns, suggested that Bracken drop in on one in July or August, when he could smell it forty rods off.[14]

Even cleanliness in killing plants, as Bracken well knew, did not guarantee table meat that was fit to eat. The New Brighton market apparently slaughtered "lumpy jaw" cattle, a fact which aroused public opinion and moved Bracken to write: "As a matter of fact this abominable business has been carried on for years in the vicinity of St. Paul, Minneapolis and Duluth, and probably other places within this state. There is no means at present for controlling such proceedings."[15]

[12] State Board of Health, *Biennial Reports*, 1897–98, p. 239.
[13] State Board of Health, *Biennial Reports*, 1897–98, p. 407.
[14] H. W. Gammell to Bracken, July 17, 1899, Minnesota Department of Health, St. Paul; J. W. Robertson, "Public Health Supervision," in Minnesota State Sanitary Conference, "Minutes," October 4, 1911, p. 13 (typescript), Minnesota Department of Health, St. Paul.
[15] State Board of Health, *Biennial Reports*, 1897–98, p. 120. For a description of butchering on the premises of a local butcher shop, see J. M. Karmany to Bracken, August 19, 1899, Minnesota Department of Health, St. Paul.

For years individual citizens, many of them unfamiliar with sanitary matters but suspicious of their meat, had written the state department for advice. "Herman Russell had a cow that suffered injuries," wrote a confused farmer in 1894. "He butchered her and sold quarter to me. I did not know of the injury. After family ate some of it children became ill. Questioned Russell about it when deposit of matter around bone was found. Mr. Russell didn't think it would hurt anyone and refused to make refund. What shall I do in this case for justice?" The anxious president of a village council said that he had been checking up on local beef and had found that diseased stock was being slaughtered. "Please advise about having our meat inspected," he wrote Hewitt. Government inspectors frequently complained to the Minnesota department about the slaughtering of diseased cattle. Hewitt invariably answered these complaints by requesting local health officers to investigate, but by then the damage usually had been done.[16]

Hewitt could only repeat what he had told meat inspectors again and again. "Your duty," he wrote a recently appointed inspector at New Brighton, "is to keep track of all live stock coming in or passing through those yards to feed or water, for sale or for slaughter there. . . . If you find any stock suffering from any form of disease or injury which unfits them for slaughter you will insist that they be isolated till Dr. [C. E.] Cotton can come and decide what is permitted to be done with them. This instruction applies only to stock stopping in Minnesota for slaughter or other purpose and not to stock going through to Chicago or other places outside the state." [17]

Bracken furnished inspectors with specific instructions about what to look for. He told them to condemn "as unfit for food, on post-mortem any carcass in which the disease is clearly evident, that is, where there is any lesion, even if local, if of any extent; also condemn where the disease is at all generalized, viz., if in more than one organ or locality, even though the several lesions be small. As for instance, a small lesion in a lobe of the lung and a few tubercles on the Pleura or Peritoneum, or elsewhere. Or where the disease affects the lung substance and any of the glands; which is pretty generally the rule, that is, when the lung is affected. The Mediastinal glands are also

[16] Letters to Hewitt from A. T. Kramer, April 11, 1894, from J. P. Mitchell, October 9, 1894, and from Richard Price, October 29, 1896; Hewitt to H. N. Avery, October 22, 1896, and to Price, October 28, 1896. Minnesota Department of Health, St. Paul.

[17] Hewitt to W. H. Witty, October 30, 1896, Minnesota Department of Health, St. Paul.

affected, almost invariably. Pass, as fit for food, a carcass where there is a small lesion and, to all appearance, incapsulated, and localized to that one place; no evidence of fever and no great emaciation being present." [18]

Even qualified inspectors, acting in accordance with specific instructions, sometimes found problems that strained their patience. C. A. Janssen was forced to tell the St. Paul health commissioner on one occasion that the problem of diseased meat was beyond his control. He complained that dealers continued to sell diseased meat because they knew they were free from prosecution unless it could be proved that the meat was used for human food. He said if he condemned meat at one place, it might be sold at another. When this complaint reached Bracken, he could only say, "There ought to be a law," and add that he hoped the next session of the legislature would pass one. Before the Minnesota legislature could provide relief, nineteen students at Shattuck School in Faribault had been poisoned, a family in Lakeville was stricken, and New Ulm was asking Bracken to go there in an attempt to persuade the city to establish a clean public abattoir.[19]

Despite innumerable cases of food poisoning attributed to diseased meat, despite the continued slaying of "lumpy jaw" cattle, despite the railroad practice of selling cattle killed on tracks to packing plants, and despite vigorous newspaper support for a state meat inspection law, the legislature of 1899 failed to act. Perhaps one reason was that the federal government was inspecting meat. But this inspection applied only to meat that was for interstate transport. National inspection did not cover cattle slaughtered to provide meat within Minnesota. Jurisdiction, in this case, rested in the individual community, not in the state. Hence Minnesota as a state had no protection. Bracken felt that Minnesota meat packers opposed the proposed law because it carried a system of fees and because it stipulated that all meats sold in the state should be inspected. Representatives of certain packing houses, he said, contended that all packers having federal inspection should be exempt from both state inspection and from the payment of inspection fees.[20]

[18] Bracken to Avery, January 25, 1898, Minnesota Department of Health, St. Paul.
[19] C. A. Jansson to Alex J. Stone, January 26, 1898; A. A. Dodge to Wesbrook, November 1, 1898; Strickler to Bracken, March 3, 8, 1899; Bracken to Stone, January 31, 1898, to John W. Sanber, January 11, 1899, and to Strickler, March 8, 9, 1899. Minnesota Department of Health, St. Paul.
[20] *Pioneer Press*, March 6, 7, September 12, 20, 1899; State Board of Health, *Biennial Reports*, 1899–1900, p. 119; George F. Wright to Bracken, September 12, 1899, W. A. Fleming to Bracken, August 26, 1899, Minnesota Department of Health, St. Paul. For a copy of the proposed law, see State Board of Health, *Biennial Reports*, 1899–1900, pp. 120–125.

TOWARD BETTER FOOD AND DRINK 157

In 1911 Bracken estimated that in the Twin Cities and Winona possibly about fifty per cent of the meat consumed had passed federal inspection, while in Duluth the percentage was probably about seventy-five. But for the entire state, he felt that only about five per cent of the meat purchased by the housewife had been approved by the federal government. Although George A. Hormel thought Bracken's estimate was too low, he did say that cattle raisers did not bring diseased stock to packing houses where federal inspectors worked. Instead, inferior cattle were sold to local slaughterhouses, which were not under inspection. It was precisely this situation that Bracken wished to eradicate and that he presented to the American Meat Packers Association at Washington, D.C., in January, 1912. He pointed out that very few municipalities in the United States had proper meat-inspection programs and said that in country districts the condition was simply appalling. He urged, as he had been doing for years, the enactment of state laws which would make mandatory the inspection of cattle before they were slaughtered. Despite his efforts, Minnesota has not yet seen fit to pass such an act.[21]

This does not mean, however, that Minnesota has no controls over meat. The State Live Stock Sanitary Board, created in 1903, together with the Minnesota Department of Health and local health departments, exercise wide jurisdiction. Diseased animals may be condemned and slaughtered; veal may not be killed when less than four weeks old; and meat dealers must protect their products from dust, flies, and vermin. The sale of horse meat for human consumption is forbidden. By 1948 the Minnesota housewife, if she patronized reliable butchers and did not purchase directly from a farm where ignorance and unsanitary methods prevailed, could be assured of clean meat. This assurance is the result of years of planning and effort on the part of public health officials. Their dramatic fight against cattle diseases and against trichinosis in hogs marked another victory in the endless battle to prevent disease.[22]

An equally exciting battle in the struggle to give Minnesota pure

[21] Bracken to George A. Hormel, December 6, 1911; Hormel to Bracken, December 4, 1911; Albert H. Veeder to G. W. Swift, December 31, 1898; Bracken, "Outline — Federal and State Inspection of Meat and Dairy Products," 1912 (typescript). Minnesota Department of Health, St. Paul.

[22] Minnesota, *Statutes*, 1945, chapters 28, 31, 35; *St. Paul Daily Press*, February 15, 1866, November 17, 1874, March 21, 1875; *Pioneer Press*, February 10, 1882, February 3, 1884; Wesbrook to R. F. Lynch, January 23, 1899, and to N. M. Cook, November 20, 1900, Minnesota Department of Health, St. Paul. For a history of trichinosis since 1913, see C. Barton Nelson, "Trichinosis in Minnesota," in *Minnesota Medicine*, 30:640 (June, 1947).

food was waged in the field of dairy products — milk, butter, and cheese. Long before pasteurization was known and before even the most advanced dairyman had heard of certified or graded milk, consumers were worried about the purity of the milk they gave their children. The farm lad of fifty years ago drank greedily from the tin bucket of milk cooling in the damp springhouse. His mother skimmed off cream and churned her own butter, the handle of the churn thumping monotonously as she pumped it up and down. Cheese, too, was manufactured on the farm according to recipes that had been handed down from grandmother to daughter and from her to grandchild. Sometimes raw milk was clean, and when it went into butter and cheese that, too, was sanitary. But on other occasions whole families using these products were taken ill and, all too frequently, another stone or two was erected in the rural graveyard.

City residents, forced to purchase milk and dairy products from farmers or from a local store which got its products from the farm, never knew what they were getting. Every Saturday morning, as regular as clockwork, their milk-and-butter man would appear at the back door, lugging a can and a dipper in one hand and carrying a brown earthenware crock of butter in the other. Up and down the street he went, supplying his regular customers. Many of these private milkmen ran clean dairies and did their best to shoo flies away from pails and to make good butter. Some were notoriously careless, never cleaning their barns, seldom washing their hands before milking, and not always washing churn and dipper. Few were sufficiently learned to recognize a diseased cow. Most were in the dairy business to make money. Anything that interfered with profits, such as a program of tuberculin testing, was opposed. This, in brief, was the problem that the state health department had to face and solve. The situation was complicated when dairy interests incorporated, purchased raw milk from farmers, "processed" it, and then dispensed it to retailers or directly to the consumer on the milk route.

The twenty years from 1870 to 1890 heard a rising cry of protest against adulterated dairy products and saw the beginning of attempts at control by both the state and municipal boards of health. In 1877 the *St. Paul Pioneer Press* was asked by a bewildered citizen how he could tell if milk had been adulterated with water or chalk. A few years later a reporter visited city dairies and returned to say that "cows which are huddled together in a yard, and which cannot get the pure air and nutritious grass of the country yield a quality of milk much inferior to the country supply — so much inferior that any physician would consider it almost poisonous as administered to a delicate babe." He suggested that milk inspectors be appointed to rudely handle milkmen who watered their product or who kept dirty and cramped dairies. So intense did public interest in milk become that Hewitt received countless letters from consumers asking how they could protect themselves. "I have read so much lately about diseased milk," began a typical inquiry to Hewitt, "that I have become uneasy and anxious to know if the milk I am using is pure and fit for human consumption. Can you tell me what will be the probable cost of analizeing [sic] some from my two cows and where I can get it done?" From Two Harbors came the complaint that many families kept from two to twenty cows on one lot fifty by a hundred and forty feet. One man had twenty-four cows, one bull, two horses, and even a hundred hens on the back half of two lots. "They all sell milk," the health officer said. "I traced four cases of sickness to one cow yard and stable where there were kept six cows on a half lot, two ending in death. . . . the cow question may be too much for the board of health unless the state board comes to our rescue." [23]

Butter was equally suspect, and sharp commercial reporters were quick to say so. "There is not one pound in a thousand made in this State," commented a journalist in 1877, "that will rank as choice fresh table butter, while much the largest portion of the product would pass as poor common and much of it only as grease and *Poor Grease At That!*" He urged cleanliness in milking, clean milk rooms, well-ventilated cooling rooms, and careful working-out and salting. Finally, he suggested that butter be packed in new, clean muslin and put in a pasteboard box. Although Minnesota-made cheese generally was cleaner than butter, the state dairy commissioner frequently found cheese that was not up to standard.[24]

In 1887 the state dairy commissioner reported improvement in the butter content of milk as the result of investigation by his office. But Minneapolis dealers objected strongly to what they called the "rigid" tests applied to their products, although an inspector examining samples from two hundred and fifty wagons in Minneapolis reported that a hundred carts were carrying adulterated milk.[25] This reaction

[23] *Pioneer Press*, January 12, 1877, November 5, 1882; B. D. Little to Hewitt, November 2, 1894, and J. D. Budd to Hewitt, September 8, 1892, Minnesota Department of Health, St. Paul.
[24] *Pioneer Press*, April 26, 1877, August 7, 1891.
[25] *Tribune*, June 28, August 24, 1887.

was understandable, for the office of dairy commissioner was a new one, having been established on April 1, 1885. W. C. Rice, the first commissioner, had to determine his policies as he met each new problem, for he had no precedent to guide him. Among his first acts was the testing of twenty-one dairy herds to determine the percentage of fat in their milk. He found that the lowest average was three and a half per cent in the milk of any herd, while the highest was four and sixty-five one-hundredths. Rice said flatly that, if the average was taken as a standard, it would be too low. The question, as he put it, was whether the standard should be reduced to the minimum in the interest of the dairyman or be raised for the protection of the consumer. This was only the beginning of the vexing difficulty centering around the highly important question of whether milk should be judged in the interest of public health or from the angle of the producer.

"It is safe to assume," said Rice with some bitterness, "that the dairyman will not sell milk that tests much above the standard, and this gives opportunity either for dilution, or for the selection of cows, or the using of those foods that produce a large flow of watery milk. When it is remembered that the human mother's milk contains five per centum of fats and that so many infants in our day must be fed upon cow's milk, which in our cities need contain but three per centum, is it any wonder that so many of the innocents die before they reach the age of five years?" Rice recommended that the standard be raised to three and a half per cent "on the ground that such a standard is as low as is consistent with the public health." [26]

Minnesota's first act to prohibit and prevent the sale or manufacture of unhealthy or adulterated dairy products was passed in 1885. This was the legislation that created the office of dairy commissioner, that caused confusion with the state health department, and that also set the low milk standard of three per cent fat, which Rice speedily sought to raise. Almost immediately the validity of the act was challenged in the case of Butler v. Chambers, but the Minnesota Supreme Court on November 11, 1886, upheld the legislation, partially on the grounds that adulterated products were injurious to public health and that the legislature was justified in suppressing or remedying this mischief by the imposition of severe penalties.[27]

Progress toward improving milk standards was infuriatingly slow, even though public opinion demanded richer and cleaner milk and

[26] State Dairy Commissioner, *Biennial Reports*, 1885–86, pp. 9, 10.
[27] Minnesota, *Laws*, 1885, p. 189; Butler v. Chambers, 36 *Minnesota*, 69–75.

the courts had upheld the act of 1885. Charles W. Drew, professor of chemistry at the Minnesota College Hospital, found that more than half the milk samples he tested were below the legal limit. Sixty-five per cent of the samples taken from Minneapolis hotels and restaurants were illegally low, as were fifty-two per cent of those taken from dairies. The situation was about the same in St. Paul, where a private detective was employed to gather samples. From a total of eighty-seven samples, only three were found to be above standard. "The adulteration of milk . . . is a heinous crime," the *Pioneer Press* said the day following this report. "Although the ingredients added may not be in themselves the least harmful, although the adulteration may consist in nothing but a judicious mixture of water, the effects are serious and far-reaching. Milk enters largely into the diet of children at a time when deficient nutriment may produce upon their systems effects less immediate but not less serious ultimately than the administering of a poison. . . . The offense is not of that supposedly venial nature which has secured it long immunity. It is most heinous in that it is directed against those who are as helpless as they are susceptible to future evil effects." [28]

The daily consumption of milk in St. Paul in 1888 was estimated at between ten and twelve thousand gallons and that in Minneapolis at a little more. The Twin Cities together used about eight million gallons annually. The bulk of this milk arrived from southern counties by way of the St. Paul, Kansas City and Omaha Railroad, the Iowa and Minnesota division of the Milwaukee Railroad, and the Omaha and Wisconsin Central Railroad. Comparatively little milk was hauled by the Northern Pacific. A local St. Paul supply from some sixty cows swelled the total. The best milk was brought into the city and the poorest milk was produced in the city itself. The St. Paul cows were considered a sanitary nuisance. That the situation was equally bad in Minneapolis is attested by the fact that at one time in 1888 twenty-seven indictments against milk dealers were pending in Hennepin County. A year later the dairy commissioner warned milk dealers that unless they cleaned up their premises they would "have to walk up to the captain's office and settle." [29]

Unfortunately threats accomplished less than was desired. All through the 1890s the sale of adulterated milk continued, although probably in a lesser degree than formerly. The state health department reported that it had found rabies virus in milk, and on October 8,

[28] *Tribune*, August 28, 1887; *Pioneer Press*, April 6, 7, August 28, 1887.
[29] *Pioneer Press*, May 20, June 8, 1888, May 8, 1889.

1901, it discussed seriously its responsibility toward the collection and care of milk. This discussion was the result of a suggestion made by Bracken in July, 1899, when he proposed that certificates be given dairymen whose cattle had been inspected and found to be free from tuberculosis.[30]

Thoroughly convinced that a safe milk supply was one of the most pressing contemporary problems and that the health department should do something immediately, Bracken began a strenuous campaign. In 1902 he read his first paper on milk before the Hennepin County Medical Society. He argued succinctly that clean milk can be secured only from nontuberculous cows and that therefore all herds should be constantly watched and tested. He also advocated pasteurization. "The commercial pasteurization of milk," he said, "can be made to supply an entire city population with milk free from tuberculous infection and this can be said of no other plan so far known. Undoubtedly some will argue that an unheated milk is superior to any form of pasteurized milk. This is not proven, but granting as much for argument's sake and recognizing the impossibility of supplying a city of any considerable size with a safe milk supply on any other plan, it would then seem that a combination of the first and second plans set forth; viz., the sale of raw milk only from dairies that are under rigid inspection, where the cows have stood the tuberculin test; and the sale of commercially pasteurized milk should be used in every city of considerable size. On the other hand the first plan might be depended upon in small cities and villages when the milk supply is taken from a small and easily inspected district."[31]

Bracken spent August of 1902 visiting dairies throughout the state, hoping to persuade their owners to put barns and milkhouses in good condition and to keep only tested cows. Meanwhile health department officials had inspected the sanitary methods used by dairymen of the Twin Cities. The dairy commissioner also had been active. Every morning inspectors left his office at daylight, each carrying a satchel containing twenty-five or thirty half-pint sample cans. Whenever they met a milk wagon they took one or two samples, registering the driver's name and the number of his license on a card. When the sample cans were filled, inspectors returned to the office to test the milk and record their findings. Returns demonstrated the effectiveness of this system. In 1896 thirty-eight per cent of the milk tested in Minneapolis aver-

[30] State Board of Health, *Biennial Reports*, 1899–1900, p. 465; 1901–02, pp. 138, 221.
[31] Bracken Papers, 2:199.

TOWARD BETTER FOOD AND DRINK 163

aged below standard; in 1897 ten per cent was below; while in 1900 only two and a half per cent was below standard. Other inspectors rode railroads that tapped milk-producing sections of the state, visiting creameries and cheese factories and making careful reports. They kept an eye out for milk in dirty cans, sour milk, tainted milk, watered or skimmed milk, milk from diseased cows, milk from cows fed on decayed or unwholesome food, and milk drawn from a cow within fifteen days before or four days after calving. The state health department, perhaps as a result of these trips, began receiving milk samples from rural areas and small towns for analysis, and requests for copies of model milk ordinances poured in. The St. Paul health commissioner addressed retail milk dealers, taking as his topic, "Death Lurks in the Dairy." [32]

Both state and St. Paul health officials were jubilant when, on April 17, 1899, the St. Paul City Council passed an ordinance to regulate the sale of milk in the city and to provide for the inspection of all cattle in herds which produced for sale in the city. There were the usual grumbles and cries of hardship, and for a time it looked as if dairymen were not going to apply for licenses under the terms of the ordinance. However, the testing program was begun. At the same time Minneapolis was compelling all who shipped milk into the city to have their cows tested. A few milkmen tried to evade testing by various tricks, but they soon were exposed.[33]

Until about 1904 most of the testing of dairy herds was confined to the Twin Cities and to areas in the southern portion of the state. At that time Duluth had 75 dairies and 1,065 cows, none of which had been tested for tuberculosis. These herds were tested as rapidly as personnel and finances would permit. With increased attention by dairy and food inspectors, by state public health officers, and by municipal health officials, the milk situation in Minnesota had improved radically by 1906. In that year only twenty-eight persons were convicted of selling adulterated milk and twenty-four of selling adulterated cream. These convictions were secured by the dairy and food commissioner. The number of convictions in counties and cities also decreased. Milk-producing farmers had learned, too, that the state health department was keeping a most watchful eye on quarantined homes that sent

[32] State Board of Health, *Biennial Reports*, 1901–02, pp. 222, 227; State Dairy and Food Commissioner, *Biennial Reports*, 1889–90, pp. 27, 28; *Pioneer Press*, July 29, 1897, February 5, 1899; Bracken to George B. Weiser, January 8, 1898, and to A. K. Norton, September 12, 1898, Minnesota Department of Health, St. Paul.

[33] St. Paul Common Council, *Proceedings*, 1899, pp. 109–112; *Pioneer Press*, April 18, 22, June 6, December 10, 1899; Norton to Bracken, May 31, 1899, Minnesota Department of Health, St. Paul.

milk to market. "It is reported to me," wrote Bracken to a farmer, "that you have had smallpox in your family and that during such time you have been sending milk to the creamery, that this has been the common custom in your township, that you are extremely careless in the methods of quarantine. They are set forth in the laws, a copy of which we send you today." It was also true, as indicated by numerous inspectors traveling throughout the state, that the old rule-of-thumb dairymen were being replaced by a new generation of creamery operators, who were erecting modern cement buildings and were learning improved sanitary methods. These men were, in general, eager to co-operate with authorities who wished to improve the quality of Minnesota's milk.[34]

Late in 1910 Bracken made two trips, one to Chicago and another to Toronto, to see for himself how those cities handled their milk supplies. He found that Chicago was not requiring the tuberculin test, but was depending solely upon pasteurization as a means of safeguarding its milk. He learned, too, that Chicago had not established any bacteriological standard for milk. A local ordinance, however, required that all milk sold in the city must be bottled. The city was being supplied with certified, inspected, and pasteurized milk, the certified milk selling at fifteen cents a quart and the inspected and pasteurized milk each at eight cents a quart. Distributing stations were unclean and bottles were being washed by hand and brush. "The place was hardly fit to be tolerated," said Bracken of one station he visited. Toronto's system was far better. There sterilizing rooms and a laboratory processed and protected more than five thousand gallons daily. All milk was delivered bottled with the exception of that which went to hotels and restaurants. A modern pasteurizing plant, running by continuous heater and intermittent holder, maintained milk at temperatures ranging from 142° to 148° F. for thirty minutes.[35] Bracken kept the most careful notes on his experiences, for he was anxious that Minnesota should develop a milk program equal to if not better than any in the nation.

H. A. Whittaker, director of the sanitation division of the state board, spearheaded the drive for sanitary milk standards. Until 1915, said Whittaker, milk production in Minnesota lacked adequate standards. He felt that only unified action on the part of federal, state, and

[34] State Dairy and Food Commissioner, *Biennial Reports*, 1903–04, p. 8; 1905–06, pp. 27, 36–64; Bracken to James Knott, May 14, 1907, Minnesota Department of Health, St. Paul.
[35] Bracken Papers, 2:218–227.

TOWARD BETTER FOOD AND DRINK 165

municipal governments could bring about a single standard for milk production. Therefore, in 1917 he approached the American Public Health Association with the problem, and a program of pasteurization standards gradually was developed. As a result of the activities of Chesley and Whittaker, a United State Public Health Service advisory board on milk sanitation was established, with Whittaker as its first chairman. The leadership of the Minnesota Department of Health in the field of sanitary milk thus is clearly established, and this department is said to be the first in the United States to consider pasteurization a public health engineering program on a par with sewage control and water pollution.[36]

Yet the mere fact that the Minnesota board had initiated a new public health approach did not mean that the state, in some magical fashion, automatically endorsed and put into operation pasteurization plants. At first Whittaker met with determined opposition from dairies, co-operative groups, and even consumers. He thought this reaction was due to ignorance and to the sturdy sense of independence which generally has marked the American businessman and farmer.[37] It was a delicate job, requiring infinite tact and diplomacy, to push a pasteurization program without making it too apparent that the state board actually was forcing an issue. The normal procedure, in those pioneer days of pasteurization, was to work with and through town officials and to co-operate with the private groups in a community that were agitating for better milk. The board has always believed that it must keep the friendly support of municipal officers. On the other hand, it has always been ready to give information to nonofficial groups interested in clean milk.

Among the strongest supporters of sanitary milk were women's clubs. Mrs. Daniel Coonan, chairman of the public welfare department of the Minnesota Federation of Women's Clubs, in 1925 issued a carefully drawn statement to each member group. This pointed out that only about a hundred of the six hundred municipalities in Minnesota had local milk ordinances and said that dangers associated with impure milk — tuberculosis, typhoid fever, dysentery, scarlet fever, diphtheria, septic sore throat — could be eliminated only by effective supervision of milk supplies. Mrs. Coonan then enumerated the services that the state health department would give local clubs: it would make surveys,

[36] Interview of the author with Whittaker, March 18, 1948.
[37] Interview of the author with Whittaker, March 17, 1948; Whittaker, "The Control of Milk Pasteurization in the Smaller Cities of Minnesota," in *Journal-Lancet*, 40:45–47 (January 15, 1920).

at the request of local officials, to determine the actual sanitary condition of any municipal milk supply, would furnish model ordinances on request to any city or village, and would issue literature.[38]

Under the inspiration of Mrs. Willard Bayliss, president of the federation, a silver loving cup was to be given to the district reporting the largest number of new, working milk ordinances before September, 1927. In addition, the clubs actively and successfully campaigned for legislative appropriations for the division of sanitation, so that its staff might be enlarged and its services increased. Through their members they enlisted the support of the state dairy and food commissioner, the State Live Stock Sanitary Board, the University of Minnesota, and the League of Minnesota Municipalities. Clubs arranged milk exhibits, raised money for traveling expenses of a milk sanitarian, and constantly kept after local authorities to adopt milk ordinances.[39]

The Hennepin County Medical Society established a special milk commission to work with the state department and to lend its support to Minnesota's women in their campaign for clean milk. Innumerable local health officers, like Duluth's commissioner, indicated that citizens were eager to start a solution of the milk question in the proper way. Beginning in 1910, Duluth officials became most anxious to see that local dairymen produced either "certified" or "inspected" milk. Eventually, of course, Duluth was to change to pasteurization.[40]

Opposition to pasteurization could be forceful, particularly on the part of legislators. "I note that you contemplate urging the passage of a bill providing for pasteurization of milk throughout the whole State," wrote Senator Joseph M. Hackney. "I wonder if you have thought of the result of such a law. In my judgment, the farmer would have no show for he could not afford to pasteurize his milk. This would result in the large centralizers doing most of the business, but this is not the meat of the nut: pasteurization of milk does no good unless it is pasteurized just before it is used or is properly conveyed from the pasteurization plant to the consumer. To pasteurize milk in the

[38] Minnesota Federation of Women's Clubs, "Campaign for Clean, Safe Milk for Every Community," 1926 (typescript), Minnesota Department of Health, Minneapolis.
[39] Minnesota Federation of Women's Clubs, Department of Public Welfare, "Report," 1927 (typescript), and "Questionnaire," 1927; Whittaker to Mrs. Daniel Coonan, November 8, 1926; A. J. Chesley, "Safe Milk for Minnesota Children," May 2, 1927 (radio script). Minnesota Department of Health, Minneapolis.
[40] Lester W. Day to Chesley, November 13, 1905; Bracken to Tuohy, December 22, 1910, to Olin W. Rowe, February 27, 1912, to Paul E. Taylor, July 19, 1912, and to E. L. Cheney, August 20, 1914. Minnesota Department of Health, Minneapolis.

country and ship it into the city would do no good as its contamination would occur after it was pasteurized as much as before." [41]

Despite such criticism, higher milk standards were on the way. Winona was among the first of Minnesota's smaller cities to drive steadfastly ahead, with the co-operation of the state health department, and to secure a clean public milk supply. It is probable that it was Minnesota's first city to have state certified milk. The story began in June, 1908, when Winona passed an ordinance providing for the inspection of milk, cream, dairies, and dairy herds. A municipal veterinarian was employed for the purpose. At the same time the city instituted an educational program designed to acquaint its citizens with the dangers of dirty milk and the need for clean milk. Commercial groups later offered prizes for clean dairies and for those showing the greatest improvement within a specified time. All cows furnishing milk to Winona were given the tuberculin test.[42] Inspectors from the state dairy and food commissioner's office were invited to check barns and herds, while members of the staff of the state health department were asked to make bacteriological counts in order to check field inspections. Results showed that "in most instances unusual precautions are being taken to eliminate bacteria from the milk" and that "dairies are fast approaching an ideal in the way of construction and cleanliness." In 1916 Winona secured the services of a local bacteriologist to make milk counts, and about the same time the editor of the *Winona Independent* asked Bracken for a statement to encourage local residents toward an even more progressive milk program. That Winona's efforts were unusual is apparent in Bracken's reply: "It has been very gratifying to this board to find a municipality taking such active measures to improve the public milk supply. This has been especially true of the city of Winona. . . . The local officials under whose direction this campaign has been carried on deserve a great deal of credit and the support of the public at large." That, for Bracken, was an exceptionally gracious and enthusiastic compliment. Early in 1917 Winona began distributing certified milk.[43]

[41] Hackney to Bracken, November 2, 1912, Minnesota Department of Health, Minneapolis.

[42] State Board of Health, "Quarterly Reports," September 30, 1914, p. 13; Bracken to R. H. Mullin, June 19, 1914. Minnesota Department of Health, Minneapolis.

[43] Division of Sanitation, "Report on the Milk Supply of Winona — Especially in Relation to the Bacterial Count," August, 1914, p. 30, and "Memorandum on Visit to Winona to Confer with Local Officials Regarding Bacteriological Counts on the City Milk Supply, February 12, 1916" (typescripts); F. W. De Guire to Bracken, April 14, 1916, Bracken to De Guire, April 18, 1916, and H. F. White to Whittaker, February 13, 1917, Minnesota Department of Health, Minneapolis. For descriptions and ratings of Minneapolis dairy farms, see the *Tribune*, November 12, 1913.

The term "certified milk" first was used by the Essex County Milk Commission in New Jersey and was copyrighted by the commission. The term was applied to milk that, generally speaking, was produced carefully and cleanly. A dairyman, wishing to produce certified milk under regulations of the Minnesota Department of Health, had to make the following agreements:

(1) That I will have my herd tuberculin tested annually by the Minnesota State Livestock Sanitary Board, and that I will not add any animal to my herd until it has been found free from tuberculosis, as shown by the tuberculin test made by the Minnesota State Livestock Sanitary Board. I further agree to notify the State Board of Health, in writing, within twenty-four hours after an animal from an outside source has been added to my herd.

(2) That I will not allow any persons to engage in milking or handling the milk or utensils until such persons have been examined by the State Board of Health and found to be free from communicable diseases. That I will notify the State Board of Health, by letter, within twenty-four hours, upon the appearance of any communicable disease, or suspected communicable disease, among any of the employees of the dairy.[44]

But that was not all. Before Winona could begin selling certified milk, dairies supplying that milk had to meet other requirements, among them proper location of privies and uniform methods of handling the product from stables to cooling rooms. Winona, however, was not content to stop there. A movement for pasteurization was begun, and in 1919 the Springdale Dairy Company and the Hardwick Milk Company could announce a pasteurized product.[45] Three years later the Winona City Council passed an ordinance providing that after October 1, 1922, all milk sold in the city must be pasteurized.

With Winona setting the pace, the better-milk movement went forward rapidly in Minnesota. To further the work, the state board added Dr. R. W. Archibald, former dairy inspector for the city of Winona, to its staff, and equipped a traveling field laboratory. Surveys were made of many dairies, some of which listed as many as seventeen recommendations for the improvement of milk supplies. The board also investigated the milk supply of the State Hospital for the Insane at St. Peter, making seven recommendations to assure a sanitary program. The division of sanitation set up an elaborate educational plan

[44] State Board of Health, "Application for Permit to Produce Certified Milk," Minnesota Department of Health, Minneapolis.
[45] State Board of Health, "Rules and Orders Pertaining to Certified Dairies, 1924"; M. J. Sexton to Whittaker, June 14, 1919. Minnesota Department of Health, Minneapolis.

to create public interest in municipal milk supplies, to survey supplies, to recommend improvements, to assist in framing ordinances, and to conduct follow-up investigations. Surveys included a study of dairy farms, milk depots, methods of transportation and distribution, and pasteurization plants, and analytical examinations of milk covering its successive stages from producer to consumer. The educational program consisted of illustrated lectures and the distribution of literature. The engineering section of the American Public Health Association was called upon for advice and guidance.[46]

Two points were hammered home constantly by Whittaker and his associates. The first defined pasteurized milk and the other insisted that the milk supply of a city is a municipal problem and must be controlled largely by municipal authorities. Pasteurized milk was defined as "natural cow's milk which has been subjected to a temperature of not less than 145 degrees F. for 30 minutes and immediately thereafter cooled to a temperature of 50 degrees F. or lower." In December, 1919, a University of Minnesota short course for operators of pasteurization plants, believed to be the first of its kind in the nation, was given on the St. Paul campus. The course made invalid the excuse given by plant owners that there was no place where operators could receive training, and it opened possibilities of future licensing of operators.[47]

By 1920 Chisholm was planning for pasteurization, and a total of about fifty pasteurization plants were in operation throughout the state. "Practically all the pasteurization plants outside of the Twin Cities have complied with the recommendations of the Division [of Sanitation] so far as their equipment is concerned; this has brought about the elimination of many mechanical defects," reported the state health department. "The municipalities are beginning to appreciate the importance, from a health point of view, while the plant owners see the commercial significance of placing pasteurized milk on a stable basis that will mean something to the consumer."[48]

[46] State Board of Health, Division of Sanitation, "Quarterly Reports," June 30, 1917, p. 5, March 31, 1919; Division of Sanitation, "Report on Certified Milk Supply from the Spirit Hill Dairy Farm at Jordan, Minnesota, November 19, 1917," and "Investigation of Milk Supply: State Hospital for the Insane at St. Peter, December 7, 1917" (typescripts); Bracken to Mrs. E. C. Gran, November 2, 1917. Minnesota Department of Health, Minneapolis.
[47] "How a City May Obtain a Safe Milk Supply," in *Minnesota Municipalities*, 4:111 (August, 1919); State Board of Health, Division of Sanitation, "Quarterly Reports," December 31, 1919, p. 7.
[48] E. H. Nelson to Whittaker, January 26, 1920, and U.S. Department of Agriculture, Dairy Division, "Recommendations to the Board of Health, Chisholm, Minnesota, March 10, 1920" (typescript), Minnesota Department of Health, Minneapolis; State Board of Health, Division of Sanitation, "Quarterly Reports," September 30, 1920, p. 5.

The situation was just a little different in Duluth and the Twin Cities. Opposition developed in these communities along several lines. First, installation of pasteurization machinery was expensive for operators; second, many dairymen had made desperate efforts to produce certified milk and did not believe further efforts were necessary; in the third place, there was a not-unusual public belief that heat destroyed the "good, old" taste of milk; and, in the fourth instance, some physicians believed that pasteurization destroyed the vitamins in milk. An investigation of the milk supply of St. Paul in 1923 revealed that five per cent of the cows within the city limits had tuberculosis and that six per cent of those outside the city were similarly infected. Some St. Paul plants were pasteurizing, but the state department said that "the present method of supervising the pasteurization of milk has no value from a health point of view" and added that "no chemical, physical, or bacteriological examinations of samples of milk have been made by the Health Department during the past six months." Two years earlier, about the time when the state department had held a conference with health officers of Duluth, Minneapolis, and St. Paul regarding the control of pasteurization plants, a Hennepin County grand jury reported that Minneapolis was obtaining defective milk from unclean pasteurization plants and recommended an amendment to the city ordinance which would result in giving Minneapolis a milk supply approved by the state board.[49]

Floyd B. Olson, Hennepin County attorney, said that the findings indicated that "a relatively small number of concerns sell and distribute most of the milk supplied to the milk consumers of the city; that these concerns are united in an association, so-called, and act more or less unitedly on matters affecting their respective businesses; that by reason thereof they should be able to standardize the conditions under which milk is handled and distributed, so as to use the highest degree of care in providing pure milk to the milk consumers of the city; that the highest degree of care is not used in that respect, but on the contrary a considerable quantity of milk ultimately consumed by residents of the city is handled by these distributors in an unsanitary manner: . . . plants . . . unclean . . . machinery defective; bottles

[49] J. D. Shearer to Whittaker, February 23, 1920, Chesley to E. W. Fahey, March 9, 1921, and State Board of Health, Division of Sanitation, "Certain Information Regarding the Milk Supply of St. Paul, January, 1923" (typescript), Minnesota Department of Health, Minneapolis; Whittaker, "The Pasteurization of Milk," in *Minnesota Medicine*, 7:681 (October, 1924); *Minneapolis Journal*, April 20, 1921; *Minnesota Daily Star* (Minneapolis), 1921.

and cans . . . not thoroughly cleaned; . . . employees handling milk . . . garbed in dirty clothing; and that on the whole the gaining of profits in the handling of milk is too primary a consideration rather than the health interests of the community. . . . that Minneapolis has the lowest standards for the pasteurization of milk of any municipality in the State of Minnesota" [50]

Reaction was swift, and Minneapolis was assured a lower bacteria count in both raw and pasteurized milk by an ordinance passed in 1922. Because of the reluctance of Dr. Francis E. Harrington, Minneapolis health commissioner from 1919 until 1944, to co-operate with the state department, Minneapolis as late as 1928 did not require that milk for pasteurization be produced from cows which had been tested and found free from tuberculosis. The Minneapolis ordinance permitted for raw milk on its delivery to the consumer a bacterial count of 200,000 per cubic centimeter. The recommendations of the Minnesota Department of Health, the State Department of Dairy and Food, the State Live Stock Sanitary Board, the Agricultural College of the University of Minnesota, and the League of Minnesota Municipalities called for not more than 50,000 bacteria per cubic centimeter. The Minneapolis ordinance permitted a bacterial count of 2,000,000 per cubic centimeter for milk to be pasteurized, while the state health board said that "no milk having a bacterial count of over 250,000 should be used for pasteurization." [51]

There was real reason, of course, why sanitary experts should wish to keep the bacteria content of milk down. A low bacterial count is not in itself an index of either the purity or the healthful condition of milk, but it is an indication of the degree of care used in the production and handling of it. Dr. Charles H. Mayo was a firm advocate of a low bacterial count, just as he was a stanch believer in pasteurization. "I am of the opinion," he said in a privately printed booklet, "that pasteurization is the only known treatment which adequately serves the purpose for which it was intended, namely, that of destroying germ cells without materially reducing the food properties. I do not contend that pasteurization will make unclean milk clean. I do contend, however, and can prove by the records, that pasteurization will and does make unsafe milk safe." Mayo had had long experience with

[50] Olson to Chesley, May 26, 1921, Minnesota Department of Health, Minneapolis.
[51] *Journal*, March 26, 1922; H. A. Whittaker, "Notes," [1921] (pencil memorandum), and Harvey Walker to Mrs. H. J. Bessesen, February 7, 1928, Minnesota Department of Health, Minneapolis.

the milk problem. As health officer of Rochester, he once had carried on a strenuous fight to secure the adoption of a pasteurization ordinance.[52]

The Minnesota Department of Health discontinued the certification of milk on July 1, 1930, after nearly thirty years of that service, because it felt that it no longer could assume responsibility for a safe supply unless milk was pasteurized before it was distributed to consumers. The public, too, was beginning to demand pasteurized products, believing rightly that the heat of pasteurization did destroy disease-producing bacteria and that milk thus treated was safer for both adults and children. The influence of the United States Public Health Service in endorsing pasteurization and in drawing up a model milk ordinance also helped the cause. To supplement this, the Minnesota board issued its own pasteurization requirements, showed how the regulations applied to various types of plants, and issued booklets explaining what constituted good milk. The report of the committee on milk supply of the American Public Health Association was distributed widely to local officials with the recommendation that health officers support vigorously effective control over pasteurization.[53]

In addition, an intensive campaign was undertaken to solve the problem of creamery waste disposal. Hundreds of creameries and butter and cheese factories throughout the state were creating nuisances by the manner in which they rid their plants of wastes. Finally, however, the division of sanitation, as the result of working with individual plants and municipalities, was able to encourage the installation of machinery adequate to care for waste in a sanitary manner. When in 1943 federal funds were being used to construct a milk-processing plant at Browersville, the state board consulted with the engineers to insure the adequate disposal of the plant waste and, to explain its action, wrote the War Production Board that it "has long been recognized in Minnesota that no public agency, person or corporation has any right

---

[52] Mayo, *Pasteurization — the Best Known of Treatments for Milk*, [2, 3], (St. Paul, 1925); Helen Clapesattle, *The Doctors Mayo*, 479 (Minneapolis, 1941).
[53] State Board of Health, "Minutes," April 30, 1929; Chesley to McC. Fischer, October 2, 1934, Minnesota Department of Health, Minneapolis; Minnesota Department of Health, *Milk in Its Relation to Public Health*, 5 (St. Paul, May, 1932), *Milk Ordinance Recommended by the United States Public Health Service, 1939* (St. Paul, 1940), *Requirements for the Pasteurization of Milk* (March, 1930), *Pasteurization of Milk: Regulation 204 and Its Application to the Most Usual Types of Plants* (St. Paul, June, 1942), *Safe Milk* (St. Paul, August, 1943), and *Sanitary Code for the Production of Milk and Cream* (St. Paul, 1944); American Public Health Association, Committee on Milk Supply, "Report," in *American Journal of Public Health*, 17:367–379 (April, 1927).

to pollute the waters of the state and no state agency has any authority to grant them permission to do so." [54]

The double-barreled campaign to decrease the unsanitary disposal of waste and to increase the amount of pasteurized milk began to bear results during the 1930s. Minnesotans were reported to be consuming 88,733 gallons of pasteurized milk and 19,252 gallons of raw milk daily in 1930. In the Twin Cities, ninety-one per cent of the milk was pasteurized. In 1933, 107,591 gallons of milk and cream were pasteurized and consumed daily, and the proportion of the entire state's population using pasteurized milk was forty-two per cent.[55]

As cleaner, safer milk appeared on the market, the number of cases of milk-borne disease were fewer than in the quarter century beginning in 1875. But they have not disappeared. Between 1911 and 1930 there were 57 outbreaks of typhoid fever involving 694 cases traced to milk; 1 outbreak of diphtheria with 105 cases; 4 outbreaks of scarlet fever with 154 cases; and 40 outbreaks of undulant fever with 43 cases.[56] Four milk-borne epidemics occurred in Minneapolis alone in 1926, caused by the use of infected milk from unsupervised raw-milk dairies. In 1941 an outbreak of gastroenteritis at Pioneer Hall on the University of Minnesota campus resulted in specific recommendations by the state health department for changes in the handling of milk and milk products. Two years later an epidemic of milk-borne septic sore throat at Forest Lake apparently was traced to a single raw-milk dairy. Acting on the advice of the state health department, the dairy installed a pasteurizing plant.[57]

[54] Whittaker to H. B. Hommon, July 23, 1919; Charles E. Smith, Jr., to Rupert Blue, July 28, 1919; Chesley to H. S. Cumming, March 1, June 22, 1921, and to War Production Board, July 23, 1943; Division of Sanitation to Charles Foster, July 15, 1943. Minnesota Department of Health, Minneapolis.

[55] Minnesota Department of Health, "Milk Memorandum on Consumption in Minnesota, August, 1930"; Whittaker to Leslie C. Frank, March 22, 1933. Minnesota Department of Health, Minneapolis.

[56] Minnesota Department of Health, Division of Preventable Diseases, "Data on Outbreaks of Communicable Diseases Traced to Milk in Minnesota, 1911–January, 1930" (typescript), Minnesota Department of Health, Minneapolis; Minneapolis Health Department, *Monthly Bulletin*, 1:1–4 (April, 1918). For a discussion of the importance of milk in the spread of communicable disease, see A. J. Chesley, "To What Extent Does Milk Contribute to the Dissemination of Communicable Diseases?" a speech delivered at Duluth on August 14, 1923 (typescript), Minnesota Department of Health, Minneapolis.

[57] Chesley to Mrs. Coonan, January 19, 1927, and to A. J. Poirer, January 20, 1943; F. J. Kilpatrick to McDaniel, October 8, 1943; Minnesota Department of Health, Division of Sanitation, "Report on the Investigation of the Source and Handling of Milk and Milk Products at Pioneer Hall, University of Minnesota, Minneapolis, Minnesota, December 19, 1941" (typescript). Minnesota Department of Health, Minneapolis.

In 1945 two hundred and fifty recognized pasteurization plants — seventeen located in the Twin Cities — were operating and were rated according to methods recommended by the United States Public Health Service. The following year twelve municipalities were operating under the United States Public Health Service milk ordinance; eight had rating ordinances; and twenty-five had one hundred per cent pasteurization ordinances. In 1945 control of pasteurization plants passed from the Minnesota Department of Health to the State Department of Agriculture, Dairy, and Food. The act of 1945 authorized the latter department to regulate pasteurization plants, prohibited the sale of mislabeled milk or of milk not meeting requirements, set a maximum allowable bacterial count per cubic centimeter of 30,000 for Grade A pasteurized milk and 50,000 for Grade A raw milk, and made provision for the establishment of production standards. The State Live Stock Sanitary Board administers a program for the control and elimination of tuberculosis and brucellosis. A most comprehensive survey of the relationship of milk to federal, state, and municipal governments was published as a joint enterprise in 1948. It says truly that "a well organized milk control program and proper pasteurization can make milk-borne disease a thing of the past for all practical purposes." In 1949 the legislature passed a state-wide pasteurization act.[58]

Meat and milk were not, of course, the only foods receiving the attention of health officials in order to protect the public. During the 1870s, when railroad refrigeration cars first began bringing perishable fruits and vegetables into the state, there was serious discussion concerning the healthfulness of those products. Controversy developed even over the use of ice in drinking water, and the purity of natural ice long was a matter for debate. Tobacco was sent to Hewitt for analysis, and requests were made that the board examine cigarettes. One of the duties of the dairy and food commissioner was the investigation of liquor dispensed in Minnesota. Physicians requested that the state health board assume the control of biologicals, and a private citizen once wrote Hewitt: "Please I would like to have this Medicine

[58] Minnesota Department of Health, Division of Sanitation, "Rating of the Milk Pasteurization Plants of Minnesota Exclusive of the Twin Cities, April 13, 1945" and "Municipality Ordinances, January, 1946" (typescripts), Minnesota Department of Health, Minneapolis; Minnesota, *Laws*, 1945, chapter 384; 1949, chapter 403; League of Minnesota Municipalities, *A Program of Municipal Milk Control for Minnesota*, 4 (Minneapolis, May, 1948). See State Board of Health, *Reports*, 1922–43, p. 97, for a discussion of brucellosis in Minnesota.

Analysed an let me no if there is any Thing in it to cause blood Poison." [59]

So intense was the opposition of dairymen to butter substitutes, particularly oleomargarine, that they argued their case on a public health basis. Substitutes were said to be adulterated food and hence detrimental to the health of the citizen. The law of 1885 creating the office of dairy commissioner also prohibited the manufacture or sale of oleomargarine or any other article designed to take the place of butter or cheese made from pure milk. As a result, inspectors for some years afterwards were busy seizing shipments of butter substitutes and securing convictions. The introduction of canned and packaged goods to take the place of bulk commodities made possible a score of threats against public health. Adulterated baking powder, containing ammonia and alum in excessive amounts, was said to be poisonous and eventually was prohibited by law. During the 1890s vinegar, flavorings, and a score of spices were confiscated and found to contain deleterious ingredients. By 1905 the Minnesota code had developed to such a degree that the average citizen was well protected against adulterated foods. A year later the federal Congress passed a pure food and drugs act, which was given additional strength in 1911 by an amendment forbidding misleading labels on medicines. These acts greatly strengthened Minnesota's fight against fraud.[60]

[59] *St. Paul Daily Press*, August 21, 1873; *Minneapolis Tribune*, June 2, 5, 1875, June 11, 1880; *St. Paul Dispatch*, August 13, 1875; *Pioneer Press*, July 7, 1877, July 6, 1878, July 6, 1890; J. S. Kilbride to Bracken, January 28, 1900, J. Landenberger to Hewitt, November 26, 1892, Bracken to J. B. McGaughey, April 30, 1897, O. E. Linjer to Hewitt, January 18, 1895, and Walter McNollen to Hewitt, July 10, 1896, Minnesota Department of Health, St. Paul. For reports of analyses of liquor, see State Dairy and Food Commissioner, *Biennial Reports*, 1889–90, pp. 303–309.

[60] *Pioneer Press*, February 26, March 28, 29, November 6, 1891, January 13, 15, 1892, November 9, 1893, April 9, 1894; State Dairy and Food Commissioner, *Biennial Reports*, 1893–94, pp. 102–116; 1895–96, pp. 13–15; 1917–18, pp. 36, 37; Minnesota, *Laws*, 1905, p. 192.

10

Moving Toward Modernity

FOLLOWING Bracken's resignation in 1919, Dr. Charles E. Smith was appointed secretary of the State Board of Health. Smith had served as assistant secretary and was fully conversant with the health department's expanding program. He was well aware of the difficulties occasioned by World War I, when the department was operating with reduced personnel and, at the same time, was attempting to carry on normal activities. Smith also had taken part in the attempts to control the war-time influenza epidemic, which had snuffed out the lives of both civilians and soldiers. He had interested himself in the creation, in 1918, of a division of venereal diseases, and had served for a time as temporary director of a newly created division of tuberculosis. In 1919 his work was complicated by an outbreak of forest fires.[1]

Unfortunately Smith was a sick man when he became executive secretary of the board. His new duties, during one of the board's most critical periods, finally proved too arduous, and in October, 1920, he took sick leave with the hope that temporary residence in the South would enable him to regain his health. He failed to improve, however, and shortly after returning to Minnesota he died. Meanwhile, on May 3, 1921, Chesley was named secretary. His selection seemed only natural.

The appointment of Chesley marked the beginning of a modern era in Minnesota public health work. He was a man well known locally, and he had already earned both a national and an international reputation. Connected with the Minnesota department for many years, he had served in a variety of capacities and had been fortunate enough to work with both Wesbrook and Hill. Indeed, he once said that he

[1] State Board of Health, *Biennial Reports*, 1918–19, pp. 7–11.

MOVING TOWARD MODERNITY 177

learned more from Hill than from any other single individual in the department.[2] Chesley's epidemiological training and experience made him an ideal person to supervise relief work abroad during World War I. In 1919 he was appointed by the American Red Cross to help the impoverished and sick of France and Poland.

The Red Cross Commission to Poland, of which he was a member with the assimilated rank of major, arrived in Warsaw on March 3, 1919. Chesley was attached to the Department of the East, a district of about six thousand square miles containing nearly three million persons. It was estimated that some thirty to fifty thousand cases of typhus were present in his district. As chief of staff, Chesley planned the attacks on this disease. Through his program food, clothing, and medical care, which included bathing, hair clipping, and delousing, were provided. In May he was put in charge of work at the front, which meant taking care of the more than three thousand refugees a day who were seeping through the lines.

Three active units comprised the Department of the East. Each was composed of a staff of about twenty-five persons, including one doctor, two nurses, a clerk, a mechanic, nurses' aids, sanitary men, and general "cleaners up." Mechanical equipment consisted of rolling field kitchens, sterilization outfits, and tractors. Whenever possible, the commission utilized equipment abandoned by the Germans. When Chesley became head of the commission, with the assimilated rank of lieutenant colonel, headquarters and warehouses for the Department of the East were established at Bialystok. A laboratory also was set up to meet urgent calls for vaccines against typhoid, paratyphoid, and cholera. Chesley's next step was the division of eastern Poland into three sections, so that relief work might be better organized. In co-operation with the minister of health, the commission made surveys of public water supplies in the cities of eastern Poland and Galicia. The Lyster bag was introduced for field work in the Polish Army, and the commission took charge of the water supply when Kiev was occupied, thus guarding the city against a threatened cholera epidemic.[3]

These experiences in France and Poland, as well as his thorough knowledge of public health problems, gave Chesley a distinguished background for the work in store for him in Minnesota. Possessed of great energy and enthusiasm, he began his new duties with vigor. Shortly after becoming secretary, he outlined the work of the depart-

[2] Interview of the author with Chesley, June 27, 1946.
[3] American National Red Cross, *Annual Reports*, 1919, p. 123; 1920, p. 103.

ment, saying that "changes for the better in living conditions among civilized people and the scientific discoveries applied in medicine and public health . . . are truly marvelous." But, he added, the main factors in the public health problem in 1922 were about the same as they had been in 1872. He thought, as had Hewitt, that one-fourth of Minnesota's sickness might be prevented "by the active, intelligent use of sanitary measures by local authorities through local boards of health." [4]

In his first report as secretary, Chesley indicated clearly that his administration was to forge ahead and not be bound entirely by the traditional pattern set by his predecessors. He called for extension of public health work into the fields of public health education, child hygiene, and industrial hygiene. "Some day," he predicted when speaking of child care, "the people will realize that every mother must be taught how to keep her children well. Then appropriations will be granted for public health education and to protect children under school age from preventable sickness and death." [5]

Administratively, the department was organized into the five divisions of records, vital statistics, preventable diseases, venereal diseases, and sanitation. Smith's administration had included a division of tuberculosis, an educational agent, and a superintendent of nurses. These had been either merged or discontinued altogether by Chesley. Oscar C. Pierson directed the division of records, which numbered among its duties the distribution of antitoxin, the licensing of embalmers and of rendering plants, and the handling of nuisance complaints. His wife, Gerda C. Pierson, was director of the division of vital statistics, a steadily growing department concerned primarily with the registration of births and deaths. She saw to it that monthly transcripts were sent to the United States Bureau of the Census. "These statistics," wrote Mrs. Pierson early in Chesley's administration, "constitute the foundation on which to base public health work, and are valuable in proportion to their accuracy and completeness. Complete and accurate morbidity statistics of preventable diseases constitute one of the pillars on which public health work rests, while for final and permanent study, nothing can take the place of birth and death registration." [6]

[4] Chesley, "How Minnesota Protects Her People," in *Health*, [2]:21 (October, 1922).
[5] State Board of Health, *Biennial Reports*, 1920–21, p. 9.
[6] State Board of Health, *Biennial Reports*, 1920–21, p. 36. For a study on gathering vital statistics and a survey of the records available, see Works Progress Administration, Minnesota Historical Records Survey Project, *Guide to Public Vital Statistics Records in Minnesota* (St. Paul, 1941).

McDaniel was director of the division of preventable diseases, and E. Marion Wade was chief of the laboratories. Whittaker continued to head the division of sanitation, having as his sanitary engineers J. A. Childs and O. E. Brownell. The staff also included a bacteriologist. The division of venereal diseases was in charge of Dr. H. G. Irvine, a pioneer worker in the field who was to achieve a national reputation. He was assisted by a staff of four, among them a field physician and bacteriologist, a social hygiene supervisor, and a chief social worker.

Chesley's key staff members, including the directors of divisions, numbered fifteen in 1921. They were almost all experts in their fields, and together they constituted one of the most forward-looking health departments in the United States. Their policy, as in early days, was to co-operate with local health officers as far as possible, and only in rare instances would they carry an issue over the heads of town councils or village health officials. The bulk of the duties performed by the department centered about epidemiological field work, laboratory analyses, and sanitary surveys, including the investigation of both water and milk. The extent of epidemiological field work is clearly apparent, for example, in 1921, when 331 investigations were carried out. These involved 341 sanitary districts located in 76 counties and required 42,334 miles of travel by railway and 13,843 miles by automobile.[7] The diseases investigated were poliomyelitis, epidemic meningitis, tuberculosis, typhoid fever, dysentery, diarrhea, scarlet fever, smallpox, and chicken pox.

The large number of investigations led Chesley to suggest a change in the reporting of rare and unusually dangerous diseases. In 1913 the board had passed a regulation requiring that certain diseases listed be reported directly to the department by telephone or telegraph. The list was amended on July 12, 1921, to include, among others, botulism, epidemic encephalitis, and epidemic jaundice. In addition, reportable diseases were divided into two groups, the first including those which must be reported within twenty-four hours by telegraph or telephone, and the second enumerating those which could be reported by mail. In the urgent category were such diseases as anthrax, cholera, septic sore throat, glanders, rabies, Rocky Mountain spotted fever, and typhus and yellow fever. The second list included dysentery, hookworm, leprosy, malaria, pellagra, and trichinosis.[8]

Another regulation provided that physicians report on special

[7] State Board of Health, *Biennial Reports*, 1920–21, p. 153.
[8] State Board of Health, *Biennial Reports*, 1920–21, p. 71.

postcards or blanks certain other diseases to local health officers, but not to the state department. These diseases included poliomyelitis, chicken pox, diphtheria, typhoid fever, and whooping cough. By 1948 rules for control measures and for reporting communicable diseases had become so extensive that they occupied some twenty-three pages of small type. Early in his career as secretary, Chesley urged upon physicians and parents the most careful reporting of contagious diseases. He seemed particularly anxious about measles and whooping cough, and he quoted a well-known statement: "No health department, state or local, can effectively prevent or control disease without knowledge of when, where and under what conditions cases are occurring."

Chesley pointed out that in 1927 only 5,618 cases of measles and 1,031 cases of whooping cough were reported. Sixty-five per cent of deaths from measles and ninety-seven per cent of fatalities from whooping cough occurred in children under five years of age. Continuing his argument, Chesley, relying mostly upon statistics, showed that the diphtheria death rate could be reduced if cases were reported and if diphtheria toxin-antitoxin was administered. He called for county-wide diphtheria immunization work through the co-operation of health officers, school authorities, family physicians, and parents. Regarding typhoid, he explained the work of the division of preventable diseases and the division of sanitation, both of which were concerned with typhoid carriers and with public water supplies and pasteurization plants.[9]

Chesley also listed the five leading causes of death in 1927. In their order of importance, these were heart disease, cancer, external causes, pneumonia, and tuberculosis.[10] This list was vastly different from lists compiled in an earlier day by Hewitt, who was concerned primarily with smallpox, typhoid, and diphtheria. It seemed as if the main fight against these earlier diseases was about concluded and that the department now could begin to turn its attention elsewhere. That, of course, is exactly what happened. Year by year, as contagious diseases were conquered or controlled, the degenerative diseases gained in importance. Heart disease became the leading cause of death in Minnesota for the first time in 1914, and continued to hold that position from then on, except in 1918 when, during the influenza epidemic, pneu-

[9] State Board of Health, *Biennial Reports*, 1920–21, p. 72, and *Minnesota State Health Laws and Regulations*, 54–77 (Minneapolis, 1948); Chesley, "Reportable Diseases in Minnesota," in *Minnesota Medicine*, 12:1–5 (January, 1929).
[10] Chesley, in *Minnesota Medicine*, 12:3 (January, 1929).

MOVING TOWARD MODERNITY   181

monia displaced it. Reasons for this change are not difficult to find: "First, improved control of the communicable diseases has been possible because of an increased interest and understanding of public health problems by the general public. Second, better equipped public health agencies with trained personnel are better able to aid in the control of disease outbreaks, advise on problems of environmental sanitation, and direct other preventive programs. Third, the aging of our population causes more of our people to be in those age groups where degenerative diseases are most apt to occur. Fourth, a better trained medical profession equipped with better diagnostic instruments can correctly diagnose a larger proportion of the degenerative conditions that do occur." [11]

As the decline of one disease has been followed by the emergence of another, new public health problems have arisen. The old-time activities of the epidemiologist have been subordinated more and more to the work of the clinician and the sanitary engineer. And, as decade followed decade, public health on the state level has been more and more identified with public health on a national scale.

Minnesota, in many instances through the active and diplomatic efforts of Chesley, became the recipient of federal funds with which to institute new programs or to carry on those already existing. In other instances, the aid was less direct. The health of the state's Indians, for example, is a joint responsibility.[12] The Venereal Disease Control Act of 1938 provided for the distribution of federal grants-in-aid to the states through the medium of the United States Public Health Service. Under the provisions of the Sheppard-Towner Act of 1921, federal funds were made available for a maternal and child welfare program, "providing such a program was conducted by an existing state department of health in accordance with plans approved by the Children's Bureau of the United States Department of Labor." Later the Social Security Act provided federal money for the same type of program.

[11] Minnesota Department of Health, "Thirty Years of Health Progress in Minnesota," dated March 4, 1941, in Minnesota State Medical Association, Speakers Library Service, *Thirty Years of Health Progress in Minnesota* (n.p., n.d.); Minnesota Department of Health, *Longer Lives* (St. Paul, 1939).

[12] For a general discussion of the role of the federal government, see United States Public Health Service, *Observations on Indian Health Problems and Facilities* (Bulletin 223 — Washington, D.C., 1936). A brief résumé of state agencies concerned with Indian welfare and their relations to federal agencies may be found in United States Senate, Committee on Indian Affairs, *Survey of Conditions of the Indians in the United States*, part 26, p. 14377 (Washington, D.C., 1932), which names the Minnesota State Board of Health as "the pioneer State agency to attempt cooperation with the Federal Government in the care of the Indian population."

The Sheppard-Towner Act also made possible the position of superintendent of nurses in the division of public health nursing. After the Social Security Act went into effect, it was possible to subsidize public health nursing services by either of two methods, one of them a direct money subsidy and the other a demonstration service.[13]

Under the Social Security Act, aid available annually to Minnesota, if all federal requirements were met, totaled $225,000. These funds were allocated for two purposes: First, they were to enable "each state to extend and improve as far as practicable under the conditions in such state services for promoting the health of mothers and children especially in rural areas and in areas suffering from severe economic distress." Second, they were to be used "in establishing and maintaining adequate public health service including the training of personnel for state and local health work." The allocation was to be made on the basis of population, special health problems, and financial needs. Money received under the first two headings had to be matched by the state, fifty per cent by existing funds and fifty per cent by new appropriations. Utilizing an allotment from these funds, the University of Minnesota expanded its training center for public health personnel.[14] Here physicians, engineers, and nurses from many states and from foreign countries come to attend the courses in public health given by the Department of Preventive Medicine and Public Health of the university in collaboration with the Minnesota Department of Health.

Chesley concerned himself also with a Civil Works Administration project which in 1934 established a nursing service to carry out a state program in child health as set up by the United States Children's Bureau. This project terminated on March 31, 1934, after a life of only a few months. The service was continued, however, by the State Emergency Relief Administration. In addition, the Works Progress Administration developed a nursing and housekeeping aid project

[13] State Board of Health, *Reports*, 1922–43, pp. 112, 158, 181; American Bar Association, Committee on Courts and Wartime Social Protection, *Venereal Disease Prostitution and War*, 5 (Washington, D.C., February, 1943); E. C. Hartley, *Sheppard-Towner Bill as Administered in Minnesota by the State Board of Health — Division of Child Hygiene* (reprinted from *Minnesota Medicine*, 6:442–445 — July, 1923); Edwin F. Daily, *Summary of Report on Maternal and Child-Health Services under Title V, Part 1, of the Social Security Act* (reprinted from *The Child*, 5:18–25 — July, 1940); United States Department of Labor, Children's Bureau, *Child-Welfare Services under the Social Security Act* (Publication 257 — Washington, D.C., 1940). Pages 46 and 47 of the last named reference contain a discussion of child welfare services in Minnesota.

[14] Chesley, *Federal Aid for Public Health Work in Minnesota*, 44, 45 (reprinted from *Minnesota Municipalities*, 22:44–47 — February, 1937).

MOVING TOWARD MODERNITY   183

which was sponsored by the state health department in 1936 and was discontinued in 1943.[15]

The federal government, also under the generous health provisions of the Social Security Act, made possible the establishment of a section of dental health education. Minnesota thus became the twenty-first state to introduce this type of activity. Following a policy advocated by the United States Public Health Service, the Minnesota State Dental Association in 1942 recommended a separate division of dental health. This division was created on July 17, "thus giving recognition to the fact that dentistry, like medicine and engineering, is a profession whose state-wide public health program should be administered by a member of the profession concerned." [16] Until 1943 funds for the division came entirely from federal sources.

The substantial financial assistance given Minnesota by the federal government for the furtherance of public health is indicated by appropriations for 1942–43. A total of $453,496 was received, of which $105,762 was earmarked for maternal and child health; $136,441 for venereal disease control; $208,293 for public health; and $3,000 for Indian nursing service. The grand total of income for the year 1942–43 amounted to $777,385, and the grand total of expenditures came to $764,134. Public health, indeed, had become big business, and Hewitt, who spent only $500 in 1872, would have been properly astonished.[17]

Hewitt would have been surprised also at the enlarged scope of health activities and at the change in the secretary's duties. Vast surveys of river pollution and complicated investigations of factory conditions had been unknown to him. He would have marveled at mobile X-ray units and a score of private and public social agencies which now were interesting themselves in Minnesota's health. He would have been interested, for example, in the co-operation of the division of dental health with the State Department of Education and other school authorities, with state and local welfare agencies, county welfare boards, and practicing dentists, with the School of Dentistry and the Department of Preventive Medicine and Public Health of the University of Minnesota, and with various state, district, and local organizations, including parent-teacher associations, mothers' clubs, and the American Legion Auxiliary.[18]

[15] State Board of Health, *Reports*, 1922–43, p. 188.
[16] State Board of Health, *Reports*, 1922–43, p. 190; American Dental Association, National Health Program Committee, *Dentistry and Government* (1940); "A Division of Dental Health," in *Northwest Dentistry*, 21:210 (October, 1942).
[17] State Board of Health, *Reports*, 1922–43, p. 294; *Annual Reports*, 1873, p. 19.
[18] State Board of Health, *Reports*, 1922–43, p. 191.

Hewitt's duties frequently had taken him into the field on routine or special investigations, but Chesley's work more and more took him into the committee room and to national conferences, where he gave his talents to getting things done unobtrusively. Hewitt could grasp every activity of the department in 1880, but in 1948 the duties of the department had become so complicated that a secretary could not begin to keep section and department details in mind. At one time Hewitt could sit at his desk and actually see the entire physical plant which housed practically all the activities of the department. The one room in which he labored had been expanded tremendously. In 1922 the executive office was located in the basement of the Capitol; in 1932 the executive and administrative offices and the division of vital statistics were moved from the Capitol to the new State Office Building. Other divisions of the health department occupied quarters in 1922 in the Psychology–State Board of Health Building on the University of Minnesota campus in Minneapolis. A few years later additional rooms were provided in Millard Hall. When expanding facilities made space too small, a five-story building was erected in 1938 on the Minneapolis campus.[19]

New and enlarged quarters both in St. Paul and Minneapolis afforded the department additional space and more modern facilities, but did nothing to decrease the amount of work that a growing state demanded. Chesley correctly pointed out that the "degree of public health" enjoyed varies according to time and place. Certainly Minnesota's over-all health program was stepped up considerably in the middle decades of the twentieth century. During the eight years from 1914 to 1921 the department's laboratories, for example, averaged somewhat more than 57,000 examinations a year. In 1938 examinations numbered 433,204, and in 1941 the war effort increased the laboratory work to 462,057 examinations, 63,865 of which were venereal disease examinations for selective service men. The total jumped again in 1942, when 644,003 examinations were made, of which 227,675 were concerned with draftees.[20]

The department first prepared and distributed typhoid vaccine in 1914 and later prepared a vaccine for preventing paratyphoid fever. From 1922 to 1941, inclusive, between 15,000 and 20,000 c.c. of vaccine were distributed annually in answer to from 250 to 300 requests. On three occasions, in 1927, 1935, and 1942, the increased demand for vaccine resulted in the distribution of 53,730 c.c., 41,010 c.c., and 72,520

---
[19] State Board of Health, *Reports*, 1922–43, p. 23.
[20] State Board of Health, *Reports*, 1922–43, pp. 24, 92.

c.c. of vaccine respectively. Poliomyelitis convalescent serum was first prepared and distributed in 1930. Later the department discontinued the distribution of this serum because its value could not be proved. But this was not all. Meningococcic serum was distributed in 1931, and each year up to 1938 from 6,000 to 12,000 c.c. were sent out. Every year since 1926 the board has made and distributed from 30,000 to 42,000 ampoules of silver nitrate as a prophylactic treatment for the eyes of the newborn.

Distribution of pneumonia serum was started in 1937, after it was found that over seventy-three per cent of patients with pneumonia due to types I, II, V, VII, and VIII could be helped by it. "The Division of Preventable Diseases," wrote Chesley, "will determine the type of pneumococcus in specimens submitted by physicians and also will check on 'typing' done in local laboratories. Prompt diagnosis and early administration of the correct serum according to the type of pneumococcus responsible for the case are essential. The therapeutic serum must be specific in character and to get results should be given before the end of the fourth day after onset of symptoms. To carry out the pneumonia program throughout the state the Board expects to develop local 'typing' services as soon as possible." Mantoux test material also was manufactured and distributed by the division of preventable diseases in 1937, and on July 1, 1943, this division took over the distribution of diphtheria biologics and smallpox vaccine. Pertussis vaccine also was made available for the immunization of children under two years of age, and pertussis hyperimmune serum for passive immunization of children under eighteen months.[21]

Tuberculosis has been one of the major disease problems of the State Board of Health ever since its founding in 1872. In that year thirteen per cent of all deaths were due to the pale killer. Building of sanatoriums for the isolation of open and infectious cases and thorough epidemiological investigation of those exposed to the disease have given the tuberculosis death rate a tremendous downward push. Today, with the mobile unit and mass X-ray of thousands of apparently healthy people, there is hope for an even more dramatic drop.

Among the special problems handled by the division of preventable diseases was the establishment of a trachoma clinic in Duluth in 1923 and the creation in 1937 of a Rockefeller influenza laboratory, which continued until 1942. Trachoma is a disease of the eye and is recognized when lids become inflamed and granular. The trachoma clinic

[21] Chesley, *Federal Aid for Public Health Work in Minnesota*, 46; State Board of Health, *Reports*, 1922–43, pp. 100–102.

resulted from a request by the St. Louis County Health Department for assistance. Chesley in turn asked the surgeon general of the United States Public Health Service for help. Officers of the public health service had previously made several surveys of trachoma prevalence in Minnesota. The most extensive had been in 1912–13, when, in three separate investigations, 52,847 people, both white and Indian, had been examined. The last survey, in 1922, covered 13,919 people in eleven counties. As a result, two surgeons were detailed to Minnesota, where they selected thirty-six cases from St. Louis County and two from Itasca County as suitable for operation. From September, 1924, to August, 1925, the United States Public Health Service, in co-operation with the St. Louis County Health Department, conducted a trachoma hospital at Eveleth which admitted 248 cases.[22]

The influenza laboratory, which Chesley was instrumental in developing, resulted from an arrangement entered into between the department and the international health division of the Rockefeller Foundation. Dr. Clara Nigg of the Rockefeller Institute became the bacteriologist in charge. The work included investigations of influenza outbreaks in the University of Minnesota, Carlton College, Willmar State Hospital, and other state and county institutions. In 1940 and 1941 a complex influenza A vaccine, prepared by the Rockefeller Foundation laboratory, was administered to 8,783 persons, most of whom were in state institutions. To secure a larger number of cases for laboratory study, an appeal was made to Minnesota physicians in December, 1942. In addition to the influenza laboratory, the division of preventable diseases was interested in the establishment of a virus laboratory for the study of equine encephalomyelitis, which was prevalent in Minnesota in 1941. The next year research was undertaken in pigeon psittacosis.[23]

One area of public health work which has expanded enormously since its legal inception in 1919 is public health nursing. The first state public health nurses were sent out by the Minnesota Public Health Association, and their primary concern was with tuberculosis. Two epidemics, poliomyelitis in 1916 and the influenza epidemic of 1918, necessitated the employment of nurses by the state board. Despite the 1919 law, which "makes possible the discovery of cases requiring attention which might otherwise be neglected with sad results, and gives rise to

[22] State Board of Health, *Reports*, 1922–43, pp. 105, 108; Chesley, "The Trachoma Problem in Minnesota," [1923] (typescript), Minnesota Department of Health, Minneapolis.
[23] State Board of Health, *Reports*, 1922–43, pp. 109–111.

MOVING TOWARD MODERNITY 187

the possibility of proper treatment," there was little development in this field until the creation of the division of child hygiene in 1922. Growth since then has been steady, except during the depression. In 1930 there were 216 public health nurses in 48 Minnesota counties, and by 1948 there were a total of 470, with 19 in Duluth, 81 in St. Paul, and 133 in Minneapolis.[24]

Meanwhile Chesley was faced with a series of problems resulting in part from the swift development of small communities after 1900 and in part from the increasing industrialization of certain sections of the state. The rapid rise of the city complicated his problems further. In addition, the department was facing a world whose tempo had accelerated because of new mechanics and a startling technological advance. The factory, filled with intricate machinery, might be a health menace not only from the viewpoint of industrial accidents, but also from that of ventilation, drinking fountains, and toilet facilities. But the problem was even broader and more fundamental than that. "Studies conducted in a number of industries," it was stated, "have shown a high incidence of certain diseases commonly considered as nonoccupational, such as tuberculosis, pneumonia, and the degenerative diseases. While it is true that much of the disease among wage earners is due to harmful dusts, vapors, fumes, chemicals, excessive temperatures, and faulty plant sanitation, yet we cannot disregard the effects of improper living conditions, hurry, strain, malnutrition, and communicable diseases." To meet these problems an industrial hygiene unit was formed in 1940, which in July, 1941, became the division of industrial health. The program was supported entirely by federal funds.[25] The modern hotel or apartment house, too, if its plumbing was not properly installed, could be the point of origin for disease. Hard roads and the automobile certainly altered the everyday living of Minnesotans, and the hundreds of fatalities and thousands of injuries caused each year

[24] Minnesota, *Laws*, 1919, p. 35; A. T. Laird, "Community Control of Tuberculosis," p. 3, a paper presented at a meeting of the Minnesota Public Health Association and the Minnesota State Sanitary Conference, Rochester, September 29, 1915 (typescript), Minnesota Department of Health, St. Paul; Mary A. Johnson, "Rural Public Health Nursing in Minnesota," in *Public Health Nursing*, 28:681–684 (October, 1936); Charles Bolsta, "The Certification of Public Health Nurses," in *Minnesota Public Health Nurse*, vol. 3, no. 5, p. 2 (May, 1930); E. C. Hartley, "An Outline of Rural P. H. Nursing in Minnesota," in *Minnesota Public Health Nurse*, vol. 3, no. 10, p. 2 (October, 1930); interview of the author with Anne Nyquist, August 9, 1948.

[25] Leslie W. Foker, "Minnesota's Industrial Health Program," in *Minnesota Medicine*, 25:970 (December, 1942), and "Health in Minnesota Industry," in Hennepin County Medical Society, *Bulletins*, 13:35 (April, 1942); Minnesota Department of Health, "Industrial Hygiene as a Function of the Department of Health" (typescript), Minnesota Department of Health, Minneapolis.

by automobile accidents have posed in a very real sense a public health problem. Sooner or later, all these things were bound to result in activity by Chesley's department.

For many years the state board, often reluctantly, had left major responsibility to local health officers. City and village boards of health were appointed by city and village councils. County health boards were appointed by the boards of county commissioners, and town boards, by the supervisors. All this seems reasonable at first glance, but, in actual practice, there was confusion over jurisdiction.[26] All too frequently the health officer was hampered either by lack of funds or by misunderstandings between him and town supervisors or county commissioners. This friction and lack of funds sometimes hindered not only the work of local health officers, but also the services of the state department. Although the state board could do little legally to alter the situation, it thought that it could, perhaps, relieve the condition in part.

Chesley felt that conditions might be improved if his department could be brought closer to the rural areas. Except for the Duluth laboratories, most of the board's services were concentrated in St. Paul and Minneapolis. When a township needed assistance, epidemiologists and engineers were dispatched to give what help they could and then they returned to the board's headquarters. This procedure, followed for many years, had worked reasonably well. But it also had its disadvantages. For one thing, it permitted of no consistent, over-all health policy, and for another, it usually operated only during emergencies or when a special problem arose which was beyond the ability of a local health officer to handle.

In an attempt to give Minnesota's rural areas consistent service, Chesley and his staff, following practice in other states, endorsed the idea of bringing several counties together into district health units. It was believed that such a program would be beneficial, because the board planned to staff each district with a public health physician as director and epidemiologist, a public health engineer, and a public health nurse who would serve in an advisory capacity to all public health nurses employed in the district. Such a staff was to be paid from public funds by the department and was to be responsible to the department. This plan, of course, actually meant the decentralization of the activities of the board. "The program," it was pointed out, was

[26] Oscar C. Pierson, "Powers and Duties of Township Boards of Health in Minnesota," in *Minnesota Medicine*, 22:390–394 (June, 1939).

"identical with the program conducted for the entire state by the Minnesota Department of Health, except that certain critical situations were to be referred to the central office for solution, and the districts depend entirely upon the laboratory facilities of the Department, none of them having laboratories of their own." [27]

On July 1, 1937, with financial aid from the federal government under the terms of Title VI of the Social Security Act, district health units were created in the northern and southern parts of the state. District 1, with headquarters at Bemidji, included the counties of Beltrami, Koochiching, and Itasca. This area was selected for experimental purposes because it was representative of northern Minnesota, containing iron mining, lumbering, small farms, and a large resort business. District 2, with headquarters at Mankato, served Jackson, Martin, Blue Earth, Freeborn, and Mower counties. District 4, consisting of St. Louis, Carlton, and Cook counties, was also created in 1937, with the St. Louis County health officer becoming the district health officer. By the end of 1942 four districts were in full operation, District 3, with headquarters at Rochester, having been established in the autumn of 1938. Eight districts were in operation in 1948. Although work varied in each district according to local problems, the activities of District 4 are fairly representative.

The staff planned for during 1945–46 in this district consisted of one nurse in Cook County, two nurses in Carlton County, and five in St. Louis County. In addition, there was an advisory nurse. A public health engineer and five clerk-stenographers completed the roll. This group was concerned with a generalized public health service, including communicable disease control, community X-ray surveys, venereal disease control, a maternity program, and an infant and preschool program. This meant the directing of expectant mothers to routine prenatal examinations and the examination and immunization of children against diphtheria, tetanus, and smallpox. Routine visits to newborns as early as possible were continued. A school hygiene program consisted of routine inspection of all beginners and all students in several grades. In order to relieve nurses, teachers were to be instructed in vision testing procedures and were to take heights and weights annually. The program also included work with crippled children, with special attention paid to all diagnosed and suspected cases of rheumatic fever. A home safety program was planned, with nurses attempting to give instruction in the prevention of domestic accidents.

[27] State Board of Health, *Reports*, 1922–43, p. 62.

As District 4 was without a public health physician, the services which he would have rendered were omitted.[28]

Although not all districts always operated in an ideal fashion, the plan seemed sufficiently successful for the department to continue it until the counties themselves could organize and finance districts of their own. Perhaps the major problem in the working of state districts was that of personnel, for lack of finances and the scarcity of public health physicians and engineers during the war years made it extremely difficult to fully staff each district. By 1947 the department felt that perhaps the time had come when counties could begin organizing their own districts, which would permit the state board gradually to diminish its districting program. But to accomplish this the legislature had to act.

On January 16, 1947, a bill was introduced in the Senate which would authorize counties to establish, or join in establishing, county or multiple-county health departments. Although it failed of enactment, the bill was one of the most progressive steps recommended in Minnesota for many years, and its provisions deserve mention. It defined a health department as one "organized and supported by one or more counties and employing qualified medical, nursing and other personnel under the direction of a full-time qualified health officer." It authorized any county or two or more adjacent counties, by resolution of their county boards, to establish a health department. It specifically excluded any city of the first or second class from coming under the jurisdiction of a county health department, but it also made provision for such municipalities to become identified with a county health department if they so desired. The bill stipulated further that every health department should be responsible to a local board of health and indicated how local board members should be appointed. Departments were to be operated and maintained from funds appropriated and fees collected within the counties, together with such state and federal funds and private grants as might be appropriated or granted. In the event that two or more counties co-operated to form a health department, the cost of maintenance was to be born jointly "on the basis of the ratio of the population of each such county to the total population served by the health department." Other sections provided for budgets, for regular meetings, for the employment as health officer of a doctor of medicine eligible to practice in Minnesota and having special training or experience in public health work, and for the issu-

[28] Leah M. Keable, "Work Plan for District Health Unit No. 4, July 1, 1945–June 30, 1946" (typescript), Minnesota Department of Health, Minneapolis.

MOVING TOWARD MODERNITY 191

ance of annual reports. The first subdivision of Section 8 stipulated that "Every health department created under this act, subject, however, to the general supervision of the state board of health, shall cause all laws and regulations relating to public health to be obeyed and enforced within its jurisdictional area." [29]

This bill, which, if passed, might have given Minnesota a more modern public health program, failed of enactment for several reasons. Although the Minnesota State Medical Association expressed itself officially in favor of it, it was said that St. Paul physicians privately were opposed to it. Some legislators from rural districts failed to support it because, although the bill did not carry an appropriation item, they felt that sooner or later the state might be asked to help support county health departments. It is possible also that those interested in its passage did not do sufficient preliminary work and that, as a result, neither the legislature nor the public really understood its intent. But Minnesota public health officials and an active committee of citizens felt that Senate File 27 was only the beginning of a campaign that some time must be successfully concluded if county residents were to have the full benefit of contemporary public health protection.

If supporters failed to achieve legislative approval of county health departments, they were most successful along other lines. One of these was a program of public health education, an approach that Hewitt certainly had endorsed in 1885 when he established his slight periodical, *Public Health in Minnesota*. Bracken, too, had taken many occasions to acquaint the public with public health facts and to try to develop an interest among both adults and children in the control of disease. But not until July, 1917, did the Bracken administration create the position of educational agent. From then until 1928 an educational program ran in fits and starts. After 1928 the program lapsed and it was not revived until July, 1937. At that time the board employed a physician with public health training as director of public health education.

The director's work, for the most part, consisted of meeting with groups interested in public health. These included colleges, parent-

[29] The bill, Senate File 27, introduced on January 16, 1947, was entitled "A Bill for an Act relating to Public Health and to the Control of Preventable Diseases; to Authorize Counties to Establish and Join in Establishing County or Multiple County Health Departments; to Provide for Financing by Local, State and Federal Governments and for Private Gifts; to Provide for Boards of Health and Full Time Health Officers; to Provide for the Suspension under Certain Circumstances of Existing Local Boards of Health and Health Officers; to Provide for Promulgation by County Boards of Regulations for Preservation of the Public Health."

teacher associations, nurses, women's organizations, service clubs, and professional societies. No consistent, long-range radio program was undertaken because the Minnesota State Medical Association already had an acceptable program upon the air. The public was reached as it had been in the past, by the preparation and distribution of pamphlets, especially a series devoted to diphtheria, smallpox, scarlet fever, measles, and whooping cough. Begun in mimeographed form in 1937, these pamphlets were issued and reissued until some 80,000 copies had been released. They were then set in type and published as a WPA art project, running through four editions which totaled 290,000 copies.

In co-operation with the Minnesota State Medical Association, the educational director assisted in the preparation and distribution of twenty-three pamphlets dealing with such subjects as immunization and vaccination, home accidents, and tuberculosis and respiratory diseases. By the autumn of 1940 the department was sending articles of public health interest to the *Minnesota Registered Nurse,* and two years later it supplied the *Minnesota Pharmacist* with brief sketches, some of which were reprinted in the *Northwestern Druggist.* Educational material was supplied also to the American Red Cross Home Nursing Program. From time to time special exhibits were prepared for showing at medical meetings, the Minnesota State Fair, the Minnesota State Conference for Social Work, the Farm Bureau, and the Minnesota Federation of Women's Clubs. The educational director in 1942 assisted the Bemidji State Teachers College in developing a course entitled an "Introduction to Public Health," and a few years later he gave similar aid to the Mankato State Teachers College.[30]

This early, pioneering period in health education was administered by Dr. Donald A. Dukelow, who in 1945 left the department to become medical director of the Council of Social Agencies in Minneapolis. He was succeeded in 1946 by William Griffiths, who had worked with Dukelow and had witnessed a few of the trying experiences that faced the development of an educational program.

Building on the firm foundation erected by Dukelow, Griffiths was able both to extend and to enlarge the division's activities. To "co-ordinate the informational and educational activities" of all sections of the department was, of course, no easy task. In addition, the educational division in 1948 was charged with providing consultant services to schools and communities, with aiding the development of community health education programs, and with developing study units for use in schools. Other activities included, as in the past, the prepara-

[30] State Board of Health, *Reports,* 1922–43, pp. 65–68.

MOVING TOWARD MODERNITY 193

tion and distribution of literature and news releases. The postwar years, which eased restrictions, made it possible for thousands of Minnesotans to benefit from the department's educational program.[31]

In January, 1947, for example, the educational division issued the first number of *Minnesota's Health,* a spritely bulletin edited by Netta W. Wilson and designed to "let you know what your Health Department is doing and planning, and also to tell you how you can help in promoting and maintaining good health for the citizens of your community." Ten thousand copies were printed and distributed free each month to professional and educational groups as well as to private citizens who requested copies. In a very real sense this bulletin carried on the spirit and traditions of Hewitt's *Public Health in Minnesota.* Members of the division also prepared a volume on personal health and human relations to be used in grade schools and compiled a bibliography of health literature available for distribution by the department.[32]

To further assist public health education in the schools, the state departments of health and education jointly began in 1947 the publication of a mimeographed bulletin called *School Health News,* which was distributed free to school health directors, school nurses, county nurses, and county superintendents of schools. A typical copy carried comments on dental health records, safety slogans, a discussion of epidemic ringworm of the scalp, and news of school medical examinations. In addition to clearly written pamphlets on contagious diseases, Griffiths' division planned and produced a most attractive booklet, *Are You Livin'?*, designed primarily for college students. Packed with good advice and filled with common sense, it was an informal guide to intelligent, healthful living in a university atmosphere. Several simply and clearly written pamphlets on sex education for children have gained very wide circulation.[33]

Chesley, in addition to departmental administration, found time also, in this modern period of the board, to interest himself in special services and to take part in community health surveys. Under his direction as executive officer, the department set up elaborate programs to

[31] State Board of Health, *The Minnesota State Board of Health — Organization and Functions,* 10 (St. Paul, 1948).
[32] *Minnesota's Health,* vol. 1, no. 1, p. 3 (January, 1947); Lillian L. Biester, William Griffiths, and N. O. Pearce, *Units in Personal Health and Human Relations* (Minneapolis, 1947); Minnesota Department of Health, *Health Literature Available for Distribution by Minnesota Department of Health* (St. Paul, 1948).
[33] *School Health News,* vol. 2, no. 2, pp. 1–8 (March, 1948); Margaret Chant, *Are You Livin'?* (n.p., n.d.). The pamphlets on contagious diseases included *Measles* (St. Paul, 1947), *Scarlet Fever* (St. Paul, 1947), *Diphtheria* (St. Paul, 1947), *Smallpox* (St. Paul, 1947), and *Whooping Cough* (St. Paul, 1947).

protect the health of troops on maneuvers in the Camp Ripley area in both 1937 and 1940. This type of work interested Chesley, an old army man. He had been complimented for his vaccination work at Fort Snelling in 1917 and, after his return from France and Poland, he had continued his interest in army sanitation. Therefore, when he learned that some forty thousand troops would concentrate in Minnesota in the summer of 1940, he set to work with a will. The division of sanitation made investigations of all municipal water supplies and of all milk pasteurization plants in the training area. A laboratory was established in the high school building at Little Falls in order that analytical results on both water and milk samples could be determined quickly. An emergency chlorination plant was also dispatched to Little Falls. Bathing beaches and other environmental sanitary factors were investigated, and an epidemiologist from the division of preventable diseases visited chronic carriers of typhoid bacilli in or near the maneuver grounds to make sure that every possible precaution was being observed to prevent contamination of milk, water, or food. The division of hotel inspection made a check on all places licensed by it, securing detailed information that would be of service if infection occurred among troops or civilians. Chesley informed army officials that the United States Public Health Service had detailed two of its staff to come to Minnesota to help him develop a venereal disease program.[34] He also asked Professor William A. Riley, chief of the division of entomology and economic zoology at the University of Minnesota, to make a survey of mosquitoes in order, if possible, to prevent malaria.

During the years 1944, 1945, and 1946, Chesley, in addition to other routine duties, took an active interest in three health surveys. The first, reported by the American Public Health Association, studied public health in St. Paul and Ramsey County and made some thirty-seven recommendations, ranging from a recommendation for the establishment of a city-county health department to the suggestion that additional facilities be provided for the diagnosis and treatment of rheumatic fever. A survey of Minneapolis had been made in 1938. Dr. Haven Emerson, professor emeritus of public health at Columbia University and many times a Minnesota visitor, prepared the second report. He investigated community organization in Minneapolis, with special

[34] Major Henry S. Greenleaf to Chesley, June 5, 1917, Colonel H. C. Gibner to Chesley, June 4, 1940, Chesley to the Commanding General, Headquarters, Seventh Corps Area, Omaha, Nebraska, July 8, 1940, Minnesota Department of Health, Minneapolis; Minnesota Department of Health, Division of Sanitation, "Quarterly Reports," June 30, 1940, p. 22.

MOVING TOWARD MODERNITY 195

reference to public health and organized care of the sick. Emerson's recommendations not only included suggestions for strengthening Minneapolis' health services, but also paid attention to psychiatric services, maternity hospital facilities, and a venereal disease clinic. The third survey that interested Chesley was conducted by the members and staff of the Blue Earth County Council on Intergovernmental Relations and resulted in a most searching descriptive report on health activities in the Mankato region.[35]

Chesley's interests ranged wider, however, than his participation in safeguarding the health of troops in training and his contributions to health surveys. From 1925 to 1945 he was professor of public health in the University of Minnesota's Department of Preventive Medicine. As if this were not enough, Chesley for many years was secretary of the Conference of State and Provincial Health Authorities of North America. Not until 1946 did he succeed in having his annual resignation as secretary-treasurer accepted. He had then held the position for twenty years. He was president of the conference for one year. The number of other offices he held seems incredible. He was a member of the board of directors of the American Child Health Association, president of the American Public Health Association in 1930, member of the board of scientific directors of the Rockefeller Foundation's international health division, and honorary fellow of Britain's Royal Sanitary Institute. He also served as a member of the American Medical Association's joint committee with the National Education Association on health problems in education. Chesley's appointments to local and state committees are too numerous to list. In 1947 he was given an honorary life membership in the American Social Hygiene Association, and was described as a "stout-hearted fellow worker in whom idealism, humor, common-sense and wisdom are equally measured and well mixed for the benefit of all with whom he has to do."[36] A year later the Minnesota State Medical Association presented him with its distinguished service medal in recognition of a half century of service.

Such honors did not deter Chesley from continuing his active interest in routine departmental business and in trying to keep abreast of modern developments. The very structure of the department was

[35] American Public Health Association, *Public Health in St. Paul and Ramsey County, Minnesota*, 1–14 (New York, 1944); Haven Emerson, *Report on Health Situation* (Minneapolis, 1945); Blue Earth County Council on Intergovernmental Relations, *A Survey of Public Health and Related Services in Minnesota with Particular Emphasis on Health Activities in Blue Earth County* (Mankato, 1946).

[36] From a folder issued by the American Social Hygiene Association in 1947 and distributed to guests of the association at the time Chesley received his honorary life membership.

altered from time to time in order that the board might better serve the people of Minnesota. The creation of new divisions was proof enough that Chesley was not content to permit administrative tradition to impede change. The division of child hygiene was established in 1922. This was followed by the transfer of the independent office of state hotel inspector to the health department as the division of hotel inspection in 1925. A rural health service was established in 1935; a public health educational service, as has been noted, in 1937; a division of public health nursing in 1938; a division of industrial health in 1941; and a division of dental health in 1942.

The most recent administrative change in the department took place on January 1, 1947, when Chesley streamlined functions and activities by abolishing the nine divisions and creating in their place five sections, each of which was further divided into divisions and units. Under the long-discussed reorganization, the sections and their chiefs were: the section of departmental administration, Dr. R. N. Barr; the section of preventable diseases, Dr. D. S. Fleming; the section of medical laboratories, Dr. Paul Kabler; the section of environmental sanitation, Dr. Herbert M. Bosch; and the section of special services, Dr. Viktor O. Wilson. The chiefs, in addition to their regular duties, served as an advisory council to Chesley.[37]

Under the new organization, Chesley hoped to co-ordinate better the activities of the department, to extend them, and thus to give Minnesotans better health protection than they had formerly had. A cancer control program was introduced, hotel inspection was placed under the supervision of a trained public health official, a mental hygiene unit was created, renewed vigor was given to a program to prevent water pollution, and increased attention was paid to conditions in lumbering and industrial camps and among Minnesota's Indians. Chesley's department indeed had modernized itself and was apparently prepared to meet the health challenges of the second half of the twentieth century.

[37] *Minnesota's Health,* vol. 1, no. 1, p. 2 (January, 1947).

11

Epidemics in the North Woods

NO DOUBT it is true, as Wright T. Orcutt said, that old-time lumberjacks were "mighty men in many ways, mighty of bone and sinew, hardy, alert, self-reliant, resourceful, and they possessed great courage and endurance."[1] Yet on more than one occasion these big men of the woods quaked with fear when smallpox, that scourge of Minnesota's pineries, forced them to flee from camps, where the disease was claiming the lives of choppers, teamsters, clerks, and cooks. Although smallpox was not unique to lumber camps, it did strike savagely at logging centers from the 1880s until the turn of the century. It was responsible for more sickness and more deaths than either typhoid fever or diphtheria.

From earliest days, when pioneers from Maine first began to swing the ax against stands of white pine, until the lumber frontier moved westward out of Minnesota, scores of stout log camps — along the St. Croix and the Rum and up into Itasca County — were burned or abandoned because of smallpox epidemics. Despite these annual visitations of the disease, the great companies continued to fell tremendous numbers of trees. The lumber manufactured from them was desperately needed in a score of prairie states for the construction of homes and frame business houses. Daniel Stanchfield, an ardent lumberman, once estimated that more than ten billion board feet were cut in the fifty-two years between 1848 and 1899. In 1880, just about the time when the Minnesota Department of Health began interesting itself in the health of lumberjacks, the St. Croix Valley produced 212,238,870 scaled feet. Anoka's figures totaled 15,116,110 scaled feet and Brainerd's, 1,996,-960. No wonder an Eastern visitor wrote with awe that Minnesota's forests were the sources of fabulous wealth and "afford a theatre for

[1] "The Minnesota Lumberjacks," in *Minnesota History*, 6:3 (March, 1925).

the lumber business excelling any thing ever witnessed in Maine or New Brunswick."[2]

The sighing of monarch trees in the wind and the thunderous crash when they tumbled ignominiously to the ground to the piercing cry of "t-i-m-b-e-r!" was a primitive drama with wide appeal. Something about the Mackinaws and heavy boots, the peavey and the saw, the bean hole and flapjacks — something about the very life of the logger cast over it an aura of romance.

> Old Wes he is a lumberman
> You ought to know him well
> He cruises around Pokegama
> Some say he's right from Hell.[3]

Twin City residents in the early winter of 1883 followed with eager interest an account of a journey to Mousseau's Camp on the headwaters of the west branch of the Rum River. Those who read that account got a graphic picture of a typical Minnesota logging center. The long, log house was put together roughly, but was securely chinked. Its eaves were not more than eight feet above the ground and the roof was made from heavy pine or tamarack slabs, weighted with sod, hay, and snow. The entire structure was low and squatty. Inside, three rooms, each about forty by thirty feet, were measured off. The first two were the jacks' living and sleeping quarters and the third was the kitchen. Two-tiered bunks lined the sides of the sleeping quarters. There were no side windows; light and ventilation came from small openings at the end of the building and from two small skylights. In the center of the living room stood "a great sheet-iron heater, which swallows up wood which is fed it with generous prodigality. Around the stove a hanging frame work, adorned very soon after the arrival of the men from the works, along towards dark, with drying socks of variegated colors, prodigious size and common odor."[4]

Sanitary facilities were most primitive. Dishwashing must have been haphazard in many camps and the washing of clothes a most difficult procedure, at least during cold winter months. Bedbugs were plentiful. Indeed, these vermin were abundant in at least one Minnesota camp

---

[2] Daniel Stanchfield, "History of Pioneer Lumbering on the Upper Mississippi and Its Tributaries," in *Minnesota Historical Collections*, 9:361; Minnesota Commissioner of Statistics, *Reports*, 1880, p. 241; J. M. Tuttle, "The Minnesota Pineries," in *Harper's Magazine*, 36:409–423 (February, 1868).

[3] Fred Kennerson, "Reminiscence of Early Minnesota Lumbering," a typewritten manuscript in the possession of the Minnesota Historical Society.

[4] *Pioneer Press*, February 3, 1883.

as late as 1928.[5] But the greatest menace to public health was a contaminated water supply. All too frequently privies were located too close to wells. Sometimes drainage from barns and manure piles polluted drinking water. A typhoid carrier with dirty hands could easily infect an entire camp. The constant drifting of lumberjacks in and out of camps could result in the spreading of the disease by one individual among several logging centers.

The erratic migrations of loggers were responsible also for the wildfire swiftness with which smallpox traveled from one camp to another. For some jacks, cutting timber was a seasonal affair. They would work for a time, collect their pay, and start for Duluth or the Twin Cities, where they loafed until their money was gone. Putting up in cheap, dirty hotels and not always paying strict attention to personal hygiene, these loggers frequently contracted infectious diseases. When they returned to the woods, alone or in tow of some company labor scout, they might expose an entire camp. In 1883 three Minneapolis hotels — the Home Hotel, the American House, and the Kramer Hotel — proved to be the sources of smallpox infections which were carried into the pineries.[6]

For years communities had been apprehensive that traffic to and from lumber camps would result in just such an outbreak. Minneapolis was concerned about the health of some four hundred loggers in camp near Pokegama Falls in 1872, and Taylors Falls said that unless immediate measures were taken to prevent the spread of smallpox "great damage will be apprehended in this vicinity in that the supply teamsters who pass through the settlement on their way to and from the pineries may spread the disease here, as was the case two or three winters ago." Concern was expressed also that a "distemper," which was killing off horses in camps, would be carried into the cities. From time to time loggers stricken with typhoid fever were brought to St. Paul or Minneapolis for treatment.[7]

Late in December, 1882, came the first startling news that epidemic smallpox had broken out at Caldwell's Camp between Grand Rapids and Leech Lake. A few days later a logger from that camp died at Grand Rapids. By the end of January, 1883, smallpox patients were filtering into Duluth for treatment. The situation was so frightening

[5] C. M. Oehler, *Time in the Timber*, 19–22 (St. Paul, 1948).
[6] State Board of Health, *Biennial Reports*, 1883–84, pp. 23, 48–51.
[7] *Minneapolis Tribune*, January 26, December 10, 1872; *Taylor's Falls Reporter*, quoted in the *St. Paul Daily Press*, February 4, 1872; *Stillwater Gazette*, April 9, 1879; *Pioneer Press* (St. Paul), October 27, 1881, November 29, 1882.

that S. C. Bagley made a special trip from the logging district to Red Wing to consult with Hewitt. He said there was a "feeling of restlessness and anxiety among the men, because of past neglect on the part of the authorities, and the gradual but certain spread of the disease, and something must be done immediately to prevent an early abandonment of some of the most exposed camps."[8]

Bagley's impatience with the health board was not entirely justified. On December 22, 1882, five days before the first case was reported in the newspapers, Hewitt had received word of the outbreak and on the same day had written Dr. E. H. Belyea, Grand Rapids health officer: "I send you copies of tracts on small pox and infectious diseases for distribution; please act for me in your town and adjacent district; inquire as to the origin of the case in your hands; if necessary, go to the camp whence he came; take such other steps as are necessary, following guidance of the circulars, to control any cases you find; have ordered thirty points of vaccine sent to you; use it on children, if there are any, first; use the 'eighth day lymph' from them for adults, as the best and quickest in operation." After receiving the vaccine, Belyea went to work. Meanwhile a physician from Duluth began treatment of patients at Caldwell's Camp. By then the first victim had died, and it was found that he had contracted the disease in the Home Hotel in Minneapolis. The difficulty was that exposed lumberjacks were fleeing from Caldwell's Camp to the little town of Aitkin, which immediately organized a board of health. By the time Bagley arrived in Red Wing, Hewitt had dispatched vaccine to Aitkin and had ordered its general use. Still Bagley was not satisfied, for he wrote on February 1 that more physicians were needed, that camps were far apart, and that "if something more than sending a preliminary surveying party is not done, we shall have one of the nicest little visitations Minnesota has had since the Sioux outbreak."[9]

To complicate Hewitt's difficulties in trying to fight an epidemic in the midst of forest country by long distance, Brainerd's mayor sent a frantic message to Minneapolis city officials that "panic-stricken" lumbermen were leaving the camps and heading toward the Twin Cities. Brainerd police were attempting to stop these runaways. The Brainerd messenger crossed Hewitt's path, for Hewitt was already at Aitkin and soon reached Brainerd, where he appointed Dr. J. C. Rosser of Brainerd as health officer in charge of infected districts and named Dr. C.

[8] *Tribune*, December 29, 1882, January 4, 25, 1883; *Pioneer Press*, January 28, 1883.
[9] State Board of Health, *Biennial Reports*, 1883–84, pp. 53, 57.

Q. Scoboria of Elk River as Rosser's assistant. Then Hewitt hurriedly returned to the Twin Cities to make a plea for vaccine, old cotton cloth, linen, towels, and other supplies for the sick. He conferred with Governor Lucius F. Hubbard, who approved Hewitt's handling of the emergency.

Hubbard and Hewitt agreed that special deputy sheriffs be appointed to keep exposed loggers in camp and to assist physicians with their vaccination. After advising his health officers to concentrate the sick as near together as possible and to burn camps which they had used, Hewitt then issued some general instructions: "Use every means to quiet the fear of the disease among the men, telling them that you represent the executive officer of the State board for their protection from infection and for their care, if sick; *prevent panic* and instruct your assistants to do so, too. As to deputy sheriffs, select them from the lumbermen themselves; men in whom they have confidence will enable you to control them. You should as far as possible detain suspected parties in their own camps, as cheaper and better every way." [10]

Quarantine hospitals were established at Aitkin and Grand Rapids, and the Northern Pacific Railroad ordered the vaccination of all its employees. Despite the best efforts of the state board, lumbermen continued to demand the assignment of a physician to every infected camp. When Richardson's Camp sent another patient into Grand Rapids this request was repeated. Hewitt knew that it was virtually impossible to station a doctor at every camp. Physicians were few in the north country during the 1880s, and many of them were acting as only part-time health officers. He was aware also that lumber companies paid little attention to the health of the men until an outbreak threatened decreased production. Had the companies insisted upon hiring only vaccinated laborers, they could have avoided smallpox in the camps and would not have needed medical attendants. Nor could the state board, in the midst of an epidemic, vaccinate all lumbermen in districts where there was no smallpox. This was recommended by Stillwater interests, who argued: "The epidemic has not as yet reached the logging regions on the St. Croix, but should it prevail to any extent on the Mississippi, an exodus of laborers from that region may be looked for with certainty, and it is equally certain that their principal point will be the camps on the St. Croix. In this way the scourge may be brought to our very doors before we are aware of it." [11]

[10] *Daily Globe* (St. Paul), January 30, 1883; State Board of Health, *Biennial Reports*, 1883–84, p. 58.
[11] *Pioneer Press*, January 30, February 1, 2, 1883; *Stillwater Gazette*, February 7, 1883.

Dr. A. P. Brackett of Minneapolis was employed by about thirty camps on the Willow, Moose, and Split Hand rivers, his salary being paid jointly by the Chase and Miller's camps and the De Laittre interests. As a contract physician, Brackett might have been expected to give the lumber companies the benefit of any doubt. Instead, he wrote of the deplorable condition in which the companies maintained camps. He said a camp which he visited had been unhealthful for over two years, with the "buildings used several winters and not renovated in the least — eight cases of varioloid there, one severe case of facial erysipelas and eight or ten are now showing signs of typhoid, one case of incised axe wound refused to unite, though I have tried everything. The camp is illy ventilated, infernally nasty, dark, damp, and the stench horrible. Shall insist upon burning both camp and bedding." Brackett met further difficulty when company officers refused to have loggers vaccinated, giving as their reason that vaccination would hinder men from working. So well known was the opposition of a few companies to vaccination and their reluctance or inability to run clean camps that the *Pioneer Press* said bluntly: "The lumber camps are distributed over a wide extent of territory, and certain habits of uncleanliness which prevail in all lumber camps, the huddled condition in which the men live, makes these winter homes exceptionally fruitful fields for the ravages of disease." [12]

Six days later, after having talked with men from infected camps and with Aitkin health officers, the *Pioneer Press* again described the unsanitary condition of logging camps, which as a rule, said the editor, were "dens of filth, wherein a person of weak gastric possessions could not exist." By then, despite rigid precautions to prevent exposed or sick men from leaving the epidemic district, at least two, and probably more, lumberjacks had made their way into St. Paul. Lewis Brown, scaler for Camp and Walker, arrived to say that the outbreak was more formidable than had been believed, and Charles Taylor was taken to the pesthouse, where he died. Hewitt himself returned from the region north of Aitkin and reported that there were only sixteen cases in the woods and four in the hospital at Aitkin. Eight cases escaped before they could be apprehended, but strict watch was being kept at Aitkin, Brainerd, Duluth, and Northern Pacific Junction for them. Major George A. Camp, a lumberman, said that smallpox figures had been greatly exaggerated, but to offset this, Rosser charged that lumbermen

[12] State Board of Health, *Biennial Reports*, 1883–84, pp. 65, 71; *Pioneer Press*, February 8, 1883.

had tried to conceal the seriousness of the outbreak. Belyea said further that lumbering interests had refused to permit physicians to visit their camps and vaccinate the men.[13]

While this bad feeling between public health officials and lumbermen was developing, another crisis in the woods demanded Hewitt's attention. For years Indians had moved in and out of logging centers. They came to do a little begging and trading, to watch with sullen eyes the destruction of the forest, and to salvage scraps of food. Sometimes jacks took squaws to bed. Their exposure to the white man's way of life resulted, of course, in disease. Indians were present in Caldwell's Camp when smallpox first broke out there. These Chippewa carried the disease to their home on Lake Winnibigoshish, where thirty-three deaths were reported early in February, 1883. Another group on Bowstring contracted the disease from sick lumberjacks who stopped at their camp. Indians roamed the woods, spreading the disease so rapidly that it was impossible to trace its course. A second outbreak among the Chippewa, which was preceded by an epidemic of measles and accompanied by an epidemic of chicken pox, occurred in August, 1883. Dr. James R. Walker, government physician at Lake Winnibigoshish, assisted by state health department doctors, vaccinated as many as he could, destroyed every article of property, except canoes, that would burn, and issued each victim a new suit and blanket.[14]

Both the outbreak in the lumber camps and the two epidemics among the Indians were under control by autumn. In September, James Caldwell, in whose camp the disease first made its appearance, said there were no more cases in the woods. He added that the epidemic had obliged him to purchase new bedding and camp equipment, to pay men extra for caring for the sick, and to hire private physicians at a cost of twenty dollars per day. His personal expenditure, he estimated, amounted to twenty thousand dollars. At the time the outbreak occurred, some two thousand men were in the woods.[15]

The epidemic of 1883, although it was not the first nor the last to occur in the pineries, was of particular public health significance because it emphasized the unsanitary condition of the logging camps, because it proved the imperative need for vaccination among lumberjacks, because it demonstrated the difficulty of providing adequate care once an epidemic had broken out, and because it showed graph-

[13] *Pioneer Press*, February 14, 18, 19, 1883; State Board of Health, *Biennial Reports*, 1883–84, pp. 73, 84.
[14] State Board of Health, *Biennial Reports*, 1883–84, pp. 86, 93.
[15] *Pioneer Press*, September 4, 1883.

ically the health relationship between logging areas and other communities. Both Minneapolis and Duluth reported small outbreaks as the result of infections brought from the camps on the upper Mississippi. At least eight patients escaped from the pineries to spread the disease in Minneapolis, and at least one victim fled to Duluth. It is possible that other exposed lumberjacks fled to northwestern Wisconsin, there to infect still others in an outbreak that seems to have stemmed from camps on the North Wisconsin Railroad and from Montgomery's Camp in Burnett County. It may have been that one source of infection arrived from Pennsylvania and another from Duluth.[16]

The cost of the 1883 epidemic in the pineries to the State of Minnesota ran to almost $3,000, of which $2,452.50 was for physicians' fees. Luckily the legislature had made a special appropriation for the relief of the pineries, and the expenses did not come from the budget of the state board.[17]

To prevent another serious smallpox outbreak in lumber camps, Hewitt took two definite steps. In November, 1883, he addressed an open letter to the lumbering interests urging vaccination of all employees. "So far as now known," he wrote, "there is no small pox in the State. But there will be constant danger in the woods, that one or more men, coming from so many and distant parts of the country may bring the infection with them. Vaccination and revaccination carefully on every one, will absolutely prevent danger from this source. Looked at as a business precaution, it will pay any person to have this done. It will save anxiety and perhaps a repetition of the sickness and death of last winter."[18]

Hewitt's second activity was the revision of a pamphlet on smallpox which originally had been issued in 1883. This revised tract of 1884 was distributed broadcast in the logging regions. It told in simple language that smallpox is a very infectious disease, characterized by a peculiar eruption on the skin, which goes through the stages of pimple, little water blister, pustule, and scab. Citizens were told that smallpox could be avoided by vaccination, and the nature of vaccine was explained. Hewitt concluded by listing seven recommendations for the care of the patient, beginning with isolation and concluding with directions for disinfection of personal belongings and the sick room.[19]

[16] State Board of Health, *Biennial Reports*, 1883–84, pp. 108, 119.
[17] State Board of Health, *Biennial Reports*, 1883–84, p. 177; Minnesota, *Senate Journal*, 1883, p. 135; *Pioneer Press*, February 9, 10, 1883.
[18] *Pioneer Press*, November 3, 1883.
[19] State Board of Health, *Biennial Reports*, 1883–84, p. 180.

This educational program, desirable as it was, did not eradicate smallpox from the north woods. Epidemics are soon forgotten, and old ways of ignorance and laziness reassert themselves. Many loggers could not see the necessity of having their arms scratched, and many lumber companies, desperately needing timber crews, felt that they could not hire only men who had been vaccinated. And the State of Minnesota had no law making vaccination compulsory for either children or adults.

The result was years of real and fancied smallpox scares. In 1885 smallpox broke out in T. B. Walker's camp on the Clearwater River, about seventy miles from Crookston. This was one of five outbreaks all traced directly to a single case entering the United States by way of Winnipeg. Hewitt dispatched Dr. Edward J. Brown to the Clearwater, where he made a searching investigation. At the same time Pierre Bottineau wrote his wife from Crookston that smallpox was prevalent there.[20] This annoyed Walker, whose lumber camps in the vicinity of Crookston already were becoming uneasy. Walker, therefore, published a brief history of the outbreak which affected his camps.

"This spring," began Walker, "a lumberman, who had worked at one of my camps during the winter, came out to Beltrami station, and went from there to Crookston, over the Manitoba road. The supposition is that he came in contact with a small pox patient who went over the road to Manitoba about that time. A week or ten days later, this man went back into the woods and commenced work building a dam. A few days later he was taken sick, could not work, and went out. He passed through Fosston and on to Crookston, and stopped at the Merchants hotel. He had an eruption on his body which he called measles; but the physician pronounced it small pox. He was taken to the pest house, where he had a light run of varioloid, being able to bring wood and water and play cards with his nurse during his detention."

Walker went on to say that the "landlord of the Merchants Hotel, believing that the man from the woods had measles only, was probably imprudent in handling him, was prostrated and had a light run. Mr. W. S. Taylor, who has charge of my lumber business at Crookston, wrote me on the 21st instant stating that there were no other cases that he knew of. These were all the cases that had occurred at Crookston up to the time I came away — one week ago. There have been five cases in the woods. When the first one occurred, Mr. Kline, who had charge of the Crookston case, sent a special messenger out to Crookston, and Mr.

---

[20] *Tribune*, May 13, 1885; *Pioneer Press*, May 14, 23, 1885; State Board of Health, *Biennial Reports*, 1884–86, p. 9.

Taylor telegraphed to me. I immediately saw Dr. Leonard, of the state board of health, and then telegraphed to Dr. Hewitt, at Red Wing, who came to Minneapolis immediately. Dr. Brown was sent north at once and found one case at Fosston, and one in a quarantine camp in the woods. Four other cases occurred in the woods and one more at Fosston. The most vigorous measures were taken by Dr. Brown to protect the towns between the woods and Crookston, as well as the drivers on the river."

"Vaccination," continued Walker, "was made general throughout the whole region when danger of communication existed. Every man coming from the woods must have a pass or be placed in quarantine for two weeks. Under date of May 15, Mr. Kline wrote me: 'The small pox has died out here, I think. There is only one case here and two at Fosston. Dr. Brown goes out tomorrow.' One of the men taken in the woods, named George Webster, got away from his nurse, and though diligent search was made for him, he has not been heard of since. Dr. Brown is of the opinion that he perished in the woods." [21]

After receiving Brown's report, Hewitt again wrote the lumber companies, urging them to vaccinate every person going into the camps. He kept a record of his correspondence in order that, "should small pox again appear in any of the lumber camps, the responsibility will be fixed where it belongs." His efforts were only partially successful, as Dr. B. J. Merrill, the health officer of Stillwater, pointed out. Merrill left Stillwater in November, 1885, at the request of a number of companies, to vaccinate camps on a line with the North Wisconsin Railroad. He described how companies urged vaccination. One firm indicated that any man refusing would be given his time; another did not insist upon vaccination, but said that if smallpox struck, it would discharge every unvaccinated individual; and a third company only "desired and urged" vaccination. Merrill visited some thirty camps, each with an average of forty men. Although he did not indicate how many lumberjacks were vaccinated, he did say that he got positive results on about ninety per cent of those treated. He thought loggers were reckless in matters pertaining to personal health and safety, and he chided the companies, "in the face of statistics and reason," for not making vaccination obligatory before sending men into the woods. "But the fact remains," he concluded, "that they are very negligent in regard to this simple business expedient, and are loth to active efforts

[21] *Pioneer Press*, May 24, 1885.

in protecting their camps against small-pox, until that unpleasant disease appears within their vicinity." [22]

Brown, later recalling his work for the board, emphasized the lack of co-operation that a state inspector received in attempting to control an epidemic. His work, he said, had been "somewhat rocky," for "between the town authorities who wished to send me out to the small pox family six miles in the woods, to sleep in a corn crib and eat with the family, but compromised on a log cabin over run with vermin, and a drunken lumber camp cookee, between these and the Irish settlers whom I had to threaten with all the pains of hell in order to get milk for my sick ones, my experiences for the first days were interesting." [23]

Annually the state board continued to press for more complete protection from smallpox in the camps. Foremen were urged to keep records of when men were vaccinated and were told to isolate any having suspicious symptoms. Minneapolis health officers, following the lead set by the state board, also circularized the camps, asking the vaccination of all laborers. Results were slow but certain. Although companies did not insist upon vaccination, they showed a greater willingness to report suspected cases to the board and to ask for assistance. At a Mitchell and McClure camp near Carlton in 1894, a foreman had instructions from his company to spare no care or expense in treating an outbreak. When smallpox broke out in camps operated by the Alger, Smith interests in 1900, Bracken drew attention to the employers' liability act. "As I understand this law," he wrote the company's general manager at Duluth, "should you import new men into this camp without advising them of danger from exposure to small-pox, or should men already in camp come down with the disease after there had been sufficient time to take steps to prevent its spread, these parties would have a case of law against you. I mention this fact simply to put you on your guard and to urge upon you the necessity of protecting yourselves in every way by insisting on vaccination among your men and watchfulness for the appearance of the first symptoms of any disease and diseased individuals." The manager replied that, after the disease became known, the company supplied a physician with over three

---

[22] *Public Health in Minnesota*, 1:54, 79 (September, December, 1885); *Pioneer Press*, September 25, 1885.

[23] Edward J. Brown, "Some Professional Recollections after Fifty Years," [2] (Minneapolis, 1926), a typewritten manuscript in the possession of the Minnesota Historical Society.

hundred vaccine points and directed him to take every step to suppress the disease.[24]

By the turn of the century a few lumber companies were hiring their own physicians on a contract basis. Sometimes the doctor was under contract to a logging outfit and a railroad at the same time. But, in at least one case, Bracken believed that contract stipulations specifically exempted the physician from caring for contagious diseases. At Nickerson the Lumbermans' Hospital not only cared for cases brought in but also furnished sanitary advice to the camps. Upon occasion companies seem to have considered that the best way to treat an infected workman was to turn him loose in the hope that he would be picked up and cared for by a local health officer. So many ambulatory patients straggled into Mountain Iron in 1901 that the superintendent of the Oliver Iron Mining Company wrote a vigorous note of protest to Bracken. "We protest against the action of the camps," he said, "in thus ridding themselves of such cases as rightfully belong to them, and probably originated with them, by sending them away to drift into our community and be cared for by us. . . . We would not for one minute think of sending a case, originating in our midst, from us, to be a menace and expense to other people, but would properly isolate and care for it." Bracken replied that he thought companies were anxious to control smallpox and said that lumberjacks were prone to move from place to place. "If any one can advise some method," he wrote, "of keeping this shiftless class of men from wandering about in the northern part of Minnesota without calling into service a few regiments of soldiers, I shall be exceedingly thankful."[25]

Soon after this reply to the complaint of the Oliver Iron Mining Company, health officers from the state board visited Duluth and Superior to see for themselves what the "runaway" situation was. They had been irritated by several reports from private citizens that smallpox was present throughout the country all the way from Bemidji to Duluth. A Minneapolis visitor to Bemidji complained that there were cases of smallpox in three houses on the town's main street, and a local resident described the manner in which his doctor took smallpox

[24] *Public Health in Minnesota*, 5:104 (December, 1889); *Pioneer Press*, September 26, 1885; *Mississippi Valley Lumberman*, 24:6 (January 4, 1894); L. A. Sukeforth to Hewitt, June 13, 14, 15, 17, 23, 25, 1894, Charles Morse and E. P. Duffy to Hewitt, June 18, 1894, Bracken to R. N. Marble, August 7, 1900, and Marble to Bracken, August 8, 1900, Minnesota Department of Health, St. Paul.

[25] Bracken to J. L. Greatsinger, July 18, 1900, to W. S. Reynolds, May 12, 1900, and to M. S. Hawkins, January 5, 1901; Greatsinger to Bracken, July 19, 1900; Reynolds to E. T. Carish, May 2, 1900; Hawkins to Bracken, January 2, 1901. Minnesota Department of Health, St. Paul.

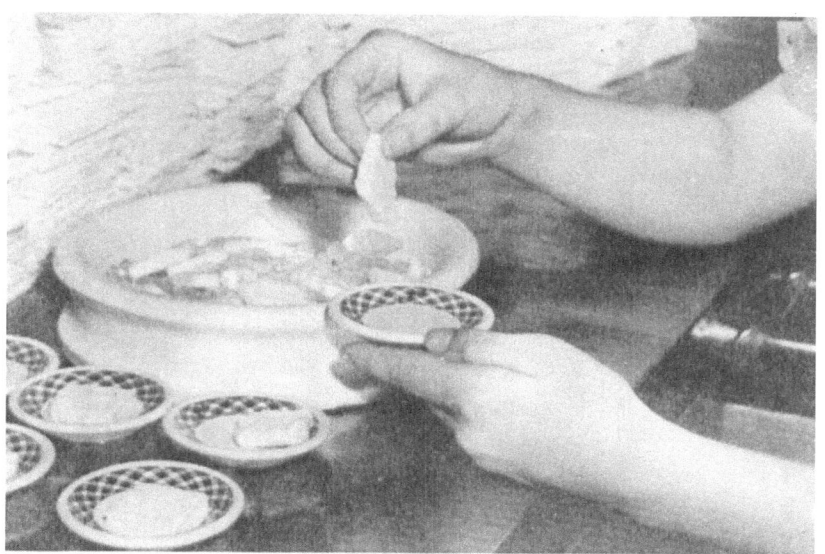

How Not to Serve Butter

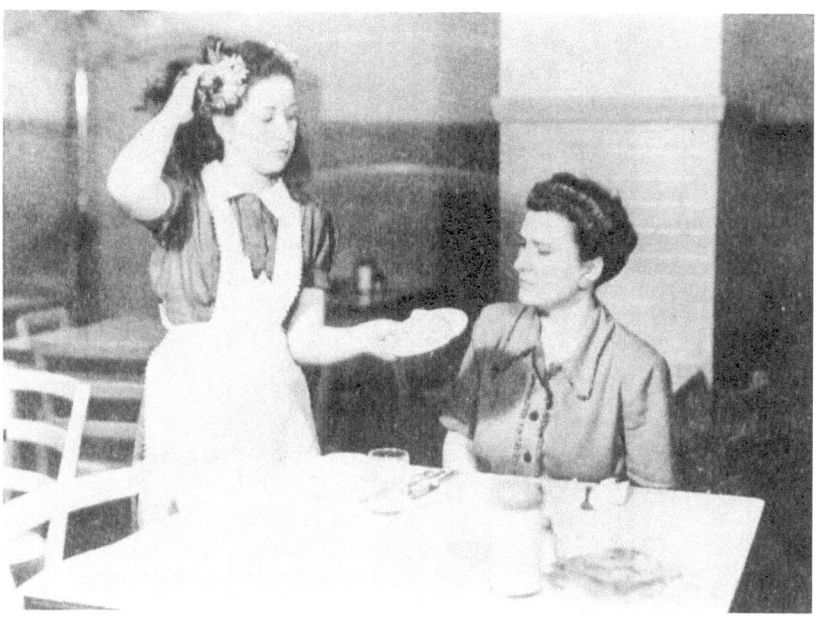

How Not to Wait on Table
Courtesy Minnesota Department of Health

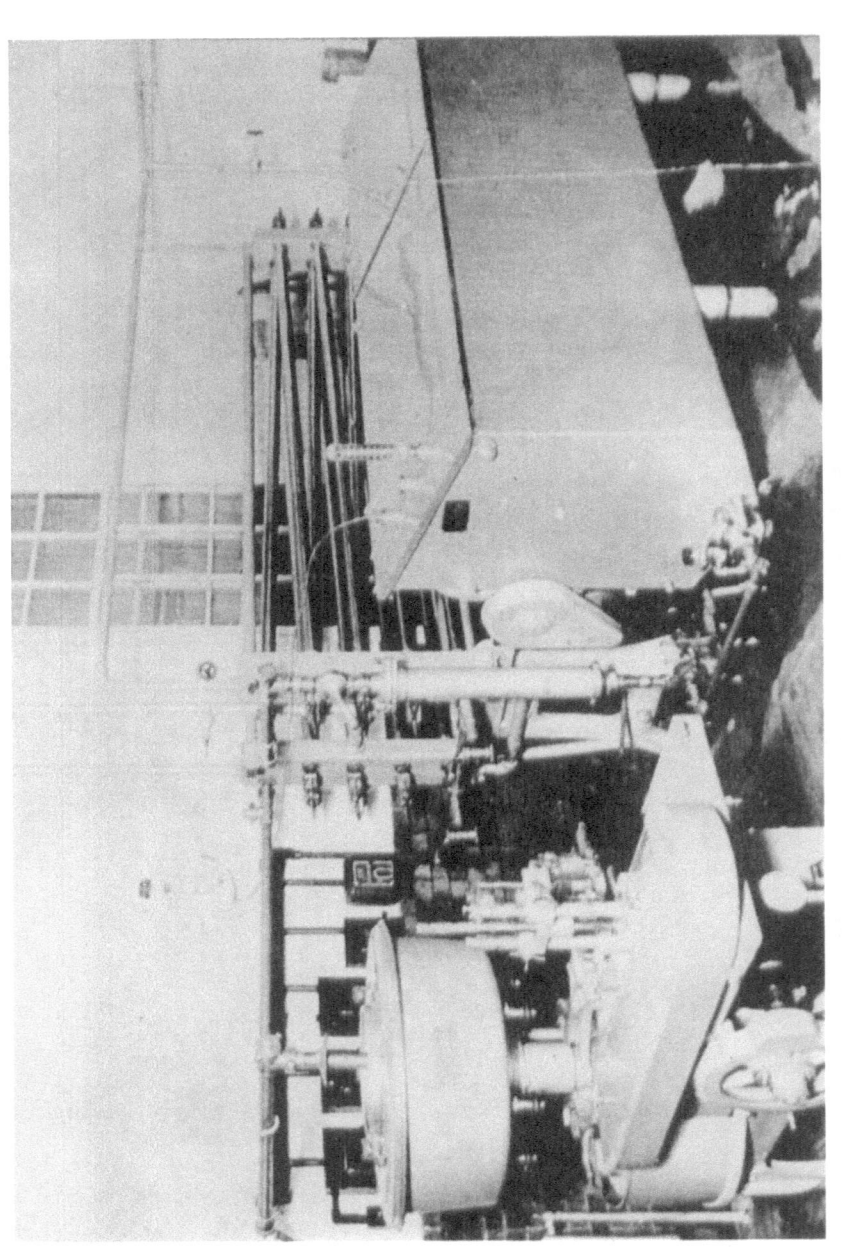

A Modern Milk Plant with Pasteurization Equipment
Courtesy Minnesota Department of Health

cases to the pesthouse: "He goes to the livery barn, hires a rig, gets robes from the same place, takes his patient out to pest house, returns, brings the rig and robes back to barn without disinfecting the same. Now is that careless or not?" [26]

Bracken met with representatives of five Bemidji lumber concerns in an attempt to formulate a control policy. Apparently the one offending camp from which jacks were fleeing was Gray's. At least a hundred had been exposed and, said a Bemidji physician, "with men now leaving the woods and bringing out old blankets and clothes I see no end of trouble." State inspectors expressed their criticism of some companies openly, saying they had a very difficult problem in handling lumber camps. Prominent men stated in open meeting that a lumber camp was no place for a sick man and added that they would dismiss any jack who had been sick for twenty-four hours. By doing this, of course, they were turning out men, who were already a source of infection, about three days before the smallpox eruption appeared.[27]

The state board protested again and again, and its files fairly bulged with letters practically begging companies to keep both suspected and active cases in quarantine. But still health officers in local communities continued to report laxness on the part of the companies. At Eveleth the quarantine hospital was filling rapidly with cases from camps, and expenses to the town for their care were heavy. It was reported that the Northern Lumber Company was sending unattended patients to town. A jack with smallpox wandered in, had dinner in a restaurant, and was in other public places. Although the manager of the company denied there had been any smallpox in his camps for two months, Eveleth physicians said specifically that James McCarroy, a teamster with the disease, had come from one of the company's camps near Sparta. While the Powers-Simpson Pine Lands and Logs Company was interested in a vaccination program, it thought that the program should be carried out during the summer months and that local health officers should have the authority to vaccinate every new arrival in town. "It is useless to ask the loggers to employ only those men who have been vaccinated," said the company. "When we want men, we want them badly and cannot discriminate between those vaccinated and those not. Men are not plentiful enough to allow us to

[26] J. P. Davison to Bracken, January 9, 1901; C. F. Schroeder to Bracken, February 19, 1901. Minnesota Department of Health, St. Paul.
[27] Bracken to S. S. Bagley, M. Gray, McCane & Gough, Cook & Giles, and Brainerd Lumber Company, February 25, 1901; D. B. Newman to Bracken, March 7, 1901; Bracken to J. M. Robinson, January 25, 1901. Minnesota Department of Health, St. Paul.

do that." Bracken replied merely that it was possible to round up and vaccinate lumberjacks if they came into town from an infected area, but that no law could compel loggers to be vaccinated under any other circumstances.[28]

There was a neat way, however, to force vaccination upon unwilling loggers. On October 8, 1901, the state board passed a resolution relative to the withholding of wages from lumberjacks ill with smallpox. It said that money in the hands of those ill with a contagious disease was to be looked upon as a source of possible infection and hence no such logger was to receive pay. Bracken was assured by legal experts that the board could authorize the withholding of money under these circumstances. He told the Swan River Logging Company that this policy would save the county, the state, and the lumber camps much expense, and he ordered the Powers-Simpson Lumber Company at Hibbing to withhold money from men in quarantine until the quarantine period had passed.[29]

Meanwhile the state board had met with the boards of health of Wisconsin and Michigan and with lumbermen, railroad officials, and others interested in the control of smallpox. Their sessions were held in Duluth beginning on August 13, 1901. When Bracken proposed that vaccination be made a compulsory prerequisite for employment in the logging industry, a representative of the Alger, Smith Company took the floor and said: "There is one thing I notice and that is that Dr. Bracken makes special reference to the lumbermen. I do not know why he should do that. There are others besides lumbermen. I have been told that there have been smallpox patients taken out of stores right here in Duluth. It seems to me that special reference is made to the business of lumbering here. I do not know much about medicine but it has never been my opinion that men get smallpox in the pine woods. I thought that was about the healthiest place to work. In my opinion smallpox visits from the cities to the woods and visits back again, and I think that the lumbermen of this district have been just as earnest as any other section of business men. Now I came here to listen and I am willing to do all I can to help, but I do not like the

[28] Letters to Bracken from W. C. Harwood, February 15, 1901, from Charles W. More, February 15, 23, 1901, from R. M. Weyerhaeuser, February 20, 1901, and from George A. R. Simpson, October 3, 1901; Bracken to Simpson, October 4, 1901. Minnesota Department of Health, St. Paul.

[29] Bracken to Robinson, November 2, 1901, to the Cloquet Tie and Post Company, November 29, 1901, to E. E. Wyman, December 6, 1901, to the manager, Swan River Logging Company, January 9, 1902, and to the manager, Powers-Simpson Lumber Company, January 9, 1902. Minnesota Department of Health, St. Paul.

tenor of this thing. It does not seem to be fair. We pay $5000 taxes on property in this city and pay more in this county and also in Lake Co. We should get something for this. This burden should not fall entirely on us. The Mayor said it had cost $2000 in Duluth. It has cost our firm twice that much. We will do all we can to help, but do not cripple the lumbermen."

Despite this protest, the conference passed resolutions providing that lumber camps and other industries require a certificate of successful vaccination before hiring laborers, that state inspectors be prepared to vaccinate at any camp at the expense of the men themselves, the employers, or the county, and that all disinfection be done by a competent disinfector. Another resolution stated that all camps in which smallpox had existed must be immediately disinfected or quarantined or burned. The expense of disinfection was to be borne by the owner of the camp. A final proposition pertained to the withholding of wages from employees infected with contagious diseases.[30]

The Minnesota board also made a long series of recommendations for the sanitary control of lumber camps, mines, and other industries. These placed responsibility for the proper enforcement of regulations on companies and their authorized agents. They also provided for at least three hundred cubic feet of air space per occupant for any dwelling occupied by employees and stipulated that a substantial floor be raised at least a foot from the ground. Dwellings were to be supplied with adequate lighting. A separate, not connected, building was to serve as cookhouse, and buckets for both solid and liquid refuse were declared mandatory if the building had no correctly constructed drainage system. Latrines were to be located at a place satisfactory to a properly authorized health officer. It was stipulated also that the printed regulations of the Minnesota Department of Health were to be posted in a conspicuous place. Regulation 12 was interesting, for it made provision for a pay deduction of not less than fifty cents and not more than a dollar to be used to pay the fees of camp physicians. This was an innovation. "The owner, manager, agent or foreman or other person in charge of any lumbering camp, or other industry in which men are employed," read Regulation 13, "shall require a certificate of recent successful vaccination of each employee when he is engaged by the Company or its agent and where evidence is not forth-

[30] "Minutes of the Meeting of the State Boards of Health of Minnesota, Wisconsin, and Michigan, also Lumbermen, Railroadmen, and Others Interested in the Control of Smallpox in the Northern Parts of These States," Duluth, August 13, 1901, pp. 5–31 (typescript), Minnesota Department of Health, St. Paul.

coming, it shall be their duty before employing any person, to obtain such evidence of such vaccination." This was an interesting regulation, for Minnesota, then and now, forbids compulsory vaccination. Other sections set forth in detail what procedures should be followed when contagious disease broke out, and provided for the proper enforcement of the regulations.[31]

These preliminary regulations, modified and amplified in the years to come, marked a step forward in the sanitary control of the logging industry. But they could not immediately rectify attitudes or correct conditions which had been present in the dirty, primitive camps since lumbering first began in Minnesota. For one thing, jacks were highly migratory. The camps themselves seldom remained long in any one place. When a district was denuded of its best timber, the old camp was abandoned and another was built closer to the new operations. Yet the fact remains that reports from health officers, in at least some instances, were more encouraging than they had been. Still the situation was far from ideal. Bracken upon one occasion considered bringing suit against a company on the grounds that it transported a smallpox case to Hibbing and then sent it to Minneapolis. Some loggers still refused to be vaccinated. To prevent unvaccinated loggers from experiencing the pleasures of St. Paul, Dr. Justus Ohage, health commissioner, prohibited them from entering the city without certificates of health and proof of successful vaccination. So many smallpox cases were arriving in Superior by way of the Duluth and Iron Range Railroad that Superior's health commissioner requested railroad officials to guard against such passengers.[32]

The early months of 1903 witnessed small outbreaks throughout the north country, especially in Beltrami County. At Chisholm's Camp, near Bemidji, sixty-five exposed men were under guard at one time. Two cases fled from Williamsons' Landing to Winnipeg, causing a Canadian health officer to comment sharply: "Will you be good enough, to let me know what steps are being taken to limit the spread of the disease, from the above mentioned place. It would appear that up to the present time, there has been, but very meagre quarantine." Camps on Black Duck Lake reported the disease and listed ninety-three exposed lumberjacks under guard to prevent their escape. The

[31] Bracken, "Suggestions Used in Formulating the Resolutions at the Duluth Meeting, August 13, 1901" (typescript), Minnesota Department of Health, St. Paul; Minnesota, *Statutes*, 1894, section 6619.
[32] Bracken to O. S. Watkins, January 8, 18, 1902; Watkins to Bracken, February 23, 1902; Ohage to Bracken, March 5, 1902; L. B. Shehan to Bracken, January 29, 1902. Minnesota Department of Health, St. Paul.

Bonne & Howe camps in Hubbard County, on the boundary of Beltrami County, reported fifteen cases, causing Beltrami's county physician to fear that some of these men might come into his district with the biweekly tote teams. The Pine Tree Lumber Company of Little Falls had some sixty to eighty cases in its camps in the southern part of Cass County.[33]

Bracken put the blame in the last instance squarely on the company. "It is stated," he wrote, "that they had this disease in their camps last winter, that they were ordered to fumigate, and burn blankets, that they did not burn the blankets, and that when the men came down with the disease this winter it was found that they were using the blankets that had been infected the winter before. . . . It is stated that when these men got to Camp No. 3 in the evening they found several men sick in bed. The foreman told them that it was the grippe, but when daylight came they found that these men's faces were all broken out with small pox." The Pine Tree Lumber Company vigorously denied these statements, although one of its officers wrote privately: "One of our camps here has had smallpox almost continuously since Thanksgiving time." The company said, however, that isolation practices were enforced, "so that the crew was practically free from infection." The blanket situation was a little different. Three-fourths of the blankets were brand new, and those used in infected camps had been disinfected. But blankets actually used by smallpox patients had been destroyed. "You certainly do not expect us to destroy all the bedding used in these camps by men who were not infected with the disease," an official wrote Bracken, who replied, courteously enough, that perhaps he had been misinformed about the use of infected blankets. But he went on to say that he did not doubt that men had been hired for Camp 3 with the statement "that there was no smallpox there, when as a matter of fact there was." [34]

For the next decade, from 1903 to 1913, lumber camp sanitation, coupled with intermittent outbreaks of smallpox, was an annual headache for health officers. Although more than six thousand cases for the state as a whole were reported in 1908, lumber centers were comparatively free. Two years later Duluth physicians reported cases in camps

[33] F. A. Blakeslee to Bracken, January [?], 8, 15, 1903; E. H. Wood to Bracken, January 6, 1903. Minnesota Department of Health, St. Paul.
[34] Bracken to A. H. Wilcox, March 19, 1903, and to B. J. Hinkle, March 31, 1903, and Hinkle to Bracken, March 24, 30, 1903, Minnesota Department of Health, St. Paul; Charles A. Weyerhaeuser to W. Hayes Laird, March 6, 1903, in the Laird Norton Company Papers, in the possession of the Minnesota Historical Society.

of the Alger, Smith Lumber Company, especially in the vicinity of Knife River. The disease also appeared in Mountain Iron camps of the Cloquet Lumber Company. At the same time a threatened epidemic of diphtheria worried health officers. After so many years of attempting to control camp sanitation and to enforce vaccination rulings, Bracken was so nearly at his wit's end that he wrote: "In dealing with lumber jacks, etc., we are in a helpless position relative to the control of communicable diseases, and this includes small pox. There is no law that compels these men to be vaccinated, and no legal restraint on them except quarantine. I realize that quarantine in a lumber camp is next to an impossibility, so nearly an impossibility that I would not urge anyone to do it. The only thing to do is to use sound judgment in the handling of these cases, and do it in the best way possible."[35]

Fortunately smallpox decreased in 1912 and 1913, with only minor outbreaks occurring in Aitkin, Polk, and St. Louis counties, where lumbering was being carried on, but these cases did not involve the pineries primarily, although they affected them. Less than two thousand cases were reported for 1914 and 1915.[36]

The decrease of smallpox gave the Minnesota Department of Health an opportunity to turn from epidemiological work to sanitation. This activity was aided by inspectors from the State Department of Labor and Industries, which had been reorganized on August 1, 1913.[37] Among its duties was the inspection of laborers' boardinghouses, railroad camps, and lumber camps. The Minneapolis Associated Charities was interested also. Strictly speaking, the health department had no legal authority to inspect camps except in connection with the outbreak of a contagious disease. Therefore, when complaints were made that lumber camps were in frightful condition, Bracken could only reply that the board lacked authority to act and that it was without funds and personnel to investigate even if it had the power. Typical charges were these: "There is no floor under the lower bunks, nothing but some poles with finish layed on them, and some hay and the hay is damp and mouldy most of the time both from the damp of the

[35] State Board of Health, *Biennial Reports*, 1909–10, p. 58; Bracken to F. J. Patton, January 20, 1910, to C. H. Clark, January 26, 1910, and to Tuohy, January 25, 26, February 28, 1910, Tuohy to Bracken, January 25, 27, 1910, and to the Cloquet Lumber Company, January 31, 1910, Alger, Smith Company to Tuohy, January 21, 1910, Cloquet Lumber Company to Tuohy, March 4, 1910, Minnesota Department of Health, St, Paul.
[36] State Board of Health, *Biennial Reports*, 1913–14, p. 184; 1914–15, p. 136.
[37] Minnesota Department of Labor and Industries, *Biennial Reports*, 1913–14. See pages 14–22 for a history of the department.

EPIDEMICS IN THE NORTH WOODS 215

ground and the leak of the roof which leaks bad enough to wet through all the blankets and hay on the top bunks and the blankets of the bottom bunks. The roof consists of poles that are split and layed on with the round side up, and covered with tar paper unsufficient to keep from leaking." [38]

One of the most extensive investigations conducted by the labor department occurred early in 1914, when logging centers in the vicinity of Boy River were visited. Everything from hospital care to menus, including wages and construction of bunkhouses, was inventoried carefully. Sanitary facilities in all the camps were inadequate, but some were better than others. The Fagan Brothers had made arrangements with the Benedictine Sisters of St. Anthony Hospital at Bemidji to care for their jacks in case of sickness or accident. For this service the hospital received one dollar monthly for each employee who was not protected by a hospital ticket. But "chronic or contagious sickness, such as scarlet fever, small pox, measles, venereal diseases and sickness arising from intoxication, or accidents arising from fighting," were excluded from this benefit.

The hospital-ticket plan, sometimes known as the ten-dollar plan, was a curious institution. Companies sometimes charged loggers a flat fee of ten dollars, deducting it from their pay. For this sum, the lumberjack, miner, or railroader received limited medical care, including hospitalization, if necessary. The difficulty, of course, was that turnover among such laborers was large. A jack might spend only a week or a month at a camp and then pick up and leave, because the food was not to his taste, because the foreman was unpleasant, because work was too heavy, because the camp was infected, because pay was too low, or merely because he became bored. When he took another job, another ten dollars was withheld from his pay. Many jacks considered the ten-dollar plan only a carefully concocted scheme on the part of companies to reduce their incomes.[39]

Except for liniments sold in company commissaries, first-aid facilities — bandages, tourniquets, splints, even stretchers — were lacking. Trainmen reported that companies did not even make an effort to transport injured men to trains, leaving that duty to their comrades. Nor did the

[38] Bracken to J. W. McCord, March 8, 1910, and to Tuohy, March 8, 1910, Minnesota Department of Health, St. Paul.
[39] Hugo V. Koch and Martin Cole to W. F. Houk, March 1, 1914, Minnesota Department of Health, St. Paul; Philip D. Jordan, "Beginnings of Minnesota Public Health," in *Bulletin of the History of Medicine*, 21:750 (September–October, 1947).

company telegraph ahead to have someone unload the patient at his destination. On one occasion lumberjacks broke into a section house, rolled out a handcar, placed an accident victim on it, and then pumped the car to Federal Dam, where they borrowed a team and drove the patient to Bena. There they managed to get him abroad a train. At other times employees made up purses to pay a patient's railroad fare. As pay was thirty dollars a month for sawyers and from thirty-five to forty for cant-hook men, with an over-all average of about twenty dollars, the jacks were not flush. The company stores around Boy River in 1914 seem to have charged a fair price, although the men constantly complained. Pipe tobacco sold at ten cents, soap at five cents a bar, underwear at two dollars a garment, German socks from twenty-five to sixty cents a pair, and overalls at a dollar.[40]

Cookhouses were fairly clean, but tin dishes and table tools were washed in sloppy water, so that they were greasy when returned to the table. Menus were adequate, with emphasis placed on fresh beef, mutton, salt pork, and sausage. Tremendous quantities of potatoes, rutabagas, kraut, tomatoes, and corn were served. Oatmeal and rice were standard. Pumpkins, apples, apricots, and raisins were used for pies. Oleomargarine was used as a butter substitute. Bread and biscuits were made from good quality flour. Water usually was secured from wells, which all too frequently were located too close either to privies or to disposal pits. Kitchen refuse was sometimes dumped on the surface of the ground not far from the kitchen door.

Inspectors described one camp privy that was only a pole enclosure, six by twelve feet, with a low roof covering an open pit filled with excrement up to the height of the seat. There was no evidence that lime had been used at any time during the season. Another privy was filled above the poles serving as seats, and "all along the paths leading into the camp were piles of excrement." It is little wonder that the inspectors said: "It is a pity one cannot go into such a camp as this, order the men to get their belongings out and then touch a match to it and burn it to the ground." A better situation prevailed in another camp, where the privy was constructed of boards; it was scrubbed weekly, and lime was applied.[41]

In 1923 the health department proposed to adopt regulations affecting logging and industrial camps. Such regulations, of course, would

[40] Koch and Cole to Houk, March 1, 1914, Minnesota Department of Health, St. Paul.
[41] Koch and Cole to Houk, March 1, 1914, Minnesota Department of Health, St. Paul.

have the full force of law and could be enforced. A meeting of interested parties was held in September, and regulations were ready by November 6. They defined a "camp" as any place where ten or more men were employed and housed in temporary quarters; specified proper location and arrangement of buildings; gave directions for the proper amount of air space in sleeping quarters; stipulated that screens no coarser than fourteen mesh be installed; said that floors must be of wood, concrete, or some equally good material; insisted that bunks be at least twelve inches above the floor and be constructed of iron; laid down rules for the cleaning and heating of living quarters; insisted that water supply meet requirements of the state health department; made detailed provision for location, construction, and maintenance of toilets and privies; and contained instructions for the disposal of refuse, garbage, manure, water waste, and slops. These regulations became effective on October 1, 1924. Revised from time to time, they still contain much of the original thinking.[42]

Slowly but surely the enforcement of these regulations had their effect on the logging industry. The Timber Producers Association at Duluth sent a form letter to its membership in 1943. "How much attention are you giving to living conditions around your Camp? How near or how far are you from reasonable compliance with the state regulations governing industrial camps?" it asked. The association went on to say that "many operators" were neglecting to make improvements required by law to make conditions more comfortable and attractive. "Some complaints have reached this office in regard to cleanliness for which there is no excuse as long as soap and water and willing elbow grease are at hand. A few operators fail to provide enough lights so that men can read or mend clothes in the evening. At another camp, which has been running two years, we are informed that there is only one washtub for the crew to use in washing clothes. . . . The reason for sending out this letter is to call the attention of our members to the fact that every reasonable effort must be made to attract and hold whatever manpower there is available to the timber producing industry at this time when competition from other industries is so strong."[43]

Ilmar Koivunen, president of the Timber Workers' Union, Local

[42] "Meeting Held September 25, [1923], Regarding Industrial Camp Sanitation" and "Regulations Relating to Industrial Camps, November 6, 1923" (typescripts), Minnesota Department of Health, Minneapolis; State Board of Health, *Regulations Relating to Industrial Camps* (Minneapolis, June 17, 1937), and *Minnesota State Health Laws and Regulations*, 90–93 (Minneapolis, January 1, 1948).

[43] Timber Producers Association to Members, January 8, 1943, Minnesota Department of Health, Minneapolis.

Number 29, wrote Governor Stassen that operators were completely disregarding state health regulations and charged that the state health department had not satisfactorily enforced the regulations. He asked the governor to appoint a representative "to see that the Board of Health's regulations on camp conditions would be enforced." As a result of this letter and because of the communication distributed by the Timber Producers Association, the division of sanitation proposed that a survey be made of all logging camps in co-operation with the Industrial Commission.[44]

Sanitary surveys proceed slowly and consume time, especially during a war period when loss of personnel and emergency demands tax the efforts of any department. An inspector was assigned to survey logging camps, but he did not work rapidly enough to suit CIO officials, who complained that he was neglecting his responsibilities and said that conditions in camps were getting worse instead of better.[45] By 1946 inspection of camps had become routine practice, with specific reports made not only of violations, but also of recommendations which would improve conditions. Violations included, for example, an insufficient number of windows in bunkhouses, lack of separate clothes-drying rooms, faulty construction of floors, walls that were too low, insufficient number of exits in bunkhouses, and unsatisfactory ventilation. Recommendations included replacement of wooden bunks with metal ones, use of mattress slips, laundering of pillow slips, and the airing of wool blankets. Other recommendations pertained to the location of the source of water supply, the construction of the water system, and the remodeling of privies. The old-time lumberjack, living in the midst of filth in the 1880s, would have been utterly astonished to know that in 1946 the health department insisted that toilet paper be placed in outhouses and that unchipped dishes be used on dining tables. He would have been equally surprised to learn that the old tin dipper no longer was acceptable, but that individual paper drinking cups were preferred.[46]

[44] Ilmar Koivunen to Harold Stassen, January 13, 1943; Whittaker to Chesley, February 1, 1943. Minnesota Department of Health, Minneapolis.
[45] Koivunen to Chesley, December 17, 1945, Minnesota Department of Health, Minneapolis; Minnesota Department of Health, Division of General Sanitation, "Quarterly Reports," December 31, 1945.
[46] Minnesota Department of Health, Division of General Sanitation, "Report No. 1 on Wisconsin Minnesota Timber Company, January 2, 1946," "Report on Slatten Logging Camp No. 1, March 1, 1946," and "Report on Investigation of the Walter Zagrabelny Logging Camp, March 3, 1948" (typescripts), Minnesota Department of Health, Minneapolis.

The old days indeed were gone, but the peak of Minnesota's logging activities had passed also. No longer do tall stands of dignified Norway pines thrust their mighty trunks straight into Minnesota's blue skies. Instead the north country, once the scene of smallpox epidemics and the home of infected lumberjacks, is now covered with a second growth of poplar and dotted with hundreds of resorts. What camps remain are tightly supervised, so that today public health is as well protected in the woods as in the cities.

12

Health Officer vs. Medicine Man

THE HEALTH of Minnesota's Indians has long been a problem. Before they were pushed from tribal hunting grounds to become wards of a government that placed them on reservations and restricted their liberty, both the Chippewa and the Sioux had felt the ravages of contagious diseases. They were sovereigns of the woods and lakes, but abject humans who cried aloud for relief when smallpox struck or trachoma blinded their eyes.

As early as 1698 smallpox created terrible havoc along the Mississippi River and, as decade followed decade, explorers and travelers noted in their journals one epidemic after another. Henry R. Schoolcraft, in particular, spoke of the prevalence of smallpox, which had appeared in the north country in 1782, and said that the Indians called it "Ma Mukkizziwin," a term which suggested the disfiguration of flesh and skin. As Schoolcraft's expedition was ordered to vaccinate as many red men as possible, he took more than the usual interest in Indian health. The report of his surgeon, Dr. Douglas Houghton, showed that he had little difficulty in convincing Indians of the efficacy of vaccination and the "universal dread in which they hold the appearance of the small pox among them, rendered it an easy task to overcome their prejudices, whatever they chanced to be."[1]

Before arriving at Lake Pepin, Count Francesco Arese passed through the remains of the village of La Feuille — probably Winona — where many unfortunates were dead from smallpox. Later, along Red Pipestone Creek, Arese and his party discovered the intermingled bones of men and horses of a band of Sioux who had attempted to flee

---

[1] E. Wagner Stearn and Allen E. Stearn, *The Effect of Smallpox on the Destiny of the Amerindian*, 33 (Boston, 1945); Schoolcraft, *Narrative of an Expedition through the Upper Mississippi to Itasca Lake*, 83, 252 (New York, 1834).

from an outbreak at Vermillion but had been overtaken by the disease. Ramsay Crooks, agent of the American Fur Company, wrote Sibley in 1834 that Indians were afflicted with "hooping" cough. Residents in primitive St. Paul in 1849 heard Indians tell of great epidemics of measles that had swept through the tribes about twenty years earlier.[2]

The most trustworthy reports of health and disease among Minnesota's Indians, however, were made in the early period by army surgeons attached to western posts. Generally these physicians were men of ability, who had some general scientific interests in addition to their medical training. They were required to submit periodical reports to the surgeon general's office, reports that dealt not only with the health of troops, but also with topographic and climatic conditions, with flora and fauna, and with disease among the tribes. "As far as I am informed," wrote a surgeon stationed at Fort Dodge, Iowa, in 1852, "the numerous Indian tribes west and north of us are fast becoming extinct by cholera and smallpox — by the latter disease in particular."[3]

Surgeons stationed at Forts Ripley and Ridgely in Minnesota agreed with their Iowa colleague that both cholera and smallpox had decimated the tribes, but they felt that the Indian population was not doomed to extinction. Indeed, Dr. David Day, attached to the Winnebago Agency, wrote positively that the Winnebago had not decreased in numbers in three years and said further that the birth rate equaled or exceeded the death rate. Day added several interesting observations. He said that the Indian did not live as long as the white man or the Negro, that infant mortality was very great among Indians, and that the proportion of births among them was greater than in any other people.[4]

Although Assistant Surgeon Head at Fort Ripley did not mention either cholera or smallpox, he did list the prevailing diseases among the Indians with whom he came in contact. They were bronchitis, dysentery, and diarrhea. He saw only one case of tubercular phthisis. Gonorrhea of a mild character was commonplace, but Head said that he had never seen nor heard of a case of syphilis. The army doctor at Fort Ridgely in 1856 listed the same diseases that Head had named, but he added scrofulous affections, rheumatism, and diseases of the ear and eye. The last, which was undoubtedly trachoma, he said was

[2] Francesco Arese, *A Trip to the Prairies and in the Interior of North America [1837–1838]*, 97, 135 (New York, 1934); Crooks to Sibley, December 31, 1834, in the Sibley Papers, in the possession of the Minnesota Historical Society; *Minnesota Pioneer*, December 26, 1849.
[3] Coolidge, *Sickness and Mortality in the Army, 1839 to 1855*, 56.
[4] Coolidge, *Sickness and Mortality in the Army, 1839 to 1855*, 63.

remarkably frequent among Indians, and he attributed it to exposure to the glare of sun and snow, the cold winds of the prairie, and the smoky atmosphere of wigwams.[5]

Neither surgeon commented upon the custom practiced by both Sioux and Chippewa of isolating patients suffering with contagious diseases and then burning their wigwams and possessions when these illnesses had run their course, but Dr. Hasson, also at Fort Ridgely, wrote at length upon the activities of the medicine man. He told of the chanting, the beating of rude drums, and the rattling of gourds, all of which were presumed to drive the evil spirits of sickness from a patient's body. Yet Hasson also said that Indians resorted to sweat baths and used herbal medicines.[6]

Dr. Thomas S. Williamson, a missionary who arrived at Fort Snelling in May, 1835, recalled that consumption was the prevailing cause of death among the Indians whom he saw. Smallpox, measles, and dysentery ranked next. Cholera infantum, dysentery, and fever attacked children during the autumn of 1845. It was during that crisp fall that Williamson moved from Lac qui Parle to Little Crow's village in order to tend the sick. Kaposia, located about six miles by river below St. Paul, was indeed an afflicted community when the doctor arrived. He treated several genuine cases of fever and ague and saw a large number of abnormal cases of paludal disease. A few years later whooping cough caused much distress. Like other physicians before and after him, Williamson competed with the medicine men. He thought these painted, yelling practitioners were quacks, but he was honest enough to admit that they administered vegetable medicines with a fair degree of success, especially as emetics, purgatives, and clysters. Indeed, the Dakota name for physician was "pay-zhe-hoo-ta-we-chasta," which meant herb-root man.[7] For purging, both the Dakota and the Ojibway used the root of the euphorbium. They also practiced phlebotomy, devising a blood-letting instrument from sharp flint fastened in a stick which, like a fleam used in bleeding horses, was driven in with one stroke.

Only a year before Williamson began practice in the Minnesota

---

[5] Coolidge, *Sickness and Mortality in the Army, 1839 to 1855*, 61, 72.

[6] William W. Warren, "History of the Ojibways Based upon Traditions and Oral Statements," in *Minnesota Historical Collections*, 5:100; Coolidge, *Sickness and Mortality in the Army, 1839 to 1855*, 71; William T. Corlett, *The Medicine-Man of the American Indian and His Cultural Background* (Springfield, Illinois, 1935).

[7] Williamson, "Diseases of the Dakota Indians," in *Minnesota Medicine*, 23:802 (November, 1940).

country, the federal government took an important legislative step which eventually resulted in the development of an Indian health program and was to involve the Minnesota Department of Health. This act of June 30, 1834, created the Department of Indian Affairs and specifically stipulated that an agency be established "for the Saint Peter's [Minnesota]."[8] Here, then, was the legal beginning of the eight Indian reservations and five Indian communities which were operating in Minnesota in 1948, one hundred and fourteen years after this act was passed.

By 1855 three regular agents, two farmer-agents, and a physician were tending to the educational, economic, and physical needs of Minnesota's Indians. Dr. Asa W. Daniels reported the appearance of smallpox, but said that a speedy and successful vaccination program prevented its spread. Two years later, when Charles E. Flandrau and other agents were concerned primarily with the Spirit Lake uprising, only one government worker commented upon health conditions. He spoke particularly of the ravages of consumption among the Winnebago. When Dr. John V. Wren, physician to the Chippewa, visited Gull and Leech lakes in 1859, he said that he was astonished "that any people could, as a whole nation, be so thoroughly saturated, if I may use the expression, as I found these Indians with that curse, the syphilis." He treated a total of 632 cases among both adults and children. Other government doctors commented upon the presence of venereal diseases.[9]

The difficulties which these government physicians faced in caring for their charges were numerous. Their primary concern, as Dr. A. Barnard indicated, was to improve the sanitary conditions of the tribes and to prevent disease if possible. But Barnard pointed out that he had charge of some four thousand Indians, that they were scattered over a wide extent of territory, some bands being a hundred miles from his house, and that the best he could do was to attempt regular visits once every three months. Practically all doctors and agents mentioned at one time or another that disease among the Indians increased as more and more white men migrated to Minnesota. Edward P. Smith, agent at White Earth, said frankly that Mississippi Chippewa at White Oak Point were "coming more and more in contact with lumbermen, who are close on the border of their reservation, and some of them are

[8] *Statutes at Large*, 4:736.
[9] Commissioner of Indian Affairs, *Annual Reports*, 1855, p. 68; 1857, p. 116; 1859, p. 72; 1862, p. 91.

learning to work in their camps, while all are learning more or less of the worst vices of civilization." [10]

Not all blame for unsanitary conditions, however, was laid to the vast hordes of people pouring into Minnesota after the Civil War. An agency physician at Red Lake blamed the tribes themselves, saying that their illnesses were caused by filthy habits of living, by exposure to cold and moisture, by meager diet, by inherited virus, and by excessive purgation. Indians were said to live in filth and among vermin, and the implication was that they enjoyed that way of life. On the other hand, the agent at White Earth pointed out that his charges were grateful for sanitary advice and eager to receive medical attention. He suggested, however, that the government send only graduates of medical colleges as physicians to agencies. "Heretofore persons have been employed who have assumed the responsibilities of physicians," the agent reported to his superiors, "and the consequences were that they met with poor success in keeping down sickness, as well as to cause the Indians to lose faith in the superiority of the white man's medicines and to return to their former methods of curing their sick." [11]

Regardless of the reasons why Minnesota's Indians fell sick, the fact remains that they did and that when Hewitt helped establish the state board in 1872, the public health of the red man already was a sizable problem. At that time agencies had been established, by various religious denominations and under the terms of several treaties, at Bois Fort, Fond du Lac, Grand Portage, Leech Lake, Mille Lacs, Red Lake, White Earth, and White Oak Point. Collectively, they occupied 7,835 square miles. Although population figures for all these agencies are difficult to obtain, it is known that the Mississippi Pillager, Pembina, and Red Lake bands of Chippewa in 1881 numbered just a little over six thousand. By then the federal government was collecting statistics showing diseases among the Indians. Thus Hewitt was able to determine that, on the reservations at White Earth, Leech Lake, and Red Lake, zymotic or infectious diseases for the year 1881 accounted for 365 illnesses; that venereal disease cases totaled 171; that diathetic diseases numbered 564; that tuberculosis was responsible for 424 cases; that parasitic diseases totaled 183; and that diseases of the respiratory tract accounted for 639. Diseases of the eye outnumbered diseases of the ear by 347 to 114. It is interesting to note, too, that afflictions of

[10] Commissioner of Indian Affairs, *Annual Reports*, 1866, p. 295; 1872, p. 209.
[11] Commissioner of Indian Affairs, *Annual Reports*, 1876, p. 83; 1878, p. 81.

the digestive tract far outnumbered diseases of the urinary tract. Births outnumbered deaths by only a slight margin of six.[12]

During the smallpox epidemic at Wadena in June, 1877, Hewitt had visited the White Earth Reservation to vaccinate the agent, the missionaries, and some of the half-breeds who were loafing about. He elicited a promise from both the agent and the physician that wandering bands of Indians would be called in and vaccinated. The agent also promised to send Hewitt reports if smallpox cases developed. Again in 1883 Hewitt was apprehensive that the smallpox epidemic which was running through lumber camps in Itasca County would spread to Indians. His fears were justified, for thirty-five Indians lost their lives in that epidemic. Dr. Ashley Thompson, agency physician at Red Lake, had to make a special trip to St. Paul in March, 1883, in order to reach Leech Lake, where smallpox had broken out among the Pillager Chippewa. A little later the Reverend Joseph A. Gilfillan, an Episcopal missionary who had worked among the Indians for years, reported that the White Earth and White Oak Point Indians had suffered severely from smallpox during the winter. From Fort Frances came word that twenty Indians had died from smallpox.[13]

On April 14, 1883, Hewitt telegraphed the secretary of the interior that word had reached him that Indians who had been exposed to smallpox were wandering about the country wearing infected clothing, and he requested that a competent person be instructed with full power to act. The commissioner of Indian affairs immediately answered that the agent at Lake Winnibigoshish had been instructed to purchase new clothing for his wards and said that a government physician had the situation well in hand. This doctor was the same Thompson who had been ordered to minister to the Pillager Chippewa. In his own defense, Thompson wrote, in effect, that he could not be everywhere at once. Then he added: "For me to leave Winnebagoshish before the fourteen Indians here and the ten at Raven's point, quarantined in their wigwams have cast away their disease-saturated clothing and blankets, would indeed look like doing the duties of a health officer in a most incompetent manner."[14]

This seemed to satisfy Hewitt, but in August he again became worried over a report from Duluth that an explorer just returned from

[12] Commissioner of Indian Affairs, *Annual Reports*, 1881, pp. 265, 280, 310.
[13] State Board of Health, *Annual Reports*, 1878, p. 8; *Biennial Reports*, 1883–84, p. 18; *Pioneer Press*, March 20, 21, April 13, 1883.
[14] *Pioneer Press*, April 15, 1883.

Itasca County had reported smallpox among the Indians. He said they were entirely without medical aid and that "this terrible disease has full sway." Hewitt immediately dispatched Dr. Vespasian Smith of Duluth and Dr. J. C. Rosser of Brainerd to the Bowstring. They found only the remains of burned bodies and wigwams. These Indians had fallen victims to smallpox the previous winter and represented no new cases.[15]

Periodically, of course, Minnesota newspapers reported that Indians were dying because of lack of food and clothing. Early in 1875 the report circulated that girls enrolled at the Winnebago Indian Agency were common prostitutes with the knowledge and approval of their parents. During the winter of 1883–84 Hewitt was upset by stories that the Mille Lacs Indians were in desperate plight and that many were dying for want of food. Again, in 1890, charges on the White Earth Reservation were reported to be destitute. It was true, as many agents frequently pointed out, that the Indian population sometimes suffered severely, especially during winter months. Older braves and squaws suffered particularly, for they were subject to infirmities that prevented them not only from gathering food but also from traveling to a physician when they became ill. Sometimes it was even impossible for younger folk, when the temperature was forty below zero, to travel to food distribution centers.[16]

Yet on February 8, 1887, the federal government had passed the General Allotment Act, which sought to make Indians reasonably independent by granting to each head of a family one quarter section of land, to every single person over eighteen years of age an eighth of a section, and to each orphan child under eighteen an eighth of a section. It is interesting to note that, only a few days later, Congress passed an act granting the Saint Paul, Minneapolis, and Manitoba Railway Company the right of way through Indian reservations in northern Montana and northwestern Dakota.[17]

The Indians were slow in taking up their allotments, even though some of them had been engaged in more or less haphazard farming for years. They seemed to prefer to harvest the wild rice and, as the agent at White Earth indicated, to collect blueberries and cranberries and to make maple sugar. He also said in 1894 that hunting and fishing

---

[15] *Minneapolis Tribune*, August 11, 1883; *Pioneer Press*, August 17, 1883.

[16] *Pioneer-Press*, May 20, 1875, February 20, 18, 1890; Commissioner of Indian Affairs, *Annual Reports*, 1894, p. 152. For a recent discussion of famine, see the *Tribune*, March 17, 1948.

[17] *Statutes at Large*, 24:388, 402.

were getting poorer every year, so that old ways of securing food would have to be replaced by new. That year a total of 2,826 allotments had been taken out on the agency, but its aggregate population was 7,132. Robert M. Allen, the agent, suggested that every Indian house have at least a half-acre garden, for he thought that produce from this, in addition to the regular annuities, would make every home almost self-sustaining.[18]

The state health department, during the latter decades of the nineteenth century, was concerned with Indian diet and housing only because of their relationship to health. Both Hewitt and Bracken knew that poor food and unsanitary homes contributed to disease, especially tuberculosis. Each felt that both state and federal governments should attempt, as a public health policy, to root out factors making for the spread of disease. Yet Minnesota's Indians were under the supervision of the national government, and the state department could take action only as a co-operative agency or only when an epidemic among Indians threatened the health of the rest of the population.

Health officers operating in both organized and unorganized northern Minnesota areas were well aware that Indian agents did not always paint a complete and accurate picture of affairs on reservations. They knew, too, that government physicians attached to reservations were not always men of high professional attainments. Both state and local health officials did their best when disease was rife among the tribes, but frequently their best was limited by ineptness and noncooperation. At other times, of course, the state department received genuine and expert assistance from agents and physicians.

Regardless of all this, the state department knew that periodic epidemics might be avoided and the general health of the Indian improved. For years individuals and the press had talked of sickness among the tribes. In 1873 the missionary Gilfillan "constantly saw children clad only in the cotton shirt, cotton leggings, and moccasins, standing in the road in the cold snowy weather, coughing violently with the whooping cough." An old trader recalled how in 1855 Indians applied salt pork saturated with turpentine to the throat when treating an outbreak of diphtheria. John H. Fairbanks, Sr., told of an epidemic of measles among the Leech Lake Indians and estimated the total deaths at 175. And Bracken was most concerned over the smallpox epidemic of 1901–02.[19]

[18] Commissioner of Indian Affairs, *Annual Reports*, 1894, p. 149.
[19] Gilfillan, "The Ojibways in Minnesota," in *Minnesota Historical Collections*, 9:98; *Stillwater Gazette*, November 27, 1878; *Pioneer Press*, April 23, 1880.

The first indication that smallpox was appearing came late in 1900, when Bracken read that the Turtle Mountain Indians of North Dakota were afflicted. Not until June of 1901 did the Minnesota department begin receiving complaints that the disease had struck in the vicinity of Cass Lake. From then until the end of the year innumerable complaints reached Bracken. The health officer at Grand Marais, for example, found two cases among the Indians and quarantined their homes. But he said that he was unable to hold the occupants very closely for these reasons: "(1) Indians are notoriously restless under restraint and when not suffering themselves seem to be careless about exposing others. (2) It is difficult to get others than Indians to act as Police and of course they sympathize and fraternize with each other. (3) There is no jail or other place where one could be confined if arrested, consequently we are almost powerless to enforce strict regulations." [20]

Bracken immediately followed his usual practice when dealing with Indian epidemics. He wrote the agency physician at Onigum asking for statistics, and, in this instance, he complained to Washington that the epidemic on the White Earth Reservation was not being properly handled. Shortly thereafter the agency doctor, W. J. Stephenson, perhaps stimulated by a letter from the commissioner of Indian affairs, wrote Bracken as follows: "I was congratulating myself that we had Small Pox suppressed on this Agency. But I received word on the 27" that there was small Pox at Squaw Point, (a remote part of the Reservation). I visited the point on the 28" and found four cases developed and placed them under quarantine. We have ordered vaccine points from the Department which we will receive next week and will revaccinate every Indian on the Reservation that has not had small pox, and will keep at it until all are immune." About a month later Stephenson again wrote to Bracken, this time reporting additional cases on Pine River and at Bear Island. The doctor added: "I am free to confess now that the Parke Davis virus we used last winter was a failure — and responsible for a great deal of Small Pox here. We are using the National vaccine virus and it is all right." [21]

Meanwhile the Aitkin County clerk had telegraphed Bracken that smallpox had broken out at Sandy Lake north of McGregor.

[20] Bracken to A. A. Harper, May 14, 1901, and to H. D. Jones, June 20, 1901; Jones to Bracken, June 16, 1901. Minnesota Department of Health, St. Paul.
[21] Stephenson to Bracken, July 8, August 29, September 27, 1901; Bracken to Stephenson, July 13, 1901, and to W. A. Jones, August 3, 1901; Jones to Bracken, August 20, 1901. Minnesota Department of Health, St. Paul.

Bracken replied that Indians are federal wards, adding: "If you will kindly advise me as to the agency these Indians are under, I will draw the attention of the Indian Agent to the fact. The Local Board of Health, or in the event of these Indians being in unorganized territory the County Board of Health can take temporary action against them. The localities can quarantine against them so that you can protect yourselves until the Indian Agent through the Indian physicians has time to act." [22]

Once again, after waiting for action by government physicians, Bracken complained to Washington, and once again the usual reply was made — that the matter had been taken up by the commissioner of Indian affairs and that instructions had been sent to Minnesota agents to take the necessary steps to control and eradicate the disease. Two weeks after Bracken received this letter of assurance a physician at Aitkin wrote that several bands of Indians were camped in different parts of the county, some near Mille Lacs Lake and others near Sandy Lake, and that these Indians had smallpox. The doctor added that Indian agents at White Earth and Leech Lake had been notified and had promised to attend to the matter, but had failed to do so. "These Indians are running around and mingling with the white settlers more or less and will probably spread the disease," continued the Aitkin doctor. "Is there anyway to compel the Government officials to take care of them? In some cases the Indians are defiant and as they are scattered, it is a pretty difficult & expensive proposition for the County to assume. Just at this season of the year this county is full of men from all over this state and others, hunting & looking up lands — they often meet and come in contact with the Indians. Please let me know what can be done." [23]

Bracken replied that the Indian problem in northern Minnesota was by no means an easy one to deal with. He said that he had corresponded with officials in Washington and that he thought some good had come from it. But he promised to "stir up" matters again if he found agents not inclined to do their duty. When the Aitkin doctor again complained that three Indian deaths had occurred and that the agency physician at Cass Lake had no authority to act other than to

[22] George W. Dodge to Bracken, July 20, 1901; Bracken to Dodge, July 22, 1901. Minnesota Department of Health, St. Paul.
[23] Bracken to Thomas Ryan, September 26, 1901; Ryan to Bracken, September 30, 1901; Carlton Graves to Bracken, November 10, 1901. Minnesota Department of Health, St. Paul.

vaccinate, Bracken promised to take the matter up with the Department of the Interior.[24]

As a result of this complaint, Bracken got a sharp answer from an Indian agent stationed at Ashland, Wisconsin. The outbreak at Aitkin seems to have spread to Ely by way of lumbering camps and thus it involved the jurisdiction of the La Pointe Indian Agency. Bracken's criticisms had been referred there. S. W. Campbell, the agent, told Bracken that Indians living off reservations were amenable to the laws of the town, county, and state in which they lived and were entitled to all the rights and privileges enjoyed by any other citizens of the state. He argued further that agencies had no right to order quarantine off the reservations and that they had never interfered in the least with state health officers. The duties of both agent and physician were to see that the Indian got fair treatment and, when he was neglected, to supply him with what he needed to make him comfortable. "You have heretofore made unfair complaint to the Department at Washington," Campbell continued, "in regard to these matters as you reported a part of the truth only. In doing so you screened your local health officers and wrongfully censured the officers of this agency. I am willing to take censure from my proper superiors when I am guilty of neglecting my duty, but I will not stand it for a moment from parties who are endeavoring to shield their own negligence." [25]

Campbell, in a later letter, also told Bracken that Minnesota lumber camps were more dangerous to health than were Indian reservations. To this Bracken agreed cheerfully, saying: "I appreciate the fact that it is much harder to handle lumber jacks than it is to handle Indians, and I am doing everything I can to bring the lumbermen themselves into line. They are after the almighty dollar however and care little for laws." [26]

This sharp exchange of letters, nevertheless, did not diminish Bracken's zeal in dealing with Indian agents and physicians. As smallpox continued to spread among Indians in Aitkin County and as Bracken continued to hear that afflicted Indians were off their reservations and were roaming without supervision over the countryside, the secretary penned a pungent note to a government physician at Frazee. "It is

[24] Bracken to Graves, November 11, December 2, 1901, and to E. A. Hitchcock, December 2, 1901; Graves to Bracken, November 30, 1901. Minnesota Department of Health, St. Paul.
[25] Campbell to Bracken, January 6, 1902, Minnesota Department of Health, St. Paul.
[26] Campbell to Bracken, January 20, 1902; Bracken to Campbell, January 21, 1902. Minnesota Department of Health, St. Paul.

reported to me that smallpox has existed on the Reservation all spring and summer," he wrote. "It seems strange that the Federal government would allow this to continue. Certainly the Indians should be rounded up and vaccinated and steps should be taken to quarantine them. We do not want the Indians spreading smallpox into the surrounding territory." [27]

The difficulties that an agency physician faced are clearly revealed by Dr. E. R. Barton's reply. He said, first of all, that he had been less than a month on the job. He told Bracken that the only way to get reliable statistics on contagious diseases was to make a house-to-house canvass, and he indicated that this was most difficult. Not only did Indians frequently live in isolated places, but they also were most reluctant to report cases. However, when cases were known, they were immediately quarantined. The doctor also reported that all, or nearly all, the population of the White Earth Reservation had been vaccinated in the fall of 1901 by Dr. J. B. Carman of Detroit. All Indian children were required to give evidence of recent successful vaccination before being admitted to school, and every Indian had to produce the same proof before he could draw his annuity. Barton said warmly that both he and the agent were most anxious to confine smallpox to the reservation. For once Bracken was satisfied. But in his annual report he mentioned the fact that the year 1901 had witnessed 8,485 smallpox cases in Minnesota.[28]

It is interesting to note that neither Captain W. A. Mercer, acting agent at Leech Lake, nor Simon Michelet, agent at White Earth, mentioned the epidemic in their reports for 1901, although superintendents of several of the reservation schools spoke not only of smallpox but also of measles. John Morrison, principal teacher at Cross Lake School at Red Lake, was the frankest of all. "Owing to the prevalence of smallpox at the present time, I fear that much trouble is in store for us during the coming year," he wrote. The next year, however, Michelet told of a large number of cases among the Mille Lacs Indians and said, with obvious pride, that 4,409 Indians out of 4,752 had been vaccinated on the White Earth Reservation.[29]

In 1905 the Office of Indian Affairs recommended that every agency

[27] Bracken to A. H. Reed, March 10, 1902, to Zack Leon, August 12, 1902, and to Edgar R. Barton, August 12, 1902, Minnesota Department of Health, St. Paul.
[28] Barton to Bracken, August 14, 1902, and Bracken to Barton, August 15, 1902, Minnesota Department of Health, St. Paul; State Board of Health, *Biennial Reports*, 1901–02, map facing 98.
[29] Commissioner of Indian Affairs, *Annual Reports*, 1901, part 1, p. 253; 1902, part 1, p. 224.

physician be furnished with a kit of simple surgical instruments and that an Indian tuberculosis sanatorium be established. Four years later tuberculosis stood at the head of diseases afflicting the Indian and was on the increase. Moreover, trachoma was spreading rapidly among the government's red wards. Although the Minnesota Department of Health had in the past assisted reservation authorities in making water and sanitary surveys, it had not actually taken part in a searching investigation of any one disease. The department had also been concerned indirectly with the use of whisky by the Indians, and Bracken had supported Minnesota's laws for prohibiting the sale of liquor to the red man.[30]

The opportunity to co-operate with the national government in a health survey came early in 1912. The previous year an extensive investigation of the White Earth Reservation had begun with government physicians making house-to-house inspections. Both Dr. William H. Abbott and Dr. Thomas T. Powell found large numbers of cases of tuberculosis and trachoma. Other statistics showed that 10.58% of the population on the reservation had tuberculosis and that 58.88% were afflicted with trachoma. When Bracken became aware of this, he requested the United States Public Health Service to send a surgeon to Minnesota to make trachoma surveys. Dr. Taliaferro Clark was ordered to the state, and during his stay he conducted three surveys. The first occupied the month of May, 1912, and consisted of a preliminary investigation of portions of the White Earth and Leech Lake reservations and the examination of a number of school children in towns close to the reservations and of miners on the Mesabi and Vermilion iron ranges. The second was made in October and November and was concerned with the Indian population. The final survey ran through March and April, 1913, and consisted of examinations of public and parochial school children, students at normal schools, and inmates of state institutions, including schools for the deaf and the feeble-minded. Hill and Chesley assisted Clark on his trip to the iron range.[31]

[30] Commissioner of Indian Affairs, *Annual Reports*, 1905, part 2, p. 6; 1909, p. 2; 1911, pp. 36–38; Charles L. Davis to Harry Snyder, March 8, 1899, Bracken to Davis, March 14, April 25, 1899, and Davis to Bracken, April 20, 1899, Minnesota Department of Health, St. Paul.
[31] *Report in the Matter of the Investigation of the White Earth Reservation*, 2:1872–1874 (62 Congress, 3 session, *House Reports*, no. 1336 — serial 6336); Commissioner of Indian Affairs, *Annual Reports*, 1911, p. 152; Taliaferro Clark, *An Investigation of the Prevalence of Trachoma in the State of Minnesota*, 1331 (Reprint 134 from United States Public Health Service, *Public Health Reports*, June 27, 1913 — Washington, D.C., 1913); State Board of Health, *Biennial Reports*, 1911–12, pp. 279-282; H. W. Hill, "Preliminary Report on Trachoma Investigation, May 6–15, 1912" (typescript), Minnesota Department of Health, St. Paul.

Stimulated by Clark's surveys, the state board on July 9, 1912, recommended that trachoma be made a conditionally quarantinable disease, that school supervision be adequate, that every trachomatous child be excluded from classes, that visiting nurses follow up infected children, and that there be systematic treatment of each case. Treatment was outlined by Clark. On the day after the board met, Bracken wrote Governor Eberhart, calling attention to the trachoma situation among the state's Indians. He also forwarded to the governor copies of the board's resolutions regarding the situation, as well as a circular distributed by the Indian service to the Indians of the White Earth Reservation.[32]

"The nature of trachoma," explained the circular, "is such that in its early stages, sometimes until it has run one, two or more years, the eye may feel perfectly well; after a time, however, there are periods when the eye or eyes feel as if sand, dust, a weed seed, or some other foreign body had lodged therein, and inflammation and pain exist for some little time, when all may pass away and the eye feel well again. This may be repeated at intervals for long periods; then more or less the eye ball and lids become affected and sight interfered with, and in many cases to the extent that complete cure is impossible.

"This disease requires a long and regular course of treatment to bring cure or even the best results. An experience extending over several years, and in treating many thousands of these cases, has convinced me that to put medicine into patient's hands for the cure of trachoma is to fail to obtain a cure; so if you who are afflicted will go to the physicians upon the reservation and repeat these visits as often as required and as long as it takes to cure the disease, you will be cooperating to that degree which will bring success to the physician's

[32] Taliaferro Clark, "Trachoma with Especial Reference to the State of Minnesota," in *Journal-Lancet*, 33:159–170 (March 15, 1913); State Board of Health, "Minutes," 1910–12, vol. 5, pp. 407–409, and Bracken to Eberhart, July 10, 1913, Minnesota Department of Health, St. Paul. Bracken for months had carried on an extensive correspondence with officials regarding trachoma. See Bracken to Robert G. Valentine, February 26, 1912, to James N. Graham, March 7, 1912, to Joseph M. Murphy, March 22, 1912, to D. R. Alaway, April 13, 1912, to the commissioner of Indian affairs, April 13, 1912, and to T. H. Beaulieu, April 15, 1912, Beaulieu to Bracken, April 13, 20, 1912, and F. C. Stevens to Bracken, April 17, 1912, Minnesota Department of Health, St. Paul. Bracken wrote Beaulieu on April 23, 1912: "Of course, looking at the [trachoma] question from a selfish point of view, my interests are only for the people who are not on the Indian reservations, for I presume that we can consider the Indian reservations as not under the jurisdiction of the State, but looked at in a broader view, if I can do anything that will be helpful to the Indians, I am ready to do it, both for their sake and for the protection of those with whom they come in contact." Minnesota Department of Health, St. Paul.

work and cure and eradication of this dangerous eye malady from your people." [33]

Trachoma investigations in Minnesota were a part of a nation-wide investigation of Indian health. When Congress on August 24, 1912, made its appropriations for the Office of Indian Affairs, it provided an additional fund of ninety thousand dollars to be used "to relieve distress among Indians and to provide for their care and for the prevention and treatment of tuberculosis, trachoma, smallpox, and other contagious and infectious diseases, including the purchase of vaccine and expense of vaccination." In addition, Congress appropriated ten thousand dollars to enable the United States Public Health Service and the Marine Hospital Service to make a thorough examination "as to the prevalence of tuberculosis, trachoma, smallpox, and other contagious and infectious diseases" among the Indians of the United States.[34]

This act ranks as one of the four outstanding pieces of legislation affecting the American Indian. The others were the act creating the Department of Indian Affairs in 1834, the General Allotment Act of 1887, and the Wheeler-Howard Act of 1934. Under the health provisions of the appropriation act of 1912, the United States Public Health Service went to work and early the following year returned the first comprehensive report on the health of the Indian. It revealed that Minnesota ranked seventeenth in the twenty-five states investigated for trachoma. Oklahoma showed the largest number of cases, with 68.72%, and Florida had no cases. The percentage for Minnesota was 15.05%. On the Leech Lake Reservation the tuberculosis rate among Indians examined for the disease was found to be 49.2 per 1,000, on the Nett Lake Reservation, 48.2, on the Red Lake Reservation, 55.4, and on the White Earth Reservation, 46.8. This was exclusive of Indian boarding-school children. The tuberculosis rate among the white population was 5 per 1,000.[35]

Sanitary conditions on reservations were found on the whole to be unsatisfactory, and United States Public Health Service surgeons said frankly that Indians were careless and dirty in their personal habits and generally ignorant of the first principles of hygiene. But that was not all. Indian personal and social habits favored the spread of disease,

[33] W. H. Harrison, "Notice to the Indians of the White Earth Reservation," (undated mimeographed circular), Minnesota Department of Health, St. Paul.
[34] *Statutes at Large*, 37:519.
[35] *The Prevalence of Contagious and Infectious Diseases among the Indians of the United States*, 24 (chart), 42 (62 Congress, 3 session, *Senate Documents*, no. 1038 — serial 6365).

because the Indians was "careless about spitting and the disposition of human and household waste." Schools for Indians were found to be generally overcrowded, to lack an adequate number of towels, and to possess obsolete toilet facilities, which frequently were in disrepair. Imperfectly screened, schools offered little protection against flies, except in dining rooms and kitchens.[36]

Insanitary conditions in Indian homes, of course, had long been recognized. Three government physicians attached to the White Earth Reservation in 1909 wrote a description that is typical. "There is a certain class of people on this reservation," they said with official caution, "whose dwellings are the crudest sort of hovels, consisting in some instances of one small room which is low ceilinged, poorly lighted, and unspeakably filthy—reeking with the accumulated dust and filth of years. In such a hovel a large family will harbor; the one room must serve all the purposes of kitchen, dining room, living, bed chamber, bedroom, and guest chamber; and right here we wish to state that such families usually have many visitors, especially when they have sickness in the home. . . . Once tubercular infection is introduced into a shack like the one described it immediately becomes a hotbed from which the army of tubercular victims is perennially recruited. It is impossible to disinfect such a chamber of horrors by ordinary methods, for it is occupied, and it would be manslaughter to turn the family out into a snow bank, while their domicile was being fumigated. Then again, if such a dwelling were kept scrupulously clean it would not be a sanitary habitation for a family, because it is lacking in every architectural detail which makes for a modern, hygienic domestic abode."[37]

Dr. Ruth Boynton, director of the division of child hygiene of the Minnesota Department of Health, found almost these same conditions among the Chippewa in 1926, and in 1932 testimony at a hearing before a Senate subcommittee on Indian affairs showed that few of the Indians at Red Lake lived in good homes; the majority still resided in wigwams and frame shacks or log houses. "The fact is," continued the report, "that they know of no other way of living and are content with low standards. Owing in part to restricted diet and overcrowding in homes tuberculosis is very common." Two years later Mark L. Burns, superintendent of the Consolidated Chippewa Agency at Cass Lake and firm friend of the state health department, told an investigating

[36] *Contagious and Infectious Diseases among the Indians*, 78 (serial 6365).
[37] *Report of the Investigation of the White Earth Reservation*, 2:1864 (serial 6336).

committee that a number of Indians, especially the old ones, lived in "very poor" homes. He said also that tuberculosis, trachoma, gonorrhea, and syphilis were most prevalent.[38]

The United States Public Health Service, in its report of 1913, had made twelve recommendations to improve Indian health and had suggested that, whenever necessary and practicable, state boards of health co-operate in their administration. Summarized briefly, these recommendations were: (1) The economic status of the Indian should be improved. (2) Education in personal and domestic hygiene and in the methods necessary for guarding against contagious and infectious diseases should be increased. (3) Housing and sanitary facilities should be improved. (4) As far as practicable, each house should be restricted to one family. (5) Sanitary privies should be provided for permanent dwellings and camps. (6) Reservations should be divided into sanitary districts. (7) An adequate census of each sanitary district, of the sanitary condition of all dwellings, and of the physical condition of each inmate, with special reference to the existence of tuberculosis and trachoma, should be made. (8) Regular sanitary inspections of reservations and their dwellings, boarding schools, and day schools should be made. (9) Reservation medical officers should become sanitary officers of their jurisdictions in fact as well as in name. (10) Reservation medical officers should be under the supervision and control of a distinctly medical bureau. (11) Illnesses and deaths on Indian reservations should be made a matter of permanent record. Transcripts should be sent regularly to the surgeon general of the United States Public Health Service and "reports of outbreaks of certain specified diseases, such as plague, smallpox, and scarlet fever, should be made by telegraph to this official, whose duty it is, under law, to keep the State and local health authorities and the country at large informed of the prevalence of sickness and the occurrence of epidemics." (12) Only competent physicians should be appointed to work on reservations.[39]

This was an ambitious set of suggestions, but one that Minnesota's health department was willing to further if it could. Both lack of complete jurisdiction and inadequate funds from the state, of course, made it impossible for the department to assume any major share of respon-

[38] Ruth E. Boynton and Hortense Hilbert, "Government Medical Care Betters Health Conditions of Chippewa Indian Tribe," in *The Nation's Health*, 8:306 (May, 1926); Senate Committee on Indian Affairs, *Survey of Conditions of the Indians in the United States*, part 26, p. 14400; part 30, p. 16152 (Washington, D.C., 1934).
[39] *Contagious and Infectious Diseases among the Indians*, 82 (serial 6365).

sibility. But there were areas where Chesley thought substantial contributions might be made.

Shortly after the division of child hygiene was organized in 1922, the department established an Indian nursing service through the Consolidated Chippewa Agency at Cass Lake. This program was financed with a gift of three thousand dollars which was matched by Sheppard-Towner funds. The original aim of this service was to secure nurses of Indian descent who were familiar with the circumstances and mode of living of Minnesota Indians. Two nurses of Chippewa extraction — Theodora Davis and Marie Broker Hoffman — were employed by the board in 1923. The following year, Elizabeth Sherer was added to the nursing staff, and in 1927 Josephine Parisien was appointed for duty at Red Lake.[40]

Within a year these Chippewa nurses had made almost three thousand home visits and had immunized more than two thousand children against diphtheria. They made house-to-house calls in order to win the friendship of Indian mothers, did bedside nursing, and gave demonstrations in infant care and feeding. Travel sometimes was slow and difficult, for in 1927 concrete roads did not penetrate the north country. The nurses would go as far as they could by automobile and continue by team or on foot. On one occasion a nurse was guided to a wilderness home with the promise that she would be conducted out. But the guide did not return. "We waited until 11 o'clock," wrote the nurse, "but no sign of his return. It occurred to me that it was taking a long time so I suggested that he was evidently not coming back. I offered to walk the two miles to find out what had happened but could find no one that knew the trail from there well enough to risk guiding me at night. We waited until 12, then by the time we got the car started it was 12:30, but no sign of anyone so we started back for Mahnomen. We had no more than left the woods when we found ourselves in a real blizzard, with the road hidden from view so much that it was unwise to try to drive. We turned in at the first decent place and stayed the night."[41]

Chesley was so enthusiastic over Minnesota's Indian nurses that he took two to Chicago in 1928, when the American Public Health Association met there. Clad in native costume, Miss Sherer and Miss Parisien captivated delegates and were the subject of numerous newspaper articles and photographs. Both girls made short talks, Miss Pari-

[40] State Board of Health, *Reports*, 1922–43, p. 186.
[41] Minnesota Department of Health, "Public Health Nursing Work among the Minnesota Indians," in *Minnesota Nurse*, vol. 1, no. 12, p. 31 (September, 1928).

sien telling of the problems of Minnesota's Indians and Miss Sherer summarizing health conditions that were faced by the department.[42]

The next big step, taken on November 16, 1935, was the establishment of the Chippewa Health Unit with headquarters at Cass Lake. This was made financially possible under Title VI of the Social Security Act. The unit at Cass Lake, wrote Chesley, had no definite territory, but was concerned with Indians wherever they were found in Minnesota.[43]

Meanwhile, on June 18, 1934, the Wheeler-Howard Act, sometimes referred to as the Indian Reorganization Act, became law. Although this act did not deal with the health of the Indian, it did stop the breaking up of Indian reservations and protected the Indian from loss of his remaining land. In addition, it restored to Indian ownership land which had originally been within reservations and had later been opened to white homesteaders, but which had not actually been homesteaded. It also enabled tribes to organize themselves for their mutual benefit, to enjoy self-government, and to incorporate for business purposes. It was hoped, of course, that indirectly the act would help improve the economic status of the Indian, as was recommended in 1913 by the United States Public Health Service. The Wheeler-Howard Act also established an educational loan fund to enable gifted Indians to receive advanced education, an Indian civil service, and a revolving fund to provide needed credit for Indian tribes, and it authorized the purchase of additional lands for Indians.[44]

The Congress that passed the Wheeler-Howard Act also provided for Indian health in its act of June 30, 1935, making appropriations for the Department of the Interior. For the support of hospitals for Chippewa in Minnesota $121,490 was appropriated. In addition, the Pipestone Hospital was granted $20,910, and another $20,000 was set aside for a clinical survey of tuberculosis, trachoma, and venereal and other diseases among all Indians in the United States. About that time also, as the result of an arrangement with the State of Minnesota and the Indian service, Indian tubercular patients were taken for care to Ah-Gwah-Ching, the state sanatorium at Walker. This institution replaced

[42] *Chicago Daily Journal,* October 16, 1928; *Minnesota Nurse,* vol. 2, no. 3, p. 14 (December, 1928).
[43] State Board of Health, *Reports,* 1922–43, p. 62; Chesley, *Federal Aid for Public Health Work in Minnesota,* 47.
[44] William A. Brophy, "Story of the Indian Service," a mimeographed address by the commissioner of Indian affairs before the employees of the Department of the Interior, August 29, 1946, Minnesota Department of Health, Minneapolis; *Statutes at Large,* 48:984–988.

HEALTH OFFICER VS. MEDICINE MAN 239

the "old, unsafe and inefficient" sanatorium formerly maintained by the Indian Service at Onigum.[45]

The great national depression beginning in 1929 affected the Indian, of course, as well as the white man. Crop failures and drouth accelerated the severity of the depression among the Indians, and the Indian service was faced with a people in destitute condition. Conditions did not improve radically during the next decade. In 1938 a special appropriation from tribal funds became necessary to help maintain a decent standard of living. A consignment of army shoes helped the clothing situation, but still many Indians were in rags. During the summer of 1938 the health department, in co-operation with the WPA, the Minnesota State Emergency Relief Administration, and the Indian service, conducted a health camp for Chippewa children. During the years from 1938 to 1941 whole or partial relief was given to over eighty per cent of the Indian population.[46]

With the tapering off of the depression, Indian economic conditions and health improved somewhat. World War II brought a certain amount of prosperity to the tribes. After peace came, it was possible to emphasize health programs. Dr. Percy T. Watson, for many years a medical missionary in China and the holder of six Chinese decorations given him for distinguished work in suppressing pneumonia and bubonic plague, was sent by the department to Bemidji, where he devoted much of his time to improving Indian health. Watson suggested to the Soroptimist Club of Minneapolis that it adopt the financial support of an Indian nurse to do public health work among Indians. The club, as a result, financed two Indian girls while they were studying practical nursing at the Vocational Hospital and the Vocational High School in Minneapolis. A third girl also was in training. All three completed the course in June, 1948, and were ready to begin work among their people.[47]

Other activities of the health department among Indians included several diagnostic clinics. In 1945, for example, a mass X-ray survey was made on the Red Lake Reservation which involved examination of 89% of the population. Tuberculosis was found in 4.1% of the Indians examined, most of it being of the early or minimal type, with a good

[45] *Statutes at Large*, 48:375–376; *Indian Truth*, vol. 13, no. 8, p. 1 (November, 1936).
[46] *Indian Truth*, vol. 7, no. 2, p. 1 (February, 1930); *Minnesota Chippewa Bulletin*, 1:3 (November 21, 1938); 2:3 (December 20, 1938); State Board of Health, *Reports*, 1922–43, p. 188.
[47] *Minnesota's Health*, vol. 1, no. 6, p. 4 (June, 1947); vol. 1, no. 4, p. 1 (April, 1947); vol. 1, no. 9, p. 1 (September, 1947); vol. 2, no. 6, p. 4 (June, 1948).

chance of cure. The percentage of Indians and non-Indians entering Minnesota sanatoriums with tuberculosis in various stages during the period 1940–46 follows: [48]

Stage of Tuberculosis	Per Cent Indians	Per Cent Non-Indians
Early	21	12
Moderately advanced	28	33
Far advanced	51	55

Trachoma has decreased among the Chippewa, not only because greater attention has been paid to it but also because the use of the sulfa drugs and penicillin has made treatment less painful and more effective. The old treatment, not always too successful, consisted of turning back the lids and scraping the membrane. Today, after treatment with the new drugs, some Indians who were partially blind are able to drive automobiles. A change has taken place, too, in the Indians' attitude toward hospitals. Once they viewed hospitals with fear and suspicion; now seventy-six per cent of pregnant women are delivered in hospitals. Consequently the infant mortality rate has decreased. An Indian population of about twenty-four hundred is cared for at the hospital at Red Lake, and the Cass Lake Indian Hospital is prepared to handle both medical and surgical cases. The latter institution is well equipped and well supplied, but understaffed. In 1946 two full-time physicians were attached to the hospital and two Indian nurses and one non-Indian nurse were on duty.[49]

Venereal disease still ranks high among diseases of Indians. Some medical observers believe that an excessive use of alcohol stimulated promiscuity and hence increased the venereal disease rate. It is said that during the depression years many Indians saved their sugar rations, purchased tomato juice, and added yeast and sugar to produce a highly intoxicating beverage. In 1947 the Minnesota legislature

[48] *Minnesota's Health*, vol. 1, no. 4, p. 1 (April, 1947).

[49] Phillips Thygeson, "The Diagnosis and Treatment of Trachoma," in *Military Surgeon*, 96:353–361 (November, 1945); Dean J. Barius, "Penicillin Treatment of Trachoma," in *American Journal of Ophthalmology*, 28:1007–1009 (September, 1945); F. S. Lavery, "Sulfonamides and Penicillin in the Treatment of Trachoma," in *British Journal of Ophthalmology*, 30:591–594 (October, 1946); United States Public Health Service, *Reports*, vol. 38, no. 9, pp. 383–407 (March 2, 1923); *Minnesota's Health*, vol. 1, no. 4, p. 1 (April, 1947); Commissioner of Indian Affairs, *Annual Reports*, 1941, p. 431; interview of the author with Dr. Percy Watson, June 28, 1946, and with Chesley, June 30, 1946; Philip D. Jordan, "Report of a Trip, June 27–30, 1946."

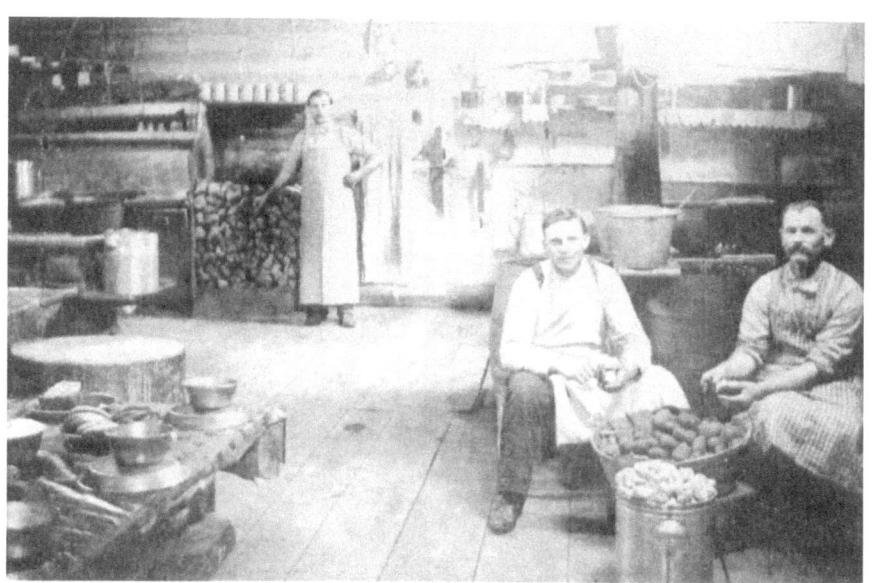

A Lumber Camp Kitchen

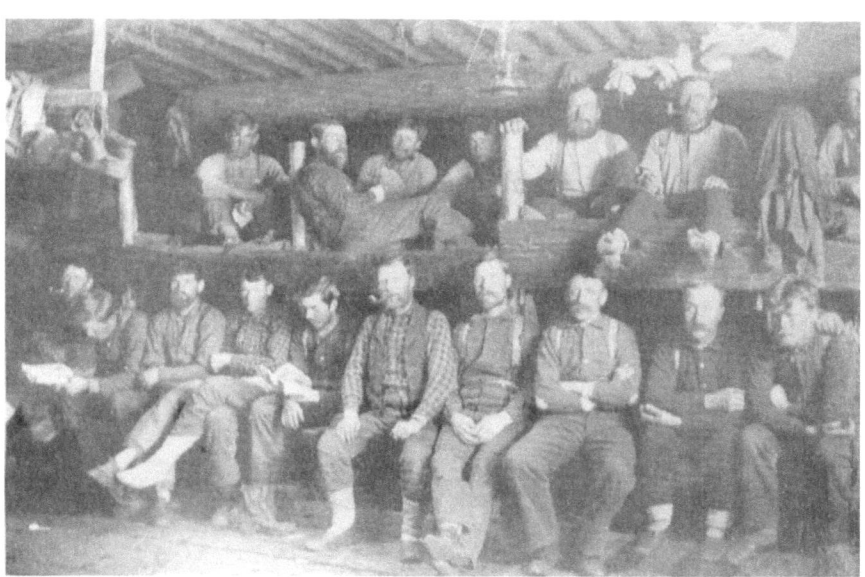

A Lumber Camp "Sitting Room"
From the collection of the Forest Products History Foundation, Minnesota Historical Society

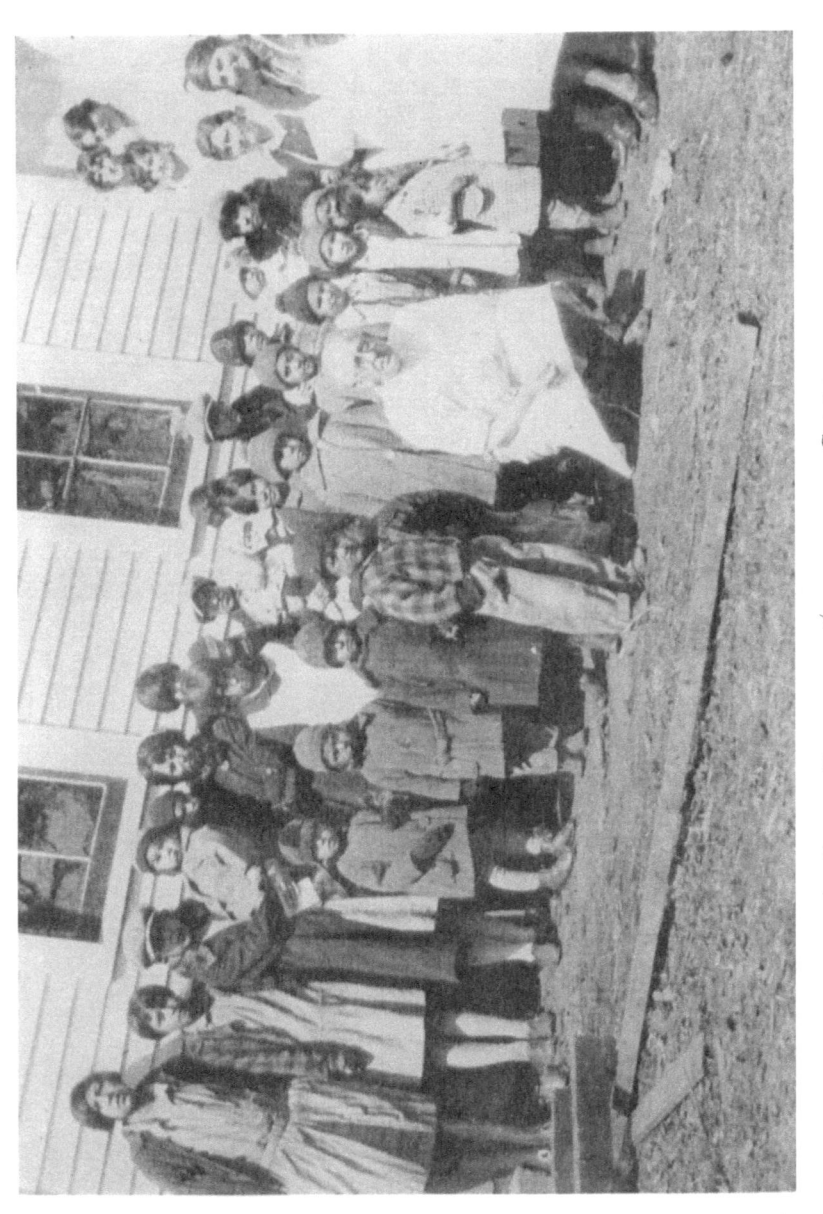

AN INDIAN DIPHTHERIA IMMUNIZATION CLINIC
Courtesy Minnesota Department of Health

amended the statutes to make the sale of intoxicating liquor to Indians legal.[50]

Low incomes, tuberculosis, and inadequate housing, however, continue to be the three great deterrents to the progress of the state's Indians. Their homes generally are of three types: tar-paper shacks, small frame structures, and rehabilitation houses. The majority are one- or two-room structures, poorly built, in need of repairs, and, in a few instances, not habitable. "The typical home," according to a Minnesota survey in 1947, "is a shack 12' x 16', 16' x 18', or 16' x 24'. Many of the structures are covered with tar paper. Some are ceiled with wallboard, cardboard, or newspaper on the interior. Practically none of the homes have cellars or foundations of any kind; all of the homes have flooring of some kind. Few of the homes have running water and even fewer have indoor toilets. While some families secure their water from nearby springs, the majority carry or haul their water from community wells." Most yards were described as overgrown with weeds and littered with broken furniture, boxes, food, and other debris. Little privacy, if any, existed for any member of a household, and inadequate heating often forced families to center all activities in one room. The housing condition of the typical Indian family "living in Indian communities near or on reservations is inadequate. Their household equipment is similarly inadequate if normal family life is considered as a criterion for these people."[51]

Yet there is reason to believe that the health of the Indian, even in the midst of insanitary and miserable housing, may continue to improve. About thirty per cent of Indians examined under the Selective Service Act were rejected for physical unfitness. Although this rate was higher than for the general population, the Office of Indian Affairs reported that Indians were in much better physical condition than during World War I. The death rate for the nation's Indians has decreased steadily, although it still is twenty-five per cent higher than for the population as a whole. On the other hand, the Indian birth rate is thirty-five per cent higher than that of the general population. It is significant, too, that physicians of the Indian service, after years of battling the medicine man, have come to realize the beneficial effects of curing ceremonials. Today they are discovering values in the Indians' medicinal herbs, massages, sweat baths, cathar-

[50] Interview of the author with Watson, June 28, 1946; *Laws*, 1947, p. 110.
[51] Governor's Interracial Commission, *The Indian in Minnesota*, 59 (Minneapolis, 1947).

tics, and cauterizations, and they are also "sensing a strong psychotherapeutic value in the songs, prayers, and ceremonials of the Indians." [52]

Progress in Indian affairs has been slow, but Commissioner William A. Brophy feels that much of this is due to the fact that, for generations, Indians have been stripped of their best lands. "A hungry and sick Indian," he said, "is not brought nearer to the day when he may have food and good health if we allow his meager resources to be further diminished or wasted." [53]

[52] Commissioner of Indian Affairs, *Annual Reports*, 1941, pp. 431, 433.
[53] Commissioner of Indian Affairs, *Annual Reports*, 1947, p. 349.

13

Control of Venereal Disease

THREE years after the great Chicago fire of 1871 another blaze started in a ragpicker's shanty, spread to a paint factory, and within minutes was roaring through one of the "worst and vilest" districts of Chicago. About twenty blocks were destroyed and more than five hundred prostitutes lost "costly fittings and wardrobes." Many of these "most notorious keepers of vile abodes" migrated, even before the embers had cooled, to flourishing St. Paul and Minneapolis. For years these rapidly growing cities had been the mecca of soldiers from Fort Snelling, trappers and hunters from the Red River, and lumberjacks. The Chicago fire of 1874, it was estimated, doubled the number of prostitutes in Minneapolis.[1]

Despite public awareness of this evil, police undertook only token enforcement of regulations. Only forty-five St. Paul madames were arrested in 1868 and only fifteen women were charged with prostitution. In June, 1871, seven operators of houses of ill fame were apprehended in Minneapolis. The influx of professionals from Chicago after the fire briefly stirred St. Paul police to activity, but this probably was due to the fact that noncity girls offered unfair competition to well-established houses and had not as yet learned how to get along with law-enforcement agencies. When a Chicago woman was picked up in St. Paul, she exclaimed bitterly: "Burned out in Chicago and jailed the first night in St. Paul!"[2]

The customary procedure — one that was rather general throughout the United States — was for police to raid houses periodically, bring the madames into court to pay a fine, and then release them to con-

[1] *St. Paul Daily Press,* July 16, 19, August 27, 1874.
[2] *St. Paul Daily Press,* April 20, 1869, July 22, 1874; *Minneapolis Tribune,* July 8, 1871.

tinue their activities. Jail sentences seldom were imposed. This system accomplished two purposes: it gave the public the impression that the law was being enforced and it brought a steady income into city treasuries. Kate Hutton, who eventually met her death at the hands of a customer, paid sixty-five dollars on January 4, fifty-five on January 18, sixty-five on March 7, and sixty-five on March 21, 1872. "The social evil," commented a reporter that month, "pays license money, or whatever else it may be called, to the amount of $292 for the month of January, with one establishment yet to be heard from." Much the same situation prevailed in Duluth.[3]

Suppression of this evil was no easy matter. All types of solutions were proposed by the clergy, legislators, and members of city councils. A bill was introduced into the Minnesota legislature which declared all houses of public prostitution a nuisance and provided that action against them might be commenced by any citizen. Early in 1873 the St. Paul City Council repealed an ordinance of 1869 entitled "Disorderly Houses and Houses of Ill Fame," and replaced it with another providing penalties not only for keepers of such houses but also for persons frequenting them. As a result the chief of police was instructed to notify all persons owning buildings used as houses of ill fame to have them vacated within thirty days. Another proposal suggested that a list be published with the names of all persons visiting brothels. A more plausible recommendation was offered by the St. Paul Council in February, 1874, when it passed a resolution calling for the selection of a police officer who should be responsible to the council for the rigid enforcement of the ordinance relating to disorderly houses. In addition, he was to furnish the Ramsey County district attorney with a "list of all houses of ill fame, their location, by whom kept, the names of all other persons who may be material witnesses."[4]

The debate on this resolution was most lively, with a wide variety of opinions expressed. One alderman believed that, if bagnios were suppressed, "it would be dangerous for respectable women to be on the streets after dark." Another thought a policeman should be stationed at the door of every house of ill fame, and others declared that brothels were located too close to schools and churches and they decreased the value of property. One irate councilman complained that for years there had been a well-known institution in the rear of his

[3] *Pioneer Press*, September 1, 1881; *St. Paul Daily Press*, January 4, 5, 18, March 7, 21, 1872; *Duluth Minnesotian*, October 12, 1872.
[4] *St. Paul Daily Press*, January 11, 1872, March 5, August 20, 1873; St. Paul Common Council, *Proceedings*, 1872–74, p. 221; 1874, p. 26.

home and that only recently another had opened directly in front. A few aldermen favored the keeping of brothels in the center of town where they could be watched. "Why, gentlemen," one said, "if these houses are out of the thickly settled parts of the city we shall have murders and rows frequently." [5]

Nevertheless, the resolution was passed and temporarily, at least, it proved effective. Several madames announced they were closing up, one to go to St. Louis and others carefully guarding the secret of their destination. "If this exodus continues," exulted an editor, "St. Paul will have cleared its skirts without any extraordinary effort." Less than a month, however, after the council's special police officer had succeeded in removing some of the city's prominent prostitutes, he was attacked by aldermen. A motion was made that the resolution of February 4 be rescinded. It was charged that the police had run the matter long enough and had made the council "the laughing stock of the city." The entire matter was referred to a special committee, which apparently did not report.[6]

Gradually St. Paul resumed its former practice of arrests and fines. The suppression of houses of ill fame was thought to stimulate streetwalking and, for some reason or other, that was considered worse than the brothel. Other Minnesota communities were facing the same difficulties. Red Wing, Hewitt's home, in 1874 had a disorderly house within its city limits, and Waseca residents knew of a house of assignation there. At Winona newspapers said a man kept a notorious brothel. By 1875 the Winona City Council was considering an ordinance that would prohibit prostitution, and at Chippewa Falls infuriated citizens burned a house of ill fame.[7]

But Minneapolis, because of its size, faced a greater problem than did smaller towns. Washington and Cedar avenues were lined with bagnios and were raided repeatedly, as was First Street North. Generally speaking, Minneapolis authorities followed the policy of arresting and fining. On one afternoon in August, 1875, fourteen persons were fined a total of $205 on charges of running a disorderly house of prostitution. A few days later another "soiled dove" paid ten dollars and costs. When soldiers on leave from Fort Snelling visited Minneapolis, police, as a matter of course, raided known houses and turned military

[5] *St. Paul Daily Press*, February 4, 1874.
[6] *St. Paul Daily Press*, February 12, 17, 24, March 20, 1874.
[7] *St. Paul Daily Press*, March 21, 26, May 16, 21, 22, June 18, 1874, April 10, 1875; *Waseca News*, quoted in the *St. Paul Daily Press*, May 22, 1874; *Pioneer-Press*, April 11, 1875.

personnel over to army authorities. The red-light district of the city grew so rapidly that parties of men and boys pelted brothels with stones.[8]

In May, 1877, the vice problem was getting so much attention that the Minneapolis City Council reframed its ordinance pertaining to houses of ill fame and prostitutes. This ordinance, much like that of St. Paul, made it illegal for persons to keep or frequent brothels and for a property owner to rent any building for use as a brothel. Later the council appropriated the fines of prostitutes and of persons resorting to houses of prostitution to the support of institutions for the care and reformation of fallen women. Yet the year after these acts were passed, 63 keepers of houses of ill fame and 192 prostitutes were arrested in Minneapolis.[9]

So great was the influence of vice in Minneapolis that no legislative methods could terminate prostitution. After several years of attempting to eradicate the evil, Minneapolis began licensing its brothels. "The experiment of prohibition," said an editor, "has practically amounted to nothing, merely scattering the women and making their detection and punishment almost impossible. Accordingly the police have received orders to arrest the offenders once a month." One result of the licensing system was to swell the income of the Bethany Home, an institution which cared for wayward girls.[10]

Meanwhile the Minnesota State Magdalen Society had been organized in St. Paul in October, 1873. This unique organization was begun when five prostitutes approached the YWCA and asked that they be helped. The association at once published a call for the Christian women of St. Paul to meet at Plymouth Church to establish a home for the reformation of fallen women. The first inmate was received into the home on November 20. Before May, 1874, girls had entered from eleven Minnesota communities, including the Twin Cities, Duluth, Brainerd, Mankato, and Red Wing. Others were received from Hudson and Eau Claire, Wisconsin. Some of these women were ill with tuberculosis and others were afflicted with venereal disease.

Mrs. D. S. B. Johnston, president of the Magdalen Society in 1875, issued a general statement to St. Paul women, in which she described

[8] *St. Paul Daily Press*, May 16, 21, 29, October 6, December 10, 11, 1874, January 29, 1875; *Minneapolis Tribune*, May 12, August 17, 1875, May 29, 1876, May 9, 1878; *Pioneer-Press and Tribune*, May 30, 1876.
[9] Minneapolis City Council, *Proceedings*, April 11, 1877–April 9, 1878, pp. 38, 198; Minneapolis City Officers, *Annual Reports*, 1879, pp. 97, 98.
[10] *Tribune*, June 29, 1881; Minneapolis City Council, *Proceedings*, April 13, 1880–April 12, 1881, pp. 28, 54, 93, 114, 126, 141, 151, 169.

the work of the society and made a bid for woman suffrage. "Christian women," she said, "did you know that the city of St. Paul licenses our sisters at ten dollars a month, payable in advance, to sell their souls and bodies to Satan, and if not paid promptly, they are liable to be shut up in the city prison until they either serve out a certain length of time, or are bailed out by some 'friend' or keeper of a 'house'? O, if for no other purpose, I would like the right of suffrage to help regulate these laws and have them enforced. We are told that nightly these dens of inquity are crowded. If so, whose sons, brothers, and husbands are these who frequent them? May our eyes be opened to see our duty, and then do all we can to stay this great flood of evil."[11]

Minneapolis took a keen interest in this society, for, it was said, disreputable houses were increasing and their "depraved inmates throwing out temptation of the most seductive nature to the youth of both sexes." It was suggested that lay groups unite with church organizations to give all support possible to the Magdalen Society. Unfortunately, members of the society greatly embarrassed St. Paul police both by their active interest in prostitution and by not watching their charges carefully enough. It was charged that girls slipped away from the home to ply their trade and, when arrested, coolly explained that they were under the protection of the society and could not be charged in court. "Under these circumstances," it was explained, "the police do not feel warranted in interfering with them, while at the same time they are absolutely convinced that the women who have placed themselves in charge of the society are practicing a fraud of the worst possible description." By 1890 the Sisters of the Good Shepherd were conducting a Magdalen department at their St. Paul convent.[12]

About the time that the Magdalen Society was organized, a St. Paul physician began lecturing on the history of prostitution and its remedies. Under the auspices of the Knights of Pythias, Dr. A. J. Stone frankly sketched the social evil in St. Paul, listing six regular houses with thirty-six inmates and six irregular houses — cigar stores and private apartments — with an estimated forty to fifty women. He recommended a system of fines but added that, in case of sickness, fines should be remitted and the girls should be treated at city expense. All in all, Stone believed, some four hundred women were engaged in the trade. In his second lecture the doctor spoke of the health aspects of prostitution. This lecture "was well attended and was even

[11] *Pioneer-Press*, October 29, 1875.
[12] *Minneapolis Tribune*, December 16, 1875; *Pioneer-Press and Tribune*, July 23, 1876; *Pioneer Press*, October 20, 1890.

more interesting than its predecessor." Two years later, Stone again took the platform to repeat and enlarge upon what he had said previously. The significance of Stone's activities lies in the fact, not that he spoke about prostitution, but that he was one of the earliest lecturers to talk frankly on the subject of venereal disease as a public health problem.[13]

Another indication of progress was the beginning of the public use of the term "syphilis." At a meeting of the Minnesota Dental Association in 1875 the members debated the question: "Do syphilitic diseases register themselves on the teeth in the second generation?" The discussion was fully reported in the public press. This airing of opinion, however, did not mean that all professional men supported a program for suppression of vice. Dr. Brewer Mattocks, St. Paul's health officer, for example, took violent issue with the objectives of the St. Paul Society for the Suppression of Vice. Mattocks argued that "each girl in a concert saloon does more harm to the morals of a community than six girls in a house of prostitution. The mere fact of shutting up a girl in a disgraceful house and giving her a disgraceful name, prevents her from creating evil to any marked degree; she merely panders to it. Not so with the concert girls, and cigar sellers, and so-called 'shirtmakers'; they are tempters, and are to be dreaded. Supposing societies for moral effort would work as boards of health to prevent and control contagious diseases, rather than to suppress pest-houses?" Another citizen summed up the attitude of his group by declaring: "I make bold to say that all municipalities should tolerate, and in that case necessarily regulate, houses of ill fame . . . moral sewers are as necessary as street sewers."[14]

No matter what course city councils adopted, they were always attacked. When brothels were fined, the charge was made that this procedure was not really a technique to deter vice, but only a shameful policy to bring easy money into a city treasury. But when houses were closed, critics said sharply that the result was the mischievous spreading of pollution over the city to sections that were unpolluted before. If fines did not go to the city proper, but were distributed to homes for wayward girls, some citizens were sure to complain that the city was losing money. On the other hand, if fines were kept by a municipality, there was complaint that welfare agencies were being deprived of a rightful source of income. Few persons argued the case on the basis

[13] *Minneapolis Tribune*, December 23, 1874; *St. Paul Daily Pioneer*, December 23, 1874; *St. Paul Daily Press*, December 23, 30, 1874; *Pioneer-Press*, March 9, 1876.
[14] *Pioneer-Press*, May 28, 1875, July 31, 1879, February 24, 1880.

of public health during those early days. Consequently a city's attitude toward prostitution was apt to vary with each change of administration. Mayors and city councils were badgered, whatever policy they might adopt.[15]

Beginning in 1878 and continuing into 1883, St. Paul constantly was agitated by impromptu crusades and by official action. A local clergyman touched the campaign off by gathering and publishing vice statistics. Although he denounced established brothels, he was more severe on cigar stores, which a newspaper said were conducted "in every instance by the lowest order of women from whom all sense of decency, all traces of beauty, and all vestige of modesty has gone." These stores were described as dirty little shanties with a beggarly display of cigars and fruits in front, "while behind is a sitting room containing some gay furniture and a wheezy organ, or jingling piano . . . while several asthmatic painted females are prepared to sing or play cards." Leading haunts were located on Third, Jackson, Robert, Seventh, and Wabasha streets.[16]

So much publicity appeared during the early days of 1878 that a special meeting of the St. Paul Council was held to hear testimony from private citizens and physicians. Mattocks appeared to argue against the licensing system and to say that known houses of ill fame were not as dangerous as "insidious semi-private" places. Another physician thought that establishments under proper regulations and proper medical attendance were "not half so pernicious, either morally or physically," as the less public ones. The police chief read a paper setting forth his experiences in ten years on the force.[17] Other sessions followed, and a special committee of the council was appointed. On March 4 this committee, of which Mattocks was a member, returned its report.

In this report, for the first time, specific mention was made of the health aspects of prostitution, although neither the term "venereal disease" nor the word "syphilis" was used. Nevertheless, the report marks one of St. Paul's first official forward-moving steps. Vice, said the committee, is divided into two questions: Shall prostitution be licensed and placed under medical surveillance? or shall what is known as the raiding, harassing, or stamping-out system be adopted? The committee found that prostitution existed in four forms: "First, prostitutes ply their vocation in the guise of cigar venders, in companies of two or

[15] *Daily Globe* (St. Paul), April 13, 1881; *Pioneer Press,* January 15, 1878.
[16] *Pioneer Press,* January 21, 1878; *Daily Globe,* January 23, 1878.
[17] *Pioneer Press,* January 25, 1878; *Daily Globe,* February 15, 1878.

more, in small shops in public streets; second, in private furnished apartments in public buildings, under the name and pretence of shop, or sewing girls; third, in houses of public prostitution on our more public thoroughfares; fourth, in houses of prostitution, on what is known as unfrequented streets."

The committee took the ground that the first duty of St. Paul was to suppress, as far as possible, all four forms and to notify owners of buildings that they would be responsible for the actions of tenants. "While it would be difficult," continued the report, "to convict or even find cause for arrest for one suspected of vice, it would not be difficult to secure the ejectment of a suspected female from a building by notifying the owner or lessor of the same of her tainted character." Yet, despite the committee's good intentions, vice continued to flourish, and in 1879 a Ramsey County grand jury returned indictments against several women. At the same time, the jury strongly condemned "the policy which prevails in the administration of the city government, whereby the so-called 'social evil' is fostered, condoned and, in fact, protected." It said that a local ordinance intended to crush out prostitution was a dead letter.[18]

Despite this blast, prostitution continued to such a degree that a country editor in 1880 pictured St. Paul as infested with prostitutes "like a swamp with loathsome vipers." Three years later a new administration came into office. One of the first moves of Mayor C. D. O'Brien was to instruct the police department to close known houses and to order their inmates to leave within three days. Some twenty left St. Paul immediately, but others preferred to remain, be arrested, and risk jury verdict. The famous test case involved Minnie Oliver and Maud Hudson, charged with visiting an alleged house of ill fame. A jury, after being out two hours, returned a verdict of guilty, but only after asking the court if they also could add that they considered the principle of the prosecution unjust. Both girls were fined twenty-five dollars and sentenced to thirty days in the House of the Good Shepherd. The latter part of the sentence, however, was suspended pending their good behavior, but the court warned that, if the women returned to prostitution, it would enforce the suspension.[19]

Shortly after this test case, merchants and politicians organized to attack O'Brien and to force the repeal of the ordinance prohibiting

[18] St. Paul Common Council, *Proceedings*, 1878, p. 17; *Pioneer Press*, March 6, 1878, May 15, 16, 17, 1879.
[19] *Martin County Sentinel*, quoted in the *Daily Globe*, February 3, 1880; *Pioneer Press*, June 8, July 26, 1883.

houses of ill fame. Business men said trade was being driven from St. Paul. In one night thirteen hacks filled with out-of-town merchants and visitors left the Merchants Hotel for Minneapolis. An alderman told the council that curtailment of vice had caused more syphilis than ever before and said this increased health menace was due directly to the mayor's action. For months the fight over repeal continued. It was solved by keeping the ordinance, but gradually and unofficially returning to the previous license system.[20]

This system, interrupted now and again by reform movements and changes of administration, continued throughout the 1890s and, to some degree, after the turn of the century. In 1890 St. Paul health officials proposed a program of medical examination for prostitutes, but this was opposed by Presbyterian ministers. Now and again a girl was sentenced to jail, but in most instances fines were imposed. Fights and robberies in brothels were numerous, and the public avidly followed stories of young girls who had fallen into a life of shame. In 1894 the council discussed a new measure to regulate vice, but failed to enact it into an ordinance. The following year, however, an ordinance was passed which was much stricter than the old Ordinance Number 10, in that it prohibited the existence of houses and made it illegal for any person to frequent such a house or to tipple, revel, riot, or engage in disturbance in a house. In 1900 fifty-four persons were arrested for visiting houses of ill fame and fourteen were arrested as keepers of disorderly houses. That St. Paul's new ordinance was accomplishing something is apparent after a contrast with arrests in Duluth, where a hundred and fifty-one keepers of brothels were arrested in a twelve-months period.[21]

St. Paul's attempts to control prostitution were fairly typical of those of other Minnesota communities. Minneapolis went through a similar cycle of reforms, followed by a return to the license system. Clergymen attacked vice there just as they did in the state's capital. Patients with venereal disease were divided between the Homeopathic Hospital and St. Barnabas Hospital. Periodic raids were frequent, with greatest attention given well-known madames with such colorful nicknames as "Swede Mary." In May, 1891, eighteen women were arrested

[20] St. Paul Common Council, *Proceedings*, 1883, p. 307; *Pioneer Press*, August 8, December 4, 1883, June 3, 1885; *Tribune*, November 24, 1885.
[21] *Pioneer Press*, February 11, May 3, June 6, 1890, January 22, 29, 1891, March 3, 1894; St. Paul Common Council, *Proceedings*, 1895, p. 197; St. Paul City Officers, *Reports*, 1900, p. 772; Duluth City Officers, *Reports*, 1891–92, report of the police chief, 13.

and charged with operating brothels. In September four others were each sentenced to thirty days in the workhouse.[22]

Although towns on the iron ranges still were considered "wide open," and although vice still was present in the Twin Cities at the beginning of the twentieth century, some very definite improvements were noticed. In the first place, the moral argument against prostitution was very gradually being replaced by a public health approach. Secondly, the Minnesota Department of Health was beginning to be interested in the venereal disease problem. Hewitt, of course, had interested himself in the vice problem, but in his day there was little that he could do as secretary of the board. Shortly before his dismissal, however, he took new interest in the problem, especially when a suspected case of leprosy was diagnosed as syphilis. Bracken, too, was troubled by reports of syphilis which were wrongly diagnosed. More and more, the syphilitic patient entered the work of the state board. When, in 1902, a physician from Anoka asked Bracken where a county patient must be cared for so as not to infect others, Bracken could only reply: "I know of no place where such an individual can be sent. Your county will have to play the best it can in the matter. He certainly should be isolated from other county inmates, and everything connected with his person or clothing thoroughly disinfected." To a person who reported a case of smallpox and one of venereal disease, Bracken answered that venereal diseases did not come under the jurisdiction of health officers.[23]

Dr. H. D. Holton, chairman of the committee on prophylaxis of venereal disease of the American Medical Association, asked Bracken a series of five questions in 1903. His queries and Bracken's replies follow:[24]

Q. Is there any law relating to prostitution in Minnesota?
A. Sec. 1299 Gen. Statutes of Minn. 1894 provides that village councils shall have authority by ordinance to restrain and punish prostitution.

Sec. 6529 provides that any one who entices an unmarried female under the age of 25 years into a house of prostitution for purpose of prostitution, or, parent who consents to the taking of a female under

[22] *Tribune,* October 1, 1886; *Svenska Amerikanska Posten,* November 7, 1893; *Pioneer Press,* November 9, 1886, April 2, 14, 24, May 1, July 3, 1890, June 10, September 6, 1891.
[23] G. Armauer Hanson to Hewitt, May 19, 1888; Martha Ripley to Bracken, April 28, 1899; C. F. Ewing to Bracken, January 13, 1902; Jens P. Anderson to Bracken, July 30, 1902; Bracken to Ripley, April 29, 1899, to Ewing, January 16, 1902, and to Anderson, August 5, 1902. Minnesota Department of Health, St. Paul.
[24] H. D. Holton to Bracken, April 3, 1903; Bracken to Holton, April 11, 1903. Minnesota Department of Health, St. Paul.

the age of 16 to any place for the purpose of prostitution, is guilty of abduction and punishable by imprisonment for not more than five years, fine of not more than $1000.00 or both.

Chap. 108 Laws of 1897 provides that any one who keeps any resort for immoral purposes is guilty of a misdemeanor and punishable by a fine of from $5.00 to $50.00.

Chap. 158 Laws of 1899 provides that any one keeping a house of ill fame is guilty of a felony and that any one renting a place for such purpose is guilty of a misdemeanor.

Q. Is there a sanitary marriage law which provides for medical examinations of the contracting parties?

A. There is no law of this nature in Minnesota. An attempt was made to pass such a law through our legislature two years ago, but the attempt failed.

Q. Is there a law against wilfully or knowingly communicating venereal diseases?

A. There is no law of this nature in Minnesota that I can learn of.

Q. What, if any, municipal regulations exist in any City in your State regarding these diseases?

A. There are various city and village ordinances prohibiting the keeping of disorderly houses, etc. In St. Paul & Minneapolis these laws and ordinances are not strictly enforced. In St. Paul they are kept under police supervision and confined to a certain district. The same measures are, I think, pursued in Minneapolis.

Bracken was correct in his answers. The Minnesota legislature, as he said, had passed a series of acts calculated to reduce prostitution, but neither the state nor municipalities had attempted to legislate on the venereal disease problem. The state health department had no such regulation and neither had any local health boards. Nevertheless, the trend was in that direction. Among the early steps taken by the state department was the distribution of circulars relating to syphilis. In 1915 the department considered the possibility of having its laboratories in Minneapolis and Duluth make free Wassermann tests. Chesley, however, raised serious doubts that such a procedure was feasible at that time. He said that, until Minnesota could require the reporting of venereal diseases and could pass regulations governing those suffering from these diseases, the laboratory could not gain anything for public health by making examinations. The situation remained the same in 1916, when Bracken was obliged to inform an attorney for the New York City health department that reporting of venereal diseases was not required.[25]

---

[25] Minnesota, *Statutes,* 1894, section 1299; *Laws,* 1897, p. 194; 1899, p. 163; State Board of Health, "Minutes," January 31, February 1, 1905, Minnesota Department of Health, St. Paul; Bracken to Fahey, August 7, 1915, and to Joseph Warren, December 19, 1916, Minnesota Department of Health, St. Paul.

Perhaps progress toward this goal would have continued to be slow had not the United States been on the verge of World War I. When war did come and almost overnight the nation was turned into an armed camp, the control of venereal disease became a pressing military as well as a public health problem. Loose women flocked to the vicinity of military areas, renting rooms in shabby hotels, leasing apartments, and boldly soliciting on city streets. Late in 1917 the state health department refused to co-operate with representatives of Minnesota medical societies, public health organizations, and social agencies who were meeting to discuss the establishment of a Minnesota social hygiene commission and bureau for the control of venereal diseases. Bracken made clear his reasons for not taking part in the deliberations. He said that unless the representatives would "recognize the State Board of Health as having an equal standing with the University of Minnesota and the social workers of Minnesota," he preferred to "keep out of the whole thing." Then he added: "As a matter of fact, I would much prefer keeping out of it, for I do not care to be mixed up in this movement." [26]

This curt refusal did not mean that Bracken was disinterested in venereal diseases; but it did signify that he believed that the department was the proper agency to supervise and control such a program. The Minnesota Social Hygiene Commission, as a matter of fact, was quite willing to recognize that the board of health had full power and so was Governor John Lind. This soothed Bracken's feelings, and, by the end of October, 1917, he was quite willing to assist in almost every possible way. He pointed out that there were three aspects to the venereal problem: the moral, the prophylactic, and the clinical. And he suggested that the attack on it might be made in four forms: social, educational, and prophylactic measures and medical care. He thought that an educational program might be worked out mutually between the board and social workers and that the state should provide free Wassermann tests and free salvarsan.[27]

Bracken had given the entire venereal disease question much thought during the previous two years and he had been in correspondence with health officers in Massachusetts and Maine. To an eastern physician who asked his opinion of the effectiveness of laws requiring the reporting of venereal diseases, he replied that he thought such

[26] Bracken to W. A. Jones, October 18, 1917, Minnesota Department of Health, St. Paul.
[27] Jones to Bracken, October 19, 27, 1917; Bracken to Jones, October 29, 1917. Minnesota Department of Health, St. Paul.

CONTROL OF VENEREAL DISEASE 255

laws were of little value until people were better educated. Alfred F. Pillsbury also had suggested to him the importance of control of venereal disease. Therefore, when Governor Lind appointed Bracken to the Minnesota Social Hygiene Commission in 1917, he was prepared to give sound advice and to make a substantial contribution.[28]

For example, Bracken was well acquainted with the recommendations of the medical advisory committee of the war council of the American Red Cross. He knew that this council, working through its bureau of sanitary service, would furnish personnel, equipment, and maintenance to public health organizations in control of civil areas surrounding army cantonments, national guard camps, and naval bases. But this assistance would be forthcoming only if requested by the United States Public Health Service, state boards of health, and local boards. Once this request was made and granted, the Red Cross would furnish a sanitary unit, consisting of bacteriologists, sanitary inspectors, public health nurses, and clerical assistants. Before Bracken had been appointed to the Minnesota Social Hygiene Commission, he had requested such a unit for Minnesota.[29]

The commission as it was organized consisted of committees on the control of venereal diseases, on law enforcement, on education, on social service, and on protective work. There was also an executive committee and a finance committee. Chesley and Bracken were members of the committee on control. A proposed budget called for $50,150. Early in 1917 the board had passed a resolution calling for an indebtedness of $35,000 to be known as the "Soldiers' Venereal Disease Fund" and to be used to prevent the spread of venereal diseases. In addition, federal aid was received as the result of the passage of the Chamberlain-Kahn Act. On January 8, 1918, the Minnesota Department of Health created a division of venereal diseases.[30]

Events moved rapidly after that. The board passed a regulation, having the force of law, stipulating that physicians report venereal disease cases. Records of these patients were to be confidential, but statistics were to be made public. Patients were required to undergo treatment until they were no longer able to infect others. In February

[28] Bracken to Frederick H. Baker, March 5, 1915, to Alfred F. Pillsbury, March 5, 1915, to F. N. Whittier, December 3, 1915, and to Jones, November 23, 1917; Pillsbury to Bracken, March 2, 1915. Minnesota Department of Health, St. Paul.
[29] W. H. Frost to Bracken, July 24, August 1, 1917; Bracken to Frost, July 27, 1917. Minnesota Department of Health, St. Paul.
[30] State Board of Health, *Biennial Reports*, 1916–17, pp. 9–13; 1918–19, p. 101; *Pioneer Press*, January 9, 1918; Bracken to Werner Hemstead, January 31, 1918, Minnesota Department of Health, St. Paul.

Bracken went to Washington to attempt to have commanders of military camps and cantonments report to the department the names of all men who, having been discharged from the service for physical reasons, were returned to Minnesota. On the same day the department received a supply of arsenobenzol, the American equivalent of Ehrlich's salvarsan, to be distributed to venereal clinics and dispensaries. A training school for women lecturers on social hygiene was being planned, and a plan for close co-operation between the state health department and the commission had been adopted. Dr. Henry D. Ulrich was hired to do the department's Wassermanns for a period of six months.[31]

To supplement the work of the commission and the newly created division of venereal diseases, Bracken requested Dr. Taliaferro Clark, director of the bureau of sanitary service of the American Red Cross, to supply Minnesota, not with a complete sanitary service, but with a sanitary inspector, a supervising nurse, and two social-service nurses. In his request to Clark, Bracken said that Colonel H. S. Greenleaf, ranking surgeon at Fort Snelling, repeatedly requested departmental help and had said that he was "unable to handle conditions satisfactorily without outside assistance." In addition, Bracken planned to have papers on venereal disease and the work of the new division read before the annual meeting of the Minnesota State Medical Association in order to acquaint physicians of the state with the program.[32]

Bracken also sent an extended manuscript, telling something of the background of the division of venereal diseases, to the *Journal-Lancet*. Written by Dr. H. G. Irvine, director of the division, this manuscript as published told the profession that Dr. Mabel S. Ulrich had been appointed supervisor of social hygiene education and that Charlotte G. Ashbrook had been selected as chief social worker. Dr. Ulrich was well known for her lectures on venereal disease, and Miss Ashbrook had had wide experience in the social-service department of the Pennsylvania Hospital at Philadelphia. The health department, continued Irvine, recognized that prostitutes were the principal carriers of venereal disease and that it therefore would work directly with law-enforcement agencies. He outlined the methods of the division as follows:

1. Education of the public as to the dangers of venereal diseases, and the problem of control.

[31] *Pioneer Press*, January 31, February 26, 27, 1918; Ulrich to Bracken, March 30, 1918, Bracken to Ulrich, June 26, 1918, Minnesota Department of Health, St. Paul.
[32] Bracken to H. Wireman Cook, April 12, 1918, and to Henry Ulrich, June 27, 1918, Minnesota Department of Health, St. Paul.

2. Education of the patients as to the treatment and prevention of other infections.
3. Education of physicians as to their duty in the plan of control.
4. Reporting of cases.
5. Provision of adequate and convenient dispensary service.
6. Social-service control of cases.
7. Diagnostic service in the State Laboratory.
8. Distribution of free salvarsan where needed.
9. Quarantine of incorrigible cases, and of carriers who are dangerous to public health.
10. Supression of prostitution.[33]

Although Irvine did not mention his own qualifications, he was well fitted for his post as director of the division. A native of Portland, Maine, Irvine was graduated in medicine from the University of Minnesota in 1903, and in 1917 he had done graduate work in Vienna, Paris, and London. He was deputy coroner of Hennepin County from 1900 to 1906, and engaged in the private practice of medicine. He was also a professor of dermatology at the University of Minnesota.[34]

Getting the division of venereal diseases under way was no easy task. Irvine put in one busy day after another, holding conferences with the Minnesota Social Hygiene Commission, speaking before various groups in the state, planning for dispensaries, and discussing Twin City prostitution with officers at Fort Snelling. He arranged with the editor of the *Minneapolis Daily News* to secure data from police blotters, and he was pleased to learn that the majority of prostitutes arrested were given jail sentences and that very few were fined or dismissed. As the result of a meeting held on May 2, 1918, with Minneapolis law-enforcement officials, all police precincts agreed to co-operate. When one of two St. Paul police officers who offered bail for professional prostitutes admitted having relations with one of the girls, Irvine insisted that he report to an official clinic and not to a private physician. In addition to all these activities, he found time to prepare materials for bulletins.[35]

These efforts bore fruit. In 47 districts 127 physicians and institutions reported in August, 1918, a total of 304 cases of syphilis, 186 of gonorrhea, and 7 of chancroid. The Minneapolis Health Department received approval from the City Council to employ additional help to

[33] Irvine, "Venereal Disease Work in Minnesota," [1918] (typescript), Minnesota Department of Health, St. Paul, and "The Warfare in Minnesota against Venereal Disease," in *Journal-Lancet*, 38:347 (June 15, 1918).
[34] Minnesota Editorial Association, *Who's Who in Minnesota*, 874 (Minneapolis, 1941).
[35] "Report of the Work before Dr. Irvine Left for California," January 23–November 14, 1918 (typescript), Minnesota Department of Health, St. Paul.

deal with the venereal disease problem, and osteopathic physicians throughout the state learned approved methods of treatment. St. Paul clinics were held at the city dispensary, at Franklin and West Ninth streets, with Drs. John Armstrong and Katherine Nye in attendance. At Duluth clinics were conducted at St. Mary's Hospital, and in Minneapolis, at the City Hospital and the University of Minnesota Dispensary. In addition, an extensive educational program, with lectures and motion pictures, was developed. The total number of venereal cases at Fort Snelling was reduced drastically, but 4,687 cases of syphilis, 6,309 of gonorrhea, and 275 of chancroid were reported for Minnesota as a whole in 1918.[36]

Two events of significance occurred in 1919. The first was a rural educational campaign conducted in thirty-seven counties, which brought to nearly all school teachers not only talks on venereal disease but also the motion picture, "The End of the Road." During the campaign more than sixteen thousand pamphlets were distributed. The second event was the amendment of the department's regulations concerning venereal disease. The new regulation, adopted on April 29, 1919, and approved by the attorney general, was far reaching. In the first place, it designated venereal diseases as contagious, infectious, communicable, and dangerous to the public health. Then it made mandatory the reporting of all cases to the state board and required that all physicians and others treating or examining persons venereally diseased keep a record of names and addresses of such patients. This regulation applied to superintendents or managers of hospitals, dispensaries, and charitable or penal institutions. Other provisions dealt with preventive measures and reporting of special cases. Local health officers were directed to use every available means to investigate known or suspected cases and were authorized to quarantine persons who had or were suspected of having a venereal disease. Prostitution was declared "a prolific source of syphilis, gonorrhea, and chancroid, and the repression of prostitution" was "declared to be a public health measure." All health officers were directed to co-operate with proper authorities to enforce laws against prostitution. Provision was made also for the posting of public notices on homes and buildings housing immoral activities.

[36] "Summary Reports of Cases of Syphilis, Chancroid, Gonorrhoea, August, 1918" (typescript), H. A. Northrop to Bracken, September 16, November 22, 1918, and Bracken to Northrop, November 19, 1918, Minnesota Department of Health, St. Paul; Minneapolis City Council, *Proceedings*, 1918, p. 330; *Pioneer Press*, October 18, December 31, 1918; State Board of Health, *Biennial Reports*, 1918–19, pp. 101–105, 108.

CONTROL OF VENEREAL DISEASE 259

Such notices read: "Warning! Venereal Disease exists on these premises." These were to be printed in black, bold-face type upon a red card with the words "venereal disease" appearing in letters not less than three inches high.[37]

By 1922 Irvine was ready to summarize the results of his program. He had made an introductory analysis in 1918 and another the following year. In the first report he said that his efforts were first centered on the army, then on the army and the community, and finally on civilians almost entirely. He pointed out also that, according to statistics of the United States Public Health Service, the percentage of drafted men from Texas who were venereally infected was 11.02% and the Minnesota percentage was 2.31. And he said that "the effect of cleaning up the streets and closing up open houses of prostitution is apparent in the marked reduction . . . of the rate for both prophylaxis and disease." He thought the treatment of prostitutes was important, but not so important as "an educational demonstration of the amount of disease among these people, and of their possibilities as carriers. The point to be emphasized is not the need of treating them, but of permanently putting them out of business as the only means of curbing their danger to health."

Then Irvine spoke more specifically of Minnesota: "Many physicians have commented on the uselessness of handling professional prostitutes and of the need of controlling clandestine prostitutes. With proper cooperation, reporting offers a big opportunity in this connection. . . . If the profession would cooperate and make a reasonable effort, the source could be reported in a large percentage of fresh cases, and most state boards of health have a social service department equipped to successfully handle this problem. We have attempted to emphasize in Minnesota the importance of this work, and our social service department is handling more than a hundred cases a month from information of this type secured from report cards."[38]

In his second report, which appeared in November, 1919, Irvine addressed himself primarily to Minnesota physicians. After briefly sketching his division's progress during the war years, he spoke of the importance of social-service work and of the necessity for laboratory

[37] L. W. Feezer to the Surgeon General, United States Public Health Service, November 10, 1919, and State Board of Health, "Amended Regulations Relating to Venereal Disease," April 29, 1919 (typescript), Minnesota Department of Health, St. Paul; *Minnesota State Health Laws and Regulations*, pp. 71–75, (January 1, 1948).
[38] Irvine, "The Venereal Disease Campaign in Retrospect," in American Medical Association, *Journal*, 17: 1029–1033 (September 28, 1918).

services, including Wassermann tests, gonorrheal fixation tests, and microscopic examination of smears. He also outlined in general an educational program. Then he listed five results which might be expected from a well-rounded program to control venereal diseases:

1. We may expect to reduce venereal diseases by reducing commercial prostitution to a vanishing point.

2. We may expect to reduce venereal disease by gaining the recognition of the medical profession and the public, to the fact that these diseases must be removed from the plane of "secret" or "shameful" diseases, to the plane of other contagious infections, which properly belong under the control of public health authorities.

3. We may expect to reduce venereal diseases by making laboratory diagnosis available to all and providing accredited hospitals and dispensaries with Arsphenamine, free of cost. Thus far the Bureau has distributed 250 ampules of free Arsphenamine, has made fifty Wassermanns, and has examined a large number of slides for gonorrhea. No one questions the value of free diagnosis and treatment in the case of diphtheria or rabies. We may safely predict a corresponding value when we apply the same course to venereal diseases.

4. We may expect to reduce venereal diseases by reducing clandestine prostitution — and thus eliminating a large body of carriers — by carefully organized social work.

5. We may expect to reduce venereal diseases by an organized system of sex education.

"We offer you then," said Irvine to the state's physicians, "the use of our machinery for investigation, for diagnosis, for social service, for education, and we ask you to avail yourselves of it. In return, we ask that you conscientiously report to the Board of Health office, every case which comes to your attention; we urge that you make every effort to trace such a case to the source of infection, and that you do not rest until you are assured as to whether or not there are other members in the family similarly diseased." [39]

This meant that venereal diseases were a peace problem and not a short-lived war activity. The effectiveness of the division's program became more apparent annually. Irvine first outlined venereal programs in twenty-five states, then discussed methods of reporting cases from physicians and hospitals, and finally tabulated as follows the work of the division for the three years 1919 to 1921, inclusive: [40]

[39] Irvine and Mabel S. Ulrich, "Program for State Board of Health for Control of Venereal Diseases and What Results May Be Expected," in *Minnesota Medicine*, 2:434 (November, 1919).
[40] United States Public Health Service, "Venereal Diseases a Peace Problem," in *Minnesota Health Journal*, 3:231 (January 9, 1919); Irvine, "Some Notes on the

Cases Reported	1919	1920	1921
Syphilis	3,326	4,451	4,815
Gonorrhea	4,622	6,020	6,277
Chancroid	197	228	202
Total	8,145	10,699	11,294
Laboratory			
Wassermann tests	5,010	14,964	23,271
Smears	698	3,234	4,975
All examinations, including dark field	5,757	18,251	28,455
Subsidized Clinics			
Patients admitted	2,087	1,639*	704
Treatments given	20,602	32,588	23,982
Arsphenamin			
Doses distributed	5,082	8,177	5,094
Social Service			
Cases handled	2,760	3,866	4,051
Number of towns in which cases were investigated	82	175	181
Educational			
Number of pamphlets distributed	198,525	167,081	52,528
Number of exhibit days	62	439	232
Attendance at exhibits	65,038	73,493	36,720
Film shows	128	132	104
Attendance at film shows	47,040	41,412	20,120
Lectures	180	108	62
Attendance at lectures	38,500	3,200	3,330
Number of towns reached		178	167

(*Does not include persons carried over into this year, but admitted last year. In all, 2,261 persons were treated this year.)

This imposing record did not indicate, except in a general manner, all the activities of the division. Inmates of state institutions in Minnesota were examined and, if infected, were treated. The State Board of Control co-operated by securing the full-time services of a woman physician and the consultation service of a specialist. A "Keeping Fit" campaign was carried on during the first half of 1920 and, in addition to previously established clinics, another clinic was opened at Virginia.[41]

Effectiveness of the Venereal Disease Program," in *Journal of the American Medical Association*, 79:1121–1126 (September 30, 1922); Chesley, in *Health*, [2]:54 (October, 1922).

[41] State Board of Health, *Biennial Reports*, 1920–21, pp. 213–221.

Once the venereal disease program got under way, received the support of most of the members of the medical profession, and was endorsed by public opinion, progress became easier and, in some instances, more rapid. Shortly after World War I, however, interest in the problem seemed to decline, and the economic recession beginning in 1929 heightened disinterest further. After October, 1929, the division of venereal diseases lost its identity as a separate administrative unit and was merged with the division of preventable diseases. Federal aid had been withdrawn the year before, but fortunately the Minnesota legislature appropriated sufficient funds to enable the health department to continue the most essential functions of the program. In 1929 clinics either were discontinued or had their administration taken over by the hospitals in which they were located.

The Federal Venereal Disease Control Act of 1938, which provided for the distribution of grants-in-aid to states through the medium of the United States Public Health Service, again stimulated interest in the problem. There were good reasons why Minnesota should avail itself of these grants. Prostitution had not by any means been eradicated in the state. It was true that the ancient profession had been driven underground in some cities, but it had not entirely disappeared. In a few communities it flourished rather openly. Had a vice commission, similar to that which investigated Minneapolis in 1911, reported in 1938, it would have found that some conditions had changed very little. Indeed, the *Minneapolis Journal* in 1937 reprinted as a pamphlet for free distribution a series of articles pertaining to venereal diseases. These were prepared by a staff writer and approved by the state health department, the Minneapolis commissioner of health, and the executive committee of the Hennepin County Medical Society. About the same time, the health department issued a short history of Minnesota's campaign against venereal disease. It concluded with the remark that the "support of every citizen of Minnesota is essential if we are to go forward in the war on syphilis and gonorrhea."[42]

The approach of World War II and the passage of the National Selective Service Act did much to renew Minnesota's interest in the problems of prostitution and venereal diseases. Some forty thousand troops gathered at Camp Ripley in the summer of 1940 for maneuvers. On April 16 at Little Falls, Governor Stassen called together health

---

[42] United States, *Statutes at Large*, 52:439; Minneapolis Vice Commission, *Report to the Mayor* (Minneapolis, 1911); Esther M. Flint, *Health Conditions and Health Service in St. Paul* (St. Paul, 1919); Arnold Aslakson, *Medical Facts That Can Save*

CONTROL OF VENEREAL DISEASE 263

and law-enforcement officers, as well as representatives of the United States Public Health Service. Officers of the armed forces also were present. This group worked out a meticulous program for the control of venereal diseases in the military area. Briefly, the plans called for the establishment at Little Falls of a branch office of the health department staffed with a venereal disease control officer, a venereal disease epidemiological worker, and clerical help; for the assignment of special agents from the State Bureau of Criminal Apprehension to ferret out prostitutes; for free diagnostic and treatment facilities; for a survey of all camps, cabins, and resorts by the division of hotel inspection; and for prompt referral through the corps surgeon's office of all information regarding known and suspected cases of infection of soldiers. As a result of these elaborate precautions, only five women were arrested, only two soldiers were reported as having contracted syphilis, and only thirty-three cases of gonorrhea were found among the military.[43]

Dr. R. R. Sullivan, who made a final report on the Camp Ripley operations, had had long experience with the problem. In 1930 he had helped organize a venereal disease clinic at the Red Lake Indian Reservation, where he was assisted by Adelia Eggestine and Ruth Young, both of the division of child hygiene. His Indian survey revealed a total of 44 cases of congenital and 111 cases of acquired venereal diseases. The usual arsenicals and bismuth were relied upon for treatment.[44]

When civilians began registering for the draft, the United States Public Health Service suggested that blood specimens for serological tests be drawn from every registrant. In Minnesota these samples were examined by the health department, the first specimens being received on November 6, 1940. By the close of the year a total of 9,326 specimens had been received and 9,992 tests had been performed. During the period from November, 1940, through December 31, 1941, a total of 68,568 specimens from 66,829 men were examined and 73,857 tests were carried out. The results indicated, but did not necessarily prove, that 0.45% were syphilitic and that 98.95% had negative findings. In

Countless Lives (Minneapolis, 1937); Minnesota Department of Health, *Minnesota's Campaign against Venereal Disease*, 15 (Minneapolis, 1937); Phyllis P. Harris and Ruth E. Boynton, *Public Health and Medical Care in Red Wing and Goodhue County*, 23 (Minneapolis, 1946).

[43] State Board of Health, *Reports*, 1922–43, p. 124; R. R. Sullivan, "Minnesota Venereal Disease Control Program in Connection with Military Maneuvers," in *Journal of Social Hygiene*, 26:371–376 (November, 1940).

[44] Senate Committee on Indian Affairs, *Survey of Conditions of the Indians in the United States*, part 26, p. 14408.

1942, from 156,840 registrants 199,809 specimens were received. Of these, only 0.6% showed a positive Kolmer reaction.[45]

The Minnesota Departments of Health and Education considered a co-operative project providing for a qualified teacher to organize and conduct classes in social hygiene in teacher-training institutions. This appointment was made on January 1, 1940. Working under the supervision of the division of preventable diseases, an instructor presented courses in eight colleges and universities during the next two years. Included were teachers colleges at Winona, Bemidji, Duluth, Moorhead, and Mankato. Similar courses were held at the University of Minnesota during a summer session, and at Hamline University.[46]

With the termination of hostilities, the department again examined blood samples from service men and women who were being discharged at Fort Snelling. From then and on through 1948 the serological laboratories also devoted themselves to examining specimens sent in by hospitals, private practitioners and doctors, and nurses attached to business houses and industrial plants. Thousands of specimens arrive yearly from railroad and mining companies and from other concerns which insist that a prospective employee have a thorough, routine physical examination.[47]

It was pointed out in 1944 that Washington, Montana, Maryland, and Minnesota were the only states above the Mason-Dixon line that did not require a physician's certificate of freedom from venereal disease before a marriage license could be obtained. "Thirty out of forty-eight states," argued an editor, "believe that parties in a marriage contract are entitled to the knowledge that their prospective partner is free from venereal disease; that the babies of the next generation are entitled to start life free from syphilis. Can these states be wrong? If not, then we in Minnesota have been remiss." [48]

Irvine promptly replied that the fact that Minnesota had no such law was not due to lack of consideration. He said that the matter had been discussed twice in the legislature and twice had been rejected. He pointed out that then, as in 1948, Minnesota had one of the lowest venereal disease rates in the entire country. His conclusion was both a

[45] State Board of Health, *Reports*, 1922–43, p. 126; Minnesota State Sanitary Conference, "Resources of the Minnesota Department of Health for the Protection of the Health of Civilians in the Civilian Defense Program of Minnesota," 2 ([Minneapolis], November 21, 1941).
[46] State Board of Health, *Reports*, 1922–43, p. 127.
[47] Interview of the author with Dr. Anne Kimball, director of the division of serology, May 4, 1948.
[48] "Premarital and Prenatal Examinations," in *Minnesota Medicine*, 27:493 (June, 1944).

tribute to the success of the program which he had inaugurated and the final answer as to why the state has not passed acts making premarital and prenatal examinations obligatory. "In any state where control has been instituted only in the past few years and rates for early cases are high," said Irvine, "such laws may be valuable and very much worthwhile, but in Minnesota at present it is surely questionable whether the cost of administration and the burden of enforcement are worthwhile. As an aid to control of venereal disease it would be nearly worthless and so far as its educational value is concerned that work is being done directly with a very complete and comprehensive program. If there is to be some such law should it not be a simple, broad one, covering a complete physical examination, and include gonorrhea, tuberculosis, or any other disease which could be transmitted by contact, as well as certain mental diseases?" [49]

[49] "Communication to the Editor," in *Minnesota Medicine*, 27:584 (July, 1944).

14

The White Plague

IT HAD many names in the pioneer period. Some settlers referred to it as catarrh, others confused it with pneumonia, and a few used the term consumption. Doctors spoke of it as phthisis. But no matter how immigrant or physician talked of this disease, they were referring to the dreaded tuberculosis, a plague as old as antiquity and one that for centuries had smothered untold lives with cough and hemorrhage. The story of the subjugation of tuberculosis in Minnesota, from 1872 to 1948, is an incredible drama involving the march of medicine, the stubborn labors of health officers, and the willing work of scores of organizations and thousands of volunteer workers. It is also a tale of patience and co-operation on the part of the patient.

Among the first activities of the Minnesota State Board of Health was an extensive investigation of the relationship of the state's climate to diseases of the lungs and air passages. Drs. Franklin Staples, G. D. Winch, and Hewitt worked on this problem for three years before publishing their findings. There was real reason, of course, why these men should wish to learn more of the nature of consumption. Minnesota was considered by many afflicted individuals to be an ideal spot to recover their health. Yet, to offset this romantic viewpoint, an opinion prevailed, and seemed to be borne out by death notices, that fatalities from tuberculosis were numerous among Minnesota residents. Citizens, worried by the prevalence of the disease, sometimes asked publicly for advice and assistance. As a result, physicians and even editors contributed to newspapers whatever knowledge was available and considered trustworthy.[1]

[1] *Pioneer-Press and Tribune,* July 30, 1876; *Pioneer Press,* December 10, 1876, July 26, October 30, 1877, June 16, 1889, June 15, 1890. On tuberculosis fatalities, see, for example, the *St. Paul Daily Press,* January 3, February 27, April 9, 27,

The three-man committee began its investigation by sending a questionnaire to Minnesota physicians. Among the queries were: "Have you in this State seen pneumonia in any of its forms result directly or indirectly in Phthisis Pulmonalis?" "Does the climate of Minnesota favor the cure of Phthisis Pulmonalis originating elsewhere?" "Have you known any cases to originate in this State in persons not supposed to be predisposed to the disease?" The questionnaires were sent out in 1874. The next year only a progress report was returned, but in 1876 Staples brought all the returns together, interpreted them, and published his findings. Without adequate means of securing vital statistics, the committee, of course, was hampered in its work. But it had been able to consult fairly reliable figures for the year 1872. These indicated that the total number of deaths from all causes was 5,228. The total number of deaths from *phthisis pulmonalis* was 499, with 260 fatalities among males and 239 among females. Most deaths occurred in August. The places of birth of the victims were: Minnesota, 58; other states, 244; Germany, 51; Norway, 37; Sweden, 22; Ireland, 35; England, 10; British-America provinces, 13; and other countries and unknown, 49. The largest number of deaths fell in the age group from twenty to forty years.[2]

Curiously enough, although Staples said that he consulted the report of the commissioner of statistics for 1873, he did not include in this first tuberculosis survey of Minnesota figures for 1870 to 1872, inclusive. Had he done so, he could have listed 459 deaths in 1870 from consumption, 445 in 1871, and 499 in 1872. The percentages of these to total deaths for the years indicated were 17.10, 11.78, and 10.73. Figures for 1873 were not available. In 1875 the total number of deaths from tuberculous diseases was 621, and in 1876, the very year that Staples reported, deaths caused by consumption were numbered at 745, leading all others by a wide margin. Staples, however, faithfully published data gleaned from the committee's questionnaire. Forty-one physicians replied to the question asking whether or not persons predisposed to tuberculous consumption were as likely to develop it in Minnesota as in the eastern or southern portions of the Union. Of these, thirty-seven answered in the negative, one in the af-

June 14, 27, July 27, September 26, October 12, 15, 17, 20, 1872, March 5, May 10, July 4, November 15, 1873, January 20, July 18, 19, August 23, 1874; the *Pioneer-Press*, May 7, 1875; and the *Minneapolis Tribune*, November 25, 1875.
[2] State Board of Health, *Annual Reports*, 1874, p. 82; 1875, p. 6; 1876, p. 67; Staples, *Report on the Influence of Climate on Pulmonary Diseases in Minnesota* (reprinted from American Medical Association, *Transactions*, 1876 — Philadelphia, 1876).

firmative, and three were undecided. A majority also believed that few cases originated in the state in persons thought not to be predisposed to the disease, and all, except two, answered that the Minnesota climate favored the cure of *phthisis pulmonalis* originating elsewhere.[3]

Despite these early valiant efforts to determine the extent of tuberculosis in Minnesota, little could be accomplished in treating it until more was known of its nature and of the way it spread from one person to another. Until then physicians and public health men could only recommend a change of climate or bed rest, or perhaps prescribe a variety of nostrums, most of which could benefit the patient only psychologically. The great change from ignorance to knowledge came in 1882, when Robert Koch discovered the tubercle bacillus and demonstrated that the disease was transmitted by contact with an infected individual.[4]

Koch's next step was the development of a method of treatment, which was first called the "lymph treatment" and later, "tuberculin." Koch announced the tuberculin treatment in November, 1890, and early in January of the following year St. Paul and Minneapolis physicians were using it. By autumn, however, the hoped-for cures had not resulted, and both the profession and the public were forced to admit disappointing and often fatal results. The *Pioneer Press* reluctantly told its readers that physicians were viewing the lymph treatment in a "cold and dispassionate" manner and, a little later, admitted that it had ceased to be the "strenuous hope" of consumptives. Hewitt had watched the increase of tuberculosis among both humans and cattle and he was much concerned when he realized that Koch's remedy was a failure. He twice warned Minnesotans against becoming too enthusiastic over the use of tuberculin, saying, first, that it would be better to "watch and wait" and, second, that "Fatal results have already followed the use of the remedy in the hands of men trained by Koch himself." He was even more cautious about the use of tuberculin in the treatment of cattle, saying that he would move only when a reliable tuberculin was available.[5]

[3] Minnesota Commissioner of Statistics, *Reports*, 1873, p. 21; 1876, p. 250; 1877, p. 119; State Board of Health, *Annual Reports*, 1876, p. 73.
[4] Wilson G. Smillie, *Public Health Administration in the United States*, 78 (New York, 1935). For a general discussion of diseases spread largely through discharges from the mouth and nose, see Milton J. Rosenau, *Preventive Medicine and Hygiene*, chapter 3 (New York, 1927). An excellent short biographical sketch of Koch may be found in M. E. M. Walker, *Pioneers of Public Health*, 178–192 (London, 1930).
[5] *Pioneer Press*, January 10, 11, 17, February 24, March 6, 15, 23, April 25, May 14, August 13, November 1, 7, 1891; *Public Health in Minnesota*, 4:94 (February, 1889); 6:103, 120 (November, December, 1890); State Board of Health, *Biennial Reports*, 1891–92, p. 25; 1893–94, pp. 15–17.

Indeed, more attention was paid to bovine than to human tuberculosis during the last decade of the nineteenth century. That did not mean, however, that the state board was disinterested in the problem. By 1898 much had been accomplished. A circular on the infectiousness of the disease had been prepared and distributed, the laboratory was making sputum examinations, and the board was considering a suggestion made by C. C. Andrews, chief fire warden of Minnesota, that land on the south shore of Cass Lake be purchased and a tuberculosis sanatorium be built on it. Hewitt constantly advocated the isolation of tuberculosis patients and wrote many letters to county health officers urging that they, too, isolate patients from well persons. He agreed in principle with the statement that the "sputa of the patients, large and small — the masses spit out and the particles thrown into the air by coughing — are the agents through and by which the bacilli are spread. If all these sputa can be arrested and disposed of before they find lodgment in quarters whence the bacilli with which they are loaded may in dried form find their way into other human systems, the disease will be 'stamped out.'" But both Hewitt and Bracken knew that this was easier said than done.[6]

No sooner had Bracken taken office as secretary of the board than he began a vigorous attack upon tuberculosis, which, before he finally resigned, was to lead him into one fight after another and was to be partly responsible for his retirement. His first step was a canvas of Minnesota state institutions to determine how many inmates were tuberculous. Most superintendents replied that tuberculosis was on the increase in their institutions and some said that they made attempts to isolate active cases. These replies prompted Bracken to encourage the incipient sanatorium movement, for he felt strongly that tuberculous patients should be entirely isolated. He thought that they should be so confined that they could not possibly do any damage to anyone else.[7]

A national American Health Resort Association already was at work encouraging restful havens in healthful climates for consumptives. At

[6] State Board of Health, *Biennial Reports*, 1897–98, pp. 64, 154, 121; W. Pfister to Hewitt, June 26, 1895, S. J. Meek to Hewitt, August 25, 1895, A. O. Lunder to H. H. Hart, November 26, 1895, James McKeon to Hewitt, January 4, 1896, and Hans A. Gulleksu to Hewitt, March 9, 1896, Minnesota Department of Health, St. Paul; *Pioneer Press*, December 27, 1896.
[7] Bracken to H. A. Tomlinson, August 3, 1897; letters to Bracken from Tomlinson, October 22, 1897, from R. A. Mott, October 25, 1897, from D. R. Greenlee, October 26, 1897, from W. H. Houlton, October 28, 1897, from Arthur T. Kilbourne, November 1, 1897, from George O. Welch, October 27, 1897, and from A. C. Rogers, November 17, 1897. Minnesota Department of Health, St. Paul.

a meeting of the Minnesota State Medical Society much attention was given tuberculosis, and a few months later a special committee reported favorably on a state sanitary resort in the pine woods. Recommendation was made that the legislative committees of the state's medical societies urge early legislation to secure a resort. In 1899 the plans were going forward and, it was said, "Hundreds of men and women in Minnesota who feel the incipient attacks of tuberculous disease are looking forward eagerly to the state legislature to see if it will put Minnesota alongside of Massachusetts in its beneficent provision for their class. Medical men from all schools have given their unanimous indorsement to the Cass lake proposal. And since our forest experts claim that the tract can be made, under careful management, to yield the state a considerable return from its forest products the proposal seems to be one which is strongly fortified by economic arguments as well as by those of a humanitarian nature." [8]

Progress was sluggish, but the state board and determined legislators pushed forward. Finally, after considerable public pressure, the legislature in 1901 passed an act appointing a committee to investigate the advisability of establishing a state sanatorium and appropriating a thousand dollars for expenses. The committee reported favorably in 1903, and the legislature appropriated twenty-five thousand dollars, which was used to purchase land on Leech Lake near Walker. Two years later fifty thousand dollars more was appropriated. Minnesota finally, in 1899, had replied to three questions asked by Dr. R. M. Phelps, assistant superintendent of the Rochester State Hospital: "First: Is it best to have any sanitarium? Second: Should the state equip and conduct such a sanitarium? Third: Should such a sanitarium be located within the borders of the state?" In 1907 the first units had been constructed and the sanatorium opened.[9]

Despite the opening of the hospital at Walker, the decade from 1900 to 1910 was one largely of planning and spade work. Bracken threw himself into an antituberculosis campaign with his characteristic vigor and bluntness. He was concerned particularly with the lack of both city and county facilities and he was annoyed by the fact that people did not understand that tuberculosis was infectious. Yet, with all his

[8] *Pioneer Press*, November 3, 1897, July 17, December 14, 1898, January 12, 16, 1899.
[9] *Pioneer Press*, February 18, 1899; State Board of Health, *Biennial Reports*, 1901–02, p. 154; *Laws*, 1901, p. 475; 1905, p. 548; Bracken to Livingston Farrand, April 4, 1907, Minnesota Department of Health, St. Paul; R. M. Phelps, "The Policy of State Sanitariums for Consumptives," in *Northwestern Lancet*, 19:348 (September 1, 1899).

eagerness, he realized the necessity of "making haste slowly." The main topic discussed by the executive committee of the board on November 14, 1901, was, "What should be done relating to tuberculosis among mankind in this state?" Bracken felt that too many organizations might result in confusion and overlapping of work and authority, but he was willing to support a district tuberculosis association. He planned also to distribute literature, to collect statistics, to devise some scheme by which counties could care for the afflicted poor, and to stimulate private individuals not only to contribute to but also to establish and maintain private institutions.[10]

The care of tuberculous patients in city hospitals was especially critical. "Although there are over 200 deaths from consumption in the city annually," said the *Minneapolis Journal*, "the city does not appropriate a dollar for the especial care of consumptive patients, where if the same number died of smallpox or diphtheria, appropriations, special staffs and special buildings would almost instantly be forthcoming." The day before, the same newspaper had charged that tuberculous patients had been refused admittance at five hospitals. Soon the situation became so bad that the Minneapolis Associated Charities proposed that lodging houses be opened to care for indigent patients.[11]

The fact, as Bracken said, that "no very important" work was being done in Minnesota and that neither St. Paul nor Minneapolis were taking adequate care of tuberculous patients resulted in two tuberculosis conferences in 1907. The first was held in February and the second in August. Bracken must have listened attentively as he heard a physician say: "The rich man . . . may go and live in tent colonies, he may go and have the experience of the world, but the poor man who depends upon his daily labor for his support and his family, what are you going to do with him? . . . We could do nothing for him but possibly he might get relief if he could go into the northern woods and stay during the summer." The establishment of a private sanatorium, at an estimated cost of nineteen thousand dollars, was the main topic of the second conference. The result was not all that was expected, but at least one tangible institution emerged. That was the Minneapolis

[10] A. G. Aldrich to Bracken, January 20, 1900; Bracken to Aldrich, January 22, 1900, to Henry Hutchinson, November 11, 1901, to H. Longstreet Taylor, January 8, August 13, 1902, to R. Leland, April 3, 1902, to L. F. Flick, December 31, 1903, to George H. Christian, August 14, 1906; Taylor to Bracken, August 14, 15, 1902; Beard to Bracken, October 2, 1903; Bracken, "Report on Minneapolis Tuberculosis Sanatorium, June, [1906]" (typescript). Minnesota Department of Health, St. Paul.
[11] *Journal*, February 12, 13, 1904; Bracken to the secretary of the Minneapolis Associated Charities, November 11, 1904, Minnesota Department of Health, St. Paul.

City Dispensary, which opened its doors on May 1, 1909. A gift from Mr. and Mrs. George H. Christian enabled Minneapolis to care for forty-five advanced cases which the dispensary could not handle.[12]

Meanwhile the legislature had not been inactive, although its efforts fell short of Bracken's hopes. An appropriation was made in 1909 for educational work relating to tuberculosis, and a bill was introduced, but not passed, that excluded tuberculous teachers and pupils from schools. Of greater significance, however, was the passage of a bill enabling boards of county commissioners to establish and maintain public sanatoriums for the treatment and care of tuberculous patients. The same legislature, however, refused to appropriate state funds to aid such patients.[13]

The passage of the act to create county sanatoriums, even though it was finally accomplished with little difficulty, was the result of years of patient activity by the state board, private individuals and organizations, and national associations. Bracken in 1907 prepared a most carefully drawn report to the legislature in which he showed that tuberculosis killed about two thousand persons annually in Minnesota and declared that it was a preventable disease. He estimated that between eight thousand and ten thousand tuberculous individuals needed treatment. "It is impossible," he continued, "to care for such a great army of patients in institutions. We must therefore provide for them in the home. To do this, we must consider the mild cases that may recover if properly cared for, and the advanced cases that will die of this disease, and who will act as centers of infection during their long illness if not properly cared for. . . . There is no other disease where so large a proportion of the patients eventually become a public charge. . . . It is impossible for the State Board of Health to carry on this work without the liberal support of the Legislature." [14]

Bracken was zealous also in acquainting the legislature with progress being made in Minnesota and abroad. He pointed out that the first tuberculosis exhibit was held in January, 1904, and was sponsored by the Maryland Board of Health, the Maryland Tuberculosis Commission, and the Maryland Public Health Association. From this exhibition developed the National Association for the Study and Prevention of Tu-

---

[12] *Journal*, February 13, 1904; Minnesota State Association for the Prevention and Relief of Tuberculosis, "Program and Minutes," February 6, 1907; "Memorandum of a Conference, August, 1907"; Elizabeth Sprague, "Tuberculosis Dispensary of City Hospital" (undated memorandum); Bracken to G. Walter Holden, February 7, 1906, and to H. W. Stone, March 7, 1911. Minnesota Department of Health, St. Paul.
[13] Bracken Papers, 3:302, 344, 354; *Laws*, 1909, pp. 398-400.
[14] State Board of Health, *Biennial Reports*, 1907-09, p. 2.

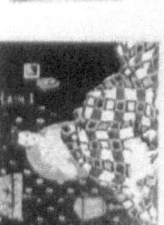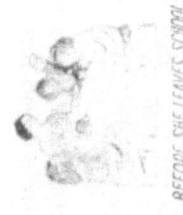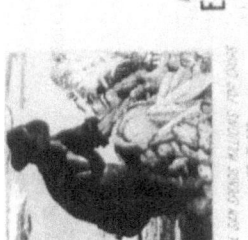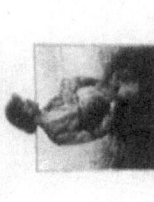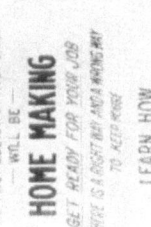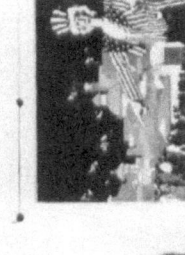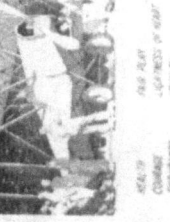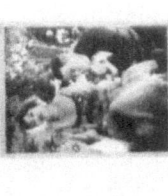

POSTERS USED IN A CAMPAIGN AGAINST VENEREAL DISEASE
Courtesy Minnesota Department of Health

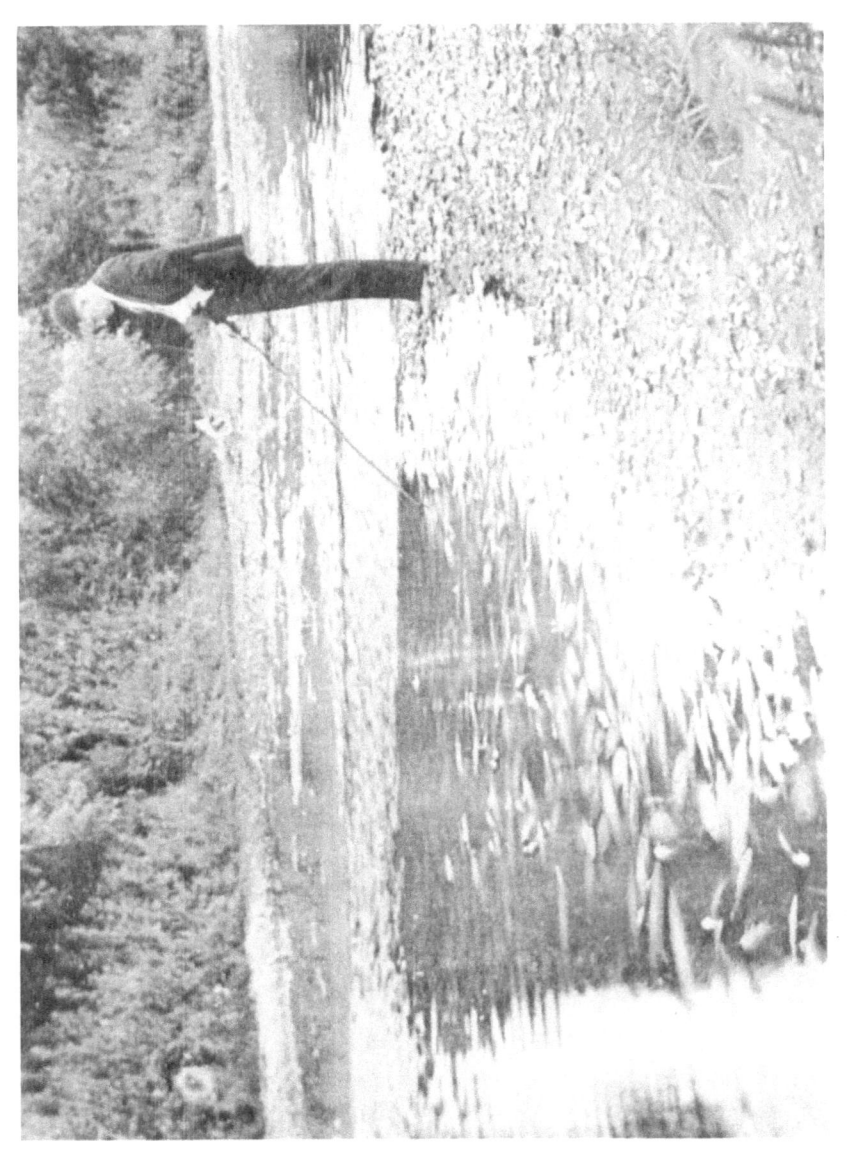

EFFECT OF STREAM POLLUTION ON FISH
Courtesy Minnesota Department of Health

berculosis, which held its first meeting at Washington, D.C., in May, 1905. The International Congress on Tuberculosis convened at Washington three years later. Stimulated by the national association, the Minnesota Association for the Prevention and Relief of Tuberculosis was organized in 1906. Then, having sketched the national history, Bracken proceeded to outline rapidly what else Minnesota had accomplished. He mentioned that St. Paul in 1907 had given land adjoining the city hospital to the state for a hospital for crippled and deformed children, including tuberculous patients; that St. Paul citizens had presented the state with land near Phalen Park and had donated money for the construction of cottages for children; that St. Paul had an active antituberculosis committee; and that Duluth also had such a committee. He pointed out, too, that private individuals in Minneapolis had maintained a summer camp for consumptives; that Hopewell Hospital maintained a twenty-bed pavilion; that the Contagious Disease Hospital had set aside twenty-five beds for victims of tuberculosis; and, finally, that both St. Paul and Minneapolis had maintained summer day camps for children.[15]

Yet, with all these efforts, plus an intensive educational program involving traveling exhibits and motion pictures, Minnesota lagged in its tuberculosis program. "While Minnesota stands in the first rank of progressive states in many matters," wrote the secretary of the Minnesota Association for the Prevention and Relief of Tuberculosis to Bracken, "it is undeniably the fact that in public measures, machinery and appropriations for the prevention of disease, its rank is by no means what it should be. This convention has been called especially to call attention to the fact that in the matter of the control of tuberculosis Minnesota is still relying upon mere educational matters and has not yet realized in any large way that a constructive state program establishing permanent agencies and institutions is required if we are to make any headway against this plague and if the educational propaganda is to bear fruit."[16]

Bracken had a ready explanation, if not a complete answer. He admitted that he had been "in the dumps" about the tuberculosis situation, but said he did not believe that the health department had a right to push things until an educational campaign had been carried on for a "long time." He indicated, too, that he found it difficult to

[15] State Board of Health, *Biennial Reports*, 1909–10, pp. 24–27.
[16] C. C. Pratt, "Report of Work of Anti-Tuberculosis Exhibition from April 1 to June 1, 1910," (typescript); National Association for the Study and Prevention of Tuberculosis, "Press Release, November 9, 1911"; Christopher Easton to Bracken, December 6, 1911. Minnesota Department of Health, St. Paul.

work with the state antituberculosis association. He admitted that the department was short of funds. Bracken had a right to be worried. Only a year earlier Hill had said that the death rate from tuberculosis during the last twenty years had diminished "in almost every state except in Minnesota, where no improvement had occurred since 1890, and we attribute this principally to a large Scandinavian population, although the Irish, of whom we have a noteworthy proportion also seem to be very susceptible." [17]

When, in 1912, Bracken attempted to explain why progress was slow in Minnesota, he again spoke of division of authority, added that financial support was difficult to secure from the legislature, and concluded by saying: "Minnesota is, in one way or another, doing considerable work along the lines of tuberculosis and we expect to introduce a bill before the coming legislature of 1913 of which I enclose a copy. The State Board of Health has done nothing practical along the lines of tuberculosis except the carrying out of its educational work through its Exhibit and compelling local officials under certain conditions to see to it that the tuberculous under their care were properly provided for." [18]

The bill which Bracken mentioned became law and immeasurably strengthened Minnesota's position. It enabled counties to establish and maintain tuberculosis sanatoriums and greatly extended the provisions of a similar act passed in 1909. The legislature of 1913 also made an appropriation for tuberculosis work, provided that reports on tuberculosis cases be made to the board of health, and, in a joint resolution, petitioned the United States Public Health Service to make an investigation of trachoma and tuberculosis among Indians on the Red Lake Reservation.[19]

Meanwhile Bracken, because of his belief that his department should have major supervisory control over tuberculosis activities, had irritated a large number of individuals and organizations working in the field. He quarreled with Dr. I. J. Murphy, executive secretary of the Minnesota Public Health Association, an organization incorporated in 1914 for the purpose of fighting tuberculosis. Bracken carried the ill feelings on to Hill, Murphy's successor. The dispute grew so heated that on April 21, 1919, the state Senate passed a resolution recom-

[17] Bracken to W. J. Marcley, December 7, 1911; Hill to C. B. Harris, August 17, 1910. Minnesota Department of Health, St. Paul.
[18] Bracken to Phillip P. Jacobs, December 9, 1912, Minnesota Department of Health, St. Paul.
[19] *Laws*, 1913, pp. 632, 634, 726–734, 914; Bracken to W. S. Leathers, November 29, 1913. Minnesota Department of Health, St. Paul.

THE WHITE PLAGUE 275

mending Bracken's resignation as secretary and executive officer. Bracken had quarreled also with the National Association for the Study and Prevention of Tuberculosis. The bone of contention there was the sale of Christmas Seals. For some reason or other, Bracken felt that the proceeds from these sales used directly for relief in Minnesota were insufficient. He made such a clamor that on March 22, 1918, the national association not only accepted his resignation as director, but also resolved that "whereas the Minnesota Public Health Association is the organization actively engaged in educational work in Minnesota, the Executive Committee instructs the office that in their opinion the Minnesota Public Health Association is the logical agent for the sale of Red Cross Seals in that state." [20]

Indeed, during the entire year of 1918 there had been a series of errors and misunderstandings. The United States was at war, and Bracken was faced with vexing, temporary problems. One of these concerned the handling of men rejected by the armed services for physical reasons. Although the department had instructed physicians on local draft boards to report promptly all tuberculous cases among registrants, results were not always satisfactory. And unless such cases were reported, follow-up investigations by the division of tuberculosis were impossible. The returned soldier presented an equally difficult problem, for, if he was tuberculous, he also needed special treatment.[21]

To help solve the problem of both the draftee and the returned soldier, a three-part policy was worked out by the American Red Cross, the Minnesota Advisory Commission, and the Minnesota Public Health Association. And on July 24, 1918, these agencies requested the health department to co-operate. Smith, head of the department's division of tuberculosis and later Bracken's successor, reacted about as violently as Bracken was in the habit of doing. "It is evident," he wrote with obvious displeasure, "that the Minnesota Public Health Association is not enough interested in harmonious work with the State Board of Health to follow up the tentative suggestions made them unofficially by a member of the Board that the Secretary of said Association and the Director of the Division confer. It is evident that the contract drawn up by the three parties mentioned was drawn with no real appreciation of the legal responsibilities of the State Board of Health, the health officer of the sanitary district, nor of the responsibility of the township for the

[20] Minnesota Public Health Association, *Journal*, 3:410 (April 24, 1919); *Senate Journal*, 1919, pp. 1305, 1636; Charles J. Hatfield to Bracken, March 22, 1918, Minnesota Department of Health, St. Paul.
[21] Division of Tuberculosis, "Quarterly Reports," June 30, 1918, Minnesota Department of Health, St. Paul.

care of its own poor. It is evident that tuberculosis workers as a whole know too little about public health as a whole. It is not denied that most health officers know too little about tuberculosis."

Smith felt that it would be most unwise for either the Red Cross or the Minnesota Public Health Association to follow up cases and to advise patients what to do. He concluded, however, by making a plea for the correlation of the work of all agencies interested in tuberculosis. Later he charged that the Minnesota Advisory Commission had assumed the legal responsibilities of the state board. Some health officers agreed with Smith and Bracken. By July, 1918, the misunderstanding between the department and F. J. Bruno, director of civilian relief of the Red Cross in Minneapolis, had grown so tense that neither was able to comprehend what the other was saying.[22]

Fearful that this feud would be aired to a horrified public, a group of those interested in the problem met on July 8 and passed the following resolution: "Whereas the interests of public health are paramount to those of any of the various organizations working individually and separately to that end; and, whereas the combined efforts of all give promise of getting the best results; and whereas the new regime contemplates complete harmony and unity of action, now, therefore, be it resolved that each of the several organizations here represented, to wit: the State Board of Health, the Advisory Committee, and the Minnesota Public Health Association pledge ourselves, severally and individually, the organization we represent, and the employees of the several organizations, to continue the harmonious beginning so auspiciously inaugurated, and go before the public with a united front to get the needed results in all public health efforts, and that any differences of policy be settled by a joint meeting of these three organizations." [23]

A joint committee meeting was held a few days later, and a ten-point program was agreed upon for the handling of tuberculous cases. The state board was given a share of the work and was made to feel that it had much to offer in the control of tuberculosis. Smith summed up the situation in a letter to a friend: "The Advisory Committee entirely repudiated the contract it had with the Red Cross, the Public Health Association reluctantly followed suit, and the State Board of Health is

[22] Division of Tuberculosis, "Quarterly Reports," June 30, 1918; Smith to Egil Boeckmann, June 29, 1918; C. L. Scofield to Smith, July 2, 1918; F. J. Bruno to Bracken, July 2, 16, 1918; Bracken to Bruno, July 5, 1918. Minnesota Department of Health, St. Paul.
[23] Joint Committee of the State Board of Health, the State Advisory Commission, and the Minnesota Public Health Association, "Minutes," July 8, 1918 (typescript), Minnesota Department of Health, St. Paul.

now engaged in the delightful occupation of showing them their contract was wrong and what they really should do." [24]

Bracken was not so encouraged. Despite this, Smith went ahead with plans for the division of tuberculosis to assume most of the duties formerly claimed by the Red Cross and the Minnesota Public Health Association. The state department was to locate, examine, classify, advise, and follow up tuberculous patients; the Minnesota Advisory Commission, through its physicians, was to give assistance; and the Minnesota Public Health Association was to visit tuberculous patients in the home. The Red Cross was to contribute whatever social service assistance was needed. This, essentially, was the plan that prevailed and that was to involve hundreds of cases. Bracken, however, still smarted, and he could not lick his wounds quietly. Unable to influence the state situation to any marked degree, he turned on the National Association for the Study and Prevention of Tuberculosis, saying to its secretary: "When you have dealings in this state you usually mess things up." The secretary's reply was to the point: "Your letter of September 16th is so deliberately offensive that I have been over my files to see if I could find any justification for it. I am glad to say that I cannot." [25]

Yet in all fairness to Bracken, it must be said that just before his resignation in July, 1919, he did attempt to co-operate harmoniously. He had taken some strenuous steps to reduce friction and to bolster up strength. His division of tuberculosis, created on April 9, 1918, demonstrated that he not only had ardently supported legislative bills, but also had called together interested persons to talk over the situation. Further, Bracken was perfectly justified in pointing out that county sanatoriums had been established at several points throughout the state during his administration. Finally, he could say honestly that no person in Minnesota had worked any harder than he had to further the welfare of the tuberculous patient.[26]

[24] Joint Committee, "Minutes," July 12, 1918, and "Proposition for an Agreement, July 14, 1918" (typescripts); Smith to David R. Lyman, July 16, 1918. Minnesota Department of Health, St. Paul.

[25] Bracken to Arthur N. Collins, July 18, 1918, and to Hatfield, September 16, 1918; Hatfield to Bracken, September 21, 1918; McDaniel to Smith, August 2, 1918; Committee of Four, "Suggestions of Dr. Smith, July 27, 1918" (typescript); Division of Tuberculosis, "Memorandum, July 29, 1918" (typescript); Charles E. Smith, "Memorandum," August 8, 1918. Minnesota Department of Health, St. Paul.

[26] Secretary, Antituberculosis Committee, "Report," April–May, 1918 (typescript), Minnesota Department of Health, St. Paul; Division of Tuberculosis, "Quarterly Reports," June 30, 1918; Bracken, "What Can Be Done for the Tuberculous in Their Homes," a paper read at the Minnesota State Conference of Charities and Corrections, Faribault, November 18, 1904; "The Present Status of the Tuberculosis Problem in Minnesota," a paper read before the Southern Minnesota Medical Association, Mankato, December 1, 1915; "The Tuberculosis Problem in Minnesota," in the *Journal-Lancet*, 37: 664–670 (October 15, 1917).

Despite all the adverse criticism, the state department had not been inactive. Free sputum examinations had been begun in 1894; in 1906 reports of cases were required by board regulations; in 1911 epidemiological investigations of tuberculosis were made routine; and in 1912 a tuberculosis survey had been undertaken. Two early reports had summarized the results of studies of the spread of tuberculosis in Minnesota families. Community control of the white plague had become a project which thousands of citizens had endorsed. Elaborate educational campaigns had fastened firmly in the public mind the fact that tuberculosis no longer was a disease that had to be endured. By 1911 most of the state's large cities and many smaller communities sponsored antituberculosis tag days. St. Paul in 1911 gave each donor a tag and an attractive pamphlet telling what the city was accomplishing and listing such pithy sayings as these: "So long as people expectorate in public places you may expect a rate from consumption"; "Consumption is a dirty-air disease. Pure air and sunshine are its worst enemies"; "To treat tuberculosis without a sanatorium for the advanced case is but continuing to care for the patients which a state manufactures by its neglect of an important preventive measure." In rural areas teachers were asked to help the sale of seals, and they participated in the sale for the first time in 1915. Seven thousand teachers raised about four thousand dollars. And in 1916 thirty-eight communities were employing visiting nurses during the school term, at least. Minneapolis had five full-time nurses for tuberculosis work, St. Paul seven, and Duluth three.[27]

The tuberculosis nurse taught the causes and symptoms of the disease and instructed both children and adults in personal cleanliness, stressing the importance of washing the hands and caring for the teeth. She impressed families with the necessity for clean, light, well-aired homes. Closely allied with the visiting nurse program were the county public health associations. These flourishing organizations, including the St. Louis County Public Health Association and the Tuberculosis Association of Hennepin County, attempted to search out in every

[27] Herbert G. Lampson, *A Study on the Spread of Tuberculosis in Families* (University of Minnesota, *Studies in Public Health—Bulletin* 1, December, 1913); Lampson, *The Spread of Tuberculosis: Report on the Spread of Infection in Certain Tuberculous Families in Five Counties in Minnesota* (*Reprint* 249 from United States Public Health Service, *Public Health Reports* — Washington, D.C., 1915); A. T. Laird, "Community Control of Tuberculosis," in *St. Paul Medical Journal*, 17:726–738 (November, 1915); St. Paul Anti-Tuberculosis Committee, *Anti-Tuberculosis Tag Day* (St. Paul, October 10, 1911); "The Seal Campaign," in Minnesota Public Health Association, *Journal*, 1:10 (July, 1916).

community each case of tuberculosis and see that it was properly cared for. They sponsored educational campaigns, demonstrated to employers the economic value of having employees examined periodically, taught parents and school boards the importance of having children examined annually, and saw that provision was made in sanatoriums for patients with active cases. When the patient was discharged, county associations followed up. Finally, they attempted to readjust the ex-patient to society and to his former life and vocation.[28]

The thirty-year period from Bracken's resignation until 1949 witnessed a steadily increased interest in tuberculosis and a gradual decrease in the number of cases reported in Minnesota. At a meeting of the Minnesota Sanitarium Association in 1924 the public health nurse was told that she should have training in a hospital affiliated with a sanatorium. She learned also that the general nurse frequently could spot possible cases of tuberculosis and that her influence in urging sanatorium care was great. In 1924 public health nurses made 1,622 tuberculosis visits in the state. The nurse who gave all her time to the tuberculosis problem was a specialist of high degree, who not only possessed a knowledge of general nursing but also was acquainted with home supervision, school contacts, treatment, and aseptic technique. Many of these girls, especially those working among the Indians, had colorful and unusual experiences. After speaking of tuberculosis among the Chippewa, Adelia Eggestine said a nurse must be prepared and willing to be "in turn a seamstress, scrub-woman, wash-woman, dietitian, sanitarian, home-demonstrator, gardener, welfare worker, mechanic; for she must be ready to do that which she finds at hand to do, and thus show how to do these things in order to demonstrate the results of cleanliness and proper care and thus win her way for further health work." [29]

Even with educational campaigns, tag days, county associations, and nurses, tuberculosis was a hard disease to conquer. There were 4,259 cases and 2,388 deaths reported in 1914; 4,841 cases and 2,157 deaths in 1920; 3,305 cases and 1,248 deaths in 1930; and 3,375 cases and 912 deaths in 1937. In 1945 deaths had dropped to 627, which is a rate of

---

[28] "The Tuberculosis Nurse" and "County Public Health Associations Combat Tuberculosis," in Minnesota Public Health Association, *Journal*, 4:443, 472, 478, (March 25, April 8, 1920); Kathryne R. Pearce, *Rehabilitating the Tuberculous in Hennepin County* (New York, 1942).
[29] State Board of Health, *News Letter*, nos. 7, 21; 5:[7] (July, 1923, May–June, 1925, August, 1928); Fannie Eshelman, "Tuberculosis Nursing in a Public Health Program," in *Minnesota Registered Nurse*, vol. 10, no. 12, pp. 6–8 (December, 1937).

25.1 per 100,000 population. In 1910 the rate had been 109.4 per 100,000 population.[30]

Undoubtedly the drop in the death rate was due in part to the establishment of sanatoriums. By 1946 one state sanatorium and fourteen county sanatoriums, with a total of about two thousand beds, were caring for the tuberculous. In addition, the United States Veterans Hospital in Minneapolis had one hundred and eighty-nine beds for the tuberculous from North and South Dakota, northern Iowa, and western Wisconsin, as well as Minnesota. The state sanatorium at Ah-Gwah-Ching, near Walker, had been opened on December 27, 1907, and the first county sanatorium, sponsored by St. Louis County, had been opened on May 22, 1912.[31]

Dr. Walter J. Marcley, superintendent at Ah-Gwah-Ching, wrote in the sanatorium's first report that two patients were admitted on the opening day. Seven months later 126 had entered. He told, too, of the beginnings of a library, noting that the State Library Commission and women's clubs of St. Paul and Minneapolis had donated light novels. Although regular religious services had not yet been established, both Protestant and Catholic had been given opportunity to worship. Marcley also mentioned a one-acre garden and spoke of the necessity for supplying patients with an "abundant daily supply of good fresh milk and eggs." The difficulties he mentioned were those due largely to the institution's remote location. He found it hard to secure supplies and domestic servants. But the establishment of a post office and a better delivery system, he added, "have greatly reduced the necessary trips to the village, thereby saving valuable time and horse flesh."[32]

Ah-Gwah-Ching grew so rapidly that in 1920 it had a capacity of 290 patients and covered 661 acres. The one-acre garden that Marcley mentioned thirteen years earlier had increased to sixty acres under cultivation. During 1919 routine X-ray examinations for the first time were made on every new case, heliotherapy was introduced, and occupational therapy became a part of the regular program. The pitiful library of 1907 had grown to 1,330 volumes. The labor question continued to be the greatest problem. During the autumn of 1913 patients began publishing the *Pine Knot*, a monthly journal in which they re-

[30] State Board of Health, *Reports*, 1922–43, p. 218; Division of Preventable Diseases, "Tuberculosis Deaths and Death Rates per 100,000 Population," mimeographed report issued March 15, 1946.
[31] State Board of Health, *Reports*, 1922–43, p. 108.
[32] State Board of Control, *Biennial Reports*, 1908–09, p. 300. This report contains contemporary photographs.

THE WHITE PLAGUE   281

corded their experiences, submitted questions for answer by physicians, and printed jokes and verse pertaining to their lot:

> At the san we spend our days,
> Fighting bugs with furious rays.
> Off we march to meet our foe,
> Peace may come and pain must go.
> Under these Minnesota skies
> We eat our beef and pies,
> Breathing the air so fresh and pure,
> Giving our lungs a right good cure.

Ching-Sing and *The Moccasin* succeeded the *Pine Knot* and first were published in March and April, 1938. "Considered as a group," said the editor of *Ching-Sing*, "we are more various and more mature than, for example, a student body. Our magazine should present us as such. We have common problems and a wide field of interests which should provide many subjects for serious discussion. Do not hesitate [to contribute] because you 'don't know a lot of big words.' Good logic is more important than good grammar." In 1946 the state sanatorium had 235 beds for non-Indians and 115 beds for Indians.[33]

Minnesota's fourteen county sanatoriums served the same purpose for smaller political jurisdictions that the institution at Walker did for the state. Although Ah-Gwah-Ching was supervised by the State Board of Control, county sanatoriums originally were under the authority of the Advisory Commission. These county institutions were located as follows: Nopeming Sanatorium at Nopeming; Otter Tail County Sanatorium at Battle Lake; Ramsey County Tuberculosis Pavilion at St. Paul; Mineral Springs Sanatorium at Cannon Falls; Glen Lake Sanatorium at Oak Terrace; Sunnyrest Sanatorium at Crookston; Lake Julia Sanatorium at Puposky; Sand Beach Sanatorium at Lake Park; Buena Vista Sanatorium at Wabasha; Riverside Sanatorium at Granite Falls; Southwestern Minnesota Sanatorium at Worthington; Oakland Park Sanatorium at Thief River Falls; Fair Oaks Lodge Sanatorium at Wadena; and Deerwood Sanatorium at Deerwood.[34]

The extent to which a county sanatorium might grow is clearly revealed by the development of Glen Lake, Hennepin County's institution. It had been in operation for fifteen years in 1931, the year it made its first printed report. The institution opened with a capacity for fifty

[33] State Board of Control, *Biennial Reports*, 1919–20, pp. 75–77; *Pine Knot*, vol. 1, no. 7, pp. 2, 3 (March, 1914); *Ching-Sing*, 1:1 (March, 1938).
[34] Advisory Commission, Minnesota Sanatorium for Consumptives, *Reports*, 1901–24, p. 16. This report contains a brief history of each sanatorium, together with financial details and photographs.

patients on January 4, 1916, and it grew so rapidly that it could care for five hundred in 1925. But the hospital that year was so crowded that it leased beds in private hospitals, and the capacity of the sanatorium itself was increased to seven hundred by converting some porches into wards and placing three patients in rooms designed for two. By 1934 the demand for sanatorium facilities had decreased so much that it was possible to transfer to Glen Lake all tuberculous patients maintained in private hospitals. In 1941 the hospital had vacancies both in the Infirmary Building and in the Christian Memorial Children's Sanatorium. The decline continued into 1943, when it was possible to use a part of the Children's Hospital for the treatment of rheumatic fever. In addition to its medical, surgical, vocational, and educational duties, the staff of Glen Lake has been noted for its extensive research and publication.[35]

Another institution dedicated to the control and treatment of the white plague was the Lymanhurst School for Tuberculous Children. This Minneapolis haven resulted from a gift of property made in 1912. The school was opened officially on May 31, 1921, and was composed of a small hospital section where children ill with tuberculosis could be treated by strict bed rest and other indicated procedures, and a day school where tuberculous children who were thought not to need bed rest could be taught as in a regular school and could be provided with special food and rest periods. The institution was a success immediately. Eight hundred and sixty-one outpatients were examined in 1925, and 1,541 a few years later. The little tots arrived at the school in the morning at 8:30. Fifteen minutes later they were served cooked cereal with whole milk and sugar. Instruction began at 9:00 and continued until 10:45, when pupils played light games. Further study took up the time until 12:30, when dinner with a caloric value of from 1200 to

[35] Sanatorium Commission of Hennepin County, *Annual Reports of Glen Lake Sanatorium*, 1931; 1937; 1940–41, p. 8; 1942–43, p. 4. Among the articles published by staff members are F. W. Wittich and Ernest S. Mariette, "Artificial Pneumonthorax — A Demonstration," in *Journal-Lancet*, 38:252–254 (May 1, 1918); R. W. Morse, "X-Ray in Tuberculosis," in *Journal-Lancet*, 42:110–112 (March 1, 1922); Mariette, "Localized Rest in the Treatment of Pulmonary Tuberculosis," in *American Review of Tuberculosis*, 11:27–38 (March, 1925); Mariette, "Glen Lake Sanatorium — Its Growth and Development," a paper read before the Hennepin County Medical Society on June 8, 1925; Mariette, "How Sanatorium Patients Are Admitted and Their Daily Schedule," in *Modern Hospital*, 28:70–74 (May, 1927); Mary Lydia Rowe and Mariette, "Occupational Therapy at Glen Lake Sanatorium," in *Occupational Therapy and Rehabilitation*, 7:229–243 (August, 1928); D. R. Hastings, "The Home Treatment of the Tuberculous Patient," in *Journal-Lancet*, 51:638–640 (October 15, 1931); and Hastings, "The Examination of the School-Child for Tuberculosis in a Rural Community," in *American Review of Tuberculosis*, 28:516–521 (October, 1933).

1500 was served. The afternoon was devoted to rest and further instruction. The day closed at 3:15.[36]

Many sanatoriums saw their populations decrease during the early 1940s. This had been expected by health authorities. Indeed, some county sanatoriums had been constructed as temporary rather than permanent institutions. The thought was that when the campaign on tuberculosis finally was concluded, there would be insufficient cases to justify further maintenance of county sanatoriums. Suddenly, however, all this changed, and once again sanatoriums not only were full but even had long waiting lists.

One reason for this was a change in attitude concerning the functions of a sanatorium. As Dr. L. J. Webster, superintendent of the Otter Tail County institution, said, "a sanatorium is not only a hospital for the care of a limited number of patients, but it should be an institution whose function is the control of tuberculosis in the area which it serves." With this in mind an extensive field investigation was begun in Otter Tail County. Results showed 698 family groups having a history of familial exposure to one or more cases of tuberculosis still residing in the areas reported upon. These groups numbered 3,867 individuals. All, with the exception of those with a previously positive reaction to a Mantoux test, were requested to attend the nearest Mantoux clinic. More than 1,500 took advantage of this invitation, and of these 765 had positive reactions. Supposedly healthy persons, as a result, were found to require sanatorium care.[37]

Health officers wondered whether or not additional surveys on an extensive scale would reveal similar conditions. St. Louis and Hennepin counties made some of these pioneer surveys. During the autumn of 1946 the state health department made a survey of South St. Paul, using a portable X-ray unit. Later the unit moved to St. Paul Park and Cottage Grove. About the same time the department ordered three mobile units. These X-ray services were free to all, and an attempt was made to popularize the project. "It is highly desirable that everyone in a community should take advantage of the opportunity to have a free chest x-ray," said Dr. Hilbert Mark, state tuberculosis control officer. "Many people have tuberculosis in the early stages, without any symptoms whatsoever. These concealed carriers can pass on the disease to

[36] Minneapolis Department of Public Welfare, *First Lymanhurst Report, 1921–23;* Jay Arthur Myers, *The Evolution of Tuberculosis as Observed during Twenty Years at Lymanhurst, 1921 to 1941,* ([Minneapolis?], 1944); Myers and F. E. Harrington, *Lymanhurst,* 64 (Minneapolis, 1932).
[37] L. J. Webster, "Preliminary Report of the Special Otter Tail County Tuberculosis Survey," in *Minnesota Medicine,* 24:145 (March, 1941).

others by common use of towels or dishes, by kissing, or even by talking, if close enough. The only way to find early tuberculosis is by x-raying people who are apparently healthy. The earlier a case of tuberculosis is detected, the greater is the possibility of a complete cure for the patient and the less chance there is for the infection to spread through a community." [38]

By the close of April, 1947, when two mobile units were in the field, Mark estimated that some forty-five thousand Minnesotans had had their chests X-rayed. In May three trailer and eight portable units set out to make a survey of the entire population of Minneapolis. The United States Public Health Service, the Minnesota Department of Health, the Hennepin County Medical Society, the Hennepin County Tuberculosis Association, and the Minneapolis Department of Health co-operated in this mass undertaking. The Ramsey County Public Health Association meanwhile had purchased a unit from funds acquired from the sale of Christmas Seals and turned over by the Ramsey County Welfare Board. Another unit was presented to Ancker Hospital in St. Paul. In April, 1947, when some eighteen thousand small X-ray pictures had been taken in St. Paul, results definitely indicated tuberculosis in about one-half of one per cent of persons X-rayed, while approximately six per cent had conditions that made it advisable for them to consult a physician.[39]

Indians on the Red Lake Reservation had been surveyed in 1946. Tuberculosis was found in four and one-tenth per cent of those examined, but generally the disease was in its early or minimal stages. All through 1946 and 1947 mobile units moved from county to county, stopping in public squares, parking under trees on shaded campuses, and pulling up before factories and office buildings. By January, 1948, ten county surveys had been completed, and a total of 214,326 persons had been examined, exclusive of those included in the Minneapolis, St. Paul, and St. Louis County surveys. One mobile unit devoted its entire time to state institutions. The program was expected to continue into 1950.[40]

The fact that having a chest X-ray was becoming "the thing to do" greatly eased the work of examiners. When Minnesotans learned that an X-ray was free, that they did not need to remove their clothing,

[38] *Minnesota's Health*, vol. 1, no. 1, p. 1 (January, 1947).
[39] *Minnesota's Health*, vol. 1, no. 4, p. 2 (April, 1947); Elizabeth A. Leggett, "The Out-patient Service for Tuberculous Indians in Minnesota," in *Journal-Lancet*, 73: 127–129, 154 (April, 1953).
[40] *Minnesota's Health*, vol. 2, no. 1, p. 2 (January, 1948).

that it took only a few minutes of time, and that everyone was doing it, they flocked to the doors of mobile units. Undoubtedly, too, a clearly written pamphlet distributed by health agencies was of great educational value. The citizen could not fail to be impressed when he learned, for example, that an estimated five hundred thousand persons in the United States were ill with tuberculosis, that three hundred thousand were under the care of physicians, and that tuberculosis causes more deaths than any other disease in persons between the ages of fifteen and forty-five years. On the other hand, he was relieved to know that tuberculosis is not inherited.[41]

Mass surveys, of course, were of little value without adequate follow-up procedure. Pulmonary findings from forty thousand consecutive survey films showed that seven-tenths per cent indicated a cardiac pathology and that two and two-tenths per cent revealed significant chest lesions. It was essential, therefore, that the sick patient be urged to go to his physician for treatment. Not until every abnormal case received clinical evaluation by the private physician could the mass surveys be said to have achieved their complete goal. Such a clinical evaluation should include a definite diagnosis and determine whether the disease is communicable; should indicate the extent of the disease and determine whether it is acute or chronic; should make a prognosis and determine therapeutic procedure; and should determine whether the tuberculosis patient requires hospital or sanatorium care or should continue under local medical supervision.[42]

[41] Lillian L. Biester and Hermina A. Hartig, *How Do Miniature X-Ray Surveys Help in the Control of Tuberculosis?*, 6 ([Minneapolis], 1946).
[42] Hilbert Mark, *Mass Chest X-Ray Surveys, Follow-Up Procedure*, 3 (reprinted from Kansas Medical Society, *Journal* — October, 1947); Mark, "Follow-up of Abnormal Pulmonary Findings Observed in Mass Chest X-Ray Surveys," in *Minnesota Medicine*, 30:1251 (December, 1947).

15

Streams That Run Filth

WITHIN sight of the pleasant village of Farmington, the Vermillion River runs placidly through rich agricultural country. At Northfield, home of two colleges, the Cannon River offers brief glimpses of shaded pools and moss-covered rocks. Years ago, when Minnesota was a little-populated, pioneer state, both the Vermillion and the Cannon were the delight of anglers. Their clear, fresh waters yielded abundant catches. Today, like many other streams in the state, these rivers are no more than open sewers.[1] The change from clean to polluted water is another chapter in the distressing tale of man's spoliation of natural resources. It is also a chapter in the long story of the attempt to preserve the public's health.

Hewitt had not been secretary of the state board long before he realized that Minnesota's natural water supply was a state treasure which must be protected against pollution. As early as 1874 he spoke of "natural and artificial" impurities and suggested that an extensive investigation be made of the population's water supplies. In his fourth annual report he published a lengthy discussion, in which he said that the waters "of our larger rivers, the Minnesota and Mississippi, if filtered, are good drinking waters." In 1877 a sanitary water survey of the state was completed. The next two years saw Hewitt become increasingly worried about river pollution. Of course, in those early days, stream pollution was caused primarily by drainage from hamlets and farms along rivers and not by waste from industrial plants and canning factories. And Hewitt was worried chiefly about the pollution of drinking water and not about damage to cattle or fish or natural environment. His major concern was with contamination of wells and creeks

---

[1] Neither Farmington nor Northfield have sewage treatment plants. On July 7, 1948, the author saw human excreta pour into both the Vermillion and the Cannon rivers.

from privies and cesspools. Not until the 1940s did the state health department undertake a well-financed, thoroughly modern attack upon rivers that run filth.[2]

Minnesota, of course, is a unique water state. Not only does it have over eleven thousand charted lakes and over twenty-five thousand miles of streams and rivers, but it also contains the headwaters of three great drainage systems: the Mississippi flowing south to the Gulf of Mexico, the St. Louis and Lake Superior flowing east to the Gulf of St. Lawrence, and the Red River of the North flowing to Hudson Bay. Hewitt recognized this, although he classified the state's waters a little differently. Until 1885 no state agency had been given supervision of this vast water supply in order to prevent its pollution. In that year, as a result in part of public clamor and in part of Hewitt's efforts, the legislature passed a bill to prevent the pollution of rivers and sources of water supply. "The state board of health," said the second section of the act, "shall have the general supervision of all springs, wells, ponds, lakes, streams or rivers used by any town, village or city as a source of water supply, with reference to their purity, together with the waters feeding the same, and shall examine the same from time to time, and inquire what, if any, pollution exist, and their causes." [3]

The passage of this bill had not been easy to secure. Indeed, the first time it was introduced it was not acted upon by the Senate, although it passed the House. Perhaps legislators could not see the necessity for the type of precaution that Hewitt urged, although he pointed out that other states, like Massachusetts, had waited too long before enacting pollution-control legislation. Before he submitted the bill a second time, Hewitt said firmly: "Now there is no such pollution which may not be easily dealt with in the interests of public health and without injury to vested interests; but it cannot be long before large amounts of capital will be invested in the class of manufactories alluded to and their methods of work be so firmly established that necessary change will involve great temporary pecuniary loss, and so create an opposition to change, which, as in Massachusetts, may involve long litigation and public expense." [4]

Minnesota's act was challenged, although not seriously, when the

[2] State Board of Health, *Annual Reports*, 1875, p. 7; 1876, pp. 27–39; 1878, pp. 57–64; 1879, p. 11. See chapter 7, above, for details of the fight to secure clean municipal water, and P. W. Riedesel, "The Water Pollution Menace," in the *Conservation Volunteer*, vol. 6, no. 35, pp. 11–14 (August, 1943).
[3] Hewitt, *Minnesota from the Standpoint of Public Health*, 3–5 (St. Paul, 1885); *Laws*, 1885, pp. 296–298.
[4] State Board of Health, *Biennial Reports*, 1883–84, p. 15.

hospital for the insane at Rochester objected to action by the local health department. Briefly, local officials charged that hospital sewage was emptied without treatment into Silver Creek, thus creating a nuisance. The matter was referred to the state board, which acted under the terms of the antipollution act. The board assumed that it had complete jurisdiction in the matter and, on July 14, 1888, ordered the hospital to abate the nuisance "by the removal of all refuse from said creek, deposited there in said sewage and that no more sewage be poured into said stream." As a result, conditions improved.[5]

In general, both township and village boards renewed their efforts to prevent the fouling of streams, and Hewitt felt that the public was paying more and more attention to pure water supplies. In 1887 he said that the growth of Minnesota industry was constantly threatening to increase stream pollution. His annual May sanitary inspection reports were filled with references to pollution, and local newspapers religiously reported nuisances that the May inspection uncovered. In St. Paul, for example, pools along the levee drained the wrong way, and contaminated material flowed back into the city. Most local health officers, however, concerned themselves more with privies, with the large number of unburied dead animals, or with the prevalence of manure piles than they did with stream pollution. Few inspectors were as competent as Dr. J. L. Adams of Morgan, who took extreme pains to describe the location of his village and to discuss its water supply.[6]

The great difficulty impeding antipollution progress, of course, was the fact that the legislative act of 1885 had appropriated no funds to carry out a program of safeguards. Then, too, Hewitt had no clear conception of what an extensive antipollution program would entail nor how it would involve not only other states, but also the Dominion of Canada. Bracken was in a similar situation. He fully understood that lakes and rivers should not be contaminated, he fought vigorously for clean municipal water, and he was most anxious to do something for the state as a whole; but he, too, was hampered by lack of funds and of engineering and technological data. Yet Bracken, like Hewitt, did his best. Local water nuisances were abated, urban water ordinances

[5] State Board of Health, *Biennial Reports*, 1886–88, p. 51.
[6] *Public Health in Minnesota*, 2:18 (May, 1886); 2:99 (January, 1887); 3:25 (May, 1887); *Pioneer Press*, June 8, 1877; letters to Hewitt from F. L. Puffer, June 5, 1892, from W. W. Freeman, May [?], 1894, from R. F. Lynch, April 5, 1894, from Frederick J. Bohland, June 1, 1896, from C. E. Hillstrom, May 4, 20, 1893, from A. J. Carpenter, May 28, 1893, from S. F. Sawyer, May 25, 1893, from F. A. Blackmer, July 15, 1896, and from J. L. Adams, May 25, 1893, Minnesota Department of Health, St. Paul.

were supported, and innumerable water analyses were made in the department's laboratory.[7]

In 1900 an extensive survey to determine the natural chlorides in Minnesota water and to gather data for an isochlor map was completed. Important as this survey was in determining chemical properties, it was even more significant from the viewpoint of pollution control. After five months in the field the chemist saw the futility of attempting to improve water conditions without additional legislation. He recommended legislation covering the following:[8]

1. Whenever a public or private water or ice supply is condemned by the state board of health, that said supply be closed at the discretion of the state board.

2. That all municipalities of the state be privileged and required to consult the state board of health as to the sanitary aspects of the location, environment and chemical analysis, of any or all, new or contemplated, sources of public water or ice supply.

3. That the enforcement of the above provisions be secured by a fine.

These suggestions revealed another weakness in the act of 1885. That law had given the state board no authority to make regulations regarding the pollution of public waters. By that time, too, Bracken himself had seen one example of pollution after another arise to vex him. On July 16, 1902, the board issued to all interested persons a circular letter calling attention to the act of 1885 and advising that towns installing new water plants or sewerage systems, or repairing old ones, consult the health department for sanitary advice. At the same time Rome G. Brown, a Minneapolis attorney, furnished Bracken with a historical summary of the law relating to pollution of waters of lakes and rivers. A large number of cases cited in Brown's report referred specifically to pollution by manufacturing plants and mining camps, to discharge of sewage by cities and individuals, and to riparian rights. Between 1900 and 1905 increased attention to pollution regulations had been paid by states, boards of health, and individuals. Minnesota's progress was slower than that of some other states.[9]

Bedeviled by increasing complaints of water pollution by waste from a starch factory at Harris and a beet-sugar factory at St. Louis Park and by dead fish cast upon the shore at Waterville, and knowing that other states had strengthened their legislation, Bracken made plans to

[7] State Board of Health, *Biennial Reports,* 1895–96, pp. 12, 44; 1897–98, pp. 55, 65, 73, 129, 137, 142, 154.
[8] State Board of Health, *Biennial Reports,* 1899–1900, p. 262.
[9] State Board of Health, *Biennial Reports,* 1901–02, pp. 236–266.

approach the Minnesota legislature. To help the antipollution cause, the board on July 9, 1902, passed three resolutions. The first provided that all villages, cities, and public institutions must submit to the board all plans for new water plants and must indicate the source from which water was to be drawn. The second stipulated the same supervision for sewerage systems. The third called upon the State Board of Control to abate a nuisance created by the discharge of sewage from the Anoka State Hospital upon the low ground adjoining the Rum River above Anoka. A large number of cases of typhoid fever in Duluth and throughout the state about the same time made it possible for the board to act a little more drastically than it otherwise might have done.[10]

There was little difficulty, therefore, in persuading the legislature in 1905, after recommendations by a law revision committee, to give the board of health authority to regulate the pollution of rivers and sources of public water supply. In addition to this, a new legislative provision read as follows: "Said board shall advise with the authorities of villages and cities concerning their water supply, and no municipality shall furnish its inhabitants with water for domestic use from a source or in a manner forbidden by such board after a full investigation, upon notice and hearing pursuant to rules by it prescribed." [11]

The cumulative effect, then, of legislative acts from 1885 to 1905 was to recognize the pollution problem, to place control of public waters in the state health department, and to protect citizens from contaminated water. In Hewitt's time the primary interest was surface water supplies. After 1905 the emphasis was definitely on all state waters. Bracken recognized this and acted accordingly. He knew, for example, that Lake Superior was being polluted by Duluth sewage. He also was aware of the increasing contamination of the Rum and Mississippi rivers.[12]

An early hearing on the pollution of these rivers was held by the state board on March 19, 1912. One of the first comments made indicated that the board was acting under authority granted by the *Revised Laws* of 1905. Testimony offered by Dr. J. F. Corbett, Minneapolis city bacteriologist, showed that he had "found evidence of three

[10] State Board of Health, *Biennial Reports*, 1901–02, pp. 145, 266–270, 317, 318.
[11] *Revised Laws*, 1905, chapter 29. For a history of the committee on revision, see *Index to Revised Laws*, 1905, pp. 3–6. In reality, the law of 1905 carried on the spirit and implied powers of the act of 1885. See also *Statutes*, 1894, p. 120, and *Revised Laws*, 1905, p. 399.
[12] Tuohy to Wesbrook, October 20, 1910; State Board of Health, "Hearing on the Question of the Pollution of the Waters of the Rum and Mississippi Rivers, March 19, 1912" (typescript). Minnesota Department of Health, Minneapolis.

sewers emptying into the Rum River" and that he had been informed of "a number of other sewers from the private houses entering into the Rum River." When pressed as to whether or not he had found bacilli, Corbett answered that colon bacilli were present in varying amounts in the Rum River below the Anoka State Hospital, at the pumping station, below all the sewers, and near the bridge. He testified further that he had undisputed clinical evidence that the raw waters of the Mississippi River contained typhoid bacilli.[13]

Although this first hearing was largely exploratory, it did establish a precedent and it helped pave the way for later extensive surveys of Minnesota waters. Each successive year saw the state health department edge closer to comprehensive investigations. In 1911, for example, public water supplies were examined thoroughly, and in 1917 Whittaker wrote that the public "is now displaying a rapidly growing interest in the improvement of the water supplies of the state as is demonstrated by the large number of requests for investigations on this subject." [14]

It was not until 1919, however, that a small-scale survey of the Mississippi was begun. This survey really was prompted by Professor E. B. Phelps of the United States Public Health Service, who in 1918 recommended that a study be made of the Mississippi with reference to its pollution and its capacity for receiving and disposing of sewage without nuisance. On January 22, 1919, Bracken requested the United States Public Health Service to furnish technical assistance. This was done, and a sanitary engineer was ordered to Minnesota to consult with the health department. The engineer and the department decided to limit activities to two problems: (1) a general study of the river within the boundaries of Minnesota to determine the important factors contributing to its pollution and their effect on the stream, and (2) an intensive study of the Mississippi between the Washington Avenue Bridge in Minneapolis and the Government High Dam.[15]

The engineer also advocated four lines of investigation:

1. The initial establishment of three points of observation in the river; one above Minneapolis, a second opposite the proposed boathouse of the University of Minnesota and a third at a point immediately above the dam. If it should prove desirable, intermediate points should be located later.

2. A systematic examination of both river water and bottom sediment at each of the three above points, at intervals not greater than

[13] State Board of Health, "Hearing on the Pollution of the Rum and Mississippi Rivers," 4, 7.
[14] State Board of Health, *Biennial Reports*, 1909–10, pp. 263–265; 1916–17, p. 364.
[15] Division of Sanitation, "Quarterly Reports," June 30, September 30, 1919.

once each week, throughout the coming autumn, winter and spring seasons, excepting at such times during which the river may be sufficiently closed with ice to render the collection of samples extremely difficult.

3. A measure of mean and bottom velocities of flow of the river in various portions of the pool during high and low stage conditions and the determination of the discharge of the river at times of sample collections.

4. The determination, by means of soundings, of the thickness of the sludge mat deposited at certain fixed points in the pool at various times, particularly at the observation point opposite the proposed University boathouse. These observations should be for the purpose of determining whether there is a progressive accumulation of sewage sludge in the channel bottom throughout a fairly long period and to what extent the natural scouring of the channel during the high water flows removes such deposits.[16]

Other suggestions included inventories of waste-producing agencies and the character of the raw water and the final effluent of water purification plants within the state. Analytical determinations of water samples were to include temperature, turbidity, color, odor, dissolved oxygen, oxygen demand, bacterial count on agar, and bacillus coli determinations. This program was carried out in part.[17]

Although little new legislation was passed between 1919 and 1927, pollution control moved forward steadily. In 1925, for example, a legislative joint interim committee of three was appointed to investigate the pollution of boundary waters between Minnesota and Wisconsin. Among the problems investigated was that of Minnesota municipalities which discharged sewage into the Mississippi. The interim committee was assisted by representatives of the state health departments of Minnesota and Wisconsin and by an engineer from the United States Public Health Service. Between 1925 and 1927 public opinion clamored for antipollution action, and state and local boards of health gave increased emphasis to the problem. In October, 1925, thirty-five representatives of legislatures, state executive departments, health, conservation, fish and game commissions, and members of the Izaak Walton League attended an antipollution conference at Red Wing.[18]

[16] H. W. Streeter to the Surgeon General, United States Public Health Service, July 21, 1919, Minnesota Department of Health, Minneapolis. The proposed boathouse site was the flats on the east river bank below the Washington Avenue Bridge.
[17] United States Public Health Service, "Program for Sanitary Survey of the Mississippi River, 1919" (typescript), Minnesota Department of Health, Minneapolis; State Board of Health, *Biennial Reports*, 1918–19, p. 95.
[18] *House Journal*, 1925, pp. 1545, 1632; *Senate Journal*, 1925, p. 748; *Pioneer Press*, August 3, 1925; *Minneapolis Tribune*, September 6, 1925; *Minnesota Daily* (Minneapolis), December 9, 1925; *Journal* (Minneapolis), October 25, 1925;

About a month earlier Chesley had outlined what the health department would like to have accomplished. "What we would like to see in Minnesota," he wrote, "is a comprehensive survey of lakes and streams for the purpose of deciding what bodies of water should be kept entirely free from all kinds of pollution, what ones might receive certain types of waste and what ones might receive all kinds of waste. At present there are only a few plants with offensive or dangerous trade wastes discharged into lakes or streams of large size. But there are a great many creameries and cheese factories where the problem of waste disposal is a very serious one." He added that, if industries increased and if there was no supervision of disposal of sewage or trade wastes, some of the finest lakes and streams would lose their attractiveness. "All this," Chesley concluded, "will be prevented by foresight if we can only get the public to understand the necessity for such a survey. The Izaak Walton League and certain other organizations strongly favor such a survey but the legislature must be induced to appropriate funds for the work. The Game and Fish Commissioner of course is anxious to have it done. But our Division of Sanitation has only $7000 per annum for Sanitary Engineering work." [19]

Chesley was fully conscious, too, of the public health aspects of stream pollution. He knew, as did others in the field, that contaminated streams not only menaced water supplies but also threatened the health of cattle, fish, and even bathers. In 1926 it was said that practically all the free oxygen was gone from the Mississippi River at the High Dam and at Hastings, and the next year the statement was made that the fact that fish were not dying in large numbers in a particular locality was no positive evidence that Minnesota had no pollution problems.[20]

Between September, 1927, and September, 1928, the health department's division of sanitation, in co-operation with the commissioner of game and fish, made twenty-three investigations of streams. These were

Pierson to Whittaker, June 17, 1925, Whittaker to Joseph H. Masek, October 27, 1925, Chesley to the Minneapolis City Council, July 28, 1925, James A. Carley to Chesley, August 4, 1925, J. C. Vincent to N. W. Elsberg, September 16, 1925, and J. K. Hoskins, H. A. Whittaker, and C. M. Baker, "To the Members of the Interim Committees of the Minnesota and Wisconsin Legislatures, December 3, 1925" (typescript), Minnesota Department of Health, Minneapolis.
[19] Chesley to James A. Tobey, September 16, 1925, Minnesota Department of Health, Minneapolis.
[20] J. A. Childs, "The Public Health Aspect of Stream Pollution," in American Water Works Association, *Journal*, 14:578–580 (December, 1925); *Pioneer Press*, December 4, 1926; State Board of Health, "Memorandum on Biological Investigations of Lakes and Streams in Relation to Pollution, [1927]" (typescript), Minnesota Department of Health, Minneapolis.

made possible by the expenditure of approximately thirteen thousand dollars from the funds of the Department of Conservation. Chesley wrote the president of the Minneapolis chapter of the Izaak Walton League: "You ought to get a good deal of satisfaction at this time for all the things you have attempted to do have been accomplished. . . . I am sure that the State Board of Health would not have succeeded either in securing the legislation or in securing the funds to carry out the stream pollution survey." [21]

The legislation to which Chesley referred, entitled "An Act relating to the administration and enforcement of laws relating to pollution of the waters of the State of Minnesota," was approved on April 19, 1927. Consisting of seven sections, this act authorized the State Board of Health to enforce laws against pollution of waters, to investigate, to co-operate with other departments, to hold hearings, to receive money or property to further its duties, and to secure assistance from other state departments. This was a far-reaching improvement, and it enabled the board to extend its activities. But the act did not carry an appropriation with it. It did, however, focus all pollution responsibility on one agency, the health department, and sportsmen were delighted.[22]

The passage of the act of 1927 and a budget of about thirteen thousand dollars made it possible to secure additional personnel and to begin an antipollution program. Assigned to the work were Eugene W. Surber, biologist; E. G. Reinhard, associate biologist; Frank L. Woodward, associate sanitary engineer; and L. S. Farrell, assistant sanitary engineer. This staff was ready to begin work by September 26, 1928, on the first comprehensive antipollution program in Minnesota's history. Earlier investigations had been handicapped by lack of funds, authority, and trained personnel. The work proceeded along the lines indicated in a nine-point preliminary program:

1. A study of the sanitary engineering investigations and biological studies conducted by other departments on stream and lake pollution work.

2. A compilation of information on stream and lake pollutions throughout the state from existing records for use as a basis in outlining a program of surveys to be undertaken.

3. The assembling of reference books and papers on pollution in-

[21] Division of Sanitation, "Investigation of Stream and Lake Pollution, September, 1927, to September, 1928, in Cooperation with Commission of Game and Fish" (typescript), and "Quarterly Reports," September 30, 1927, Minnesota Department of Health, Minneapolis; Chesley to Judson L. Wicks, June 6, 1927, Minnesota Department of Health, St. Paul.
[22] *Laws*, 1927, p. 390; *Owatonna Journal-Chronicle*, March 4, 1927.

vestigations, and the preparation of an index covering the information that would be needed in connection with the sanitary engineering and biological studies.

4. The preparation of outline maps for field and office use, covering lakes and streams under consideration and of charts and outlines for recording field and laboratory data.

5. The preparation of small-scale plans of municipal sewage treatment plants for the use of the sanitary engineers when in the field to assist them in their observations on existing sewage treatment plants.

6. Studies to determine the best field and laboratory equipment and apparatus which might be used in the investigation work.

7. The selection and ordering of field and laboratory equipment and apparatus which would be needed for the sanitary engineering, biological, bacteriological, chemical, and biochemical studies.

8. Conferences with officials and representatives of organizations interested in the stream and lake pollution studies for the purpose of obtaining their views on certain phases of the work.

9. The coordination of the work on the pollution investigations with the administrative and technical activities of the Minnesota Department of Health.[23]

This approach, together with a proposed plan for stream and lake pollution investigations, was approved by J. F. Gould, commissioner of game and fish. Members of the Izaak Walton League's commission on pollution also endorsed the proposed investigations. Among these were surveys of the Mississippi River, of Lake Superior and the harbor adjacent to Duluth, of Detroit Lakes, and of a series of smaller bodies of water, including Chisholm Creek, Straight River, and Lakes Agnes and Minnewaska. By the close of 1928 many of the surveys were begun, although not all were completed.[24]

Preliminary work demonstrated clearly that water pollution was a vast problem, for it was tied in with innumerable specific nuisances and was associated with many of man's daily activities. For example, engineers found that pollution investigation must concern itself with water used for public consumption, with water used for commercial purposes, and with water used by the individual. It was also associated with ice supplies, both for human consumption and for refrigeration. It was

[23] Minnesota Department of Health, "Progress Report on Stream and Lake Pollution Investigations, [1927–1928]" (typescript), Minnesota Department of Health, Minneapolis.

[24] H. A. Whittaker, "Memorandum of Conference with Mr. J. F. Gould, Commissioner of Game and Fish, Relative to the Proposed Cooperative Work on Stream and Lake Pollution Studies in Minnesota, November 17, 1927" (typescript), Chairman of the Commission on Pollution, Minnesota Division, Izaak Walton League, to E. W. Backus, November 25, 1927, and State Board of Health and Commissioner of Game and Fish, "Progress Report on Stream and Lake Pollution Investigation, 1928" (typescript), Minnesota Department of Health, Minneapolis; *Journal*, December 16, 1927.

concerned with livestock, for animals drank water and there was danger of infection from animal to animal. Many forms of aquatic life depended for successful living upon safe water. Antipollution experts pointed out, too, that their surveys involved bathing, boating, fishing, and the aesthetic appearance of Minnesota's lakes and streams. But the far-reaching implications of pollution control did not stop with these factors. Control involved both hydroelectric and condensing power, and it was of significance to navigation. Impure water could be offensive both to boat crews and to passengers, and boat engineers were concerned with the type of water used in boilers. Water also influenced property values and, in some cases, involved riparian rights. Finally, of course, water was affected by domestic sewage, industrial waste, and storm and farm drainage.[25]

With this sort of a score card to check against, sanitary engineers and bacteriologists went to work. They collected data on industrial waste systems and disposal plants and, in co-operation with the State Live Stock Sanitary Board and the State Department of Agriculture, brought together statistics revealing whether or not a given stream constituted a menace to livestock. Antipollution experts attempted to secure co-operation from paper companies and steel plants. Meanwhile other specialists were dissecting fish and identifying parasites found on bass. It was not forgotten that in 1929 some 1,600,000 tourists were attracted to Minnesota by the beauty of its countryside and by their desire to fish or hunt. Polluted streams and lakes would not exert much drawing power for vacationists.[26]

By the close of 1929 pollution control was well under way. By then the departments of botany and zoology of the University of Minnesota were co-operating and the Mayo Foundation had made financially possible the creation of two fellowships in sanitary engineering. The United States Public Health Service was giving technical advice, and the Dominion of Canada, through its Ministry of Health, offered to co-operate on pollution studies undertaken on boundary waters between Minnesota and Canada. Nor was this all. Minnesota had entered into mutual-benefit agreements with other states having common pollution problems. Among them was the Great Lakes Drainage Basin Sani-

[25] State Board of Health, "Progress Report on Stream and Lake Pollution Investigations in Minnesota, [1928]," (typescript), Minnesota Department of Health, Minneapolis.
[26] Division of Sanitation, "Quarterly Reports," March 31, June 30, 1928; Minnesota Department of Health, "Special Laboratory Examinations on Fish and Game, [1928]," and Wicks to George W. McCullough, December 24, 1929, Minnesota Department of Health, Minneapolis.

tation Agreement.[27] In addition, state boards and departments of health of Iowa, Minnesota, and Wisconsin entered into a triple agreement on dairy waste disposal. The City of Duluth and the Wisconsin State Board of Health co-operated in 1929 on a pollution study of the St. Louis River, the Duluth-Superior Harbor, and that portion of Lake Superior adjacent to Duluth.

Since the passage of the act of 1927, not only had these interstate agreements been negotiated, but also the general plan for stream and lake pollution studies outlined then had been carried through. A summary of the work done reveals this clearly. During 1920, 10 streams and 16 lakes were investigated or observed, 175 sewage and industrial waste problems were investigated, and plans for 28 sewage disposal projects were examined and recommended for approval. Laboratory work included the examination of 133 biological, 687 bacteriological, 302 chemical, and 249 biochemical samples of water, sewage, and industrial waste. An extensive special report was made also on Minnesota sewage treatment plants. Of the 111 municipal and large institutional sewage treatment plants in the state, the survey showed that 86 provided for preliminary treatment consisting of sedimentation units alone and that only 25 provided for secondary treatment, including some form of oxidation such as trickling filters or activated sludge units. The investigation also revealed that "municipal officials and plant operators had practically no conception of the processes that were taking place in their plants, what results to expect, or how to operate them." Most operators, however, expressed a desire to learn.[28]

By 1930 stream pollution control, although still inadequately financed, had met with public approval and had demonstrated its validity. Special studies, such as that on the Straight and Cannon rivers, had convinced scores of persons that these activities actually resulted in the improvement of Minnesota. Sportsmen were especially gratified when Minnesota's legal department, on December 29, 1930, said that the responsibility for taking the initiative in cases of water pollution injurious to fish life "is placed squarely upon the State Board of Health by the 1927 act, which enjoins the board to cooperate with other state departments and officers, and authorizes the board to request them to furnish funds and other assistance in carrying out the purposes of the

[27] For the text of this agreement, see State Board of Health and Commissioner of Game and Fish, "Progress Report on Stream and Lake Pollution, 1929" (typescript), Minnesota Department of Health, Minneapolis.
[28] State Board of Health and Commissioner of Game and Fish, "Report of Special Investigation of Sewage Treatment Plants in Minnesota, June 15 to September 15, 1929" (typescript), Minnesota Department of Health, Minneapolis.

act." Lovers of the out-of-doors were also pleased by mounting newspaper editorials commenting upon pollution and by articles in conservation journals.[29]

Although the legal picture of pollution control did not change from 1927 to 1945, the scope of the work was enlarged annually. The decade of the 1930s witnessed an increase in the number of investigations and a corresponding increase in biological examinations. Special studies were completed on the problem of creamery waste disposal, on institutional sewage treatment plants, and on the Minneapolis-St. Paul sewage disposal situation.[30] Whittaker, director of the division of sanitation, took a keen interest in these problems. He had represented Minnesota at the Lake Michigan Sanitation Congress in 1928, had worked to negotiate the Great Lakes Drainage Basin Sanitation Agreement, and had been a member of the Great Lakes Board of Public Health Engineers in 1929.[31] During 1930 and 1931 he supervised generally pollution studies of the upper Mississippi, although much of the work was done by Woodward. In 1933 and again in 1935 special surveys of the Mississippi were undertaken. Indeed, the Mississippi and its tributaries have been almost constantly under investigation since 1926, as have the Red River of the North and the St. Croix.[32]

[29] State Board of Health and Commissioner of Game and Fish, *Report of the Investigation of the Pollution of the Straight and Cannon Rivers*, 1928–30 (Minneapolis, [1930]); H. A. Whittaker, "The Lake and Stream Pollution Problem in Minnesota," in *Fins, Feathers and Fur*, 91:12, 21 (November, 1930); Judson E. Wicks, "Pollution: A Problem We Must Solve," in *Minnesota Conservationist*, 3:3, 16 (August, 1933); *Journal*, December 10, 1930; Chester S. Wilson to Chesley, December 10, 1927, December 29, 1930, Minnesota Department of Health, Minneapolis.

[30] Whittaker to William D. Stewart, September 16, 1932, Minnesota Department of Health, Minneapolis. On the Minneapolis-St. Paul sewage disposal situation, see chapter 8, above.

[31] Whittaker to L. S. Finch, October 14, 1929; Whittaker, "Memorandum of Attendance at Lake Michigan Sanitation Congress, Gary, Indiana, March 7 and 8, 1928," "Memo of Meeting of Great Lakes Board of Public Health Engineers, Gary, Indiana, December 11–12, 1928," and "A Brief Report of the Second Annual Meeting of the Great Lakes Board of Public Health Engineers, Cleveland, Ohio, December 9 and 10, 1929" (typescripts). Minnesota Department of Health, Minneapolis.

[32] Division of Sanitation, "Pollution Studies of the Upper Mississippi River, [1930–1931]," "Progress Memorandum on Pollution Survey of Upper Mississippi River above Minneapolis, 1930 and 1931," and "Report of Special Investigation of the Pollution of the Mississippi River, May and June, 1933" (typescripts), Minnesota Department of Health, Minneapolis; Minnesota and Wisconsin State Boards of Health and Minnesota Department of Conservation, *The Pollution of the St. Croix River from the Dam at St. Croix Falls to the Junction with the Mississippi River* (Minneapolis, 1935); Minnesota and Wisconsin State Boards of Health and Minnesota Water Pollution Control Commission, *Report of the Follow-Up Investigation of the St. Croix River from the Dam at St. Croix Falls to the Junction with the Mississippi River* (Minneapolis, 1946); E. V. Willard, "Upper Mississippi River Problems," in *Conservation Volunteer*, vol. 7, no. 38, pp. 19–24 (January–February, 1944).

STREAMS THAT RUN FILTH

Among the really intricate and vexing pollution problems that faced Whittaker and his staff was one that concerned the Rainy River, a beautiful stream running between International Falls and Wheelers Point on Lake of the Woods. This river, marking the boundary between the United States and Canada, was for years an anglers' paradise. Shortly after the act of 1927 was passed, sporting organizations and health officials began receiving complaints that the Rainy River was being contaminated by industrial waste. It was said that paper mills at International Falls and Fort Frances "have been dumping their sulphite and other waste into the Rainy River for the past twenty years." Conservation officials told Whittaker that the great spawning grounds for walleyed pike in North America at one time were in the waters of the Rainy River and suggested that this stream should be among the first to be investigated. At Baudette, a little village north of the Red Lake Indian Reservation on Rainy River, local residents complained bitterly of the stream's pollution, saying that the water tasted bad and smelled bad and that all the fish had been driven away. "We people living along the shore of Rainy River," said an irritated citizen, "have had to put up with the river being polluted, by the paper mill at International Falls, for a long time, we have from time to time taken this matter up with the State board of health, and the Game and Fish Department, but nothing was ever done about it. The river was so badly polluted this spring that not even the minnows would come into the river from the lake, and it was so bad that wall-eyed pike were driven about 45 miles away from the river, this is not guess work on my part, I have made a study of pollution, and I hope you people will investigate the thing for your own information."[33]

Shortly after the first complaints were received Harvey G. Rogers, engineer attached to the division of sanitation, was sent to Baudette "to obtain a general idea of the situation . . . in anticipation of the investigation to be made next year." Accompanied by a local individual who had made several complaints about the pollution of the Rainy, Rogers not only found "no evidence of excessive pollution at that time," but also was "unable to find any appreciable deposits of an objectionable nature" when the river bottom was stirred. Apparently a recent storm had cleared the channel of offensive waste. From local residents Rogers learned that the main damages to the Rainy were the de-

[33] A. M. Sanderson to Wicks, March 13, 1928; Thaddeus Surber to Whittaker, April 12, 1928; Joseph C. N. Rowell to the State Board of Health, June 11, 1928; Rowell to the State Conservation Commission, July 11, 1933. Minnesota Department of Health, Minneapolis.

positing of wood pulp on the river bottom in the spring, which destroyed spawning grounds; the nuisance from odors created by decomposing of wood pulp; and the prevention of proper conditions for bathing.[34]

There seemed no doubt, however, that the Rainy was being contaminated by both industrial waste and municipal sewage. With this in mind, the health department went ahead, but with extreme caution. The pollution of the Rainy River made a delicate problem. It involved two governments, the United States and Canada. It also involved several wealthy and influential American and Canadian industries. In October, 1929, a little more than a year after Rogers made his exploratory trip, Whittaker called together a few interested persons, including the chief engineer for the Department of Health of the Dominion of Canada and the director of sanitary engineering of the Ontario Department of Health. The purpose of this conference was to "discuss a general plan for organizing the co-operative program between the Canadian and Minnesota Departments of Health." The most tangible result of the meeting was an agreement to meet again the following year. It was also "suggested that the various departments might establish contact with the industries and municipalities discharging waste into the river at that time, with the view of securing their co-operation."[35]

During the next few years progress was exasperatingly slow. Tremendous amounts of industrial waste continued to pollute the Rainy, threatening fish life and decreasing landowners' sport. Yet Minnesota's health department was not inactive. Plans were made for a co-operative survey of the river with Canada in 1929, but early the following year Whittaker and the Minnesota Department of Conservation received word that the Province of Ontario could not assist because of too many projects already begun. A few days later Whittaker wrote Ontario's deputy minister of health: "Our people feel that the relationship of these studies to fish life is so important that we should have the co-operation of your Department of Marine and Fisheries when the investigation is undertaken." He then postponed the investigation until some future time. Once again one of the worst pollution problems facing Minnesota was laid aside.[36]

[34] H. G. Rogers, "Memorandum on Trip to Baudette, Minnesota, August 14 and 15, 1928," Minnesota Department of Health, Minneapolis.
[35] Whittaker, "Memorandum on Conference with Messrs. Ferguson & Berry Relative to Co-operative Studies on the Rainy River, October 3rd, 1929" (typescript), Minnesota Department of Health, Minneapolis.
[36] Whittaker to George H. Ferguson, March 2, 1920; H. H. Mackay to Surber, January 15, 1930; Chesley to John A. Amyot, January 29, 1930. Minnesota Department of Health, Minneapolis.

But the situation was not forgotten by either residents in the vicinity of the Rainy River or by the health department. Early in 1934 Whittaker again approached Ontario health officers, but first he took the matter up with Minnesota conservation officials. "If you feel that a survey should be undertaken in the near future," he wrote the commissioner of conservation, "we will communicate with the proper [Ontario] health officials and request their co-operation in this work. . . . It is our understanding that if such a cooperative investigation is made and a report prepared, the matter will then have to go before the International Joint Commission for their consideration since the Rainy River is an international boundary stream over which the Commission has jurisdiction by a treaty agreement between the United States and Canada. In other words, the information contained in the report would constitute the basis for such further action as the Commission might feel disposed to take." [37]

Being assured that the conservation department was eager for a survey, Whittaker then opened negotiations with Dr. R. E. Wodehouse, deputy minister of health for Ontario. He pointed out the problem, said that on several occasions the matter of a joint survey had been discussed, and suggested a meeting of all interested parties. About the same time Whittaker wrote the United States Public Health Service, outlining the problem and asking for support. The conservation department was stimulated by a petition signed by ninety-five members of the Lake of the Woods Sportsmen's Association, which, after recounting the injurious effects of industrial waste on marine life, requested the abatement of this nuisance and pledged the organization to assist any "practical solution of this serious problem" for the good of all.[38]

These efforts resulted in a meeting of representatives of the Department of Pensions and National Health of Canada, the United States Public Health Service, the Province of Ontario, and the State of Minnesota. When Minnesota's delegates arrived at Toronto on April 16, 1934, they found Canadian enthusiasm for the survey at low ebb and came home without completing plans for the joint investigation. About a year later, Governor Floyd B. Olson, somewhat annoyed, judging by the tone of his letter, wrote the Honorable Mitchell Hepburn, prime

[37] Chesley to E. V. Willard, January 20, 1934, Minnesota Department of Health, Minneapolis.

[38] Chesley to R. E. Wodehouse, February 27, 1934, and to H. S. Cumming, March 9, 1934; Lake of the Woods Sportsmen's Association to the Minnesota Conservation Commission, May 25, 1934 (carbon copy). Minnesota Department of Health, Minneapolis.

minister of Ontario. Olson said that when Minnesota representatives met at Toronto they were surprised to learn that no complaints had been presented to Canadian authorities relative to the alleged pollution of the Rainy River, either by riparian owners on the stream, by commercial fishing interests, by anglers, or by municipal authorities. He continued: "Observations made by the State of Minnesota in August, 1928, May, 1929, May, 1933, and May, 1934, have given evidence that the allegations are based on facts. The Minnesota Department of Conservation and the Minnesota State Board of Health are of the opinion that a thorough investigation of the Rainy River should be made in order to ascertain whether the pollution does affect public health and fish life, such investigation to include (a) a study of the sources, quantity and the pollutional characteristics of the sewage and industrial waste discharged into the streams, (b) studies of the condition of the water and the river bottom, and (c) observation on fish life, to include tests with live fish to determine the effects of pollution upon the migration of fish."[39]

Almost continuous pressure of this type finally resulted in a meeting at Detroit on June 3, 1937. Ontario agreed to co-operate, and the details of the survey were tentatively agreed upon, but not before Chesley had urged Ontario authorities to act "before something disastrous occurs" and not before he had told the United States Public Health Service that no answer had been made to Olson's letter. Chesley added, however, that correspondence with the Ontario Department of Health indicated an interest in joining in a pollution survey. This interest was made concrete in the Detroit meeting.[40]

Details of the survey were worked out early in July, 1937, at International Falls. Work on the river was divided between the Ontario and Minnesota health departments, which established a bacteriological and chemical laboratory in the high school at Baudette. A total of 1,020 water samples were collected and 903 chemical and bacteriological examinations were made during the six-weeks period of the survey. In addition, plankton and bottom samples were obtained and a thorough study was made of the sources and quantity of wastes discharged from the Minnesota and Ontario Paper Company at International Falls.[41]

[39] Olson to Mitchell Hepburn, February 1, 1935, Minnesota Department of Health, Minneapolis.
[40] Division of Sanitation, "Quarterly Reports," June 30, 1937; Chesley to J. T. Phair, February 18, 1937, and to Thomas Parran, February 18, 1937. Minnesota Department of Health, Minneapolis.
[41] Division of Sanitation, "Quarterly Reports," September 30, 1937.

The results, signed jointly by Whittaker and A. E. Berry, director of the sanitary engineering division of the Ontario Department of Health, may be summarized briefly: (1) The major sources of pollution of the river are the untreated or partially treated sewage and wastes from the municipalities located along the river and the wastes from the wood-products industries. (2) The effect of this pollution is felt throughout the entire length of the river, from Ranier to Lake of the Woods. (3) The bacterial pollution in Rainy River has increased markedly during the interval between the 1913 survey by the International Joint Commission and this survey in 1937. (4) The bacterial concentration in the river, from the dam at International Falls and Fort Frances to Lake of the Woods, now exceeds recognized standards of pollution in raw water acceptable for treatment by chlorination alone or by filtration and chlorination combined. It also creates a hazard in the use of the river as a source of ice supply. (5) The water in the river between the dam and Lake of the Woods is polluted to such an extent that it is objectionable for bathing purposes, and the bacterial concentration in the water exceeds usually accepted standards for bathing. (6) The wood-products wastes discharged at the river create extensive deposits throughout the stream and suspended material in the water; both conditions are inimical to fish and other aquatic life and interfere with the operation of waterworks systems. (7) The discharge of sewage and other wastes, particularly wood-products wastes, has resulted in extensive deposits and floating stumps and islands, which interfere with the use of the stream for recreational purposes. (8) The pollution of the stream makes the water undesirable for the use of livestock. (9) In order to correct the situation in the river it will be necessary to provide relatively complete treatment of the sewage and to bring about exclusion or a substantial reduction in the strength and amount of industrial waste.[42]

This report certainly marked a definite forward step, but it did not solve the pollution problem along the Rainy River. Another decade of slow, patient work had to pass before that was accomplished. In the first place, representatives met at Detroit on February 9, 1939, to work out the details of the final report. Then it was necessary to enlist the co-operation of the Minnesota and Ontario Paper Company. This was attempted on August 24, 1939. But representatives of Minnesota's health department were told that the company was in receivership, that plant changes were limited to necessities, and that any extensive

[42] "Rainy River Pollution Survey, 1937" (typescript), Minnesota Department of Health, Minneapolis.

program of waste elimination would be difficult to undertake. The company did say, however, that improvement was being made in reducing the quantity of waste discharged into the river and hope was held out that, after the company was relieved of receivership, something more definite might be accomplished.[43]

The situation, then, was relatively static until November, 1941, although Minnesota had continued to press the general aspects of the problem all through the preceding year. On November 26, 1941, the Minnesota and Ontario boards of health conducted a public hearing at Fort Frances on the pollution of the Rainy River. This was an informal hearing which was not conducted for the purpose of taking testimony under the legal rules of evidence. Delegates represented townships, counties, and towns, as well as paper companies, the United States Bureau of Fisheries, the Minnesota Department of Conservation, the Minnesota Live Stock Sanitary Board, the Minnesota Department of Agriculture, Dairy, and Food, the Social Security Board, the Minnesota Resources Commission, and, of course, the boards of health of Minnesota and Ontario.[44]

Although no definite action was taken, the hearing did give the interested groups an opportunity to talk together and to learn how serious was the pollution of the Rainy. This was accomplished by photographs showing waste material found in the river, the nature of the fibers in bottom material, and plankton and fibers suspended in the water below International Falls. Legal phases were also discussed, as were the problems of municipal water and sewage plants. Shortly after the Fort Frances hearing, Chesley addressed letters to the city councils of Ranier, International Falls, Spooner, and Baudette, saying that the "logical first step in the solution of your portion of the problem lies in the making of engineering studies and the preparation of plans for adequate treatment of sewage." He added that there should be no delay. In a letter to the Minnesota and Ontario Paper Company he pointed out that the company's first step lay "in the preparation of plans and the installation of methods or equipment to remove all bark, and to reduce the amount of ground wood fiber discharged into the

---

[43] "Memorandum of Conference [on] Rainy River Survey, Detroit, Michigan, February 9, 1938"; H. G. Rogers, "Memorandum of Conference with Minnesota & Ontario Paper Co. Officials, August 24, 1939." Minnesota Department of Health, Minneapolis.

[44] Whittaker to Berry, September 19, 1940; Chesley to L. A. Fullerton, October 16, 1940; Chesley, "Notice of Public Hearing"; Minnesota and Ontario Departments of Health, "Agenda of Informal Hearing re Pollution of the Waters of the Rainy River at Fort Frances on the 26th Day of November, 1941." Minnesota Department of Health, Minneapolis.

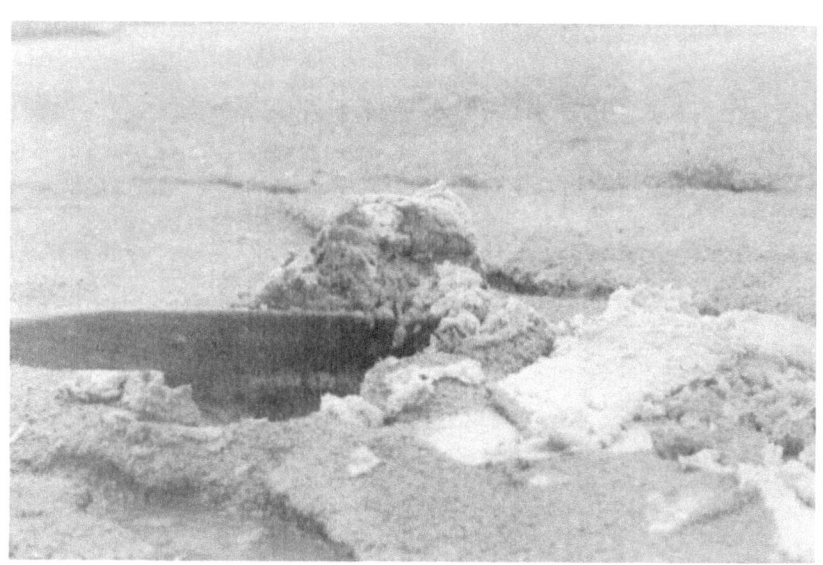
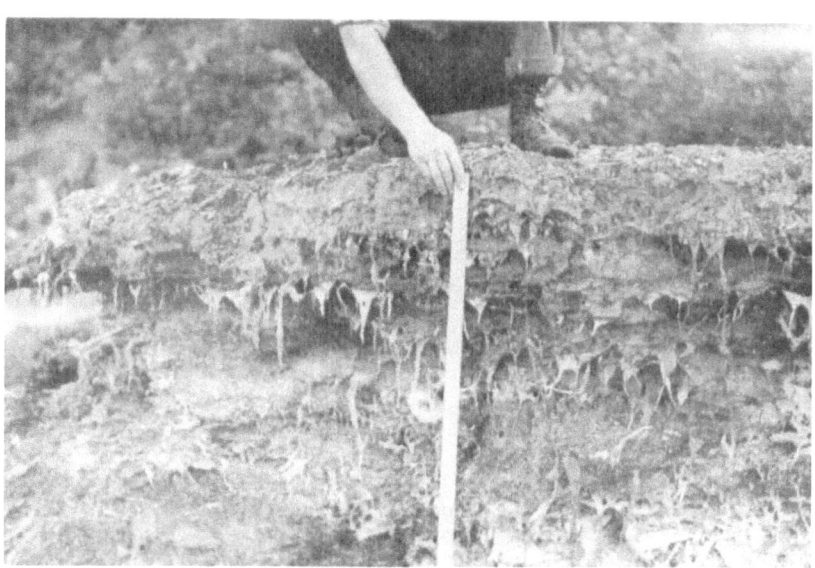

POLLUTION OF RAINY RIVER FROM PAPER MILL WASTES
Courtesy Minnesota Department of Health

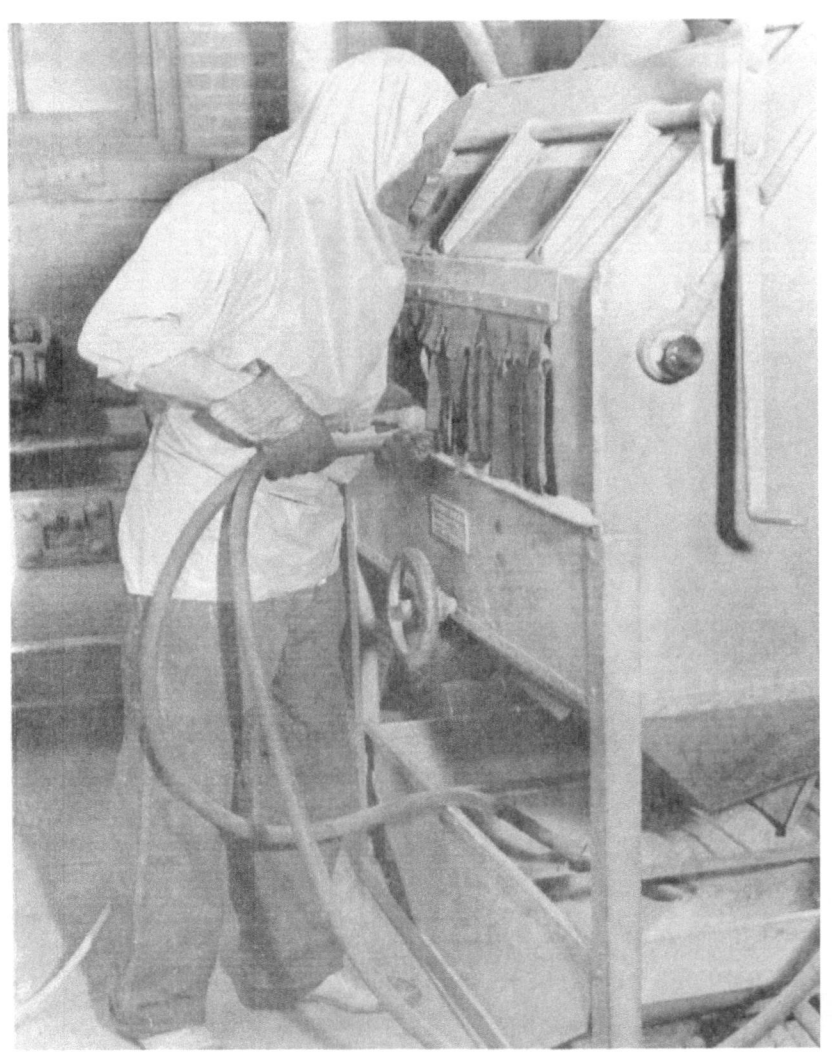

A Sand Blaster Protected According to
Public Health Standards
Courtesy Minnesota Department of Health

river to approximately 1.0 per cent. The next step is the elimination or material reduction of the strong sulphite waste." [45]

By 1942 municipalities on both the Canadian and the United States sides of the Rainy River were beginning to plan for modern sewage disposal plants, but World War II considerably hampered their efforts. Some improvement was noted also in the disposal of industrial waste. But in 1946, at International Falls, it was said that "the condition of the river had not changed materially since 1941 and there has been no material reduction in waste discharged from the paper company." [46]

Minnesota was in a little better position to handle pollution problems after 1945, for in that year the legislature passed the Water Pollution Control Act creating a water pollution control commission. The commission was given authority to administer and enforce all laws relating to the pollution of any of Minnesota's waters and, among a long list of its powers, was the right to "assist and cooperate with any agency of another state, of the United States of America or of the Dominion of Canada or any province there in any matter relating to water pollution control." The Minnesota Department of Health does the technical work of the commission and the secretary and executive officer of the State Board of Health is ex officio the secretary of the commission.[47]

Among the first official acts of the commission was the consideration of the Rainy River pollution problem. It sponsored a meeting at International Falls before the International Boundary Commission, which heard progress reports, but also learned that industrial waste was too prevalent. The results of this meeting may best be summed up by Rogers, who later was made director of the division of water pollution control and sanitary engineer consultant to the State Water Pollution Control Commission: "Following the meeting at International Falls, the Minnesota and Ontario Paper Company announced that their directors had authorized the expenditure of $500,000 to deal with their waste disposal problem. The principal towns along the American

[45] B. A. Westfall and M. M. Ellis, "Pulp-Mill Pollution of the Rainy River near International Falls, Minnesota" (United States Bureau of Fisheries, *Special Scientific Report* 7 — Washington, D.C., March, 1940); State Board of Health, "Public Hearing on Pollution of Waters of Rainy River, Held at Town Hall, Fort Frances, Ontario, November 25, 1941" (typescript); Chesley to the City Councils of Ranier, International Falls, Spooner, and Baudette, Minnesota, December 2, 1941, and to the Minnesota and Ontario Pulp and Paper Company, December 3, 1941. Minnesota Department of Health, Minneapolis.

[46] Berry to Whittaker, December 4, 1944, April 9, 1945; Whittaker to Wilson, January 29, 1945; Division of Sanitation, "Quarterly Reports," December 31, 1942, June 30, 1946. Minnesota Department of Health, Minneapolis.

[47] *Laws*, 1945, pp. 761–770.

side of the Rainy River, including Baudette, Spooner, International Falls, and South International Falls, have all had plans prepared and approved for adequate sewage treatment facilities. Work on disposal facilities is now in progress at Baudette and at the paper company's plant at International Falls. Control of pollution on the Canadian side of the river is under consideration through the Ontario Board of Health. On the whole, the prospects are good for a very substantial improvement in pollution conditions all along the Rainy River in the near future."[48]

With the long-standing Rainy pollution problem finally near abatement, the commission turned to other pollution nuisances. Between 1945 and 1947, for example, the commission considered 218 projects for improvements in sewage and waste disposal facilities throughout the state and approved plans for 148 projects, including 11 municipal sewer systems with treatment plants, 141 additions to existing systems, 17 new sewage treatment plants, major improvements at 5 existing plants, 2 industrial waste disposal systems, and 1 connection to an existing system with a sewage treatment plant. In addition, it had interested itself in 21 engineering studies, including 12 new systems with treatment plants, 14 new plants, and 1 major improvement. Field investigations were made of 6 streams, including the St. Croix and the Minnesota from New Ulm to Mendota. In co-operation with the division of preventable diseases, the commission investigated an unusually large number of cases of swimmer's itch at Camp Ajawah on Linwood Lake, and also investigated waste from canning factories. The commission also held hearings in the matter of the application of the Reserve Mining Company for a permit to discharge industrial waste into Lake Superior, and on November 8, 1947, made a follow-up investigation at the Minnesota and Ontario Paper Company at International Falls to observe the progress made and to discuss plans for installation of waste disposal facilities.[49]

In 1947 the legislature appropriated $731,000 to be used by the commission in co-operation with the division of state institutions for providing treatment facilities for all state institutions where existing provisions were inadequate. It is estimated that the cost of the construc-

[48] Division of Sanitation, "Quarterly Reports," June 30, 1946; Rogers, "Progress in Water Pollution Control," in *Conservation Volunteer*, vol. 11, no. 60, p. 45 (January–February, 1948). The author attended this meeting on June 28, 1946.
[49] Minnesota Water Pollution Control Commission, "Report, January 30, 1947," "Chairman's Report of Hearings, December 16, 1947," and "Quarterly Reports," December 31, 1947. The Water Pollution Control Commission is housed in the Department of Health Building on the university campus, and its reports are available there.

tion program already approved by the commission will exceed seven million dollars and that additional projects under consideration will total another eight million. Certainly Minnesota has gone a long way toward protecting the public's health by controlling water pollution. Had the state organized the commission a few years earlier, the health department might have been able to solve more quickly the pollution of both the Rainy River and the Red River of the North. Minnesota nature lovers and sportsmen, as well as public health officers, know now that the state's natural resources will not be permitted to deteriorate and that every attempt will be made to keep streams and lakes clean. But, as Rogers points out, "there is still much to be done before pollution from sewage and industrial wastes is sufficiently reduced to achieve standards of stream cleanliness expected by the people of the state." [50]

[50] Rogers, in *Conservation Volunteer*, vol. 11, no. 60, p. 45 (January–February, 1948); North Dakota State Department of Health, Division of Sanitary Engineering, *Red River of the North Research Investigation* (Fargo, 1941); Minnesota and North Dakota State Boards of Health, "Report of the Investigation of the Pollution of the Red River of the North, 1931, 1932, 1933," and Rogers, "Water Pollution Control in Minnesota" (typescripts), Minnesota Department of Health, Minneapolis.

16

Keeping Workers Fit

ALTHOUGH the man with the tin dinner pail was considered the backbone of Minnesota manufacturing and industry, his health, for many years, was totally ignored by his employer. If the factory worker fell ill or was injured on the job, he was left to his own resources to regain his strength as best he might. Bosses paid little attention to healthful, happy working conditions. Indeed, foremen frequently thought a man lucky to have work and would have fired an individual bold enough to complain that machines were not properly safeguarded or that ventilation was inadequate. Sanitary conditions were atrocious, not only in wilderness lumber camps and on the iron range, but also in the heart of the state's rapidly growing industrial cities.[1]

No adequate statistics are available for 1872, the year Minnesota's health board was established, but business was booming in both St. Paul and Minneapolis. Six years later 233 St. Paul manufactories were employing 3,117 persons and producing goods valued at more than $6,000,000. The Minneapolis Board of Trade reported 63 firms with a total sale of somewhat over $10,000,000 and said it was impracticable to arrive at the amount of retail trade. At Red Wing, Hewitt's home town, although lumber yards employed the greatest number of persons, the manufacture of carriages and wagons was the leading industry. Wages throughout the state ranged from $10 a month for a butcher to $82.30 for a steam engineer. The average wage probably was around $25 a month.[2]

Long before 1887, when Minnesota created its Bureau of Labor Statistics — an agency designed to study the commercial, industrial, social,

[1] See chapter 11, above, for a discussion of conditions in the lumber camps.
[2] Minnesota Commissioner of Statistics, *Annual Reports,* 1878, pp. 215, 221, 232, 253.

KEEPING WORKERS FIT

educational, and sanitary conditions of the working classes — Hewitt had announced an almost perfect industrial health policy. It is true that he was not referring specifically to workers, but his principles certainly were apt. He said that everybody needed "pure and abundant Air; pure and abundant Water; abundant sunlight; good sufficient, varied and properly prepared Food; Healthy Work; Healthy Recreation; Healthy Rest and Sleep." Previously Hewitt had suggested the need for proper ventilation and other essentials for health in public buildings; Hand had prepared a long report on ventilation; and in 1876 Hewitt himself wrote extensively on the principles of heating and ventilation. The modern industrial engineer and health officer still are concerned with these problems.[3]

Workers, too, complained of poor ventilation in shop and factory. A Minnesota shoe operative said: "I attribute the loss of my health to the fact that the factory in which I first worked was not properly ventilated. I have worked so hard that my health is broken. I must often take spells of rest. My expenses then eat up my earnings, so I get no further ahead from year to year." Another girl, a hotel worker, said that the management lodged her in a room partitioned off from the barn, and that when the doors were closed "there was no ventilation unless we raised the 4 x 8-inch skylight." Others complained of unsanitary living quarters in homes where they worked as domestic servants.[4]

Mrs. Charlotte O. Van Cleve told the commissioner of labor statistics in 1888 that the majority of women working as servants were untrained and ignorant of their business, but she ignored the responsibilities of mistresses to provide healthful surroundings for cooks and maids. She did, however, furnish a detailed description of the very girls who were complaining of poor ventilation and inadequate quarters. Saying that perhaps the largest number came from Scandinavia, Mrs. Van Cleve continued: "They came here utterly ignorant of our ways, knew nothing of cooking, cannot make a bed properly and have no skill even in sweeping and dusting. Some have acquired only a few words of our language, but nearly all of them can say 'tree dolla,' which is their usual demand for a week's work. Some learn readily and soon become efficient in the different kinds of housework. Some are dull and *cannot* be taught to do the work satisfactorily; this class often drift into laundries, or become scrubbing girls in hotels. They are usually strong and generally willing. The training of such girls is very wearing on the

[3] *General Laws,* 1887, pp. 199–201; State Board of Health, *Annual Reports,* 1876, pp. 12, 43–54; 1876 [*1877*], pp. 35–43, 53.
[4] Minnesota Bureau of Labor Statistics, *Biennial Reports,* 1887–88, pp. 173, 179.

mistress of the house and not very many of them have the patience and forbearance necessary for the task; but those who persevere in teaching them faithfully and kindly are amply rewarded. One can soon find out whether the girl has capabilities for the work; if she has not, all efforts will be fruitless. The difficulty in the way of taking all this trouble is that as soon as a girl learns how to work, she is very apt to demand greater wages than her patient teacher is able to give. So she leaves her, and goes where *fifty* cents will be added to her weekly income. The Scandinavians are generally reliable and faithful, thrifty and economical, and very desirous to get as high wages as possible."[5]

In many ways it was better for immigrant boys and girls to seek employment in shops and factories than to hire themselves out to private families as stable helpers or maids. The legislature had attempted to regulate working hours and to assure the bodily comfort of workers in industry, but it had done nothing to protect the domestic. In 1878, for example, a ten-hour day had been established for women and children; in 1885 an act regulated the labor of locomotive engineers and firemen; and in 1889 the legislature passed a long bill for the control of convict labor at Stillwater. But not until 1889 were employers of women required to furnish seats "to such an extent as may be necessary for the preservation of their health."[6]

The legislature of 1889 passed other acts fixing the wages of laborers, protecting wages, and giving liens for the better security of mechanics, material men, laborers, and others, but it did not legislate as specifically in matters of health as did other states. The commissioner of labor statistics pointed out, for example, that Massachusetts had acts forbidding the employment of women and minors in manufacturing establishments between ten o'clock at night and six o'clock in the morning; prohibiting the employment of children to clean dangerous machinery; forbidding the employment of minors who could not read nor write and who were not regular attendants of day or evening schools; and providing for the preservation of the health of working females, for uniform and proper meal times for children, young persons, and women employed in factories and workshops, and for the inspection of factories. Other Massachusetts laws related to sanitary appliances and proper ventilation.[7]

So great, indeed, was public interest in legislation of this type that

[5] Bureau of Labor Statistics, *Biennial Reports*, 1887–88, p. 160.
[6] *Statutes*, 1878, chapter 24; *General Laws*, 1885, p. 277; 1889, pp. 54, 430–435.
[7] *General Laws*, 1889, pp. 196, 313–322, 325; Bureau of Labor Statistics, *Biennial Reports*, 1889–90, pp. 164–185.

KEEPING WORKERS FIT

both the Republican and Democratic parties, in their national platforms for 1892, called upon state legislatures to pass factory inspection laws. Minnesota's penal code provided that any person who, by any act of negligence or misconduct, caused the death of a human being, was guilty of manslaughter in the second degree. In a sense, this made an employer criminally liable, but it was far from satisfactory. This section of the penal code, as the commissioner of labor statistics indicated, "does not embody the best conception of the purpose of law. It partakes too much of the nature of the wisdom which 'locks the stable door after the horse has been stolen.' Instead of trying simply to punish a man for killing his fellow by carelessness, legislation should endeavor to prevent the killing." [8]

There was abundant evidence that factories were unhealthful places in which to work. Faulty fire escapes and internal stairways were constant hazards, as were open hatchways, hoistways, and elevators. In 1892 Minnesota had no law to force management to repair defective or unguarded machinery. Loose pulleys and belt shifters and projecting setscrews annually injured workmen. Planers, saws, frizzers, jointers, ironing mangles, flywheels, power presses, stamping machines — all these continually jeopardized the health and safety of Minnesota's laborers. In a two-year period industrial accidents caused twenty-six deaths, ten amputations of hands or arms, sixty-seven partial amputations of hands, two amputations of legs or feet, seventeen fractures of limbs or bones of the trunk, six injuries to heads or faces, and one hundred and forty-six lacerations. Translated into human terms, these figures mean that in Anoka County, for example, one worker in a sash, door, and blind factory cut off four fingers on a jointer, another was slightly injured by a knot flying from a machine, and a third had his finger taken off by a ripsaw.[9]

In 1893 the legislature passed an act calculated to reduce industrial accidents and thus better preserve workers' health. It provided that machinery be properly safeguarded and gave the commissioner of labor statistics and factory inspectors the power to enforce compliance with the safety code. Section 7 was concerned with health. "Every factory, mill or workshop or other building," it read, "in which two or more persons are employed, shall be provided, within reasonable access, with a sufficient number of water closets, earth closets or privies for the reasonable use of the persons employed therein. And whenever male and

[8] Minnesota, *Penal Code,* 1886, section 166; Bureau of Labor Statistics, *Biennial Reports,* 1891–92, p. 41.
[9] Bureau of Labor Statistics, *Biennial Reports,* 1891–92, pp. 105, 107.

female persons are employed as aforesaid together, water closets, earth closets or privies, separate and apart, shall be provided for the use of each sex, and plainly so designated, and no person shall be allowed to use such closet or privy assigned to the other sex. Such closets shall be properly screened and ventilated, and at all times kept in a clean and good sanitary condition. In factories, mills and workshops, and in all other places where the labor performed by the operator is of such a character that it becomes desirable or necessary to change the clothing, wholly or in part, before leaving the building at the close of a day's toil, separate dressing rooms shall be provided for women and girls whenever so required by the factory inspector." [10]

Hewitt was tremendously interested in the factory act of 1893. However, Section 4, which referred to the sanitation of bakeries, hotels, and public restaurants, troubled both him and the commissioner of labor statistics. Neither felt that this section was sufficiently strong or stringent. Their concern was stimulated further late in 1894 when the editor of the *Bakers' Journal* wrote the labor commissioner suggesting six changes in the section. The letter was forwarded to Hewitt, who said in his reply: "I wish the act could be amended as to insist that all employees of such establishments, who have themselves or their families been exposed to or suffered an infectious disease, should discontinue their work until such time as the local board of health has declared them free from any danger of carrying infection. A sufficient reason for this is the fact that the infection of disease is often carried upon the clothing or persons of those who are themselves well, and one can readily see how this might happen in these establishments as it has happened to other producers and manufacturers of human food." [11]

Three factory inspectors were appointed to carry out the law of 1893. In a period of eighteen months they issued 2,402 orders for the installation of safety devices of all types. These included recommendations that separate toilets for women be installed, that toilets be properly marked, cleaned, ventilated, and disinfected, and that they be removed from bake rooms. Seven orders called for more adequate ventilation and 15 for cleaning and whitewashing workrooms. A few years later 158 orders were issued in St. Paul, 175 in Minneapolis, and 37 in Duluth. Many of them dealt with sanitary problems, although most of them were concerned with accident prevention and fire protection. A few were drawn to safeguard children. Inspectors in Duluth, for ex-

[10] *General Laws*, 1893, pp. 99–106.
[11] Bureau of Labor, *Biennial Reports*, 1893–94, part 2, p. 26.

KEEPING WORKERS FIT 313

ample, ordered a firm to discharge a boy under fourteen years of age and asked that school excuses be provided for minors.[12]

These orders relating to children stemmed from an act of 1895, amended in 1897, which prohibited the employment of children under fourteen years of age in any factory, mine, or workshop. Minors could be employed during vacation periods in mercantile establishments and by public messenger or telegraph companies for not more than ten hours in any one day and for not more than sixty hours a week. On Saturdays and for ten days before Christmas children over fourteen could work until ten o'clock at night, provided they did not work more than ten hours in any one day. Children under sixteen who could not read or write simple English sentences were also debarred from employment, except during vacation periods. In 1900, 577 children under sixteen were employed in the state. The number had jumped to 1,075 two years later. That employment of children resulted in ill health was clearly apparent to both labor officials and health officers. The commissioner of labor said frankly: "Factory life for children, we have been told by some of the best authorities, is dangerous to the physical development of the child, and we all admit that the chance for intellectual development in a child who is tired, overburdened by long hours of employment, and exacting duties is not what is to be desired."[13]

Both Hewitt and Bracken realized this, but there was little they could do, for their authority as health officers did not extend to the working child. They could only hope that family incomes might be raised sufficiently to make it unnecessary for children to work and meanwhile they could try to improve sanitary conditions in home and school. They could also impose sanitary regulations on certain types of plants, such as slaughterhouses, where children were employed. But, at the turn of the century, most working children were employed in such industries as printing, brickmaking, cigar making, and barrel-making, which were not under the board of health's jurisdiction. The annual May sanitary inspections by local health officers sometimes turned up conditions affecting children that could be rectified.[14]

If the health department had little authority over children in in-

[12] Bureau of Labor, *Biennial Reports*, 1893–94, part 2, p. 124; 1899–1900, pp. 158–169.
[13] *General Laws*, 1895, pp. 386–389; Bureau of Labor, *Biennial Reports*, 1901–02, pp. 410, 419.
[14] *Public Health in Minnesota*, 1:46–48 (August, 1885); 2:25–28 (May, 1886). See also chapter 9. above, and Bureau of Labor, *Biennial Reports*, 1901–02, p. 417.

dustry during these early years, it did have an interest and a responsibility in two other labor problems. The first was the health of men in the mining camps and the second concerned railroad sanitation. When the commissioner of labor in 1899 said that the development of the iron ore industry in northern Minnesota had been truly marvelous, he was referring in part to a public health problem that directly concerned the state health board.[15]

The first physicians on the iron range — Isaac van Dusen at Tower, John Alden at Ely, Robert and William Hutchinson at the Soudan Mine — found a primitive society that lived hard and was exposed to both industrial accidents and disease. By 1894 these doctors had been joined by others, some of whom became health officers and reported conditions directly to Hewitt. At first they were concerned primarily with the prevalence of typhoid, not only in Duluth but also in the jerry-built mining towns. Some of them were troubled by insanitary milk. From Mountain Iron a citizen complained that the local health board would do nothing, adding: "Our blooming M.D. here refused to act as chairman of the Bd. and we appointed one, James Reed to take his place, but he is as bad as the other." Reed, former warden of the prison at Stillwater and a central figure of a legislative investigation, was no physician. He told Hewitt frankly enough that he was appointed in the absence of any doctor, although the latter was not strictly true as Dr. D. C. Gilbert was practicing at Mountain Iron. Reed was soon replaced by Dr. Robert L. Brown, a competent individual who compiled a mining tract and then translated it into French and Scandinavian for distribution to miners.[16]

Scarlet fever, diphtheria, an epidemic of measles, and accidents complicated the duties of Virginia and Hibbing health officers. At Hibbing contaminated meat caused much sickness among mine workers who ate in boarding houses. "There is but one way for you to prevent the sale of unwholesome meat in your city," advised Bracken, "and that is for your council to appoint a meat inspector to act under your direction, or to authorize you to appoint one. A city with the population that you have should employ such a man." This advice, although

[15] Bureau of Labor, *Biennial Reports*, 1899–1900, p. 243.
[16] O. W. Parker, in *Minnesota Medicine*, 21:332 (May, 1938); *Daily Globe* (St. Paul), November 25, 1878; *Pioneer Press*, January 25, February 2, 6, 14, 26, 1879; letters to Hewitt from H. B. Richardson, June 26, October 25, November 25, 1894, from W. G. Goffe, August 7, November 13, 26, 1894, from J. A. Reed, October 19, 1894, from C. F. McComb, November 3, 1894,. from Robert L. Brown, April 17, 1895, and from W. W. Routh, December 5, 26, 1895, August 18, 1896, and Hewitt to Routh, December 20, 1895, Minnesota Department of Health, St. Paul.

sound, did not materially assist range health officers, who were working under adverse conditions.[17]

Dr. W. de la Barre, thoroughly wrought up by a malpractice action which involved him, penned a realistic sketch of Soudan in 1899. "The entire population of Breitung (Soudan) is composed of employees of the Minn. Iron Co. & their families," he wrote Bracken. "There are no stores here at all. All supplies etc. being procured at Tower — 2 miles distant. The people here are mostly Austrians, Italians, Finns & Swedes — of the lowest type of intelligence and civilization. The houses stand close together, are small, usually of 3 rooms, from 6 to 15 children in each family, and all living in the most unsanitary surroundings." It is little wonder that tuberculosis, diphtheria, measles, and typhoid fever were almost constant visitors on the range.[18]

"Typhoid fever is our worst enemy," complained an Eveleth physician in July, 1900. Within a month after he wrote, Sparta, a small community three miles from Eveleth, had a typhoid epidemic of such serious proportions that water samples were rushed to the health department's laboratory for examination. This water was classified as "probably good," but specimens from Eveleth wells were found to be unsatisfactory.[19]

So many complaints reached Bracken between 1900 and 1910 that he finally decided to appoint a special sanitary inspector for the range if the Oliver Iron Mining Company and St. Louis County would share the expense with the department. The usefulness of an inspector, said Bracken, "could be demonstrated and we would be in a position to go before the Legislature with a strong argument in favor of such an inspector; and, secondly, in some of the new towns connected with the mining company's work it would give a chance for sanitary policing of certain parasitic towns that does not now exist." This suggestion was prompted in part by the Hibbing dysentery epidemic of May, 1910, caused by the city's water supply. State health engineers found that water was being taken from what they described as "mining shafts, for while they have been driven for water supply purposes only, still they

[17] Letters to Bracken from Z. K. Brown, May 11, 1898, February 28, 1899, from D. C. Rood, July 3, 1898, and from G. F. Smith, February 9, 1899; Bracken to Rood, July 7, 1898. Minnesota Department of Health, St. Paul.
[18] De la Barre to Bracken, May 14, 1899, Minnesota Department of Health, St. Paul; *Hibbing News*, December 23, 1898; *Duluth News Tribune*, February 17, 1900; *Times* (Minneapolis), February 18, 1900.
[19] C. W. More to Bracken, July 30, August 23, 1900, Minnesota Department of Health, St. Paul; State Board of Health, *Biennial Reports*, 1899–1900, p. 239.

are almost wholly in the ore body, and the form of construction is identical with that of the ordinary mining shaft." [20]

Bracken pushed the appointment of a special sanitary inspector with his customary vigor. A meeting of health officials and representatives of the various mining companies and railroads on the range was held in Duluth. The companies expressed interest, but they failed to endorse the project. The assistant general manager of the Oliver Iron Mining Company told Bracken that the Interstate Steel Company, the Great Northern Railway Company, the Pitt Iron Mining Company, and the Alger, Smith interests would not contribute financially. "They claim," he said, "that the burden of taxation is so high now that they feel the state can well afford such an inspector without additional expense to them." The matter held fire until January 9, 1912, when the board voted to do nothing further toward securing a range sanitary inspector.[21]

Failure to secure an inspector was a sad blow to the board. This was especially true because Bracken had followed the inspection reports made by the Minnesota Bureau of Labor. In 1898, for example, of the twenty-seven mines that were inspected, sanitary conditions of twenty-five were declared good and two were marked fair. The same rating held for ventilation. Proper safeguards were a different matter. Two mines were said to be good in that respect, twenty-two ample, and two insufficient. Mines with inadequate safeguards were the Franklin and the Zenith. At the Hale Mine on June 14, 1900, five men were crushed to death by caving ore following a blast, and at the Clark Mine on July 18, ten men were blown to bits by an accidental powder explosion in an underground chamber.[22] In 33 mines employing a total of 6,929 men in 1900, there were 39 fatal accidents, 41 serious accidents, and 363 minor accidents.

"The chances for injuries in a mine are manifold," said the commissioner of labor, "and they come, in most instances unforseen and in spite of all watchfulness and care. A very small quantity of falling ore or rock will suffice to crush a person's limbs and the careless handling of explosives has to account for a number of minor accidents. The system of contract work, it seems, has also something to do with a great number of fatalities and injuries incidental to mining. The desire to

---

[20] Bracken to More, October 28, 1910, Minnesota Department of Health, St. Paul; State Board of Health, *Biennial Reports*, 1899–1900, p. 239; 1909–10, p. 270.
[21] State Board of Health, "Minutes," October 10, 1911, January 9, 1912, Minnesota Department of Health, St. Paul.
[22] Bureau of Labor, *Biennial Reports*, 1899–1900, pp. 258, 287.

KEEPING WORKERS FIT

make big wages is an inducement for workmen to take chances, which under other circumstances they would not assume."[23] Fatal and nonfatal accidents in 1910 totaled 4,057 and were partly responsible for a most comprehensive research project on the general subject of mine accidents. The next year an intensive safety campaign was begun by the labor bureau in an attempt to reduce the 10,463 industrial accidents that had occurred in the state during 1909 and 1910.[24]

Meanwhile the health department forged ahead, with what personnel and finances it had, to try to improve general sanitary conditions among the miners. "In Minnesota we have an enormous amount of typhoid fever," Chesley told the American Civic Association. "In certain localities we have had year after year 'fly outbreaks.' The most notable ones have been on the Iron Range. There the little cities are well built and, as a rule, well sewered with excellent city water supplies, but on the out-skirts of the organized territory there are many cabins and shacks with out-door privies or none at all and at the camps where the men (mostly foreigners) live who do the common labor in the mines, the conditions are pretty bad. We have had typhoid and dysentery spread by flies many times. The city authorities and the mining companies favor all practical measures for the prevention of the spread of disease. It is extremely difficult to enforce sanitary regulations among the people who make up the large class of laborers on the Iron Range."[25]

A few months later Whittaker made a special trip to the range to consult with water superintendents and mining companies concerning water supplies. Upon his return, Bracken wrote the president of the Oliver Iron Mining Company: "we are willing to assume responsibility for the quality of a water supply only when we have had the necessary field examinations made and the data has been secured by one in our employ who is thoroughly familiar with our methods." The company replied that it had a standing sanitary committee, "the object of which is to make a careful study of all the conditions at the various points where operations are being conducted and to see that every reasonable precaution is taken to secure and maintain the most thorough sanitary conditions."[26]

[23] Bureau of Labor, *Biennial Reports*, 1901–02, p. 366. An excellent account of conditions surrounding mine workers may be found on pages 361–366.
[24] Bureau of Labor, *Biennial Reports*, 1909–10, pp. 198–244; Bureau of Labor, Industries, and Commerce, *Safety Bulletin*, 2 (St. Paul, July, 1911).
[25] Chesley to Watrous, March 28, 1912, Minnesota Department of Health, St. Paul.
[26] Bracken to W. J. Olcott, August 12, 1912, and Olcott to Bracken, August 14, 1912, Minnesota Department of Health, St. Paul.

The health department was glad to co-operate. In 1912 the department examined twenty-seven different water supplies on mining property. It recommended, among other things, that individual wells be entirely eliminated and said that underground water was preferable to surface water. It also gave directions for selecting and protecting water sources. In 1913 and 1914 the department aided the Oliver Iron Mining Company in providing bubbling fountains at Zenith, Sibley, and Ely, approved installation of filters, supplied plans for sanitary privies, and furnished free typhoid vaccine. During July, 1915, another thorough investigation was made and engineers found that progress had been made as to both water supply and sewage and garbage disposal.[27]

An investigation to determine if the public water supply on properties of the Pickands-Mather Mining Company was potable was concluded late in 1916. Although water of the Elba Mine was found satisfactory, that from the Mohawk Mine was not. The company itself suggested that eight separate water sources be studied. All were located in a stratum of rock or ore body in the underground workings of nearby mines. Of the eight investigated, four needed protective construction at the source and four were satisfactorily protected against contamination and therefore suitable for public use. This pattern of assistance by the department to the mining industry was not to change radically until a quarter of a century later, when an industrial hygiene unit was created.[28]

Meanwhile both the labor bureau and the health board were wrestling with the industrial complications occasioned by the rapid extension of railroads throughout the state. Labor officials were interested primarily in disputes, such as the strike of switchmen at Brainerd in October, 1888, and in legislation to prevent accidents, such as an act of 1887 defining the liabilities of railroad companies in relation to damages sustained by their employees.[29] The health department, on

[27] State Board of Health, Laboratory Division, "Report on the Sanitary Quality of the Water Supplies of the Oliver Mining Company on the Minnesota Iron Range, November 5–14, 1912" (typescript); letters to Bracken from Ayres and Parker, October 27, 1913, from S. S. Rumsey, December 15, 1913, and from S. W. Tarr, March 25, 1914, Minnesota Department of Health, St. Paul; Division of Sanitation, *Report on the Water Supplies and the Sewage, Excreta and Garbage Disposal at Certain Locations of the Oliver Iron Mining Company on the Minnesota Iron Range, June 22–27, 1915* ([Minneapolis], 1915).

[28] Division of Sanitation, "Report on Water Supply for the Elba Mine Location, October 24, 1916," "Report on Water Supply for the Mohawk Mine Location, October 24, 1916," and "Report on the Water Supplies at Various Properties Controlled by the Pickands-Mather Mining Company in the Mesaba District of the Minnesota Iron Range, January 19–22, 1916" (typescripts), Minnesota Department of Health, St. Paul.

[29] Bureau of Labor, *Biennial Reports*, 1887–88, p. 253; *General Laws*, 1887, p. 69.

the other hand, wanted to see that railroad camps and cars were sanitary. Bracken was particularly interested in this problem, for he knew, as did Hewitt, that trains carrying passengers with contagious diseases could easily sow epidemics. This was particularly true in a state being flooded by persons from both home and abroad who sometimes had not the slightest conception of personal hygiene.

The problem, therefore, had to be attacked from two angles. Railroad employees must be kept fit and free from accident hazards, and passengers must be protected and also prevented from spreading disease. The major threat to railroad employees was faulty switches, which injured or took the lives of many. To remedy this evil, the legislature in 1887 passed an act providing for the better protection of switches to safeguard the limbs of employees. As a result the State Bureau of Labor, during 1893 and 1894, inspected 22,836 switches. Of these, 15,800 were found to be good, 3,723 fair, 1,880 bad, and 1,434 blocked. Minnesota was the first state in the Union to provide such inspection, just as it was the first to insist that street railway employees be protected from the inclemencies of the weather. Yet with all these precautions, the number of accidents on railroads and in allied industries in 1900 exceeded those in any other type of activity. Forty years later this situation had changed radically, for only nine switchmen were then injured in a two-year period.[30]

During the same period great emphasis had been placed on the problem of smallpox and vaccination. Bracken early urged vaccination of all railway employees, and in 1902 he called a conference of railway surgeons to discuss its advisability. As a result it was agreed that "general managers shall require all men in train service . . . to be vaccinated, or show a certificate of having been vaccinated within the preceding five years, and that no new employees be accepted in their service without such certificate or other evidence of immunity." But the mere passing of such a resolution did not automatically solve the matter. Objection was made by both individuals and companies. A mail clerk complained, and Bracken said that the Northern Pacific "has offered more opposition and seemed willing to do less than any other of our Minnesota railroads."[31]

[30] *General Laws*, 1887, p. 73; 1893, p. 176; Bureau of Labor, *Biennial Reports*, 1893–94, pp. 41, 48; 1899–1900, p. 180; Department of Labor and Industry, *Biennial Reports*, 1939–40, p. 191. The office of commissioner of labor was abolished in 1921. For a history of the department, which had several changes of name, see Minnesota Industrial Commission, *Biennial Reports*, 1927–28, pp. 16–21.

[31] State Board of Health, *Biennial Reports*, 1901–02, p. 303; John Marti to Bracken, January 18, 1902, and Bracken to Ohage, December 11, 1902, Minnesota Department of Health, St. Paul.

Once Bracken interested himself in railway sanitation, he attacked it with vigor. Declaring himself to be kindly disposed to railroads, he nevertheless said that constant complaints were coming to him on railway sanitary problems. Most of them concerned improper construction and inadequate cleaning of shipping pens for cattle, the insanitary condition of stations and depots, the dirt of sleeping cars, and the miserable filth in parlor cars and day coaches. He was particularly acid when he described the day coach. "We all know," he wrote, "that its toilet closet is avoided by all respectable people, even to the point of marked personal discomfort; we all know that such coaches have by no means an attractive appearance after a service of a few hours, for passengers are permitted and even encouraged by the goods hawked through the cars, to cover the floor with the remnants of lunches and fruit, in a way that would never be permitted in a hotel or private residence. If one has a wish to learn how undesirable a day coach may become, speaking from a sanitary point of view, he has only to enter one about five o'clock in the morning after it has been in service all night and fairly well filled with passengers." [32]

Bracken criticized also supplies of drinking water on trains, saying that some water came from questionable sources. Finally the board passed a regulation which covered this situation to some degree, but in 1912 water served on trains was still under suspicion. "I think it is true that as a rule the water supplied in day coaches is taken from the public water supplies of the various cities where the railroads have their cleaning yards, or sometimes from certain stations at which trains take on supplies," said Bracken. "There is a danger of this general water supply being unsafe, for many, many of our municipalities have not a safe water supply. For the diners and sleepers, however, there is less criticism. On many of the dining cars we find either spring or distilled water carried. The railroads certainly should be sure that the spring waters are safe and as for distilled water, there should not be any question as to its purity." [33]

The matter of proper ventilation of both railway cars and streetcars was another source of annoyance. Bracken thought that railway ventilation perhaps was better than that of streetcars because coaches were not so crowded, because doors were opened at both ends of railroad cars from time to time, and because roof ventilators were better

[32] Bracken Papers, 3:9.
[33] Bracken to More, April 24, 1912, Minnesota Department of Health, St. Paul.

constructed. He dismissed streetcar ventilation with a bit of doggerel verse:

> Did you ever in riding in cars 'round the town —
> This town —
> Where most folks stood up while a few sat them down —
> Way down —
> Did you ever get squeezed till your face was sky blue,
> And find that the fellow pressed closest to you —
> Had an annual bath that was long overdue? 34

At a meeting of the National Association for the Study and Prevention of Tuberculosis in 1905, Bracken read a lengthy paper on the dangers of infection in transportation. He emphasized all the needs for sanitary inspection of rolling stock and then spoke specifically of the general habit of Americans of spitting in public places. He quoted nine recommendations made the previous year by the Conference of State and Provincial Boards of Health and urged that state legislatures pass laws of a similar nature. Three years later Bracken made the blunt statement that "there is no such thing as railway sanitation in the United States." Minnesota, he added, was in much the same position as Missouri and Florida, because the legislature failed to pass a bill covering railway sanitation — "regulations which were carefully formulated in conference with representatives of all the railways operating in Minnesota and therefore presumably practicable." 35

Bracken and Whittaker were so thoroughly convinced that insanitary railway facilities were health dangers to both employees and passengers that they made strenuous attempts at a conference of the American Medical Association on medical legislation and education to have these evils corrected. Whittaker showed that of twenty-one railroad water supplies tested by the department, thirteen were condemned. Bracken commented upon unsanitary conditions prevailing in railroad construction camps. He knew what he was talking about, for these camps had long been a scandal in Minnesota.36

"There are employers in Minnesota who house their workmen in boarding camps who seem to have no regard whatever for the health

[34] Bracken Papers, 3:13.
[35] Bracken Papers, 3:39, 60, 67.
[36] Bracken Papers, 3:111, 113. See also Northwestern Sanitation Association and American Medical Association, Committee on Railway Sanitation, "Regulations Relating to Railway Sanitation," February 24, 1913 (typescript), Minnesota Department of Health, St. Paul. These thirty-three regulations include fourteen relating to boats, railroad cars, and stations, and nineteen attempting to control conditions in industrial camps.

of their employees," said the labor commissioner the year that Bracken and Whittaker attended the American Medical Association conference. "Their workmen are herded together in dirty bunk houses, where they contract various diseases, and are then returned to the cities to associate with their fellowmen and to spread the diseases they have contracted. No laws regulate these camps and no department of the state has any authority over them. The owners of the camps have continued their practices for years without let or hindrance and often use up the vitality of strong, healthy men in one season and send them back to their homes a menace to the communities."[37]

Complaints concerning industrial camps were investigated either by the Minnesota Department of Labor or the State Board of Health. In 1913, for example, health officers inspected a boarding camp run by the Chicago Commissary Company for the Chicago Great Western Railroad. Among the recommendations made were those calling for the screening of commissary cars, kitchen cars, and dining cars; for receptacles with tight covers for all food; for an approved incinerator; and for flyproof pits and privies. Other camps investigated by labor inspectors were found to be in equally miserable condition.[38]

For years the matter of jurisdiction over industrial camps was disputed. In 1918 the labor department definitely said that the health board should be given the authority, but legislation accomplishing this was not passed until 1923.[39] Other significant progress was made in railway sanitation in general. The United States Public Health Service was given supervision of drinking water on railroads. Acting for this federal health service, the Minnesota department inspects water supplies of both trains and airplanes within the state. Sanitary conditions of depots, outhouses, and other station facilities were regulated by Minnesota's Railroad and Warehouse Commission. By 1932 a decided improvement was noted over the "old-time carelessness as to sanitary conditions and neglect of the facilities provided for heating, lighting,

[37] Department of Labor, *Biennial Reports*, 1913–14, p. 188.
[38] Koch to Houk, August 2, 1913, Minnesota Department of Health, St. Paul; Department of Labor, *Biennial Reports*, 1913–14, pp. 190–194.
[39] Department of Labor, *Biennial Reports*, 1917–18, p. 117; *Statutes*, 1941, section 157.01; *Laws*, 1923, pp. 260–262; *Minnesota State Health Laws and Regulations*, 90–93 (January 1, 1948); Chesley to R. W. Clark, July 13, 1923, Minnesota Department of Health, St. Paul. While the federal government controlled the railroads during World War I, a committee, of which Bracken was a member, was appointed to "conduct a survey of, and submit recommendations in connection with, the proper protection of the health of employees and patrons of the railroads under Federal control." See United States Railroad Administration, Office of the Director General of Railroads, *Circular* 58 (Washington, D.C., September 25, 1918).

KEEPING WORKERS FIT 323

etc." Other health and safety conditions were supervised by the United States Interstate Commerce Commission. In addition, railroad surgeons themselves improved both toilet and ventilation facilities.[40]

Inadequate working conditions for domestics, lumbermen, miners, and factory laborers in general led the Minnesota State Planning Board in 1936 to recognize the dangers of occupational diseases and hazards and to say that preventive measures were necessary. The epidemiological method was declared applicable to industrial problems. "The epidemiologist," maintained the commission, "with special training in relation to the industrial diseases as well as communicable diseases, assisted by the clinical laboratorian and the bacteriologist, should make the approach, find the cause, determine the diagnosis. He should at all times cooperate with the industrial engineer, the chemist, the attending physician, the worker, and the employer. Routine examinations of workers, including special investigations and laboratory tests pertinent to the actual and possible hazards of the occupation concerned should be made at frequent intervals. The prevention of occupational disease is truly as much a duty of the health department as that of the prevention of disease in the school room." Health department members who helped prepare this report were Chesley, Whittaker, and McDaniel.[41]

Four years after the planning board's recommendations were made the health department created an industrial hygiene unit within the division of preventable diseases and in co-operation with the division of sanitation. A year later, in July, 1941, the unit became the division of industrial health, with a seven-point program:

1. To receive and investigate reports of occupational disease.
2. To promote more adequate medical services within industry.
3. To encourage the use of ethical pre-employment and periodic physical examinations, including the use of routine serologic tests for syphilis.
4. To confer with industrial physicians with regard to special problems or general industrial health programs.
5. To provide engineering personnel who are especially trained and equipped to make studies of plant environment and to make recommendations for the control of health hazards found.
6. To promote adult hygiene programs within the industrial groups; such as, the control of tuberculosis, syphilis, and other communicable diseases.

[40] Railroad and Warehouse Commission, *Biennial Reports*, 1931–32, p. 383; Otis B. Kent, *A Digest of Decisions under the Federal Safety Appliance and House of Service Acts* (Washington, D.C., 1915).
[41] Minnesota State Planning Board, *Report of the Committee on Public Health*, 52 ([St. Paul?], December, 1936).

7. To prepare and disseminate information on various toxic materials and processes, and methods for their control.[42]

This ambitious and much-needed program had been planned with extreme care. A fact-finding survey was made to evaluate industrial health problems. From a list of 5,000 industries, 561 plants were investigated in regard to safety and medical provisions, water supply, sewage disposal, accident and sickness records, number of persons employed in each occupation, the nature of the occupation, the materials and by-products handled, the control devices in use, the number of workers exposed to toxic substances, and such other data as was needed to evaluate individual exposures and to establish means for their control. Major hazards found in this preliminary survey were, in the order of their importance: organic dust, metal (exclusive of lead, zinc, chromium, magnesium), petroleum products, silicate dusts, and extreme temperature changes.

With these facts at hand, the work of preventing disease in industry went forward as fast as war conditions would permit. Fortunately the legislature in 1939 had passed a bill requiring physicians to report occupational diseases. Indeed, it was this act that enabled the health department to set up its program of industrial hygiene, for it authorized the health board to investigate and make recommendations for the control of industrial health hazards. Realizing that Minnesota was of "sufficient industrial importance" to require the services of an industrial hygiene division, the health department nevertheless moved with good sense and caution. Dr. Leslie W. Foker, the first director of the division, indicated that it would take time to develop a program that could be built upon for years to come. He realized, as many did not, that there were in Minnesota many small plants that had no medical organization and that therefore were dependent upon industrial health services offered by the health department. Larger industrial units, such as the Pillsbury Mills, had developed their own medical services.[43]

Foker knew that from time to time studies had been made of infectious diseases in industry, but he also realized that during the war period his activities would have to center largely about health problems arising from defense plants and war industries. These, he said, were of three types: "those attributable directly to the working environ-

[42] State Board of Health, *Reports*, 1922–43, p. 129.
[43] *Laws*, 1939, pp. 343–345, 457; Minnesota Department of Health, "A Preliminary Survey of the Industrial Hygiene Problem in Minnesota, 1941" (typescript), Minnesota Department of Health, Minneapolis; Foker, in Hennepin County Medical Society, *Bulletins*, 13:36 (April, 1942). Among Minnesota's pioneer industrial physicians was Dr. A. E. Wilcox.

ment; those that are the result of the changing nature of the working force itself; and those that originate in the workers' home and community environments." Therefore, in consultation with the Quartermaster's Corps and consulting engineers and architects, the health department helped develop sanitary requirements for the munitions plant near New Brighton. Water supply and sewerage investigations were made, as were studies in environmental sanitation in the area immediately surrounding the plant. Representatives of the Ramsey County Planning Board consulted the industrial hygiene division regarding the regulation of trailer camps in the vicinity. Some twenty-six defense plants were inspected during the first quarter of 1941. In addition, a special study was made in a brass foundry.[44]

The extent and thoroughness of these wartime studies in environmental sanitation may be demonstrated by department investigations at the Gopher Ordnance Works in 1942. Samples of water were collected for bacteriological examination from the plant distribution system at two-weeks intervals; an investigation was made of the methods of transporting and transferring drinking water in barrels to work areas that were not served by the plant distribution system; suggestions were made for the elimination of possible sources of contamination in the procedure and equipment used to supply and store drinking water in the work area; an investigation was made of dishwashing procedure and of the mechanical dishwasher used in the cafeteria, and suggestions were made for the improvement of dishwashing technique. From 1940 to 1944, 874 man visits were made to 240 plants manufacturing war materials, and 5,771 determinations were made from 5,152 field and laboratory samples collected during these visits. These investigations, resulting from real or imagined occupational hazards, were brought about in some instances by the handling of new materials. Some problems were so critical that had they not been solved they might have impeded seriously Minnesota's part in the nation's war preparations. In addition, forty-three plants which were not manufacturing war materials were visited.[45]

Peace brought changes in the division's personnel and opportunities to focus attention entirely on normal industrial health problems.

[44] Lucy S. Heathman, "A Survey of Workers in Packing Plants for Evidence of Brucella Infection," in *Journal of Infectious Diseases*, 55:243–265 (November–December, 1934); Foker, "Changing Attitudes Toward Industrial Hygiene," in *Journal-Lancet*, 65:76 (February, 1945); Division of Sanitation, "Quarterly Reports," March 31, September 30, 1941.

[45] Division of Sanitation, "Quarterly Reports," December 31, 1942; State Board of Health, *Reports*, 1922–43, p. 130.

George S. Michaelsen became acting director of the division. He emphasized the role of the industrial health nurse, encouraged sound maternity policies in industry, distributed literature concerning medical service in industry and outlines of industrial hygiene programs, and he personally investigated factories and manufacturing plants. The division also began publication of a mimeographed bulletin entitled *Nursing in Industry*, and in 1947 it distributed a manual for industrial health service. Encouragement was given industries to provide adequate medical care and nursing service to employees.[46]

Industry was urged to provide these facilities because an industrial health program paid management in increased production by cutting down man-hours lost from work, by keeping skilled workers on the job, and by keeping employees satisfied and therefore efficient. Labor also was told that an industrial health program helped it by preventing the misery of sickness and injury, by protecting the worker, his family, and his community. The division told both management and labor that industrial health hazards — eye strain, respiratory diseases, dermatoses, gastrointestinal disorders, bone destruction — could be controlled with the help of experts from the state's health department.[47] The Minnesota Society for the Prevention of Blindness also co-operated with the health department and other agencies interested in the health of the worker by distributing literature discussing especially the prevention of eye hazards.[48]

Michaelsen recognized, of course, that in many ways the industrial nurse was in an unusually good position to take an active part in eliminating occupational disease hazards. "She has the opportunity," he said, "to see early signs of chronic poisoning due to dusts, fumes, gases, vapors or mists." In 1946 about 160 industrial nurses were employed throughout the state. These girls received every encouragement from the health department. They were given courses at the University of

---

[46] *Nursing in Industry*, vol. 1, no. 10, p. 2 (July 25, 1945); Charlotte Silverman, "Maternity Policies in Industry," in *The Child*, 8:20–24 (August, 1943); American Medical Association, Council on Industrial Health, "Medical Service in Industry—Industrial Health Examinations," in American Medical Association, *Journal*, 125:569 (June 24, 1944); United States Public Health Service, Division of Industrial Hygiene, *Outline of an Industrial Hygiene Program* (*Public Health Reports, Supplement* 171—Washington, D.C., 1943); Minnesota Department of Health, Division of Industrial Health, *Suggested Form for a Manual for Industrial Health Service* (Minneapolis, 1947).
[47] Minnesota Department of Health, Division of Industrial Health, *At Your Service* (Washington, D.C., 1945). Although imprinted with the name of the health department, this publication actually was prepared and distributed by the United States Public Health Service as its *Miscellaneous Publication* 33.
[48] Minnesota Society for the Prevention of Blindness, *An Ounce of Prevention!* (St. Paul, 1946).

KEEPING WORKERS FIT 327

Minnesota Center for Continuation Study in April, 1947, and were urged to enroll for the annual course in industrial health problems. The division of industrial health saw to it that nurses received the latest bulletins of interest to them, and frequently the division of public health nursing supplied them with specially prepared reports dealing with home safety. The division of preventable diseases kept industrial nurses informed of the nature and spread of infantile paralysis. Irvine wrote a special article in response to requests for information about the employment of workers with syphilis.[49]

The variety and scope of the activities of the industrial health nurse were well expressed by a nurse employed by Powers Dry Goods, Inc., in Minneapolis. She told of the difficulty of getting new workers to understand the meaning of the industrial health program and of introductory talks that explained the uses of medical and nursing service, the advantages of the in-plant food service, the opportunities for recreation, and the high cost of sickness and its attendant worries. But, she continued, "the nurse's most effective educational work is done in her daily contact with individual workers. In these the nurse is not obliged to generalize at all. She can get down to facts pertinent to the one person in the picture at the moment. His interests, abilities, peculiarities, religious and family background, and anything else that goes to make up his particular set of circumstances can be given due consideration. He is receptive because he has come seeking information or counsel, and because he receives the undivided attention of a specialist in the health field."[50]

Gradually Minnesota industry learned to appreciate the work of the division of industrial health and to request assistance when a particularly difficult situation arose. Of course, some industries were a bit suspicious at first, but as time went on management more and more came to consider the division a helpful, friendly consulting agency. Certainly the division did everything in its power to dispel the notion that it wanted to step in and ride roughshod over the rights of either the employer or his men, and it exerted itself to prove by tactful conduct that its primary business was to work with both management and labor.

The variety of investigations made was amazing, and they demon-

[49] *Nursing in Industry*, vol. 2, no. 2, p. 5 (February 4, 1946); vol. 2, no. 5, p. 3 (May 1, 1946); vol. 3, no. 3, pp. 1–4 (March, 11, 1947); vol. 3, no. 11, p. 2 (November 25, 1947); *Minnesota Eye Health*, 2:1–4 (March, 1947); Division of Public Health Nursing, *Home Safety*, a mimeographed bulletin issued in December, 1945; Division of Preventable Diseases, *Poliomyelitis*, a mimeographed bulletin issued July 22, 1946.
[50] Bethel J. McGrath, *The Nurse's Role in Health Education in Industry* (reprinted from *American Journal of Public Health*, 37:298–302 — March, 1947).

strated that the health department could definitely improve the worker's industrial environment. During a three-months period in 1947 fifty per cent of the services to industry originated with plant managers, physicians, the department of labor and industry, and others outside the health department. Many of these bids for assistance involved some form of ventilation problem. A metropolitan newspaper, for example, was studied to determine the ventilation needs of its classified advertising telephone room, and a Duluth foundry was investigated to determine atmospheric dust concentrations. A significant study of the relationship of sound to workers' health was carried out in a noisy factory manufacturing nuts and bolts. Although information regarding sound levels that are harmful to the human system was quite meager, researchers came to some interesting conclusions. Their findings indicated that continuous exposure to sound levels of from eighty to ninety decibels caused impairment of hearing and that there is considerable variation in individual tolerances of sound. In addition to causing impairment of hearing, "excessive noise also places excessive strain on the nervous system of persons exposed, producing a very significant fatigue factor." Once these data were determined, recommendations were made for correction. Noise producers were to be controlled by totally enclosing them in insulated boxes or tubes. The benefit to plant workers, of course, was tremendous.[51]

As the division of industrial health continued its work, it was able to improve conditions in a dry-cleaning plant where atmospheric carbon tetrachloride was so excessively high that it exposed cleaners to poisoning. Three recommendations, when followed, removed all danger and resulted in better health for labor and more efficient operation for management. Another gas problem was solved in a manufacturing company where carbon monoxide was threatening men in the motor-testing department. An unusual industrial problem occurred in seed-treatment plants in the Red River Valley. This business was seasonal and consisted of treating seeds chemically for the control of fungi. A study was undertaken to determine whether the atmospheric mercury concentrations were sufficiently high to be considered harmful from a health standpoint. A hazard was found and six recommendations, from the use of toxic dust respirators to a program of good housekeeping, were made. Once again, Minnesota workmen had received a type of protection utterly impossible a century earlier.[52]

[51] Section of Environmental Sanitation, "Quarterly Reports," September 30, 1947; "Reports of Engineering Studies," nos. 4, 11, 25, 65.
[52] Section of Environmental Sanitation, "Reports of Engineering Studies," report dated April 11, 1947, and reports nos. 9, 33–45.

KEEPING WORKERS FIT 329

Not all studies uncovered health hazards. In 1947, for example, trainmen on the Iron Range Division of the Duluth, Missabe, and Iron Range Railway wondered if dust produced by crushing sand for increased traction while negotiating grades and dust accumulation on the roadbed might not be harmful to their health. Industrial engineers made a most comprehensive investigation, taking samples from locomotives and cabooses of trains using sand on hills, in an attempt to observe the amount of dust arising from the roadbed and the load. Samples also were collected in parlor cars and day coaches between Duluth and Ely. "In spite of the fact," concluded Michaelsen, "that the results indicate a hazard to the health of the trainmen does not result from the dust, an objectionable or nuisance dust condition does exist." This, he continued, could be eradicated by the installation of local exhaust ventilation at a point where sand, wheels, and track come together. Dust in cabooses could be reduced by weather-stripping doors and windows. These findings pleased both management and labor.[53]

It must not be thought, however, that the division of industrial health concerns itself exclusively with the health hazards that occur within industry. Specific occupational diseases cause only a small fraction of the total disability and loss of time by wage earners because of illness. Industrial hygiene activities, therefore, are extended to attempt to safeguard the health of the worker against disease of all causes. This means, of course, that the division should "act as a central, fact-finding, coordinating, educational body, receiving reports of diseases of employees, making studies of actual and potential health hazards, determining the effectiveness of control measures, correlating environmental conditions with health, and finally, disseminating the information at hand for all groups."[54]

This is why industrial nurses and physicians, as well as health officials, concern themselves with maternity programs, with care of the eyes and teeth of the worker's family, with adequate housing, domestic discord, and even recreational facilities. Minnesota's laborer today, unlike his father only a few decades ago, is the focus of a score of agencies determined to keep him both happy and well. Yet the industrial hygienist knows that much work remains to be done. New inventions and technological advances carry with them new health hazards. Many old

[53] Section of Environmental Sanitation, "Reports of Engineering Studies," no. 56.
[54] Department of Health, "Preliminary Survey of the Industrial Hygiene Problem in Minnesota, 1941"; Thomas A. C. Rennie, Gladys Swackhamer, and Luther E. Woodward, *Toward Industrial Mental Health—An Historical Review* (reprinted from *Mental Hygiene*, vol. 31, no. 1, pp. 66–88 — January, 1947); National Committee for Mental Hygiene, Inc., *Mental Hygiene and Industry* (New York, 1944), and *Industrial Mental Health* (New York, 1945).

factories could improve their ventilation, reduce noise, better their lighting. Sanitary facilities in some have not caught up with modern design. And the Minnesota legislature, despite repeated requests by the state health department, has not yet appropriated a single penny for industrial health. All financial aid has come from federal funds. Foker was correct when he said: "To both management and labor the mutual advantages of good industrial health programs have been so well demonstrated that these programs will not be discontinued. Management can evaluate its benefits in a very tangible way, and the interest of labor is well evidenced by participation in case-finding surveys, by advocacy of health and hospital insurance coverage, by the appearance of health clauses in employment contracts. All these facts lead to the belief that interest will not fall off in any of these groups, but that industrial health programs will reach a stage of development commensurate with industry itself, and will constitute a major part of medicine and public health." [55]

[55] Foker, in *Journal-Lancet*, 65:78 (February, 1945).

17

Eternal Vigilance

AN UPSTATE farmer brought his family to the Minnesota State Fair, saw the fish in the Conservation Building, admired prize winning hogs, watched racing from the grandstand, and during the day stopped at several concessions for hamburgers, potato salad, and a piece of pie. A St. Paul schoolteacher celebrated her birthday by inviting friends to dinner at a popular restaurant. Two traveling salesmen, sample cases in hand, registered at a small-town hotel. Vacationists from Iowa rented a boat for a day's fishing on the St. Croix. A Boy Scout troup, off on a hike, stripped for a quick swim in one of Minnesota's cool lakes, and a group of Brownie Scouts went into camp on the banks of the Mississippi. During the summer hundreds of visitors to the North Star State registered at motels, tourist camps, and a wide variety of resorts. Down in cheap urban districts old men in faded work clothes asked for lodging in flophouses. Near by, colorful neon lights marked hotels boasting of the utmost comfort in beds, fine cuisines, floor shows, and glittering bars. On a plane flashing through the sky overhead an air-line hostess gave a drink of water to a little girl.

All these persons, sleeping, eating, drinking, enjoying Minnesota's abundant resources for sport and relaxation, no doubt were unaware of the necessity for eternal vigilance by local and state health officers, who saw that beds were clean, food was prepared in sanitary kitchens, drinking water was pure, that boats were safe, that resorts, motels, and even flophouses met specific health regulations. They did not know, for example, that during the ten days of the State Fair two state health inspectors were watching constantly to see that the food served was fit to eat. Neither did they know that the boats they rented had been inspected and approved. The little Brownie Scout had no idea that her romantic camp, with its canvas-covered barracks and rustic main lodge, had been gone over thoroughly by sanitary engineers, who took water samples, tested the refrigerator, asked questions about the milk supply, scrutinized the privies, took the temperature of the dishwater, and noted where and how garbage was disposed.

Not until recently in Minnesota were these services and others available on a fairly efficient level to citizens and visitors. It took years of patient endeavor to bring hotel inspection, for example, in line with modern health practices. The old-time inn, developing gradually into the contemporary hotel, was managed by an individualistic keeper, who gave small thought to sanitary practices. A guest took what came his way and was expected to be thankful for any sort of shelter from the weather. But by the end of the nineteenth century, when Minnesota agricultural towns and lumbering communities were flourishing, a slowly awakening traveling public began urging the legislature to pass acts calculated to bring hotels under some sort of supervision. In response the legislature in 1903 approved an act providing for primitive types of fire escapes for hotels, inns, and public boarding houses. But this act did not apply to communities with populations of less than ten thousand, nor did it provide for any inspection to see that its provisions were carried out.[1]

Two years later the act of 1903 was amended to include all hotels with twelve or more sleeping rooms and to create the position of hotel inspector, whose "duty it shall be to visit and inspect annually, so far as possible, every building or structure kept, used or maintained as, or advertised as, or held out to the public to be an inn, public lodging house or place where sleeping accommodations are furnished to the public, whether with or without meals." The inspector was ordered to keep a set of books showing "sanitary condition, the number and condition of fire escapes and any other information for the betterment of the public service." Hotels which complied with the law were to be given a certificate stating that fact. A provision that thoroughly exasperated hotel managers provided that they must pay each time an inspection was made. These fees ranged from fifty cents for a building with twelve, but less than thirty rooms, to three dollars for buildings with two hundred rooms or more.[2]

The 1905 act was so poorly enforced and so strenuously opposed by

[1] *General Laws*, 1903, pp. 531–533.
[2] *General Laws*, 1905, pp. 594–597.

hotel managers who resented the fee schedule that sanitary conditions remained about the same. Traveling salesmen in particular complained of lack of fire escapes, dirty roller towels, filthy toilets, unclean beds, and poor food. Most salesmen were members of the Order of United Commercial Travelers, and drummers living in Minnesota belonged to a district which included the Dakotas, Manitoba, Saskatchewan, Alberta, and Minnesota. In 1910 this membership numbered more than five thousand, and about half of them made their homes in Minneapolis or St. Paul. Thoroughly weary of the state's slow progress in remedying hotel conditions, members of the order brought the matter to the attention of their district grand council in 1911. They fully realized that Minnesota was none too friendly to the idea of hotel inspection. Yet they were aware also that the legislature in 1911 again had strengthened the law governing hotels by providing for a hotel inspector to be appointed by the governor and by appropriating six thousand dollars for salaries and expenses. Soon after this act was passed two members of the United Commercial Travelers, A. W. Crozier and B. M. Lennon, were appointed inspectors. "Every member of the Order," said the grand executive committee, "owes it to himself, his brethren and the State to lend every assistance in his power to make the new department a shining success. It is again on trial and no effort should be spared to make it an ideal department, in which case future state aid will be freely extended, and result in eliminating the evil conditions that have vexed our craft during the past."[3]

Despite the endorsement of the hotel law by the United Commercial Travelers and despite the fact that a hotel manager said that the day was past when a hotel "should combat just and equitable legislation for the betterment, protection and comfort of his patron," the grand council maintained a standing committee on hotel legislation. This was a wise precaution, not only because traveling men still were making numerous complaints, but also because by 1914 fear was expressed that the Minnesota Efficiency and Economy Commission might recommend the abolishment of the position of hotel inspector. This is exactly what happened, and it is probable that the recommendation would have been followed had it not been for the vigorous intervention of the traveling salesmen. The hotel inspector had also been criti-

[3] Interview of the author with Henry C. Capser, St. Paul, September 7, 1948; Grand Council, Order of United Commercial Travelers of America, *Proceedings*, 1911, pp. 47, 55, facing p. 174; *General Laws*, 1911, pp. 265–268.

cized indirectly by Dr. Charles V. Chapin, who in 1915 reported on state boards of health throughout the nation and said that hotel inspection was not enforced as well in Minnesota as in other states.[4]

That probably was true, but it must be remembered that Minnesota's first hotel inspectors were not sanitarians, but former traveling salesmen; that they faced opposition on the part of some hotel owners; and that not until 1913 did the legislature pass an really comprehensive law, which went far beyond any previous act. Among its provisions were those regulating plumbing, lighting, and heating and requiring that all hotels furnish each bedroom with at least two clean towels daily, that sheets be at least ninety-nine inches long, and that sheets and pillow slips be made of white cotton or linen. The bill also carried an appropriation of sixteen thousand dollars.[5]

Although Chapin's criticism was apt, Crozier had not been idle after the law of 1913 went into operation. Within a year 989 inspections were made, resulting in the closing of 12 hotels, in the refurnishing and redecorating of 2 others, in the compliance of 737 after they had been issued orders, and in the attempt by 252 to bring their establishments up to the level demanded. In order to make inspection more efficient, Governor Winfield S. Hammond suggested in May, 1915, that staff inspectors of the dairy and food and oil departments co-operate in making surveys of hotels. Such a program was worked out. With the part-time assistance of some ninety investigators from these departments, work went ahead more rapidly than before. Only six hotels in 1916 were closed because of noncompliance with the law. The extent to which hotel inspection could go was clearly apparent when inspectors forced a hotel to close and insisted that all furniture and equipment be removed from the building, that all wallpaper be stripped off, that the structure be fumigated for forty-eight hours, and that the place be repapered, painted, and refurnished with new equipment. Only after this was done was a license issued.[6]

Meanwhile the United Commercial Travelers, through its legislative committee, supported an even more stringent law. W. A. Wittbecker, hotel inspector in 1919, complained of lack of funds and inadequate personnel. The legislature responded by raising the salary of the hotel

[4] United Commercial Travelers, *Proceedings*, 1912, p. 83; 1913, pp. 19, 56–59; 1914, p. 75; Minnesota Efficiency and Economy Commission, *Final Report*, 30 (St. Paul, 1914); Chapin, *A Report on State Public Health Work Based on a Survey of State Boards of Health*, 183 (Chicago, [1916]).
[5] *General Laws*, 1913, pp. 840–846.
[6] United Commercial Travelers, *Proceedings*, 1914, p. 78; 1915, p. 68; 1916, p. 56; 1918, p. 98.

inspector, by regulating the type of dishes used in restaurants, and by stating conditions under which food handlers should work. It also provided that "No person known to be suffering from any contagious disease shall be employed in any capacity in any hotel, restaurant, lodging house, boarding house or place of refreshment." The act was significant if only for the section pertaining to food handlers. The number of deputy inspectors was increased to three, but the act did not appropriate any sizable sum of money.[7]

Wittbecker said he was able to cover the ground more thoroughly as a result of the act of 1919, and he submitted a report showing that his staff had made more than 4,000 inspections and had issued 2,123 orders. A major problem, he said, involved foreigners who entered the restaurant and lodginghouse business. "Many of these people can neither read, write nor speak the English language, [they are] without any conception of sanitation and utterly unfitted by nature for this business, which makes it incumbent on this Department to keep up a constant campaign of education."[8]

By 1922 two other factors, which made Wittbecker all but forget the irritating foreign element, had developed. The first was the extensive use of the automobile for commercial purposes and the improvement of highways. These, Wittbecker wrote, were "slowly but surely working a revolution in the hotel business, outside of the large cities. The commercial traveler is the mainstay of the small town hotel, and the landlord who formerly was too busy playing cards with his local cronies to show his guests to their rooms, is fast disappearing, for the next town is only a half hour's drive away." The second factor was the rapid development of Minnesota as a resort state. Visitors to the state "must be adequately housed," continued Wittbecker in unusually glowing terms for him, "if we are to reap the full benefit of the wonderful attractions of Minnesota as a summer playground. Minnesota has scenery and recreational attractions second to none. Our highways are marvels of smoothness and reach to the remotest corners of the State, furnishing easy access to the vast forest and lake region of Northern Minnesota." Then he told of careless, dirty resort keepers, who not only jeopardized their guests' health but also jeopardized some fifteen million dollars that tourists spent annually in the state. Only a few years later Wittbecker spoke of the advent of bus lines, which were "playing havoc with the small town hotel and will eventually put many of them

[7] United Commercial Travelers, *Proceedings*, 1919, p. 51; *Laws*, 1919, pp. 661–670.
[8] United Commercial Travelers, *Proceedings*, 1920, pp. 48, 111, 112.

out of business and I believe will put many of the smaller towns themselves out of business and will result in the establishment of the chain store and the chain hotel in the more prominent towns." [9]

But Wittbecker had more to worry him than hard roads, automobiles, and bus lines. A movement was under way to reorganize the state government. Among the suggested changes was one that proposed the abolishment of the office of hotel inspector and the transfer of his activities to the Minnesota Department of Health. For some years health officials had been unhappy about the entire hotel inspection problem. In the first place, they believed that only a trained sanitarian could direct health activities satisfactorily. They also thought it unwise for the office of hotel inspector to be politically controlled. Perhaps they resented what might be considered interference by the United Commercial Travelers.

No sooner had word got about that hotel inspection might lose its identity as a separate state function and be merged with another department than the United Commercial Travelers, now thoroughly organized, took steps to prevent the merger. On June 7, 1923, its grand council for Minnesota and North Dakota unanimously passed and sent to the interim legislative committee a resolution strongly protesting any change in the status of the hotel inspection department, saying that it should "remain unmolested and be given the recognition and financial support to which this Department is so justly entitled." Henry C. Capser, chairman of the group's hotel legislative committee, worked valiantly to accomplish this, but he reported that "As soon as the Legislature convened we found the 'Cards stacked' to either obliterate entirely our Hotel Law which we have so guardedly fostered or place it in obscurity by merging the same with other departments." Publicly Wittbecker was content merely to say that his department was passing through a period of readjustment, "the final outcome of which is hard to foresee." [10]

The end came more suddenly, perhaps, than he believed possible. Under the reorganization of 1925 the hotel inspection department was abolished and its functions were transferred to the health department. After the first shock of disappointment had passed, and perhaps because they had to make the best of it, both Wittbecker and the United Commercial Travelers kept their resentment at a minimum. Wittbecker, indeed, said that affiliation with the state health department was

[9] United Commercial Travelers, *Proceedings*, 1922, p. 97; 1924, p. 65.
[10] United Commercial Travelers, *Proceedings*, 1923, pp. 30, 124; 1924, p. 65.

a great help and gave hotel inspection the "benefit of the prestige which this organization enjoys among the people of the State of Minnesota." The United Commercial Travelers was a bit more outspoken, saying that the "amalgamation is not conducive of any advantage nor in keeping with the desired results to be produced by the State Hotel Inspection Department, in the interest of not only the membership of our Order but the general traveling public." [11]

When Wittbecker became a member of the staff of the state health department his actual status changed very slightly. Hotel inspection continued as a separate department, but reports were made directly to health officials. They, however, did not appoint either the chief inspector or his deputies. No doubt this arrangement was not as satisfactory as it might have been, and perhaps health officers considered the division of hotel inspection a particularly vexing stepchild. Nevertheless Wittbecker and his successors continued their duties as best they could.

Among their first obligations, after the reorganization, was the inspection of county and state fairs. These annual celebrations had been a sanitary disgrace for years. An inspector reported in 1925 that at both Rochester and Mankato "it was a difficult matter to find their meat on account of flies as no effort was made to cover anything and in no case did I find garbage under cover." He also described toilets at the Mankato fairgrounds as a "disgrace and menace to the public." Much the same conditions prevailed at the Hennepin County Fair, but there, after recommendations were made, the place was cleaned up and the hamburger was "well taken care of in crocks and covered." [12]

The Minnesota State Fair revealed insanitary conditions on a large scale. Wittbecker found inadequate water and sewerage systems, complained that garbage was not removed frequently enough, described some eating places as having no floors, and said that ice wagons and ice-cream wagons were permitted to stand for long periods while dripping water formed nasty pools of mud. He told Chesley that a sanitary survey of the grounds should be undertaken by a competent engineer and added that he thought specific regulations should be drawn up to cover fairs. More than seventeen hundred pounds of spoiled meat — wieners, hamburger, chicken, and fish — were condemned on the fair-

[11] *Laws*, 1925, p. 768; State Board of Health, *Reports*, 1922–43, p. 155; United Commercial Travelers, *Proceedings*, 1926, pp. 65, 89.

[12] O. E. Kittleson to the State Hotel Department, August 22, 1925, and C. A. Ehlers to W. A. Wittbecker, August 31, 1925, in Minnesota Department of Health, "Reports and Hearings," 1925, pp. 366, 367, Minnesota Department of Health, St. Paul.

grounds in 1925.[13] By persistent effort some sanitary evils have been eradicated from Minnesota's fairgrounds, but in 1948 a careful sanitary survey made of many permanent refreshment stands revealed the need for further improvements.[14]

Another duty of the division of hotel inspection, one that Wittbecker had foreseen, was the investigation of tourist resorts, a new type of housing problem brought about by the automobile and hard roads. Some 550 of these resorts were scattered throughout Minnesota in 1927. Four inspectors, driving cars, were assigned to resort inspection, but Wittbecker made it plain that they were not engineers and therefore were not competent to deal with engineering problems. He said that Whittaker had volunteered to "find some advanced engineering students to whom he could give a short course of instruction that would fit them for this work." The primary problem, as Wittbecker saw it, involved water supply. "We found places," he said, "where the water was taken directly from a lake with an intake pipe extending only fifteen feet into the lake. Some took the water from open springs which are subject to flooding at every rain and also subject to pollution by animals and birds."[15]

A year later, after resorts had been checked by engineers from the division of sanitation, Wittbecker wrote that something must be done about tourist camps, which, he said, could not continue without serious menace to the health of people. "Many of them," he continued, "are in a most insanitary state and much criticism is being leveled at the State Health authorities, unjustly it is true, but the public simply sees the condition and naturally blames health authorities for the continuance of these conditions." He pleaded for extra funds with which to engage a sanitary engineer for eight months to check tourist camps. At the same time he reported to the United Commercial Travelers that tourist-resort keepers "have entered into the spirit of our work with a willingness that is certainly commendable and the time is not very far distant when we can say to the world that the tourist resorts of Minnesota stand pre-eminent in the front rank of summer play grounds."[16]

[13] Wittbecker to Chesley, September 18, 1925, to Harry J. Frost, September 28, 1925, and to Chesley, October 3, 1925, and Division of Hotel Inspection, "Report of Activities in Connection with the 1925 State Fair," in Minnesota Department of Health, "Reports and Hearings," 1925, pp. 353, 356, 357, 359, Minnesota Department of Health, St. Paul.
[14] Interview of the author with Harold S. Adams, September 9, 1948. During August, 1948, the author spent much time with hotel inspectors.
[15] Division of Hotel Inspection, "Quarterly Reports," March 31, 1927, Minnesota Department of Health, Minneapolis.
[16] Division of Hotel Inspection, "Quarterly Reports," September 30, 1928; United Commercial Travelers, *Proceedings*, 1928, p. 79.

By 1930, when A. W. Lindberg had succeeded Wittbecker, the hotel inspection staff consisted of an inspector, six deputies, a stenographer, and two clerks. Lindberg reported 3,786 inspections and 355 orders issued. Of these, 99 were complied with. From then until 1947 the general pattern of the division of hotel inspection remained the same. E. H. Berg followed Lindberg as director. He, in turn, was succeeded by Mrs. Laura E. Naplin, who cited the accomplishments of an insufficient number of inspectors, spoke of increased efficiency in inspection methods, said that the number of places requiring inspection was rapidly growing, and declared herself pleased that her division was taking in greater receipts. Her report in 1938 showed that 10,906 licenses were issued in 1929 and 19,856 in 1937; that 757 orders were issued in 1929 and 2,274 in 1937; and that appropriations or resources in 1929 were $41,752.97, compared with $45,000 in 1937. The last politically appointed inspector was Theodore T. Wold, who had previously been in the hotel business. He made his first report in 1939 and served until August, 1947. The only significant laws concerning hotel inspection to be passed between 1925 and 1943 were two acts of 1935; one dealing with the use of original containers for food or drinks and the other relating to the equipment and regulation of hotels, restaurants, lodginghouses, boardinghouses, and places of refreshment. In the latter, the term "enclosure" was incorporated in the description of places subject to inspection, thereby bringing within its scope every dining and sleeping car within the state.[17]

The first nonpolitical appointment of a hotel inspector was made in 1947 and marked the beginning of a new era. On September 16 Harold S. Adams, trained in public health and having had wide experience both in the United States Public Health Service and in municipal health work, became director of the division of hotel and resort inspection. This division was an agency of the section of environmental sanitation, as were the divisions of municipal water supply, water pollution control, industrial health, and general sanitation. When Adams began his duties the field inspection staff consisted of nine men, three of whom had full civil service status. The remaining six were provisional appointees. This staff obviously was insufficient to make an annual inspection of all hotels and public eating places in the state and to supervise the safety of small boats used for hire, a task imposed upon the division by the legislature in 1945. A certain amount of assistance, of

[17] Division of Hotel Inspection, "Quarterly Reports," March 31, 1930; United Commercial Travelers, *Proceedings*, 1934, p. 163; 1936, p. 100; 1938, p. 107; 1939, pp. 91–93; *Laws*, 1935, pp. 171–173, 495–498.

course, came from municipal hotel inspectors with whom a co-operative working agreement was arranged.[18]

To the general public perhaps the most interesting function of a hotel inspector, and one which is an important safeguard of health, is the supervision of food, food handlers, and eating places. The Minnesota resident and visitor both are anxious to have clean food served them in a sanitary environment. The act of 1919 placed the supervision of restaurants in the hands of the division of hotel inspection. For several years eating places that Wold's inspectors found satisfactory were given a certificate to display publicly, but this practice was discontinued in 1947. "Until rigid sanitary standards can be established, and consistently met, and until our staff has been expanded to allow for more frequent inspections, the issuance of such an award has been deemed inadvisable," wrote Adams.[19]

He knew what he was talking about, for milk and food sanitation practices were his specialty. During 1944, three years before he became director of the hotel inspection division, Adams, then a reserve captain in the United States Public Health Service, was sent to Minnesota to assist the division of sanitation. Much of his work was concerned with food. He made an investigation of the commissary of the Northwest Airlines at Wold-Chamberlain Field, reported on the food sanitation program of the Minneapolis Division of Public Health, and recommended sanitary improvements for forty-eight food establishments in Duluth.[20]

There was real reason, of course, why these surveys were undertaken. From January 1, 1935, to September 1, 1943, the division of preventable diseases had traced 2,005 cases of food poisoning with 13 deaths to foods other than milk and dairy products. The health department had requested assistance from the United States Public Health Service to develop and promote a program in restaurant sanitation. To meet this request Captain Adams was ordered to Minnesota. The program, which

[18] Minnesota Department of Health, "Organization Chart, March, 1948"; Division of Hotel and Resort Inspection, "Quarterly Reports," September 30, 1947; *Statutes,* 1945, chapter 157.
[19] *Laws,* 1919, pp. 661–670; Division of Hotel and Resort Inspection, "Quarterly Reports," September 30, 1947; Adams to Chesley, December 7, 1944, Minnesota Department of Health, Minneapolis.
[20] Adams, "Report on Investigation of the Commissary of the North West Airlines at Wold-Chamberlain Field . . . Minneapolis, Minnesota, June 28, 1944," "A Report on the Food Sanitation Program in the Minneapolis Division of Public Health, October, 1944," and "Suggested Inspection Points to Be Observed and Sanitary Improvements Recommended for Forty-Eight Food Establishments Surveyed in Duluth, Minnesota, July, 1944" (typescripts), Minnesota Department of Health, Minneapolis.

was directed primarily toward improving the local control of establishments handling food and drink, was well accepted. Courses of instruction for food handlers were given in Minneapolis, Duluth, and elsewhere. Early in September, 1944, Winona enacted the United States Public Health Service's "Recommended Ordinance and Code for Regulating Eating and Drinking Establishments," and thus became the first Minnesota city to take this commendable action.[21]

Minneapolis also moved forward with a food sanitation program. Early in 1945 officials of the Minneapolis Restaurant Association met with the health commissioner to discuss plans for the organization of a course in sanitation for hotel, tavern, and restaurant employees. Some 450 managers, owners, and operators of such establishments attended a meeting in February, at which definite plans were made for a course to begin later in the month. More than 2,000 Minneapolis food handlers attended at least one two-hour class, and 792 completed the course and received certificates. Soon Minneapolis bakers asked for instruction in bakery sanitation. Lectures were given to 125 bakers in March, and later fifteen bakeries were investigated at their owners' request. Other surveys and meetings were held in Moorhead, Mankato, and Bemidji. Investigations also were made of three restaurants operated by the Minneapolis park commissioners, of the kitchen and cafeteria at the University Farm School, of the cafeteria of the Butler Ship Building Corporation in Duluth, and of the Williams Box Lunch Company in St. Paul. All these surveys were requested by responsible officials who were anxious to improve their service in any possible manner.[22]

The Minnesota Junior Chamber of Commerce became vitally interested in the restaurant sanitation program and made sanitation one of its major projects for the year. So much enthusiasm was created that a number of municipalities requested surveys and ratings of their food establishments. At Fergus Falls in 1946 food handlers attended a school to prepare restaurant owners and employees for the operation of the United States Public Health Service ordinance soon to go into effect. Courses for hotel inspectors had been presented in the past, but not until the 1940s were schools for restaurant employees held in Minnesota.[23]

[21] Division of Sanitation, "Quarterly Reports," March 31, September 30, 1944.
[22] Division of Sanitation, "Quarterly Reports," September 30, 1944; Clare Gates to Whittaker, January 28, 1946, Minnesota Department of Health, Minneapolis.
[23] Division of Sanitation, "Quarterly Reports," March 31, 1931, September 30, 1945, September 30, 1946.

The basic principles of food establishment sanitation, employees were told, require that the customer's health be protected against contaminated foods and communicable disease organisms; and how well customers are protected depends upon how well an establishment, whatever its size, conforms to the following sanitation points:

1. The safety of the food and drink served.
2. The personal hygiene and food-handling practices of the food worker.
3. The safety of the water supply.
4. The sanitary disposal of sewage and water-carried wastes.
5. The protection of food from contamination during processing, display, and storage.
6. The washing, sanitizing, and storing of utensils and equipment.
7. The sanitary maintenance of the premises, including general arrangement and upkeep, refrigeration, light and ventilation, toilet and handwashing facilities, housekeeping practices, and the disposal of garbage and refuse.[24]

These were fundamentals upon which rested the safety of Minnesotans who ate away from home. Inspectors knew that generalizations would be of little help to chefs and waitresses; general principles must be made specific. Therefore they demonstrated, for example, how butter patties should be served with a butter fork, how glasses should be held by the bottom or the side instead of by the rim, and how pastries should be picked up with tongs or individual pieces of waxed paper. It was explained why food handlers should wear hair nets or bands and why all workers — dishwashers, bus boys, kitchen help — should remove street clothes and don clean, washable, light-colored outer garments when on duty. A crisp list of twelve practices to be avoided was made available. These included: "Don't go on duty with a severe head cold, sore throat, or any acute illness." "Don't report for duty if you have any skin infection or sores. . . . Consult a doctor." "Don't leave the toilet room without thoroughly washing your hands. . . . Keep nails trimmed and clean." [25]

These admonitions seem obvious enough, but hotel division inspectors knew how many, many times in scores of public eating places they were violated daily. They realized, too, that many restaurant managers had no idea that water for rinsing dishes should be at least 170°; that flies, cockroaches, ants, mice, and rats carry disease; that careful scraping of dishes before washing means less contamination of the dishwater; that proper racking of dishes is necessary to enable wash and

[24] Adams, *Milk and Food Sanitation Practice*, 164 (New York, 1947).
[25] Adams, *Milk and Food Sanitation Practice*, 164, 172.

rinse water to reach all surfaces; and that five approved rules had been established by sanitarians for the proper storing of utensils. The problem of food handling and serving was tied up, too, with engineering. Toilet plumbing and cesspools must not be too close to the source of water supply. These and a hundred more significant details were hammered home in order to protect the public's health.[26]

Even with such a strenuous campaign — one in which the United States Public Health Service was interested on a national level and one that drew articles in nationally popular magazines — disease outbreaks resulting from contaminated foods were far too numerous in the United States. They were traced to fruitades, precooked hams, salads, cream puffs, ground beef and hamburger, potato salad, chili, chicken fricassee. This list is long. In a northern Minnesota town in 1948 six persons ate baked ham sandwiches at a local cafe and each became ill. Laboratory analysis revealed hemolytic staphylococci present in the ham, and, after long investigation, the source of the outbreak was surmised to have stemmed from an ear infection of an employee. The worker worried his ear with a finger and then, without washing, sliced ham and prepared sandwiches. Another food handler was found to be a typhoid carrier. In 1946 sixteen persons fell ill after eating chow mein. Two years later six other persons reported food poisoning after they had eaten at the same restaurant. Unless managers and food handlers are taught sanitary practices and unless inspections are frequent, it is possible for such incidents to be repeated again and again in Minnesota.[27]

The division of hotel and resort inspection realizes that only constant watchfulness, education, and strict inspection procedures can make public eating places safe. There can be no halfway measures. That is why inspectors, when they go into a dining room, check carefully on a printed form ten items, including conditions behind and underneath counters, window screening, beer coils, linen, dishes, silverware, and ventilation. In kitchens they note the condition of floors, walls, and ceilings, of piping and light fixtures, of sinks, washbowls, stoves, canopies, coffee urns, pots, warming tables, and plumbing. They

[26] Adams, *Milk and Food Sanitation Practice*, 173–231; *Minnesota State Health Laws and Regulations*, 113 (January 1, 1948).

[27] Howard Whitman, "Disease a la Carte," in *Woman's Home Companion*, vol. 73, no. 12, p. 34 (December, 1946); United States Public Health Service, *Disease Outbreaks Conveyed through Foods other than Milk and Milk Products in the United States in 1945 as Reported by State and Territorial Health Authorities* (Washington, D.C., 1946); Adams to Dean Fleming, August 4, 1948, C. Barton Nelson to Adams, April 15, May 4, 1948, and Fleming to T. T. Ross, April 15, 1948, Minnesota Department of Health, Minneapolis.

look at toilet facilities, note the type of towels furnished, examine basements, backyards, stocks, and stores, and inspect water supplies and sewage disposal systems.[28]

If either water supply or sewerage system is inadequate, notation is made and the problem is referred to the division of general sanitation, which dispatches an engineer to make recommendations. If the condition is an immediate danger to public health, an inspector, under the law, may close an establishment. He may also issue an order, having the force of law, requiring that certain evils be corrected within a reasonable period of time. The degree to which the sanitary engineer assists the hotel inspector is well illustrated by the following example.

The wells of a Ramsey County restaurant upon inspection were found to be below the health department's standards, for they were situated within ten feet of the basement and were not provided with protective outside casings. These faults constituted health hazards. Engineers, following the usual practice of the department, which is based upon friendly helpfulness rather than brusque use of legal machinery, surveyed the restaurant. They recommended that the wells be provided with double protective casing and with a concrete platform sloped to drain away from the wells and placed at an elevation of at least six inches above the outside ground level, and that they be disinfected after repair work was completed. On the other hand, a small-town drugstore received orders to discontinue at once the use of water from its well for human consumption, and the well was condemned. The owner was further informed that the location of a new well site and the construction of the new well must be approved by the state health department. Yet some health officers affirm that inspection on the state level never can be as satisfactory as a program of vigorous local inspection.[29]

The mere mechanics of food supervision alone could keep the entire staff of the division of hotel and resort inspection constantly busy, but the division is charged with other equally significant responsibilities. Among them is the supervision of camp locations, a constantly growing problem since the advent of the automobile age. Generally speaking, these camps first were inspected to determine adequacy of water supplies, of toilet facilities and sewage disposal, and of garbage and refuse disposal. Camps were classified into two groups: overnight camps

---

[28] Data taken from inspectors' report form, 1948. This form was in process of revision and will be more detailed.

[29] Division of Sanitation, "Report on Investigation of Sanitary Facilities of the [name withheld] Restaurant, Mounds View Township, Ramsey County, Minnesota, July 31, 1942" and Division of Hotel and Resort Inspection, "Notice of Orders to [name withheld], May 18, 1948" (typescripts), Minnesota Department of Health, Minneapolis.

where tourists stopped only for a night's rest while en route to vacation centers and vacation camps where tourists remained to fish and hunt. In 1929 fully ninety per cent of Minnesota camps were owned and operated by municipalities or civic organizations. In general, these camps were not self-supporting. Of 127 camps investigated, 62 were supplied with water from municipal supplies; 49 had unsatisfactory wells or well constructions; 75 were equipped with unsanitary pit privies; and only 9 were using gas for cooking, only 2, electricity, and 52 used wood or coal.[30]

It was so difficult for inspectors to locate all the tourist camps that on January 22, 1930, the state board passed a regulation requiring that every person, organization, or municipality establishing or controlling a camp must register its name, location, ownership, person in charge, and such other data as might be required. This, then, was the legal beginning of supervision to protect the tourist's health. Eight years later the board interested itself in city and village ordinances covering trailer camps, and it found that none included every item of sanitation that was believed imperative. As a result, a model ordinance was worked out which guided innumerable Minnesota communities toward better camp control. This meant, of course, greater health safety for travelers.[31]

Camps increased rapidly between 1940 and 1948. The war years in particular saw the mushrooming of industrial and semi-industrial trailer camps that sprang up almost overnight in defense areas. These constituted a special problem for sanitarians and hotel inspectors. An assistant sanitary engineer of the United States Public Health Service was ordered to Minnesota early in 1942 to assist local and state health authorities. Within three months twenty trailer camps were inspected in the vicinity of the Twin City Ordnance Plant near New Brighton. The Village of New Brighton co-operated admirably in 1942 by passing a trailer-camp ordinance which not only was a model, but which also was enforced. Considerable work was done also in the vicinity of the Gopher Ordnance Works at Rosemount and near the Northern Pump Company at Fridley. The construction of cabins on trailer-camp sites offered unexpected problems. All in all, ninety-one camps with an es-

[30] Division of Sanitation, "Quarterly Reports," June 30, 1929; Divisions of Sanitation and Hotel Inspection, "Report of an Investigation of Tourist Camps in Minnesota, June–September, 1929" (typescript), Minnesota Department of Health, Minneapolis.
[31] Minnesota State Board of Health, "Regulation 247," January 22, 1930 (typescript), and George O. Pierce to Carl E. Green, September 8, 1938, Minnesota Department of Health, Minneapolis; *Minnesota State Health Laws and Regulations*, 115 (January 1, 1948).

timated population of 2,125 were surveyed and sanitary investigations were made of two prisoner-of-war camps and one foreign-labor camp.[32] After peace came, attention turned once more to surveys of private and municipal camps.

In 1948 approximately twenty-eight hundred resorts of varying types were operating in the state, with the bulk of them located in twelve northern counties. Summer hotels and resorts, as differentiated from trailer camps, offered the same type of sanitary problem. In 1927 the division of sanitation was authorized to spend about six thousand dollars from the balance of the hotel inspection fund to conduct a sanitary survey of summer resorts and tourist camps. Then approximately four hundred summer resorts were operating throughout the state. A staff of four sanitary engineers, one laboratory assistant, a laboratory attendant, and a stenographer was created for the survey, which began on June 16. The results were sent to the division of hotel inspection to be relayed to resort owners with orders from that division. During the years that followed, periodic inspection by hotel inspectors was supplemented by special investigations made by the division of sanitation. In 1936 the St. Louis County Board of Commissioners passed a resolution requiring that all applications to sell nonintoxicating malt liquors be approved by the county health department before permits were issued. But not until 1944 were St. Louis County dispensers of nonintoxicating malt liquors required to comply with regulations of the state health board relating to hotels and public eating places.[33]

Although conditions had improved in rural taverns between 1936 and 1944, an engineer said that no such progress could be ascertained in resorts. He proved his point by compiling a table of comparisons that clearly revealed indifference on the part of resort owners in St. Louis County. On every count — water supply, sewage disposal, garbage disposal — resorts lagged behind taverns. By 1946 country clubs as well as resorts were investigated.[34]

[32] Division of Sanitation, "Quarterly Reports," March 31, June 30, September 30, 1942, September 30, 1945; Village of New Brighton, "Ordinance No. 4 — An Ordinance for the Construction, Maintenance and Operation of Public Automobile and Trailer Camps within the Village of New Brighton, Requiring Permits for the Construction and Maintenance Thereof, and Providing Penalties for the Violation of Said Ordinance," in *Ramsey County News*, March 12, 1942.
[33] Division of Hotel and Resort Inspection, "Quarterly Reports," June 30, 1948; Division of Sanitation, "Quarterly Reports," June 30, 1927; E. C. Slagle to Whittaker, June 23, 1944. Minnesota Department of Health, Minneapolis.
[34] E. C. Slagle, "Memorandum on Status of Water Supplies and Excreta Disposal Facilities at Various Resorts and Taverns in the [4th Health] District, January 1, 1944" (typescript); Division of Hotel Inspection, *Reports*, 1946, no. 80. Minnesota Department of Health, Minneapolis.

Closely connected with resort life and a part of Minnesota's recreational pattern is the summer camp. Hundreds of camps, sponsored by churches and youth organizations, operate annually. In the 1930s Whittaker saw his own son return from a Boy Scout camp with impetigo. About the same time Whittaker learned of equally poor conditions in Girl Scout camps. When he investigated, a leader insisted that her girls should rough it and maintained that pasteurized milk was not a necessity. Whittaker then invited her to visit the cow barn and the dairy. They were unutterably filthy, so filthy indeed that the leader took one look and hastily retreated.[35]

Summer camps, although there were only about a hundred of them in 1935, presented a most difficult problem. Many were located in out-of-the-way places and housed young people from all parts of the nation. The health problem, then, was of interstate as well as intrastate concern. In order to meet requests from national organizations whose charters demanded an annual inspection of their camps and in order to furnish groups with some guide to proper camp sanitation, the state health department in 1934 issued an eleven-page mimeographed manual of suggestions. This was revised and elaborated four years later, and another entirely new bulletin dealing with camp nursing services was also issued. From 1934 to 1937 the divisions of sanitation and preventable diseases prepared minimum standards for summer camps in order that, when the Camp Directors Association met, a full report might be made. Directors were then told that camp surveys would include an investigation of water supply, sewage disposal, milk supply, and garbage disposal. Twenty-two summer camps were thus surveyed, some of them in co-operation with the division of state parks of the Minnesota Department of Conservation, and reports were made to camp directors and to the committee on health and safety of the Boy Scouts of America.[36]

Whittaker then conferred with James E. West, chief scout executive, and with Captain Fred C. Mills, director of the Boy Scouts' health and safety committee. An agreement was made that the Minnesota health

[35] Interview of the author with Whittaker, March 19, 1947.
[36] George O. Pierce, "Improving Protection of Health in Summer Camps," typescript of a paper presented before the public health engineering section of the American Public Health Association in Milwaukee, October 8, 1935; Minnesota Department of Health, *Suggestions Regarding Sanitation and Medical Supervision of Summer Camps* (Minneapolis, May, 1934), *Suggestions Regarding Sanitation and Medical Supervision of Summer Camps* (Minneapolis, June, 1938), and *Suggested Policies and Standing Orders for Camp Nursing Service* (Minneapolis, June, 1938); Division of Sanitation, "Quarterly Reports," June 30, 1934; June 30, September 30, 1937.

board and the Boy Scouts of America would co-operate in a sanitary survey of camps maintained in the state. Two scout officials arrived in Minnesota and were joined by Dr. Ralph Sullivan, epidemiologist, and Herbert Bosch, sanitary engineer. These four inspected thirteen camps. All the camps were using pasteurized milk, but only four had satisfactory refrigeration for the milk, only seven complied with sanitary standards for drinking water, only four dispensed drinking water in a satisfactory manner, only four had good sources of water for washing and bathing, only five had approved methods of excreta disposal, only nine had an adequate garbage disposal system, and only one had a satisfactory method for disinfecting dishes.[37]

Results of this survey became apparent in 1939, when twenty-eight approved privies were erected and when installation of new wells, dishwater disposal systems, sewage disposal systems, and purification equipment for swimming pools was completed. Special surveys were made of Camp Lawrie and Camp Williamson, and each year thereafter summer camps were reported upon.[38]

A particularly irritating and annoying health problem which sometimes arises in summer camps and resorts is popularly called "swimmer's itch," although its technical name is *schistosome dermatitis*. This shows itself on the bather's body as a smarting skin eruption, resulting from the penetration of the skin by the larvae or young of a certain species of parasite. It is particularly common, it seems, in the vicinity of Duluth, Bemidji, Ely, Brainerd, above Taylors Falls, and in the Twin Cities area, including lakes in Anoka, Hennepin, Ramsey, and Chisago counties. In 1941 this little plague manifested itself at the summer camp of the St. Paul Boys' Club of the Union Gospel Mission; a year later it appeared in Turtle Lake; and three years later it made life miserable for scouts at Camp Ajawah on Linwood Lake. Health officials have achieved good results in preventing the itch by using copper salts in the water over a limited area, but they also have warned against indiscriminate use of copper salts since they are dangerous to fish and other aquatic life. Swimmer's itch developed so rapidly in Minnesota that the health department issued a public warning about it in 1947[39]

[37] Division of Sanitation, "Quarterly Reports," September 30, 1938.
[38] Division of Sanitation, "Quarterly Reports," June 30, 1939; Section of Environmental Sanitation, "Quarterly Reports," September 30, 1947; Chesley to Harry Bartelt, May 24, 1938 [*1939*], Minnesota Department of Health, Minneapolis.
[39] John N. Wilson, "The Control of 'Swimmer's Itch,'" in *Conservation Volunteer*, vol. 10, no. 58 pp. 43–46 (May–June, 1947); Division of Sanitation, "Quarterly Reports," June 30, 1941; Chesley to John A. Moga, August 26, 1942; Division of

This concern with bathing, of course, was no novelty to the sanitation division, which in 1917 had made a sanitary survey of the public baths in Minneapolis, had established rules for operating swimming pools, had investigated the artificial outdoor swimming pool at Fort Snelling at the request of medical officers, and had reported upon a swimming pool constructed as a Civil Works Administration project in the Otter Tail River. It had also helped make safe for public use a beach on Silver Lake, as well as many other beaches and indoor and outdoor pools.[40]

Besides offering swimming facilities, many beaches rented boats for the enjoyment of patrons, and not until 1945 were adequate provisions made to protect persons who rented them. In that year the legislature passed an act providing that owners of boats rented for use on the state's public waters must secure licenses from the division of hotel and resort inspection and must see that the boats complied with certain safety standards. Among the regulations pertaining to small boat safety were the following: Boats should be marked with a capacity number. No boat not free from spilled gasoline and oil should be rented, nor should one be rented to a person obviously in an intoxicated condition, nor for the purpose of breaking ice. Rear transoms must be strongly constructed and capable of standing strains imposed by full reversing motors, and all oars, oarlocks, and paddles must be free of cracks, splits, and breaks at the time of rental. The license fee was fifty cents per boat. In 1948 thirty thousand boats were licensed and tags for them were mailed to boat livery and resort operators.[41]

Not all measures to protect the public health are directly administered by the Minnesota Department of Health, although frequently the department is vitally concerned. Through the years much significant legislation has been passed to help insure the public's safety. Its administration, in many respects, is as much a part of the program of

---

Sanitation, "Report on Investigation of 'Swimmers' Itch' at Turtle Lake, Mounds View Township, Ramsey County, Minnesota, July 20 and 25, 1942," and "Memorandum on Investigation of Outbreak of Swimmers' Itch on Linwood Lake, Linwood Township, Anoka County, Minnesota, June 25, 1946," Minnesota Department of Health, Minneapolis; *Minnesota's Health*, vol. 1, no. 5, p. 3 (May, 1947).

[40] Division of Sanitation, "Quarterly Reports," June 30, 1917, September 30, 1928, June 30, 1934; *Minnesota State Health Laws and Regulations*, 89 (January 1, 1948); Section of Environmental Sanitation, "Investigation of the Public Bathing Beach on Silver Lake, June 17, 1947" (typescript), Minnesota Department of Health, Minneapolis.

[41] *Laws*, 1945, p. 583; Theodore T. Wold, "Boat Inspection under Way," in *Conservation Volunteer*, vol. 8, no. 48, p. 14 (September–October, 1945); *Minnesota State Health Laws and Regulations*, 110 (January 1, 1948); Division of Hotel and Resort Inspection, "Quarterly Reports," June 30, 1948.

ceaseless vigilance as is the work of the section of environmental sanitation or its division of hotel and resort inspection. A Basic Science Act, for example, was passed in 1927, which, generally speaking, makes it illegal for unauthorized and nonlicensed persons to engage in the practice of healing. Other acts, passed between 1887 and 1927, established a board of medical examiners with authority to prescribe rules and regulations for the examination of applicants for licenses to practice medicine, surgery, and obstetrics. Similar acts were passed regulating the dental profession and pharmacists. Closely allied with the latter were restraints upon the sale of harmful drugs and the establishment of standards of purity for drugs. A board of pharmacy also was created. Dean Frederick John Wulling, pioneer pharmacist at the University of Minnesota, was a leader in every crusade to improve his profession.[42]

Protective legislation went still further. The Minnesotan who patronizes a chiropodist, the man who drops into a barbershop for a haircut, and the woman who phones her beauty parlor for an appointment — all these can be fairly well assured of the services of licensed operators and of sanitary conditions. The first bit of legislation bearing upon chiropody was passed in 1917. Others followed which defined terms and phrases and set up a board of registration in chiropody. Barbers first were regulated in 1897, and beauticians in 1927. Other laws bearing upon health regulated the University of Minnesota hospitals. In 1945 the legislature, in order to make "possible a wider and more timely availability of medical care, thereby advancing the public health," passed an act providing for the incorporation of voluntary nonprofit medical service organizations, such as the Blue Shield plan.[43]

The University of Minnesota also assisted in the protection of public health by training future health officers and nurses. Hewitt, of course, had advocated this type of instruction and, indeed, had taught courses in hygiene to university students. Not until 1922, however, did the university establish a separate Department of Preventive Medicine and Public Health. A course in public health nursing had been organized in 1918, one of the first such courses in the nation. Under the terms of

[42] *Laws*, 1885, pp. 179–184, 264–267; 1887, pp. 46–49; 1891, pp. 172–177; 1895, pp. 209–211; 1911, pp. 296–299; 1913, pp. 854–858; 1921, p. 67, 241–244; 1923, p. 22; 1927, pp. 153–160, 228–237, 282–285; 1925, pp. 197–204; 1937, pp. 485–493; 1939, pp. 162–164; Emerson G. Wulling, ed., *Pharmacy Forward* (La Crosse, Wisconsin, 1948).

[43] *Laws*, 1897, pp. 346–349; 1917, pp. 541–545; 1921, pp. 622–630, 655–660; 1927, pp. 349–355, 426–435; 1929, pp. 321–331; 1933, pp. 336–340; 1935, pp. 482–485; 1941, pp. 896–906; 1945, pp. 430–435; *Statutes*, 1923, paragraph 4577; 1927, paragraph 4577–4598.

the Social Security Act, the university developed a curriculum for the training of health officers and public health engineers. The final step was taken in 1944 when a School of Public Health, now accredited by the American Public Health Association and by the National Organization for Public Health Nursing, was established.[44] Under the leadership of Dr. Gaylord W. Anderson, the school grew rapidly. By 1949 students from more than thirty states and fifteen foreign countries were enrolled, and the school was recognized throughout the country as one of the best of its kind for the preparation of workers who, in the future, would keep professional vigilance over the public health of the state.

[44] State Board of Health, *Annual Reports*, 1873, p. 15; University of Minnesota, School of Public Health, *Announcements for the Years 1948–50*, 11 (Minneapolis, May 14, 1948).

18

Blue Cap and Black Bag

"THE FACT is there are but few regular nurses in St. Paul," said the *Pioneer Press* unhappily in 1883, "and it is asserted upon good authority that there have been many incompetent nurses in the field here and consequently a good deal of bad nursing." [1]

This less-than-tolerant attitude toward the nursing profession was not uncommon during the quarter century following the Civil War. At a time when women slowly were forcing an entrance into the business world as secretaries and when many men believed vigorously that "woman's place is in the home," it was difficult for a girl to enter nursing without strong opposition. Sisters of Charity might be expected to minister to the sick, but many folk considered it unthinkable for a respectable young woman to become a professional nurse. Of course, she should tend her husband and children when they fell ill and she might carry jellies and smooth brows if the nation was at war, but she certainly should not expect to make a career of nursing. Yet the trained nurse rapidly superseded the old untrained volunteer who sat by the bedside and all too frequently made life miserable for the patient.

Only five years after the *Pioneer Press* spoke despairingly of local nurses, it changed its attitude entirely. Professional nursing, it said, had undergone a great change in the last few years. "From the professional nurse of the Sairy Gamp order, with her unsatisfiable thirst for tea, if not for something stronger, who took possession of the house from turret to foundation stone and brought a despair to the victim which made death easy — from all this, by gradations of poor relations in gowns of brown mohair, and old ladies with side curls and sympathetic airs and whispers that drove the patient half insane, and old

[1] *Pioneer Press*, July 22, 1883.

352

maids with manners sharp as their noses, who went out 'nussing,' we have arrived at the trained nurse of today. Now she is herself not troubled with 'the misery'; she is tactful, well educated, cheery, thoroughly competent, sympathetic but not tearful, and often actually pretty!"[2]

This transformation so graphically described by the St. Paul press did not happen without planning and energy. Minnesota was reflecting a national trend when it began to train nurses in hospitals. The movement began in the large eastern cities. As early as 1879 the New York Ethical Society had sent trained nurses into the homes of the poor; Boston organized the Instructive District Nursing Association in 1886; and Philadelphia had a Visiting Nurse Society at the same time. Chicago followed three years later. In 1897 John Wanamaker employed nurses to help his employees in New York and Philadelphia.[3] By then many hospitals were graduating girls from schools of nursing. Indeed, the American Nurses Association had been organized in 1896.

The first graduate nurse in the United States finished her training in September, 1873 — only a year after Minnesota's state health board was created — at the New England Hospital for Women and Children in Boston. Ten years later the first nurse to be graduated west of Chicago completed her training at the Northwestern Hospital for Women and Children in Minneapolis. The first class to graduate as such from Northwestern Hospital received certificates in June, 1889. Class instruction included ten lectures on surgery, fifteen on materia medica, ten on gynecology, ten on obstetrics, and others on the practice of medicine and the diseases of children. On September 8, 1898, the Ramsey County Graduate Nurses Association was formed. By then four schools of nursing were operating in St. Paul. These were connected with St. Joseph's, St. Luke's, Bethesda, and Ancker hospitals. Louisa Parsons came from Baltimore in 1892 to assume the superintendency of the training school at Ancker Hospital; St. Luke's Hospital graduated its first class of two young ladies in 1894; and the school at St. Joseph's Hospital received a class of nineteen in February, 1894. At Rochester the first commencement at the Second Minnesota Hospital for the Insane was held in April, 1892.[4]

[2] *Pioneer Press*, May 13, 1888.
[3] Mazÿck P. Ravenel, *A Half Century of Public Health,* 441 (New York, 1921). See also James H. and Mary Jane Rodabaugh, *Nursing in Ohio* (Columbus, 1951).
[4] Bertha E. Merrill, *The Trek from Yesterday: A History of Organized Nursing in Minneapolis, 1883–1936,* [11] (n.p., n.d.); Margaret L. Hauenstein, "History of Public Health Nursing in St. Paul, Minnesota," 12 (St. Louis University thesis, January, 1948); *Pioneer Press*, March 18, 1889, September 22, 1891, April 30, August 16, 1892, January 25, February 2, 1894, August 13, 1898.

Hewitt had long recognized the value of the trained nurse. He watched with interest the increase in the number of training schools and, no doubt, smiled when naive nurses published their experiences. From his St. Paul office Hewitt followed the annual attempts of Dr. A. B. Ancker to provide better quarters for twenty-one probationers. Ancker and Hewitt agreed that the training school had contributed greatly to the material prosperity of the hospital and the general comfort and happiness of patients. But Hewitt knew that most training school graduates were planning on either remaining in institutional nursing or going into private duty. The need for trained public health nurses, especially in rural areas, was so great that Hewitt twice emphasized the imperative necessity for securing nurses. "Nurses trained to the care of infectious diseases are not to be had," he told the board, "and those of the average sort find better wages, accommodations and facilities in villages and cities, so that they are difficult to secure in townships even for greater wages than poor people can — or Local Boards are willing to — pay." Then he added: "Common humanity and public safety demand that no time be lost in making the needful arrangements for providing a supply of competent women nurses, willing to serve in the care of infectious diseases in country districts, and arranging, in part at least, for their compensation."[5]

The achievement of this goal meant long years of work and it was dependent upon a score of factors that developed after Hewitt had left office. In 1889 the Associated Charities of St. Paul began to send student nurses into the homes of the poor, and graduate nurses were made available to care for cases of infectious diseases within the city. Despite the fact that the trained nurse had proved herself superior to the untrained nurse, controversy raged in 1900 when a St. Paul post of the Grand Army of the Republic recommended that graduate nurses be used in the Soldiers' Home at Minnehaha Park. When the question was put to Bracken, he side-stepped, saying only: "It would seem as though in case of sickness, the old soldiers should have as good nursing as that which would be given at all general hospitals in good standing. In a general way it may be stated that a trained nurse would be better than one not trained. However, many nurses who are nongraduates may be very capable." On May 15 the trustees of the home authorized the surgeon in charge to "employ one competent woman nurse to be placed in charge of the Hospital nurses, who will consist

---

[5] *Pioneer Press*, September 20, 1896, April 4, 1899; St. Paul City Officers, *Annual Reports*, 1899, p. 986; 1892, p. 464; 1893, p. 878; State Board of Health, *Biennial Reports*, 1891–92, p. 10; 1893–94, p. 8.

of not more than four women 'noviciates' besides the men necessary for the heavy work." [6]

By that time five hospital training schools in Minneapolis — Northwestern, Asbury, St. Barnabas, Minneapolis City, and Swedish — were graduating nurses. Schools at St. Mary's and Abbott hospitals were established shortly after 1900. A Hennepin County Graduate Nurses Association was organized during the late summer of 1901, and three years later it assumed control of a nurses' registry. The Ramsey County Graduate Nurses Association had been incorporated on September 8, 1898, and in that year it began a registry which was still operating in 1948.[7]

No sooner had Minnesota nurses become well organized than they began to push for legislative recognition. In particular they wished to have a legal distinction made between the graduate and the nongraduate nurse. A trained nurse stated her case forcibly. After arguing that specialized education made a nurse more valuable, she denounced physicians who recommended practical nurses as "just as good" and said further that "just as good" was not good enough for a sick patient. She thought registries should concern themselves only with graduate nurses, for, she said, "Is it right to educate the non-graduate by lectures and books to take the place of the nurse who has had three years' of experience in a hospital. . . . When the doctor can educate the non-graduate by means of books, lectures, and private supervision on cases to be 'just as good' as the graduate, the need for training-schools is past." [8]

In answer to the graduate nurse's plea for protection the legislature in 1907 passed a bill providing for state registration of nurses and the licensing of persons as registered nurses. A board of examiners, appointed by the governor, was created to enforce the provisions of the act. Among the board's duties was the examination of prospective registered nurses. The act also stipulated that only graduates from training schools or persons with special qualifications could register. It also provided that "A person who has received his or her certificate according to the provisions of this act shall be styled and known as a 'Registered Nurse.' No other person shall assume such title or use the

[6] *Pioneer Press*, April 11, 1899; Bracken to J. N. Schaak, August 17, 1899, and to George R. Lewis, April 28, 1900, and Lewis to Bracken, April 27, May 16, 1900, Minnesota Department of Health, St. Paul.
[7] Merrill, *The Trek from Yesterday*, 19, 21; *Pioneer Press*, August 13, 1898; Ramsey County Registered Nurses Association, "1898–1948" (St. Paul, 1948).
[8] "The Graduate vs. the Non-Graduate Nurse," in *Northwestern Lancet*, 23:384 (November 1, 1903).

abbreviation 'R.N.' or any other letters or figures to indicate that he or she is a registered nurse."[9]

Here then was the beginning of registered nurses in Minnesota, a legal description based upon professional qualifications that laid the groundwork for the certification of both private and public health nurses. Minneapolis employed the first public health nurse in Minnesota in 1902 and two years later added a tuberculosis nurse to the staff. In 1905 St. Paul established a public health nursing service, including such specialties as tuberculosis, infant welfare, and school nursing. This was managed first by the United Charities and then was taken over by the Wilder Foundation, which by 1909 employed five visiting nurses and at least two clinic nurses. A school nurse was added to St. Paul's educational system in 1909.[10]

Meanwhile state and national movements were afoot which by 1912 were to influence Minnesota nursing. The National Organization for Public Health Nursing had been formed to stimulate responsibility for the community health by the establishment and extension of public health nursing, and, in Minnesota, an official from the United States Public Health Service recommended that the state be divided into no fewer than twenty sanitary districts, each staffed with a physician trained in sanitary science and with public health nurses. Although the state health board had no regular visiting nurses on its staff in 1912, it did have the services of two nurses loaned by the Minneapolis Associated Charities. These girls — Meta Mettle and Agnes Trinko — lectured throughout the state and were the means by which visiting nurse work began to have state-wide effect.[11]

"Our uniforms were very different from those we are now wearing," remembered a Minneapolis United Charities nurse. "Our coats for winter were heavy, tight-fitting, dark blue, double-breasted ones with high, stiff, stand-up collars. They were warm as they were padded and lined throughout, but heavy and uncomfortable. The V.N. insignia was in gilt letters worn below the left shoulder. The hats were not of the soft and comfortable styles of the last few years. The summer hats were stiff, black sailors with wide brims and small crowns and were exceedingly hard to keep on the head if there was the slightest

[9] *Laws*, 1907, pp. 167–171.
[10] State Board of Health, *Reports*, 1922–43, p. 176; Hauenstein, "History of Public Health Nursing," 14.
[11] Ravenel, *A Half Century of Public Health*, 442; Fox, *Public Health Administration in Minnesota*, 79; Visiting Nurse Association of Minneapolis, *The First History of the Visiting Nurse Association of Minneapolis, 1902–27*, 8 (n.p., n.d.).

breeze. I was forever holding on to mine frantically. Our nursing bags, first used in 1907, were of the kind physicians all carried a few years ago, much heavier than the ones we carry now." [12]

By 1915 Chesley, then director of the division of preventable diseases, was advocating the creation of a field nurse corps, which would be fully instructed in the principles and practices of communicable disease work and thoroughly trained to execute quickly and efficiently the many details of intensive epidemic work. He thought such a corps would be a "most economical investment for the state." This program did not develop as Chesley had hoped, although Bracken attempted in 1916 to develop a supervisory staff of nurses. Had that been accomplished, a Minnesota community contemplating hiring a nurse would have been expected to consult with the board first. After approval was secured, a nurse from the board would introduce a local nurse to her work. The legislature, however, did not appropriate sufficient funds, and the program died before it was born.[13]

Nevertheless the board created the position of superintendent of nurses in 1916, but two years elapsed before it was filled. The delay was caused by lack of finances. When Frances V. Brink was appointed on July 9, 1918, she was well acquainted with preventable disease work. She had been in the employ of the board and had been concerned with the organization of baby clinics and with the selection of community and school nurses, and she had taken an active part in rural health education. She was acquainted with Anna Mae Coleman, Hennepin County public health nurse, and knew that Thief River Falls was planning to hire a full-time nurse. Unfortunately World War I interfered seriously with Miss Brink's activities, although she did have the assistance of one other nurse. The influenza epidemic, beginning in October, 1918, also crippled normal nursing activities. Miss Brink nevertheless found time to engage in educational activities and to play a role in an investigation of maternity hospitals made jointly by the health board and the State Board of Control. She resigned on July 1, 1921, and the position remained vacant because of lack of funds. The future of public health nursing looked dark indeed during those days. Exclusive of public health nurses in Minneapolis, St. Paul, and Duluth, there were only fourteen village community nurses, forty-four village school nurses, and sixty-five county nurses in the state in 1919. The

[12] Visiting Nurse Association of Minneapolis, *The First History*, 8.
[13] State Board of Health, *Biennial Reports*, 1914–15, p. 121; Bracken to C. A. Harper, December 1, 1916, Minnesota Department of Health, St. Paul.

resignation of Miss Brink left these nurses without state leadership or supervision. It looked as if public health nursing was on the wane. But, just in time, two factors altered the situation entirely.[14]

The first was a legislative act authorizing city and village councils, boards of county commissioners, and town boards to employ public health nurses. The state health department was interested because the act specified that nurses should make written reports to it. Furthermore, boards of county commissioners could legally detail any public health nurse to act under the direction of the county superintendent of schools, the county child welfare board, or the county health officer. This bill, sponsored by the lay section of the State Organization for Public Health Nursing, was approved on February 27, 1919, and it stimulated increased interest in public health nursing.[15]

The second beneficial factor came two years later, when the Sheppard-Towner Act was passed in November, 1921. This made possible the use of federal funds. A third encouraging development had occurred in 1918, when the University of Minnesota, in co-operation with the Minnesota Public Health Association, the Red Cross, the extension division of the university, and the state health board began instruction in public health nursing. In 1925 the legislature provided that public health nurses be registered and certified and that "such nurses shall receive, upon request, the aid and advice of the State Board of Health in regard to nursing problems." [16]

The Minnesota public health nurse during the 1920s was a pioneer. Not only was she introducing a new service to scores of communities, but she was also braving innumerable hardships to reach patients. In many counties, still studded with timber, the nurse stumbled on foot along forest paths. With her black bag slung over a shoulder she sloshed through mud during rainy seasons and broke trail on snowshoes in winter. She warmed her cold hands at rustic stoves and, when she stepped from her rooming house on a frosty morning, she smelled the tantalizing odor of wood smoke. Highways were not always ribbons of concrete, but pitted, rutted affairs which at times became so primitive that the nurse left her temperamental automobile to continue on foot. Then, too, the nurse had to cope with a confusion of foreign tongues, with ignorance and prejudice, and with Old World super-

[14] State Board of Health, *Biennial Reports*, 1916–17, p. 14; 1918–19, pp. 53–56; 1920–21, p. 9; Anna Mae Coleman, "The County Nurse," in *Northwest Farmstead*, vol. 20, no. 24, p. 21 (December 15, 1919); Huenekens to Mrs. H. W. Froelich, September 14, 1918, Minnesota Department of Health, St. Paul.
[15] *Laws*, 1919, p. 35.
[16] *Laws*, 1925, p. 222.

stitions. Before she could nurse, she had to win the confidence of skeptical patients and relatives. This was not always easy. Frequently nurses were so busy that they neglected to make reports. When they did have time to write, their accounts, during the 1920s, indicated clearly the daily hazards of the profession.

"We had a very wild trip this month," wrote a St. Louis County nurse. "It was not so very far but what there was of it was thrilling. Was going out to have a Home Nursing Class about 60 miles north of Duluth. I had always made this trip by car so I started. Good roads lasted the first 25 miles but the next 13 miles had only been traveled by team and the next 12 miles had not been traveled at all, but after getting that far I was sure that my Dodge sure would see me through the rest of the drifts and any other difficulties that we might encounter so we traveled on. We finally arrived much overheated and in time for the class. They were all glad to see us arrive as they knew that we were on the way. They insisted that I wait until the next day to come back but I did not because of the weather, so after class we started back. . . . We made the trip both ways without getting stuck or having to shovel once — having faith in our car is great." Other nurses described their difficulties in transporting patients from homes to hospitals. One Indian lad was carried a half mile in a rowboat, twenty miles by car, and the last two miles in a motorboat.[17]

Conditions like these improved somewhat during the next twenty years, but rural nursing never has been an easy job. A somewhat typical county nursing program in 1939 included seven specialized activities. The success or failure of each depended largely upon the professional skill and the personality of the nurse. It was she who inspected pupils in rural and village schools and who made follow-up visits to children with serious handicaps. The nurse planned a vision-testing program for teachers, encouraged dental care, and interested herself in obtaining hot lunches for school children. But school activities were only the first in her seven-point program. The second was maternal and infant care. This meant visiting prospective mothers and mothers with newborn infants, distributing form letters and literature, organizing and perhaps teaching maternity and infancy classes, and introducing mothercraft classes for high school girls. Yet this was not all. The rural nurse played an important role in the control of communicable disease, co-operating with health officers, physicians, teachers, and parents. She

[17] St. Louis County Nursing Service, *Reports*, 1924–25. All county public health nursing service reports cited are filed in mimeographed form at the Minnesota Department of Health, Minneapolis.

urged immunization, organized immunization clinics, and encouraged the early isolation and care of sick children. She took part in annual tuberculosis chest clinics and followed up tuberculous cases as well as suspects and contacts. She was expected, too, to help with an annual orthopedic clinic for crippled children and to make follow-up visits. In addition to all this, the nurse had regular meetings with her nursing advisory committee, made monthly reports to county commissioners, met with various health committees in the community, and co-operated with all other organizations interested in health.[18]

For activities like these, complicated by public demands upon her personal time, a rural nurse in 1938 received an annual salary of $1,700. The budget for one county totaled $2,860.80, of which $1,800 came from the county commissioners, $400 from Social Security, $486.08 from the Minnesota Public Health Seal Fund, and $174.72 from the county Red Cross. Total expenses, including the nurse's salary, amounted to $2,779.85. In 1949 the cost of supporting one county nurse was $5,000. A nurse earning $1,260 a year reported in 1939 that she had made a total of 1,273 visits, had inspected 98 schools, had helped examine 2,230 children, and had referred 786 to private physicians.[19]

Perhaps the nursing service in Isanti County offers a typical story of public health nursing throughout the state, although each county, of course, has problems peculiar to itself. Rural nursing in Isanti County receives advice from the Minnesota Department of Health. The local service, however, stems directly from the county commissioners and through them to three committees: a county public health committee, a medical advisory committee, and a dental advisory committee. The nurse works directly with these committees. But she, in turn, is responsible for the supervision of five subcommittees representing various townships. This organization was begun in January, 1939, and has progressed with some difficulty. Before 1939 the only nursing service in the county had been financed by the Red Cross. A child welfare nurse had been employed for about two months, and in 1938 a Red Cross nurse taught a class in home hygiene. Her enthusiasm and the interest of the superintendent of schools led to the formation of an advisory nursing committee and the employment of a nurse trained in public health. To support the program, funds were appropriated by the county commissioners, the state, and the Isanti Public Health Association. Village and rural schools were to contribute

[18] Jackson County Public Health Nursing Service, *Annual Reports*, 1939.
[19] Martin County Public Health Nursing Service, *Annual Reports*, 1938; Kandiyohi County Public Health Nursing Service, *Annual Reports*, 1939.

according to their population. But, since only about half of the schools paid their share, it was necessary to borrow money from the Red Cross. The commissioners increased their appropriation in 1940, but just about that time the county nurse resigned. A demonstration nurse was then furnished by the state for three months. By the end of that period another county nurse had been hired.

This nurse practically had to start an overall program anew. Beneath the statistical cloak which covers her first report lies the very human story of what rural nursing means to Minnesota. "During 1940," she wrote in the objective third person, "914 rapid inspections were given the school children; also, 636 individual inspections and 124 partial inspections were made. One hundred forty parents were present at these inspections. Vision testing, height and weight checking, inspecting of the skin, mouth, and throat, and checking for any physical deformities makes this quite a satisfactory examination for the child. Out of 35 children with defective vision, 29 were fitted with glasses. . . . Fourteen children have had tonsillectomies. The Red Cross furnished funds for six of them. . . . In control of communicable diseases, the Nurse can be numbered in the first line of defense. She visits the schools, makes rapid inspections of the pupils, recommending exclusion from school of those pupils presenting any suspicious symptoms; visits the homes of sick children, and whenever necessary demonstrates bedside care, attempts to enlighten the family of isolation technique, and state health quarantine rules; and reports any case of communicable diseases to the local and state health officers if they have not already been reported." [20]

Perhaps no one in the entire field is as intimately acquainted with public health as it is practiced as the rural nurse. Engineers, epidemiologists, and laboratory technicians may be sent into the county for a brief period by the state health department, but individuals, even though highly trained and willing, cannot learn to know the daily, intimate problems of the people as does the nurse. The county is her home, and she knows its townships as well as she knows the palm of her hand. She understands economic conditions and has learned to recognize family or domestic troubles. She is the on-the-spot representative of an organization too complicated and too vast for most persons to comprehend. The nurse symbolizes in her person what the state department stands for. She deals with handicapped children and with ill adults. She is the person at hand who is called. And her experiences are apt to be complicated and arduous.

[20] Isanti County Public Health Nursing Service, *Annual Reports*, 1940.

At Bemidji one snowy, cold February day in 1943, the nurse got news that premature twins had been born in an isolated district. An inexperienced neighbor woman had delivered them. For several days the nurse waited for roads to be cleared sufficiently so that she could make the twenty-mile trip to where mother and babies waited for help. Finally great drifts were pushed aside, and the nurse opened the door of a miserable hut. "The family of eight," she said, "lived in a one room fishing cabin where the snow seeped in the cracks of the walls. The other 5 children, all under 7 years, were bare-footed, scantily clad, cold and undernourished. One broken down bed with ragged covers accommodated all the children. The only food in the house was that given by the neighbor lady who was present at the delivery. The father was unemployed." The smaller of the twins was already dead when the nurse arrived, and it was apparent that both the mother and the remaining baby could not live long without heat, food, and medical attention. It was up to the nurse to see that these were furnished. The four-pound infant was placed in a cardboard box heated with hot-water bottles. The box and the mother were carried to the hospital in Bemidji by bobsled and by car. A week later the child died.

Because some families in Beltrami County lived as much as sixty miles from the nearest physician and even farther from a hospital, it fell to the rural nurse to give instructions as to what to do until the doctor arrived. In nearly every home, said a nurse, at some time or other, questions such as these arise: "How can I give a bath to somebody that is sick in bed? How can I get the sheets changed? My boy is supposed to have a hot pack on his hand. What shall I use and how shall I put it on? I'm supposed to take Mary's temperature and report it to the doctor. How do you read a thermometer, anyway?" [21]

Just when county nursing seemed to be getting on its feet in Minnesota, World War II not only prevented the establishment of new programs but also seriously crippled those already in existence. The armed services drained off physicians who had assisted with nursing activities and, in some instances, reduced the number of nurses, too. Despite these and other handicaps, county nursing forged ahead with the slogan "Health for Victory." In Blue Earth County it was impossible to hold regular subcommittee meetings because of gas rationing, and quarterly meetings were discontinued. During this period students in public health nursing from the University of Minnesota were sent into counties for field experience, a practice that had begun some twenty years earlier.

[21] Beltrami County Public Health Nursing Service, *Annual Reports*, 1942–43.

BLUE CAP AND BLACK BAG 363

Rural nurses assisted many young mothers whose husbands were in the service. These nurses planned for home or hospital delivery, guided the mother to such agencies as the Red Cross, and acquainted women with the benefits available through the Emergency Maternal and Infant Care Program.[22]

During war years rural nurses continued to give classes in home nursing whenever possible. "In this day when fewer doctors, nurses, and hospital facilities are available," wrote a mother after taking the course, "it behooves us all to fortify ourselves with all the training and information possible to assist us in meeting emergencies, epidemics, etc., usually prevalent during any war." [23] These emergencies did arise, and the rural nurse had to face them. In Beltrami County the winter of 1943–44 brought with it an unusually large number of cases of communicable diseases. This general increase was attributed by the nurse to wartime conditions — "people moving from one part of the country to another, and crowded living conditions in defense areas and around army camps."

To illustrate her point the nurse related a story. A nine-year-old girl, she said, was taken to a hospital and found to have typhoid fever. Although she was acutely ill she recovered. "Investigations were conducted by the State Board of Health to determine the source of Mary's infection," said the nurse. "Her grandmother, who came to live in the household before Mary's illness, was found to be a typhoid carrier and it was revealed that previously two other relatives with whom the grandmother had lived had been ill with typhoid fever, one thirteen years ago, and one twenty-five years ago. Grandmother is ninety-one years old and had difficulty understanding the need for taking precautions to prevent the spread of the disease. Since it was impossible to give safe care in a one room house where she was living with her daughter's family, arrangements were made by the State Department of Health and the County Welfare Board, to have her returned to the home for the aged where she had lived previously." [24]

The state health board created a division of public health nursing in 1938. From then until the present time this division has provided advisory services to all Minnesota public health nurses. It sees that standards are maintained, aids in placing certified nurses, and acts as a clearinghouse for reports of all public health nursing services. It also corre-

---

[22] Martin County Public Health Nursing Service, *Annual Reports*, 1943–44; Blue Earth County Public Health Association, *Annual Reports*, 1943–44; Isanti County Public Health Nursing Service, *Annual Reports*, 1944, 1945.
[23] Blue Earth County Public Health Association, *Annual Reports*, 1942–43.
[24] Beltrami County Nursing Service, *Annual Reports*, 1943–44.

lates these services with the programs of other official and nonofficial agencies. The division disseminates information to the public, describing both public health nursing and the public health nurse. A public health nurse is defined as "a graduate nurse, registered to practice nursing, who teaches public health practices to individuals, and demonstrates home nursing care. Besides having an interest in people and an ability to work with them, she has completed special courses in public health to prepare her to do this work." In co-operation with the division of health of the Minnesota Department of Education, the public health nursing division in 1946 prepared and distributed an abstract of regulations for communicable diseases. This was sent to public health nurses and to school health directors. In addition to hundreds of pieces of miscellaneous literature, the division has also compiled an elaborate manual for nurses, which not only gives such specific details as what should go into a nurse's black bag but also describes fully the political make-up of counties and the legal obligations of county commissioners.[25]

The public health nurse also is expected to co-operate with other state and local welfare agencies. Indeed, she can scarcely escape contact with the division of social welfare of the Minnesota Department of Social Security. Nurse and welfare worker frequently must work harmoniously to achieve the goals of each. For example, the public health nurse and the welfare worker almost automatically join forces when women and children are concerned. Both are interested in crippled children. In 1943 the Minnesota Bureau for Crippled Children had 10,322 children on its register. Activities in behalf of these children included hospitalization and treatment at the Gillette State Hospital or at private hospitals; field nursing and physiotherapy; field clinics throughout the state; medical-social services; defective speech services; a heart plan; and the Michael Dowling cerebral palsy project. These services were augmented by clinics, by lectures to nurses of the Minneapolis General Hospital and the University of Minnesota Hospital, and by university courses on the care of the handicapped child.[26]

Nurse and welfare worker co-operated also during the war years, as they had in the past, in the particularly vexing problem of children born out of wedlock. Public health nurses frequently handled medical details, while the social worker concerned herself with the domestic problems

[25] State Board of Health, *Reports*, 1922–43, p. 22; Division of Public Health Nursing, *Facts on Public Health Nursing in Minnesota*, [1] (Minneapolis, 1941); Minnesota Departments of Health and Education, "Health Regulations for Certain Communicable Diseases" ([St. Paul?], 1946); Minnesota Department of Health, *Manual for Public Health Nurses* (Minneapolis, 1946).
[26] Minnesota Division of Social Welfare, *Annual Reports*, 1943, p. 41.

involved. In 1947 there were 1,959 illegitimate births in Minnesota, and a total of 2,209 children, born out of wedlock either in Minnesota or elsewhere, were referred for services. The total of 873 unmarried girls admitted to the six maternity homes in the state in 1947 represented an increase of twelve per cent over the previous year. Girls seeking care at maternity homes in the Twin Cities had to be turned away because of lack of accommodations.[27]

For many years public health nurses assisted with the work of the Infant Welfare Society of Minneapolis. This organization began its work in 1910, but it was not incorporated until two years later. Its major purpose was the prevention of infant mortality by educating women to prepare them for motherhood. Emphasis was placed also upon breast feeding and regular examination of babies by clinic physicians.[28] In 1935 the Infant Welfare Society merged with the Visiting Nursing Association under the name "Minneapolis Community Health Service." In the same year the Baby Welfare Service of St. Paul became the Family Nursing Service. Such agencies, still working in 1948, have contributed much to better health in the Twin Cities.

The public health nurse plays such an important role in so many activities that it is difficult to enumerate them all. From the time when nursing became a recognized profession, the trained nurse has been a consistent contributor to peacetime programs and has taken an important part in wartime activities. Many emergency nursing plans have been worked out in co-operation with the American Red Cross. In 1909 the American Red Cross Nursing Service was affiliated with the American Nurses Association at a meeting in Minneapolis. This relationship grew stronger with the years. When trouble on the Mexican border developed early in the twentieth century, emergency detachments of Minnesota nurses were mobilized for service. In December, 1917, Base Hospital Number 26 at the University of Minnesota was ordered to Fort McPherson, Georgia. This hospital, with its chief nurse and sixty-five nurses from Minnesota, sailed for France on June 4, 1918. At home, four naval station hospitals were organized in Minnesota. These were located at Minneapolis, Duluth, and St. Paul. The chief nurse of each was a Minnesota girl. A four-months course for naval corpsmen was given at the University of Minnesota, and nurses served as instructors. During World War II innumerable Minnesota nurses enlisted in various branches of the service. A University of Minnesota base hospital unit again was or-

[27] Division of Social Welfare, *Annual Reports*, 1947, p. 8.
[28] Helen Presley Peck to [the Division of Public Health Nursing], [n.d.], Minnesota Department of Health, Minneapolis.

ganized and it served in England and in the African and Italian campaigns.[29]

The great influenza epidemic of 1918 could not have been fought as successfully as it was had it not been for the nurses who worked in close co-operation with the American Red Cross and the state health department. The demand for nurses in afflicted areas was so great that Bracken despaired of even beginning to supply the requests that flooded his office. And the girls themselves, scattered throughout the state, found that they could scarcely meet the demands made upon them. From Aitkin a nurse wrote that she was terribly discouraged, and she added: "Then there is a queer system of requisitions here. You cannot take an aspirin tablet out of the bottle and give it without filling out a blank, later entering it in a book, and then checking back." The pressure under which public health nurses were laboring in influenza areas is clearly apparent in a report from a nurse in Dilworth. "A hasty report," she wrote. "We are very, very busy, have 24 patients in hospital now. Have dismissed about 15, two have died and perhaps one or two died last night. I didn't think they could live through the night. . . . Cannot say when we will get away. They want us to stay as long as they need us." [30]

Except during emergency periods, the nurse confined herself to normal duties. Yet these "normal" obligations had grown tremendously by 1948. No longer was the nurse an isolated entity who labored alone or under the direction of a local physician, as she had been a quarter of a century earlier. And the cost of a public health nursing program had more than doubled. The mere organization of a county nursing program had become so complicated that it approached big business.

Rural Hennepin County in 1947 was a classical example of the development of a modern nursing service. Within the county thirteen administrative agencies were employing nurses for public health work. These included the Glen Lake outpatient department, tuberculosis associations, school boards, and a Community Health Service. The total annual Hennepin County budget amounted to $53,515.72. This budget, according to a survey, secured the services of seventeen graduate professional nurses employed for public health nursing activities and two auxiliary nurses trained for bedside care in a more limited capacity than the graduate professional nurse. Five of the seventeen nurses were employed

[29] Mary Pruitt, "The American Red Cross Nurse in Minnesota" (typescript), Minnesota Department of Health, Minneapolis.
[30] Bracken to Mrs. Jennie B. Johnston, November 7, 1918, Emma C. Moynihan to Frances V. Brink, November 27, [1918], and Louise L. Christensen to Brink, October 19, 1918, Minnesota Department of Health, Minneapolis. See also chapter 20, below.

by rural Hennepin County; one school board employed two nurses; and eight other school boards employed one nurse each. Two nurses devoted their entire time to tuberculosis control. For this type of service, assisted by an advisory nurse from the state health department, citizens of rural Hennepin County annually paid $.535 per capita. Tax funds supplied $.452 of this amount. Of the $.452 from taxation, $.255 was derived from funds collected for school purposes. "It has been estimated," said a report, "that a per capita expenditure of from $1.50 to $2.00 will supply an adequate amount of the various types of public health personnel, for a community. This estimate should be compared with the 53½c now spent for service for public health nurses unequally distributed both in regard to population and responsibilities." [31]

Public health authorities estimate that fairly adequate nursing service can be assured if there is one nurse per 5,000 population. In rural Hennepin County the population per nurse ranged from 47,000 to 4,000, and the agency with the widest responsibility had a population range of from 47,000 to 17,000 per nurse. School enrollment for the fourteen nurses involved in the school health program ranged from 263 to 2,775 per nurse. One nurse, the report continued, "served 20,000 population for maternity and child health including preschools and children from parochial schools, crippled children not in the St. Louis Park School, acute communicable diseases occurring in the general population, health teaching and other services for the adult population. This nurse also provides similar service for another 26,981 population." [32]

The Hennepin County survey, with the eight general recommendations which it contains, indicates the degree to which modern public health nursing has grown. The various agencies, it suggests, should not overlap one another either geographically or organizationally; maternity and infancy programs need to be further stimulated; closer contacts should be maintained with physicians throughout the county; and a "more uniform understanding [should] be developed in philosophies in public health nursing and terminology such as 'community nursing.'" [33] Last, but very certainly not least, communities must spend more per capita if they want a complete and an up-to-date public health nursing program.

[31] State Board of Health, Division of Public Health Nursing, "Survey of Public Health Nursing in Rural Hennepin County, 1947," part 1, p. 4 and table 14 (typescript). Minnesota Department of Health, Minneapolis.
[32] Division of Public Health Nursing, "Survey of Public Health Nursing in Rural Hennepin County, 1947," part 1, p. 5; part 2, p. 1.
[33] Division of Public Health Nursing, "Survey of Public Health Nursing in Rural Hennepin County, 1947," part 3, p. 1.

Meanwhile the public health nurse does her best. She never has sufficient time to take care of all routine matters, and frequently she must deal with the unexpected. When she makes out regular reports she must fill in eleven different categories — communicable disease control, venereal disease work, maternity care, care of the infant, preschool activities, school visits and activities, cancer and heart cases, work with crippled children, public health education, and administration. In addition she submits a "narrative" of her work for the month. Copies of her reports are sent to the Minnesota Department of Health.

The director and the staff of the Hennepin County Public Health Nursing Service in a single month do a tremendous amount of work, ranging from dealing with the problem of scabies in schools to giving bedside care and demonstrations to seventy-one heart patients. A Carlton County nurse traveled 621 miles within a thirty-day period. During her tours she uncovered a new case of tuberculosis, made a home visit to a seventy-nine-year-old woman who had pneumonia and refused to be hospitalized, assisted at an outpatient clinic, and made trips to dress the burns of an old Indian woman. Visits were made also, the nurse said, "to a fifteen year old boy who chopped off the middle toe of his right foot while visiting at Grand Portage. Medical care was given in Grand Marais and the mother was advised that the boy use crutches until the physician ordered otherwise; but, on the spur of the moment, or while under the influence of liquor, as was reported, the mother threw the crutches away and with the boy boarded a bus for Superior, Wisconsin. They finally returned to Sawyer the latter part of May when the nurse came across them at the maternal grandparents. The boy walked with a definite limp and the stump of the toe was apparently infected. There was no bandage on the injury, the only covering being the heavy leather shoe the patient wore. First aid care was given by the nurse and sterile dressings left. The boy absolutely refused medical care, and the mother evidently has no influence over him whatsoever." [34]

Practically all rural nurses aided in Mantoux testing programs as a part of a campaign against tuberculosis, many nurses worked with parent-teacher associations, and others attended clinics for crippled children. A Chisago County nurse showed two motion pictures dealing with reproduction to school children in grades six through twelve. "I do not feel that this is a successful way to handle the young people and their desire for knowledge," she wrote afterwards. "But I believe we

[34] Hennepin County Public Health Nursing Service, *Reports*, May, 1948; Carlton County Public Health Nursing Service, *Reports*, June, 1948.

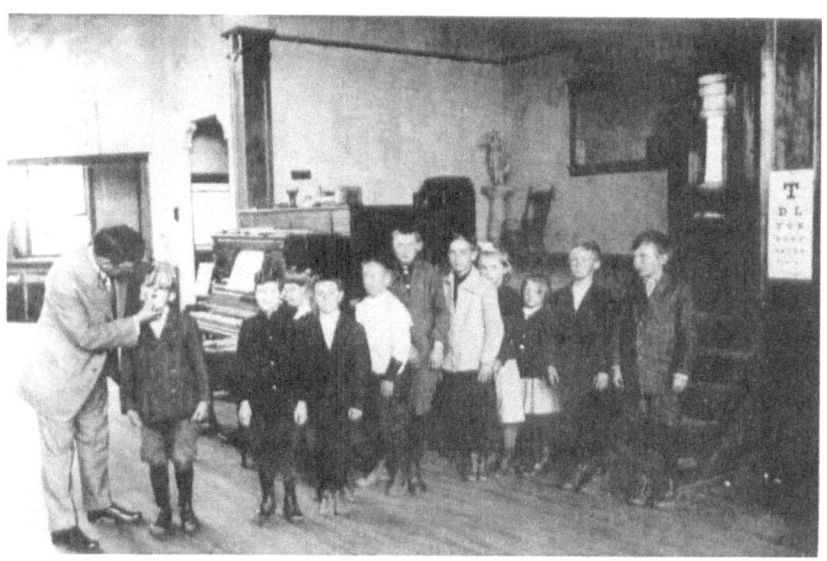

E. B. HOAG EXAMINING SCHOOL CHILDREN

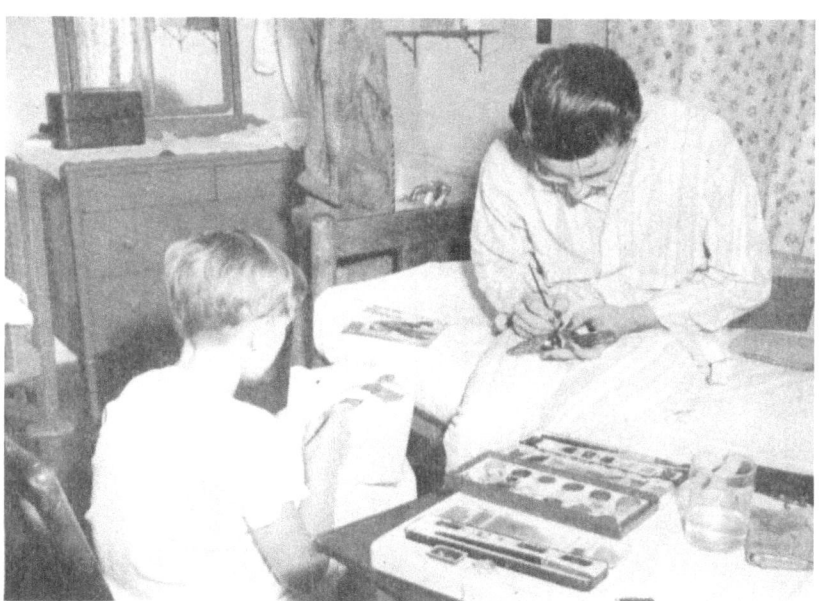

THERAPY FOR YOUNGSTERS
Courtesy Minnesota Department of Health

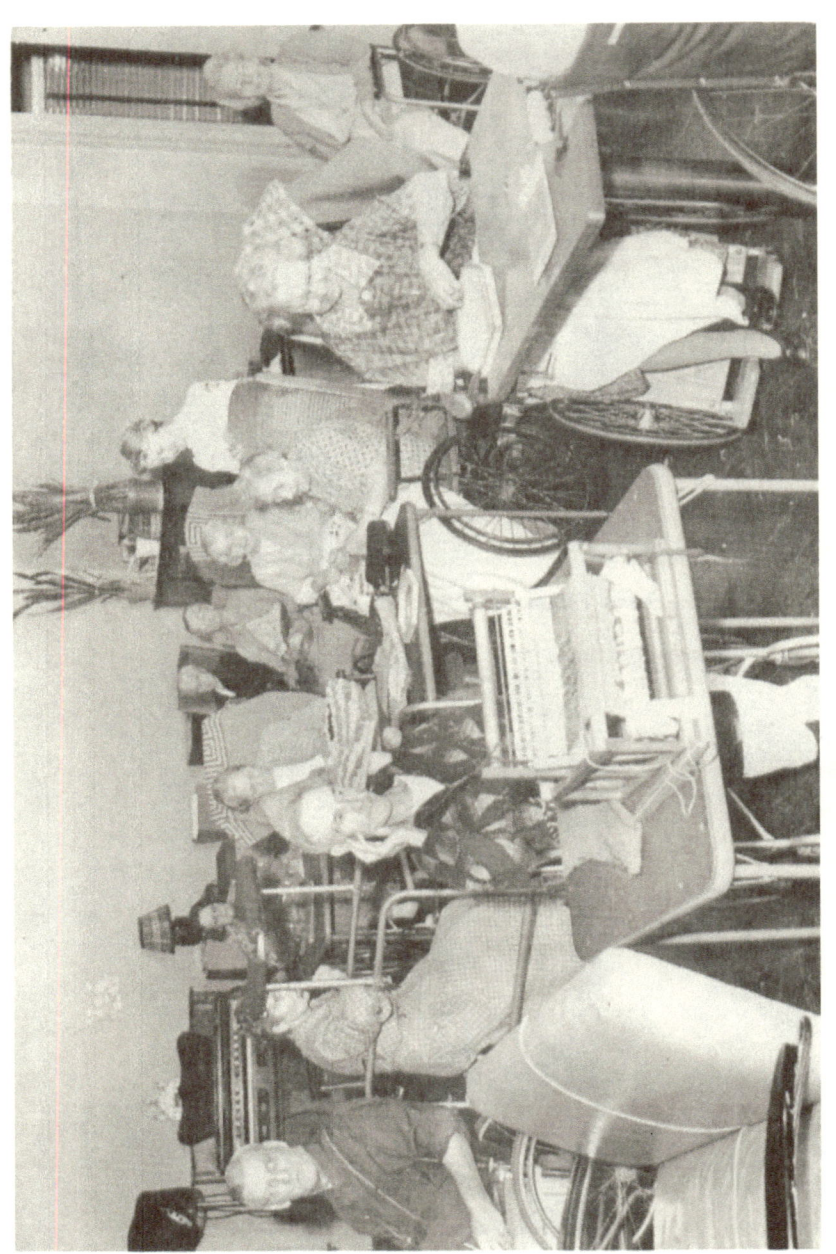

Modern Care for the Aged
Courtesy Minnesota Department of Health

made a start, and I think the teachers are more interested than ever in working human relations into their courses." Elsewhere nurses showed films relating to the Mantoux program and to cancer.[35]

Nurses were keenly aware also of social and economic conditions, and they frequently made pertinent comments upon the relationship of these conditions to health. When, early in 1948, newspapers were printing stories of the dreadful plight of the Indians in Mille Lacs County,[36] the local nurse gave her view of the situation. "In the past month Mille Lacs County has received much publicity as far as the Indian problem is concerned," she wrote. "Having talked to several people in the county the general sentiment seems to be the following: 'It isn't only the Indians who are in the same straits this time of the year. It isn't only this year that the Indians have been in need, this has been the situation for the past several years.' Also you will hear the following remark made. 'Why should Mille Lacs County Welfare and the people of Mille Lacs County support the Indians entirely? Shouldn't there be some federal aid given to them?' According to the article in the paper it would seem that no one up here has any interest in their welfare."

Then the county nurse went on to tell a little more specifically what the situation was: "On the 10th of February a home visit was made by the nurse to the Shaugobay family, the ones who were said to be 'starving' in the paper. This call was made by request, the family had left word with the teachers to tell the nurse when she came. Two children were found in bed. . . . The nurse telephoned the physician and told him the symptoms of the other children. He informed the nurse that they were in a state of malnutrition. Hospitalization was emphasized but the nurse was not in favor of this. There would not have been any charge as the Fond du Lac Hospital at Cloquet offers free medical service to the Indians. The mother asked me to inform the Welfare Office to send a food order up. This I did as soon as I reached Milaca that evening February 10th. A $25 food order was sent the next day. The publicity in the paper came out on the 16th of February, a week after the situation had been taken care of. The nurse emphasized to the family that they should apply directly to the Welfare Office for relief when they are in need. Then the situation could be investigated."[37]

[35] Chisago County Public Health Nursing Service, *Reports*, January, 1948; Mille Lacs County Nursing Advisory Committee, *Reports*, April 1948.
[36] See, for example, *Minneapolis Tribune*, February 16, 1948.
[37] Mille Lacs County Nursing Advisory Committee, *Reports*, February, 1948. For an explanation of the interrelationship between health and welfare services in Minnesota, see Minnesota Division of Social Welfare and Minnsota Department of Health, *Minnesota Manual of Health and Welfare Services* ([St. Paul?], March, 1948).

Even though the public health nurse constantly comes into most intimate contact with the actual day-by-day health problems of a community, and even though she has proved her worth again and again, there are too many sections of Minnesota without nurses. In 1947, for example, twenty-two counties lacked organized nursing services and several organized counties had no nurses. On the other hand, six counties organized public health nursing services during that year.[38] This situation had not changed materially a year later, when sixty-three counties were organized, although some had vacancies, and twenty-four counties were not organized.[39]

The failure of some Minnesota counties to provide public health nursing services is not the fault of the state health department, which has done everything possible in the way of encouragement. In the first place, the need for nurses has grown faster than the supply. This is complicated further, moreover, by the fact that some counties feel that they cannot afford the services of a nurse. Of course such an attitude reflects in some degree that of the public. If public opinion insists upon the employment of a nurse, undoubtedly the need can be filled, providing, of course, a nurse is available. In 1947 there was one nurse to every twenty thousand people in Minnesota. The goal of the division of public health nursing has been announced as one nurse to every five thousand people. In order to acquaint nurses with both the possibilities and the problems of rural nursing, the School of Public Health at the University of Minnesota assigns students to county public health nursing services for periods of from four to six weeks. Industrial nursing services are also used for special assignments. These assignments, say directors of public health nursing, give a student the "feeling of being a part of a community force that is charged with the serious responsibility of safe-guarding the health and lives of a given community." Undergraduate nurses have also been attached temporarily to rural hospitals in order to observe public health, welfare, and educational services.[40]

The success of this program has been manifested again and again. "This has been a very busy month in Isanti County," wrote an undergraduate nurse who had been assigned there. "As a student under Miss

[38] Division of Public Health Nursing, *Public Health Nursing in Minnesota*, [2] ([Minneapolis?], 1947).
[39] Interview of the author with Ann Nyquist, September 6, 1948; "Minnesota Needs Many More Public Health Nurses," in *Everybody's Health*, vol. 31, no. 4, pp. 8, 15 (April, 1946).
[40] Minnesota Department of Health, *Public Health Nursing in Minnesota*, 5; Jackson County Public Health Nursing Service, *Annual Reports*, 1940–41; Norman County Public Health Nursing Service, *Annual Reports*, 1940–41.

[Frances] Holley, I observed her during the first week in her home visits and school inspections. Later, under her supervision, I did several home visits and school inspections. . . . This consisted of height and weight measurements, vision testing, and inspection of throat, teeth, and skin. This work was very interesting, and I was glad of the opportunity to meet the mothers and discuss with them their children and their problems. . . . I was fortunate enough to be present at a 'prenatal shower' that one of the subcommittees held for an expectant mother. Dressings and pads were made for the mother and shirts and diapers for the baby. . . . I received a clearer picture of how the service for crippled children is carried out. . . . Although the county nursing program is fairly new, I feel that I have derived a great deal from working under Miss Holley, and I have been able to correlate my theoretical knowledge with the practical knowledge obtained in the field."[41]

Minnesota public health nurses early learn that they should reach the parents of young children in order to improve the health status of older children and young adults. Results from this approach have been gratifying, yet "it has been difficult for many public health nursing services to reach the younger age group in an effective manner because the pressure of local opinion keeps their few nurses working on the back-log of health problems among school children — and to assist with special programs promoted by different health interest groups."[42] Preschool health activities, of course, mean more than helping to get a child ready for school. Nurses find that many parents desire help with understanding their younger children while trying to adjust to a new baby. Parents frequently are eager to learn how to present new foods to a two-year-old and how to train for toilet. They need instruction also in when to immunize against smallpox, diphtheria, and whooping cough.

Fortunately the legislature in 1947 recognized the beneficial services of public health nurses and arranged to give financial assistance to any county interested in developing a public health nursing service. The act directed that fifteen hundred dollars a year be paid from the appropriation of the state health department to any county that met certain requirements. These included the provision that only approved and certified public health nurses be hired and that certificates of expenses be made to the state auditor.[43]

Calling the nurse the "key person" in a really effective health cam-

[41] Isanti County Public Health Nursing Service, *Reports*, October, 1939.
[42] Minnesota Department of Health, *Public Health Nursing in Minnesota*, 7.
[43] *Laws*, 1947, p. 73; *Everybody's Health*, vol. 32, no. 4, p. 2 (April, 1947).

paign, the Minnesota Department of Health, shortly after the act of 1947 was passed, made it clear that a county nurse is immediately responsible to the county's official advisory committee, of which a local physician is a member. The department's division of public health nursing is ready at all times to advise nurses in the field. With an increased awareness on the part of communities of the worth of a nursing program, and with state funds available, health officials hope that all Minnesota's eighty-seven counties may organize nursing services. Until that time, Minnesota's health will not be completely protected in rural areas.

19

Health of Mother and Child

THE DEATH rate in 1871 of Minnesota children under five years of age was astonishingly high and it accounted for a high percentage of the state's total deaths. Fifty years later the rate was dropping. By 1947 deaths among children under five years old had decreased to 8.8% of the total deaths in the state.[1]

This dramatic reduction resulted in part from an extensive public health program, introduced by Hewitt and continued until today, which gave guidance and safety not only to infants but also to mothers. Gradually, but surely, the maternal death rate fell. For many years childbearing was considered casually, and an old granny midwife was believed to be perfectly capable of delivering a woman. So little was known of diseases of children that whooping cough, diphtheria, scarlet fever, and typhoid took a fearful toll of lives. If a child lived to enter school, he learned his ABCs all too frequently in badly ventilated, inadequately heated buildings. The pupil with defective hearing or sight was at an obvious disadvantage. No school nurse made periodic visits to check teeth or to suggest posture changes. Times have changed indeed since great-grandfather heard the tune of the hickory stick in the little red schoolhouse.

The program of maternal and child hygiene, which still has a long way to go, began when the farsighted Hewitt suggested that public hygiene be made a subject of special study in teachers' institutes and urged that school boards interest themselves in it. Horace B. Wilson, superintendent of public instruction in 1873, agreed thoroughly with Hewitt and outlined what he thought pupils should learn about health matters. "They should know enough of their own physical and mental organizations to enable them to take proper care of both their bodies and

[1] State Board of Health, *Annual Reports*, 1873, p. 36; *Biennial Reports*, 1920–21, p. 63. Figures for 1947 were obtained from the division of vital statistics of the Minnesota Department of Health, September 16, 1948.

brains," Wilson wrote. Then he added: "To this end they should know when, how and what to eat and drink; when and how much to sleep; the uses and abuses of clothing; the laws of healthful labor, exercise and rest; the functions of the brain; the more obvious relations of body and mind; and the tokens and penalties of disregarding the laws of health, whether of body or mind." [2]

This was good as far as it went, but Hewitt believed that it did not go far enough. He was vitally interested, of course, in having children taught something about hygiene, but he also was concerned with their school environment. He believed, as did his associates on the board, that qualified public health men should protect the child by seeing that schools were properly heated and ventilated. The superintendent of public instruction, after Hewitt had talked with him, became so enthusiastic that he asked the board to prepare an essay on school ventilation that could be distributed to institutions throughout Minnesota. The first tract was published in 1876.[3]

No doubt public instruction officials were somewhat inclined to secure Hewitt's advice because of a survey they had made which showed schools to be in a deplorable condition. This survey, a most unscientific affair, showed that 116 schools had no ventilation, that 907 had outhouses in bad condition, and that 840 had no privies. Ventilation was exceedingly bad. "In the estimation of three-fourths of our trustees," wrote the superintendent of public instruction, "a school house is well ventilated if the windows can be opened when the room becomes uncomfortably hot. Yet several hundred of our school houses do not admit of even such ventilation. The windows are nailed, up and down, to keep the boys out in summer, and the cold out in winter." The very subjects on which the superintendent sought information from Hewitt indicate the health problems in schools during the 1870s. They included:

Expedients for ventilation in school rooms where no provision was made in their original construction.
How seats should be arranged to secure health and comfort, especially for small children.
Proper positions in sitting and standing, with special reference to the lungs and preservation of the eyes.
Means of securing pure water for use in the schools.
Sanitary and moral importance of out houses, kept in good condition.[4]

[2] State Board of Health, *Annual Reports*, 1873, p. 15; Minnesota Superintendent of Public Instruction, *Annual Reports*, 1873, p. 45.
[3] Superintendent of Public Instruction, *Annual Reports*, 1876, p. 84; State Board of Health, *Annual Reports*, [1877], appendix, 33–53.
[4] Superintendent of Public Instruction, *Annual Reports*, 1876, pp. 81, 84.

HEALTH OF MOTHER AND CHILD

Such queries, together with others, led Hewitt to begin an extensive investigation into the health of the school child. He was prompted in part by disheartening reports from many county school superintendents. From the superintendent in Blue Earth County in 1877 came a typical letter: "If a modicum of information relative to heating and ventilation could be injected into the mental tissue of the average school house builder, there would be fewer little graves made on our prairies, and the indefatigable President of the State Board of Health would feel that he has not lived in vain. . . . If Malthus could send a message from the tomb, he would doubtless say to us, 'Your public schools with their poor sanitary arrangements and infant pupils, are well calculated to keep down the surplus population of the world.'" Other schoolmen spoke of the prevalence of measles and scarlet fever.[5]

Had Hewitt's survey concerned itself primarily with the health of students in relation to their school environment, it might have revealed some significant facts. As it was, Hewitt attempted a correlation between scholastic methods and health. He was not equipped for such a task, and his research, interesting as it was, failed to be particularly impressive. Nevertheless it was important, not only because it was the first study of its kind in Minnesota but also because it drew public attention to the school health problem. A continuation report made in 1879 was concerned with the health of college students, and it presented physical data, such as height, weight, mean girth of chest, and chest expansion.[6]

Perhaps Hewitt's greatest contribution to child and maternal welfare lay, not in his studies of school ventilation and his measurement of pupils, but in his almost daily efforts to give youngsters every possible opportunity to survive and be healthy. He persisted in this until he closed his desk as secretary. In 1881 he urged that tired mothers and their infants be given an opportunity to enjoy a summer vacation in the country and he spoke out boldly for increased attention to nursing mothers and ailing children of day laborers and the very poor. He insisted upon one point which, he said, should be kept constantly in mind by everyone — "that little children are the most sensitive to the influence of unhealthy surroundings, and that their ailments are often the first clue we have to the presence and character of disease causes lurking around or in the house which is the home." He insisted that it was the parents' duty to examine the house to find the cause of illness.[7]

[5] Superintendent of Public Instruction, *Annual Reports*, 1877, pp. 110, 161.
[6] State Board of Health, *Annual Reports*, 1878, appendix, 71–108; 1879, pp. 116–125.
[7] State Board of Health, *Biennial Reports*, 1879–80, p. 122.

Emphasis on vaccination was another Hewitt contribution. He was always pleased when he could say that more and more persons were being vaccinated. He thought it a misfortune when parents and physicians neglected vaccination "till the danger of Small Pox brings them to a sense of duty." Had Hewitt's determination triumphed, Minnesota would have had a compulsory vaccination law. Such an act, however, was not in force as late as 1948. No unvaccinated child, for example, may be excluded from public school except during a smallpox epidemic. Hewitt's attitude toward compulsory vaccination was not shared by some twentieth-century health officials, who felt that compulsion by legal means was not as effective in the long run as a program of persuasion and education. Smallpox, of course, was not the only illness that kept pupils from school and took lives.[8]

During the 1870s and 1880s cholera infantum was perhaps as dangerous as any disease. The newly organized health board heard constantly that cholera infantum was striking at children. From St. Paul, Minneapolis, Duluth, and Red Wing came reports that little ones were stricken and dying. A St. Paul health officer said that the principal disease during July, 1880, was cholera infantum, and a year later Chatfield reported an epidemic. During a one-week period in Minneapolis thirty-three deaths were posted, and of these, twenty-four were of children under five years of age who had been sick with cholera infantum. More than a hundred deaths from the disease were reported in Minneapolis during July, 1887. The next year health departments were troubled by an unusual outbreak of "winter cholera," which struck down adults as well as children. Hewitt was so concerned that he assisted with a post mortem on a victim and ordered that samples of St. Paul water be sent to his laboratory at Red Wing for examination.[9]

Despite the ravages of cholera infantum, the less dramatic diseases of children took a greater toll of lives. Among them were measles, scarlatina, diphtheria, and croup. Typhoid fever was responsible for 643 deaths in 1888, many of them among children. Diarrheal diseases accounted for 7.74% of deaths from all causes in the nine-year period from 1887 through 1895. By 1897 measles was affecting so many children that Bracken said it was a more serious disease than was generally recognized and urged that a child with measles have the services of a physician.

[8] State Board of Health, *Annual Reports*, 1878, p. 9; *Public Health in Minnesota*, 3:90 (January, 1888); *Laws*, 1917, p. 490; 1923, p. 262; *Minnesota State Health Laws and Regulations*, 12, 63, 158 (January 1, 1948).
[9] *St. Paul Daily Press*, July 22, August 17, 1872, July 25, 1873; *Minneapolis Tribune*, August 7, 1872, August 3, 1880, July 30, 1882, August 2, 1887; *Pioneer Press*, August 12, 1881, January 29, February 1, 11, 12, 21, March 3, 13, 1888.

HEALTH OF MOTHER AND CHILD

However, Bracken did not feel that strict quarantine was desirable. Chicken pox, on the other hand, was rigidly quarantined. By the turn of the century significant work was being done with diphtheria, particularly in the public schools. Bracken early in 1899 took throat cultures from school children at Elbow Lake. Other investigations were made at Faribault, Owatonna, and Mankato. McDaniel played a significant role in these surveys.[10]

Gradually the work of Hewitt and Bracken to improve school sanitation and the health of pupils bore fruit. By 1904 superintendents of public instruction were paying considerable attention to heating and ventilation and were realizing that a healthy student learned better and was happier than a sick one. Yet a state school inspector wrote that small children frequently were "shoved" into inadequate rooms to receive inferior instruction. Little ones, he wrote, should have more personal attention, not less. He complained also that probably over half of Minnesota's school buildings were inadequately ventilated. Most local superintendents spoke of "steady progress," but a close reading of their reports reveals woeful deficiencies. Goodhue schools, for example, still used jacketed stoves, which were unsatisfactory because "the jacket has not been provided with a sufficient amount of air for securing good circulation and because the fresh air flue and the ventilating flue frequently have been too small." Although Houston boasted of a new building, it was not constructed on a modern plan. "Some law ought to be passed," wrote the disgruntled superintendent, "to keep districts from wasting money in building schoolhouses on plans which cannot give comfort or convenience." [11]

The twenty years from 1890 to 1910 showed greater progress in remedying construction evils, such as inadequate lighting and heating, than they did in caring for the health of the individual child. Yet shortly after the turn of the century health officers and educators began to consider the handicapped pupil. The movement really stemmed in part from a resolution passed by the American Medical Association, which recommended that health boards, school boards, and school authorities look to the examination of children's eyes and ears. This resolution was endorsed by the Minnesota State Medical Association. The Blue Earth County Medical Society also approved the resolution and reported its action to Bracken. These three resolutions, one by a national body, an-

[10] State Board of Health, *Biennial Reports*, 1889–90, p. 6, charts following p. 24; 1895–96, p. 20; 1897–98, p. 83; 1899–1900, pp. 65, 525–533.
[11] Superintendent of Public Instruction, *Biennial Reports*, 1903–04, pp. 308, 310, 378, 381, 437–453. See also Crane, *Report on . . . Sanitary and Sociologic Problems*, 151–176, for a description of the hygiene and sanitation of schoolhouses in 1909.

other by a state association, and the last by a county society really started eye and ear examinations in Minnesota schools.[12]

A state committee of five physicians was formed in 1904 to submit a plan which would, they said, result in the comfort and success of the child and in his future well-being. A simple examination of the ears was proposed: "If conversational tones can be heard at twenty feet, whispered tones at six feet, or watch tick at two feet, with each ear, for all practical purposes the hearing is perfect." With this report before him, Bracken decided to examine the eyes and ears of school children throughout the state. In April, 1904, the health board completed final details. Examination would first be undertaken of school children in villages and cities having a population of a thousand or more. When this was completed communities of less than a thousand and country districts would be visited. Meanwhile Bracken was trying to get statistics from the superintendent of public instruction as to the number of children in school. He also queried local superintendents by mail. Toward the close of 1904 a circular letter, which described the plan in full, was sent to schools throughout the state, and early the next year a follow-up form was mailed.[13]

The program was only partially successful. Minneapolis refused to co-operate, but results from other communities were sufficient to prove the worth of the project. The survey revealed a significant fact: the state board should leave future examinations to local health and educational agencies. Both groups were showing increased interest by 1907. The Minnesota superintendent of public instruction thought that physical examinations were a necessity in all schools. "The extent to which medical inspection may be carried on will depend upon the number and character of the school population," he said, "but in no school, however small, is it impossible to find some of the physical defects that mar childhood, and 'to the afflicted child,' it makes no difference whether he is one of ten in school or one of fifty. His need is his own and should be considered."[14]

The medical profession echoed these sentiments and in 1907 suggested that a health survey of Minneapolis school children might reveal some interesting figures. It was pointed out that the percentage of children

[12] Minnesota State Medical Association, *Transactions*, 1903, p. 12; J. S. Holbrook to Bracken, December 2, 1903, Minnesota Department of Health, St. Paul.
[13] Bracken to C. E. Lum, May 13, 1904, and to J. W. Olsen, April 14, 1904; State Board of Health, "Circular Letter, September, 1904," "Circular Letter, April 15, 1905," Minnesota Department of Health, St. Paul.
[14] Bracken to Margaret Curtis, March 7, 1906, Minnesota Department of Health, St. Paul; Superintendent of Public Instruction, *Biennial Reports*, 1907–08, p. 18.

needing corrective treatment was remarkably high. This generalization was borne out in 1908 when the Minneapolis Woman's Club and the Associated Charities persuaded the school board to make a physical examination of pupils. A single school was selected and 354 children were examined, with startling results. Of the total number examined, 170 were found to have enlarged cervical glands, 113 had defective teeth, 112 had enlarged tonsils, 115 were undernourished, 58 had defective vision, and 23 had defective hearing. There were 46 pupils with postnasal growths and 2 with trachoma. "This preliminary work alone demonstrates the urgency of medical inspection, and emphasizes the necessity of health and normal physiologic growth before education is crammed into children," said a medical journal. "These children have failed to pass their grades 284 times! This fact alone is an object lesson for unbelievers. If defects are responsible for failures it is time that medical inspection is put on a proper basis, and made compulsory in all schools, particularly in children who show a backward tendency." [15]

Minneapolis was convinced that the child's health should be watched. In 1909 the Board of Education created a department of hygiene and physical training. Its work, said Dr. Charles H. Keene, the first supervisor of the department, included the medical inspection and physical examination of children. This was a real step forward, and soon it was repeated by St. Paul and Duluth. Keene's successor, Dr. Earnest B. Hoag, estimated that adenoids in Minnesota school children cost the state about a million dollars, "as there are at least forty thousand children so affected, and the cost of educating a school child is about twenty-five dollars per year, and a child with adenoids usually requires nine years to finish eight grades." Hoag believed that an allowance of fifty cents per pupil at least was necessary for a competent examination program in Minneapolis schools.[16]

During 1911 the state health board employed a physician who gave his entire time to examining children. This work became so important that in 1916 the superintendent of education suggested that "the county should be fixed as a health unit, or several school districts, independent of county lines, should be permitted to unite to carry out this service in an effective manner and without unnecessary duplicate cost." Hoag had helped to formulate this recommendation, not only because of his enthu-

[15] "Examination of School Children," "Defects in School Children," and "Medical Inspection in the Public Schools," in *Northwestern Lancet*, 27:493, 535; 28:81 (November 15, December 15, 1907, February 15, 1908); Minneapolis Board of Education, *Reports*, 1908, p. 69.
[16] Minneapolis Board of Education, *Reports*, 1910, p. 97; Hoag to the Minneapolis Board of Tax Levy, September 13, 1912, Minnesota Department of Health, St. Paul.

siasm and competence but also because of his close co-operation with the state health board. As a matter of fact, he had left his position in the Minneapolis school system to become a member of the state health department with the title of special director of school hygiene. "You see," he wrote shortly after accepting the appointment, "I am located at St. Paul at last, and am under way with my new work. The Minnesota people are giving me splendid cooperation in every respect, and I am finding my work very agreeable and profitable." [17]

Hoag's appointment marked the beginning of formal work in child hygiene by the state health department in that he was the first person to be engaged especially for that purpose. He began his work on August 1, 1912, but he remained with the board for only a short time. He spent most of his time traveling about the state, talking with superintendents and teachers, giving demonstrations, picking out certain defective children, and instructing teachers in the methods of detecting defects. Frequently he addressed public meetings, stressing the need for physical examination of pupils. His object, said Bracken, was to show teachers how easy it was to detect the ordinary physical handicaps from which children suffer. Hoag also gave to the senior class of each of Minnesota's five normal schools a short course of five lectures on the physical observation of children, and he wrote an outline for the health grading of the school child, which was distributed free by the board throughout the state. His work received such attention nationally that the editor of *Youth's Companion* wrote Bracken asking for complete details.[18]

It was Hoag who prepared the preliminary outline for a division of child hygiene and school sanitation with the joint co-operation of the University of Minnesota and the Minnesota Department of Public Instruction. Such a division was at least tentatively established in 1913. Hoag included the words "school sanitation" in the title of the division for a definite purpose. He was convinced that improper ventilation was a menace to public health. He was acquainted with the miserable condition of school buildings a quarter of a century earlier, and he could have learned from correspondence of the state board that innumerable complaints were still received concerning insanitary school conditions. A schoolteacher's letter from Pillager is typical: "In behalf of my pupils,

[17] Superintendent of Public Instruction, *Biennial Reports*, 1911–12, p. 20; Minnesota Department of Education, *Biennial Reports*, 1915–16, p. 30; Hoag to W. S. Hall, October 8, 1912, Minnesota Department of Health, St. Paul.
[18] State Board of Health, *Biennial Reports*, 1911–12, p. 7; Hoag to W. S. Scherer and to the Chicago Board of Education, October 8, 1912, and Bracken to the department editor of *Youth's Companion*, October 31, 1912, Minnesota Department of Health, St. Paul; Hoag, *An Outline for the Health Grading of the School Child* ([St. Paul, 1912]).

I write to let you know of the unhealthy water we have to drink, and if you will please investigate the matter. . . . The children and myself nearly die of thirst before touching it." [19]

As Hoag talked with his colleagues in the health department he found that shortly after the turn of the century the department had begun to advise architects on the proper construction of school buildings. But the board assumed no responsibility for seeing that schools were properly built. It did, however, report on construction details and, when necessary, recommend that plans be altered. This service was not satisfactory to schoolmen. Indeed, C. G. Schulz, superintendent of public instruction in 1913, complained to Bracken that the board was too slow in its reports upon school construction and inferred that some other state department should take over the work. Schulz seemed dissatisfied with Bass's activities and suggested strongly to Bracken that it might be better if the health department entirely relinquished its jurisdiction over school sanitation. Bracken replied in a far more reasonable tone than was natural for him. He admitted that someone should be in Bass's office during office hours, but he disagreed with Schulz that authority should be removed from the health board. He thought that all sanitary matters should be under the board's supervision. Hoag, of course, agreed with Bracken. Fortunately the dispute was clarified by a legislative act placing responsibility for water supply and the disposal of sewage in public school buildings upon the health department.[20]

Schulz, although he accepted this solution, was not entirely convinced of its merit. At a meeting of the Minnesota State Sanitary Conference later in 1913, he again spoke in favor of placing health work under the control of school authorities. Then he continued: "In Minnesota, whatever our convictions on this point may be, we must in all fairness give credit to the health authorities, to the state health supervisory authorities — and in the first instance to Dr. Bracken as the Executive Officer of the State Board of Health for having initiated, having set in motion and brought under way the keener appreciation and the better understanding in regard to health conditions as relate to public schools. Now, whether

[19] Hoag to Samuel Hopkins Adams, April 14, 1913, and to George E. Vincent, May 1, 1913, A. Siemens to Hewitt, November 10, 1896, and Marie F. Lawrence to Bracken, March 29, 1898, Minnesota Department of Health, St. Paul; *St. Paul Daily Press*, October 16, 1872.

[20] Bracken to P. M. Olson, October 26, 1907, and to C. G. Schulz, January 7, 1913, and Schulz to Bracken, January 2, 1913, Minnesota Department of Health, St. Paul; F. H. Bass, "Report on School Building for District No. 27, Waseca County, September 1, 1909," and "Report on Heating and Ventilating Plans for St. Cloud Domestic Science School, December 9, 1909," and J. A. Childs, "Report on Plans for Grade School at Chisholm, St. Louis County, February 9, 1911" (typescripts), Minnesota Department of Health, St. Paul; *General Statutes*, 1913, section 2874.

or not the educational authorities shall assume a larger responsibility in regard to health work in Minnesota or not, I think that is a fair subject for intelligent and unbiased discussion and consideration."[21]

Bracken admitted that perhaps in the larger cities the boards of education should supervise medical work in schools — an opinion contrary to that which he had expressed two years earlier when he told the conference that school supervision was a part of public health work, "most decidedly a part and a most important part, because it is the supervision of the child from the beginning to the end of its school career." This controversy concerning jurisdiction over school sanitation was finally settled by the legislature, which passed a bill stripping the health department of its power to make regulations covering school hygiene except those setting standards for toilets, water supply, and the disposal of sewage. All other authority was vested in the state superintendent of education. That left the health department in a position to deal only with communicable diseases. This act, together with a lack of funds, led the health department to discontinue Hoag's services after August 1, 1913. By that time Hoag himself was convinced that health work in schools should be in charge of boards of education rather than boards of health. "It is a matter," he said, "of child study rather than medical inspection."[22]

In 1914 Dr. Carroll Fox of the United States Public Health Service made a penetrating survey of public health administration in Minnesota and found much that was not right in the child hygiene program. He said that, except in a few isolated cases, the Minnesota State Board of Health had taken little action recently toward establishing any system of school medical inspection; that it was the duty of the health department to study infant or child welfare, including prenatal care of mothers, and to institute measures to conserve human life and health during the earlier periods of existence; that if the "medical inspection of schools is placed in the hands of school authorities there is lost to the health department a most valuable period, namely, during the school age of the child, in which to carry on valuable studies and follow up the previous work in infant welfare." Fox demolished the argument that the average health department is neither sufficiently well endowed nor sufficiently well organized to carry on such work properly. He said such an argument was an excellent reason why the department should be so strengthened as to enable it to do the work and do it well. He recommended that in

[21] Minnesota State Sanitary Conference, "Proceedings," October 1, 1913 (typescript), Minnesota Department of Health, St. Paul.
[22] State Sanitary Conference, "Proceedings," October 4, 1911 (typescript), and Hoag to A. A. D'Ancona, March 24, 1913, Minnesota Department of Health, St. Paul; *Laws*, 1913, p. 796; State Board of Health, "Minutes," April 29, 1913.

HEALTH OF MOTHER AND CHILD

cities local health departments should carry on school work, while in rural communities the state department should do it. He pointed out the "great discrepancy" existing between appropriations for public health work and for school work in Minnesota, saying that the state board would receive during 1915 only $67,000 — "a totally inadequate amount"— while the state aid to public schools would be $4,300,000. He spoke with obvious dismay of Minnesota's sparse interest in conserving child life and said that school hygiene and child welfare were subjects of "such vast importance that it is to be hoped the coming legislature will appropriate sufficient money to continue this and similar work." [23]

This stung, especially since Fox had spoken approvingly of earlier attempts by the board to inaugurate a modern school program. When, in 1914, Bracken was asked for assistance by a New Yorker, he could only reply: "Minnesota is a new state and, while some work is being done along the line of infant welfare in the larger cities, it is not yet in organized form." But the seed had been sown, and in 1918 it sprouted. On April 25 a group of pediatricians met with state health representatives to discuss the need for a division of child hygiene in the state health department. Plans were made to present an appeal for the establishment of this new division to the Minnesota Public Safety Commission, and support was secured from more than a dozen influential organizations, including the State Federation of Women's Clubs, the Council of Jewish Women, the Children's Protective Society of Minneapolis, the National Association for the Prevention of Infant Mortality, and the American Red Cross. The Department of Pediatrics of the University of Minnesota became interested, as did the Northwestern Pediatric Society and infant welfare organizations in St. Paul, Duluth, and Little Falls. Bracken wrote each of these organizations that the "death rate in children under one year of age is very largely due to ignorance, first, as to the care of the child, second, as to the necessary surroundings, and it is very possible to dissipate this ignorance by careful supervision in matters especially relating to infant feeding and the proper care of the child; and this can only be brought about by the close contact of specially trained physicians and nurses." [24]

Organized activity got under way in May, 1918, when Mrs. James G. Swan, state chairman of the women's division of the Council of National Defense, announced "The Children's Year Campaign." All but twelve

[23] Fox, *Public Health Administration in Minnesota*, 66–69 (Washington, D.C., 1914).
[24] Bracken to Mildred Ashland, October 13, 1914, Minnesota Department of Health, St. Paul; form letter from Bracken to the organizations named, April 27, 1918, Minnesota Department of Health, Minneapolis.

of Minnesota's eighty-seven counties were organized, and state committees exerted political pressure where it would do the most good. In July the health department created an advisory committee on child conservation. By that time the Children's Bureau of the United States Department of Labor had become interested in the program. Dr. E. J. Huenekens was named the first director of the division of child conservation. The advisory committee was composed of two distinguished physicians, Dr. J. P. Sedgwick and Dr. J. C. Litzenberg, and of representatives of the State Board of Control and women's clubs.[25]

Despite the efforts of the interested groups, the wished-for state financial help was not forthcoming. Bracken became so desperate that he wrote Governor J. A. A. Burnquist, saying: "Must the State Board of Health give up an effort to establish such a Division at the present time? During the past few months, recognizing the greater demand on the preservation of child life, several states have created such a division." Bracken pointed out that Massachusetts, long a leader in public health, had started a child conservation division by securing five thousand dollars from the Red Cross and a like amount from the governor's contingent fund. He asked Burnquist for aid so that "we could go ahead and organize our Division and carry it through the legislative session."[26]

No sooner had word of the new children's division seeped through the state than a score of communities asked for help in establishing clinics. A nurse in Yellow Medicine County requested assistance, as the need was great; Granite Falls and Canby asked aid in establishing infant welfare clinics, where instruction could be given in food and general hygiene; and in Duluth the Scottish Rites Masons asked help for a program they already had begun. Examinations of children were made in Ramsey and Morrison counties. Indeed, so many requests for assistance came to Huenekens that he deplored his lack of facilities to care for them. Only children below the age of five years were received at clinics, and the emphasis was placed on the control and prevention of communicable diseases.[27]

Two factors brought the program to an abrupt halt. The first, of course, was lack of funds, but that might have been overcome in the course of time had it not been for a second factor — the great influenza epidemic

[25] *Pioneer Press*, September 15, 1918; Bracken to C. W. Gordon, August 2, 1918, Minnesota Department of Health, St. Paul.
[26] Bracken to Burnquist, July 1, 1918, Minnesota Department of Health, St. Paul.
[27] Bracken to Huenekens, August 12, 1918, and to William W. Hodson, October 14, 1918; Huenekens to G. A. Eisengraeber, September 11, 1918, to F. W. Hugo, September 13, 1918, and to J. P. Sedgwick, September 13, 1918; State Board of Health, Division of Child Conservation, "Report," October 8, 1918. Minnesota Department of Health, St. Paul.

HEALTH OF MOTHER AND CHILD   385

of 1918. The epidemic obviously made it unwise to continue public clinics for children. The University of Minnesota delayed the opening of its fall quarter for a week, and early in October at least a thousand cases were reported in Minneapolis. Some public schools were closed on October 14. Three days later the United States Public Health Service recommended the closing of all theaters, churches, and schools. This epidemic really put an end to the health department's first formal attempt to create and keep going a division devoted to child care. In 1919 the work was taken over by the Northwestern Pediatrics Society in co-operation with the Minnesota Public Health Association.[28]

From 1919 until July 1, 1922, Minnesota was without a state-wide children's health program sponsored by the state board. Tremendous interest still existed in many communities, but the legislature failed to see the needs of the state's children and did not appropriate the funds necessary to renew the work. The health department, therefore, was forced to look to the federal government for monetary assistance. By that time other states had made far more progress in the protection of children. Enlightened educators, social workers, and health officials had all recognized the paramount importance of well-planned programs. They were becoming concerned not only with school construction and sanitation, but also with school clinics and maternity and infancy programs.

Minnesota, through the years, had had a score of evils that needed correction. Newspapers throughout the 1870s, for example, said openly that some physicians were none too careful when they delivered women; women's diseases were declared to be inadequately studied; and the activities of midwives were an open scandal.[29] Complaints were made that midwives engaged in abortion, failed to report births for statistical purposes, and were notoriously unclean. During 1885 "baby-farming" flourished in St. Paul. [30] The situation was not completely black, however, for after the turn of the century the legislature passed two significant acts concerning children and hospitals. The first was entitled "An act to

[28] "The Influenza Situation," in *Journal-Lancet*, 38:602 (October 15, 1918); *Pioneer Press*, September 28, 1918; *Tribune*, October 4, 13, 1918; the Surgeon General, United States Public Health Service, to Bracken, October 17, 1918, Minnesota Department of Health, St. Paul; State Board of Health, *Reports*, 1922-43, p. 158; *Biennial Reports*, 1918-19, p. 9.
[29] *St. Paul Daily Press*, May 2, 25, 1872; *Pioneer Press*, May 1, 11, 1878, June 19, 1886; F. B. Norin to Hewitt, March 18, 1894, Minnesota Department of Health, St. Paul.
[30] W. G. Goffe to Hewitt, March 31, 1894, A. H. Clark to Hewitt, August 31, 1895, G. W. Smith to Bracken, May 4, 1903, and W. W. Shrader, "Report," March 1, 1898, Minnesota Department of Health, St. Paul; *Pioneer Press*, July 30, August 30, 31, 1885; *Tribune*, June 24, 1885; E. J. Huenekens, "The Minnesota Plan for the Establishment of Infant Welfare Clinics in Smaller Towns," in *Archives of Pediatrics*, 35:718-722 (December, 1918).

promote the health and welfare of infants born or cared for in places not the home of their parents," and the second, passed in 1917, required every maternity hospital in a county containing a city of the first or second class to be incorporated in order to obtain a license from the State Board of Control.[31] Much had been accomplished, of course, by both local and state health officers in dealing with infectious diseases of children and with school health and school sanitation.

Not until 1921 did Minnesota develop a public health program for expectant mothers and for mothers and their infants after childbirth. Two legislative acts — one national and the other state — formed the legal foundation upon which the board erected its division of child hygiene. This division probably would not have come into being had it not been for the generous financial provisions of the Sheppard-Towner Act of November, 1921, which made federal funds available to the states for maternal and child health programs conducted by existing boards of health in accordance with plans approved by the Children's Bureau of the United States Department of Labor. Realizing that the Sheppard-Towner bill would be passed, the Minnesota legislature authorized the state health board to develop a maternal and child welfare program and to co-operate with other agencies, including the Children's Bureau. Chesley set up a program, and the division of child hygiene was formally created on July 1, 1922.[32]

Federal funds were matched with money donated by state organizations, including the Minnesota Public Health Association, and $47,199.31 was available for the fiscal year ending on June 30, 1923. The legislature appropriated $15,000 for the fiscal year beginning on July 1, 1923. Federal aid was withdrawn in 1929, when the Sheppard-Towner Act passed out of existence, and Minnesota was forced to finance the program itself until the Social Security Act was passed during the depression years. In 1936, a year after the Social Security Act made financial assistance possible again, the legislature empowered the state health board to train personnel for maternal and child welfare work. That same year a superintendent of dental health education was appointed to the staff. In 1937 a nutritionist became a member of the division to aid mothers and children with diet problems.[33]

[31] *Laws*, 1901, p. 111; 1916–17, pp. 301–308; Bracken to J. A. Hielscher, August 28, 1902, and to More, March 13, 1918, and More to Bracken, March 8, 1918, Minnesota Department of Health, St. Paul.
[32] State Board of Health, *Reports*, 1922–43, p. 158; *Laws*, 1921, p. 599.
[33] *Laws*, 1923, p. 681; Emily Child, "What Price Mothers and Babies," in *Minnesota Public Health Nurse*, vol. 2, no. 1, pp. 5, 14 (January, 1929); *Statutes*, 1945, section 144.10; State Board of Health, *Reports*, 1922–43, p. 161.

Headed by Dr. Ruth E. Boynton, the maternity and infancy program sought to extend its services directly to the expectant mother. This was accomplished in several ways. A correspondence course, consisting of fifteen lessons, was prepared by E. C. Hartley in collaboration with the University of Minnesota's Department of Obstetrics and Pediatrics; a series of nine monthly prenatal letters was sent to expectant mothers; and prenatal clinics, through co-operation with local physicians, were held throughout the state. Sterile obstetrical packages were made up and distributed where needed in rural communities. Hartley and Boynton also surveyed the midwife situation. They found that midwives, licensed and unlicensed, numbered 118, of whom 48% had been trained for six months or more in a school for midwives, 15% had had less than six months of schooling, 27.9% had had practical experience with a midwife or physician, 1.9% had taken a correspondence course in midwifery, and 6.65% had had no training of any kind.[34]

Two other factors contributed to the success of the division of child hygiene. The first was the work of nurses connected with the division, and the second was the emphasis placed on child-health days throughout the state. A nursing advisory committee, consisting of the county superintendent of schools, the county health officer or a physician appointed by the county commissioners, a county commissioner appointed by the board of county commissioners, and two residents of the county also appointed by the commissioners, encouraged the administration of county nursing services and stimulated co-operation between the nurse and the medical profession. Child-health days were enthusiastically endorsed by the medical profession as of "vast importance to the community as well as to the individual."[35]

Maternal health was benefited further in 1942, when the program of maternity hospital licensing was transferred by law from the division of social welfare of the Department of Social Security, in co-operation with the State Board of Health, to the board exclusively. This law extended licensure to all hospitals, convalescent homes, and similar institutions. This additional obligation, however, did not hinder the division's distribution of literature nor its policy to extend its aid directly to the people. In 1941, for example, 512,534 pieces of literature and 1,287 pre-

[34] E. C. Hartley and Ruth E. Boynton, "The Minnesota Maternity and Infancy Program," in *American Journal of Obstetrics and Gynecology*, 10:863–869 (December, 1925), and "A Survey of the Midwife Situation in Minnesota," in *Minnesota Medicine*, 7:440–446 (June, 1924).
[35] Mary A. Johnson, "Rural Public Health Nursing in Minnesota," in *Public Health Nursing*, 28:681–684 (October, 1936); "Child Health Day," in *Minnesota Medicine*, 6:189 (March, 1923).

natal letters were distributed. Several postgraduate courses in obstetrics and pediatrics for physicians were held at the Center for Continuation Study of the University of Minnesota, beginning in 1937, and demonstrations to hospital groups were held in 168 cities. Nurses distributed thousands of pieces of specialized literature, which carried such titles as: *The School Lunch; Milk in Your Daily Meals; Diet of Expectant and Nursing Mother;* and *Hot Lunches at School.*[36]

The division aided in two important surveys of maternal deaths. A report on the first, which was made in co-operation with the Children's Bureau, appeared in 1933. As a result, recommendations were made to the medical profession and to the general public. Both were told that the high maternal death rate was due largely to controllable causes and that it was "necessary for all women to have adequate supervision and medical care during pregnancy, labor, and the postpartum period, such supervision and medical care to begin early in pregnancy and to be continuous through the postpartum period in order to safeguard the health of both mother and child and especially in order to control the infections, toxemias, and hemorrhages that this study and others have shown to be real menaces to life." [37]

A few years later a special study of maternal mortality in Minnesota was made by a committee of physicians under the sponsorship of the Minnesota Department of Health and the State Medical Association. This investigation began on July 1, 1941, and continued through June 30, 1942. The committee's report revealed, among other findings, that forty per cent of mothers losing their lives in association with pregnancy and childbirth were more than thirty-four years old; that failure of coroners "to request or demand postmortem examinations on those patients dying under circumstances suggestive of violence is outstanding"; and that eighty-two per cent of the cases studied had no pelvic mensuration or had less than the minimum requirements for adequate prenatal care specified by the committee. The office records of physicians, in the great majority of cases, were found to be "of very little value" in providing accurate information, "if indeed there were any records." It was discovered that, measured by the requirements adopted by the committee, adequate obstetrical care "was given in only 1.8 per cent in the prenatal period, 6.3 per cent in labor and for delivery, and 3.6 per cent in the postpartum

---

[36] Minnesota, *Statutes,* 1941, sections 144.50–144.58; State Board of Health, *Reports,* 1922–43, pp. 162, 165.

[37] State Board of Health, *Reports,* 1922–43, p. 171; United States Department of Labor, Children's Bureau, *Maternal Deaths — A Brief Report of a Study Made in 15 States,* 59 (*Publication* 221 — Washington, D.C., 1933).

period." The report stated that, while a blood Wassermann had "long been considered an absolute essential . . . 73.2 per cent of these cases did not have venapuncture for Wassermann test at the first prenatal visit; and 62.5 per cent had no Wassermann test in association with pregnancy." Seventy-three per cent of the deaths were preventable, the committee agreed, and "in all but four instances the physician was wholly or partially responsible." The committee concluded that "it would seem that charity patients received the better care"; that "deaths due to infection and to shock and hemorrhage make up 53.3 per cent of all the maternal deaths in this series"; that a "surprising revelation is the general inadequacy of the therapy used to combat puerperal infection"; and that it "appears that place of residence (urban or rural) does not materially affect the obstetric results."[38]

The work and activities of the division of child hygiene were reported to the profession in a small publication entitled the *News Letter*, which first appeared in 1923 and terminated seven years later. This periodical also printed pertinent comments from nurses engaged in the maternal health program, as well as comments from mothers. A young mother, for example, wrote of a grandmother's interference and quoted the old proverb: "Time makes ancient good uncouth." Helen McGillivray, a nurse at Austin, submitted a typical report of her activities among children. Her comments revealed how far some schools had traveled since the primitive days of the 1870s. "Ramsey Rural School has electric plates for hot lunches — The only rural school in Mower County with electric lights, Ramsey District 44, where Miss Virginia Scott is teaching her third year, is now serving hot lunches from two electric plates. . . . Some of the other features of this school are a basement, furnace, pump in the basement, and a piano. Last year the school was 100% for Diphtheria Toxin-antitoxin, having the doctor come out there to give it. They likewise had two of the winning posters in the Mower County Health Poster Contest, and none of the children were as much as 10% underweight. This school has a very active Parent Teachers Association. It is indeed encouraging to visit such a progressive rural school."[39]

Although activities of the division have expanded tremendously with

[38] Minnesota State Medical Association, Maternal Mortality Committee of the Committee on Maternal Health, "Minnesota Maternal Mortality Study," in *Minnesota Medicine*, 27:475–481, 557–562 (June, July, 1944).
[39] *News Letter*, vol. 1, no. 7, p. 1 (July, 1923); vol. 6, no. 1, p. [5] (January–February, 1929); Blue Earth County Council on Intergovernmental Relations, *A Study of Public Health Administration in Blue Earth County, Minnesota*, 40–45; Harris and Boynton, *Public Health and Medical Care in Red Wing and Goodhue County*, 15.

the years, the concept of service still remains. Earlier pamphlets have been revised and new ones have been prepared. A manual for physicians, issued in 1948, explained the maternal and child health services which were available, including an emergency program that provided care for wives of enlisted men in the four lowest pay grades of the armed services during World War II. It also assured vaccinations and immunizations for their infants during the first year of life. The entire program was completed in 1949. The division was interested also in the crippled children services of the social security department's social welfare division and the education department's vocational rehabilitation division. This orthopedic-plastic program consisted of four types of services — hospitalization of patients, field clinics, field nursing service, and medical social service. A register was maintained of all known children under twenty-one years of age diagnosed as having orthopedic or plastic disabilities. The same organization also supervised a rheumatic fever program. In 1946 the Community Health Service in Minneapolis sponsored classes for expectant mothers at the Maternity Hospital and the YWCA. These included instruction in the physiology of pregnancy, personal hygiene, nutrition, family relationships, and child management. About the same time Viktor O. Wilson, director of the division of child hygiene, formulated a seven-point industrial maternity policy.[40]

Minnesota children became the subject of unusual attention during 1947 and 1948. In September, 1947, an advisory committee of twenty-one members was created to aid the work of the diagnostic clinic for rheumatic fever in the St. Paul Wilder Dispensary. This disease was said to be the leading killer of children between the ages of five and nine. It was responsible for thirty-five per cent of all heart disease at all ages and for ninety per cent of all heart disease in children. With these facts in mind, Junior League members in Minneapolis staged a follies to raise funds for a heart hospital, which had been proposed in 1945 by the Variety Club of the Northwest — an organization of theater and entertainment men who made handsome financial gifts. The Junior League contributed five thousand dollars to the hospital and promised a yearly contribution to make possible the employment of a permanent social worker. On November 15, 1947, the American Legion Foundation announced that it would offer more than five thousand dollars to the University of Minnesota for the establishment of a heart research professor-

[40] Division of Child Hygiene, *A Study Course on Maternal and Child Hygiene* ([Minneapolis?], 1939); *Mothercraft Manual* ([Minneapolis?], 1943); *Handbook for Physicians*, 24 ([St. Paul?], 1948); *Nursing in Industry*, vol. 1, no. 14, pp. 4–7 (December 13, 1945); vol. 2, no. 2, p. [3] (February 4, 1946); vol. 2, no. 6, p. 2 (June 5, 1946).

HEALTH OF MOTHER AND CHILD 391

ship. During 1948 plans were made to enlarge the activities of the maternal and child hygiene program. These called for additional effort in 1949 to maintain the state's low maternal death rate, for steps to reduce infant deaths in the first year of life, for additional control of communicable disease by immunization and vaccination, for an expanded school-service program, and for an accident-prevention program.[41]

Intimately allied with the general well-being of mother and child is the care of their teeth. School physicians knew this, and nurses made the examination of teeth a routine procedure. Yet in many country schools, far removed from adequate professional care, interest in dental health was slight. Fortunately, as in so many other instances, the United States Public Health Service became interested in the problem after it learned of the large number of rejections in World War I because of dental deficiencies and dental disease. It was estimated also that ninety-four per cent of the nation's school children suffered from dental decay. Among the provisions of the Social Security Act was one that made possible the establishment of state dental health programs. Minnesota took advantage of this, and on October 1, 1936, established a section of dental health education in the division of child hygiene, headed by Dr. Vern D. Irwin. By 1948 dental health had become a full division in the section of special services with Dr. W. A. Jordan as director. This development followed the philosophy laid down by the Children's Bureau of the United States Department of Labor when it said that adequate provision to assure satisfactory growth, development, and protection of child health was a public responsibility. Yet every person interested in the welfare of the child knew that this, indeed, was "a long road to travel." [42]

Despite this realization, plans went forward for state dental supervision and the training of children in the care of their teeth. The immediate and long-range objectives in Minnesota were to prevent loss of teeth and serious dental disease, to encourage the replacement of teeth lost through neglect or other causes, and to promote the prompt and efficient treatment of dental diseases when they do occur. These objectives were to be accomplished by research, by education, by co-operation with other

[41] *Pioneer Press*, September 9, 1947; *St. Paul Dispatch*, November 11, 1947; *Minneapolis Star*, February 10, 1948; *Tribune*, November 15, December 4, 1947, October 17, 1948; Cecil J. Watson, "On the Founding of a Variety Club Heart Hospital at the University of Minnesota," in *Journal-Lancet*, 65:402 (November, 1945).
[42] State Board of Health, *Reports*, 1922–43, p. 190; Children's Bureau, *Facts About Child Health*, 9 (Washington, D.C., 1946), *Standards of Child Health, Education, and Social Welfare*, 3 (Publication 287 – Washington, D.C., 1942), and *Proceedings of the Conference on State Child-Welfare Services*, 138 (Maternal and Child-Welfare Bulletin no. 3 – Washington, D.C., 1938).

agencies, by school programs, by adult projects, and by the distribution of literature.[43]

Irwin contributed to professional journals and thus maintained a close relationship between his division and practicing dentists. "Perhaps our aim," Irwin wrote on one occasion, "to save teeth, conserve health, and contribute to the general well-being of individuals and communities can be more readily accomplished by pointing out to the public the *economy* of early and frequent dental care. . . . If such economy were general, most of the boys and girls of Minnesota could grow up to adulthood without losing even one permanent tooth." Of course, achievement of this goal depended upon three factors: the willingness of parents to take their children to dentists, the ability of parents to pay fees, and the availability of dentists. In 1940 the ratio of dentists to the general Minnesota population was 1 to 1,260; in 1944 it had jumped to 1 in 1,678. The ratio of dentists to the school population in 1944 was 1 to 337, but that of dentists to the school population outside of the Twin Cities was 1 to 474. In Kanabec County the ratio for the entire population was 1 to 4,825, and for the school population, 1 to 1,067. In Hennepin County, on the other hand, the ratio was 1 to 811 for the whole population and 1 to 178 for the school population.[44]

Assisted by officials from the United States Public Health Service, Irwin set up three specific problems for investigation:

(1) The use of an index of extractions of permanent teeth in school-age children as a means of evaluating dental health programs.

(2) The effect of caries incidence of topical application of fluorine on children's teeth.

(3) Lactobacillus acidophilus counts in relation to caries in children.[45]

Irwin also, with Netta W. Wilson, made an extensive survey of dental health literature. Short courses for dentists, nurses, and teachers were offered, and in January, 1942, dental health advisers were sent into the field. Their work resulted in a great increase in dental work among

[43] Children's Bureau, *Federal and State Cooperation in Maternal and Child-Welfare Services under the Social Security Act*, 25 (*Maternal and Child-Welfare Bulletin* no. 3 — Washington, D.C., [1937]); *Grants to States for Maternal and Child-Welfare under the Social Security Act*, 7 (*Maternal and Child-Welfare Bulletin* no. 1 — Washington, D.C., 1935); State Board of Health, *Reports*, 1922–43, pp. 191–195; "Dr. Jordan Urges Extension of Dental Plan for Children," in *Minnesota Welfare*, vol. 3, no. 3, p. 9 (November, 1947).

[44] Irwin, "Dental Economy for the Public," in *North-West Dentistry*, 20:119 (April, 1941), and "A Money-Saving Dental Health Program," in *Minnesota Welfare*, vol. 1, no. 2, pp. 4–6 (August, 1945); "Dental Health Education," in *North-West Dentistry*, 23:98 (April, 1944).

[45] State Board of Health, *Reports*, 1922–43, p. 195.

HEALTH OF MOTHER AND CHILD 393

children. The Minnesota Congress of Parents and Teachers sponsored a preschool dental program, and the state education department aided materially in the development of a program which was carried on in public, private, and parochial institutions. School programs were further accelerated when the state health department published a booklet for teachers on children's teeth, and when state educational authorities included specific units on teeth in their curriculum bulletins for both grade and senior high schools.[46]

This ambitious program was endorsed by the Minnesota State Dental Association through its dental health education committee. There was need for such a program. Examinations of 3,304 Minnesota school children in 1947 revealed that the average child five to nine years old had at least three teeth needing immediate attention. At about the same time, fifty dental health experts met at the Center for Continuation Study at the University of Minnesota to plan for further health services. They deplored the shortage of dentists in the state and urged the extension of state aid. When the Minnesota State Dental Association met early in 1948, it paid particular attention to preventive dentistry, and later in the year Minnesota dentists contributed thirty thousand dollars for a research program to improve the dental health of the public. Meanwhile experiments in fluoride applications were going forward on a large scale. Dean W. H. Crawford estimated that this treatment would cut decay by forty per cent.[47]

Although the many activities of Minnesota's maternal and child health program have not solved all problems in the few short years since the Social Security Act was passed, they have secured innumerable benefits. Minnesota is on its way toward the continued improvement of the health of its people.[48]

[46] Irwin and Wilson, *An Evaluation of Dental Health Literature* (St. Paul, 1942); State Board of Health, *Reports*, 1922–43, p. 192; W. A. O'Brien, "What the Schools Can Do," in Minnesota School Board Association, *Proceedings*, 131 (Minneapolis, 1942); Minnesota Department of Health, Division of Dental Health, *Dental Health for Children* (Minneapolis, 1947); Minnesota Department of Education, *Growing Up for Efficient Everyday Living*, 35 (St. Paul, 1946); *Individual and Community Health — Efficiency for Living*, 57–60 (St. Paul, 1946).
[47] "Dental Health Education," in *North-West Dentistry*, 22:44 (January, 1943); 22:144–146 (July, 1943); *Minneapolis Star*, September 18, 1947; *St. Paul Dispatch*, September 18, 23, 1947, January 22, July 7, 1948; *Pioneer Press*, September 22, 1947, August 29, 1948; *Tribune*, September 23, 1947; *Minnesota's Health*, vol. 1, no. 10, p. 1 (October, 1947); vol. 2, no. 7, p. 1 (July, 1948); *Educational Helper*, vol. 41, no. 1, p. [2] (September, 1948); *School Health News*, vol. 2, no. 3, p. 1 (May, 1938).
[48] Children's Bureau, *White House Conference on Children in a Democracy, Final Report*, 315 (Washington, D.C., 1940).

20

Old Plagues Don't Die

BRILLIANT flags fluttered from turreted towers. From a band shell a rollicking popular tune blended with the hoarse cries of side-show barkers, peanut venders, and loud-speakers. Avenues were jammed with sight-seers, who were braving the intense summer heat to see Chicago's Century of Progress. Off to the east, behind scores of white exhibition buildings which caught up the hot rays of the sun and reflected them in the faces of the perspiring crowds, the blue waters of Lake Michigan slapped lazily at the beach. Visitors, come to see the sights, jammed Chicago hotels. After a day at the fair they dragged themselves back to their rooms intent upon a cooling shower and a pitcher of ice water. This abnormal demand for water put an unusual strain upon the city's water department and caused a decided drop in pressure. Here was the beginning of tragedy for some of the guests in two hotels.

Before anyone realized what was happening, visitors became sick. Guests in the two hotels experienced symptoms surprisingly like those of appendicitis. Indeed, some of these cases were diagnosed as appendicitis. Many guests did not actually fall ill until after they had returned home from Chicago. At first their home-town physicians did not know what was wrong. They, too, thought in terms of appendicitis. The number of Chicago cases mounted so rapidly that they soon caught the attention of the city's dynamic health officer, Dr. Herman Bundesen. The outbreak was declared to be amebic dysentery. Water carrying contaminated feces is instrumental in spreading the disease.[1] This is what happened in Chicago, and, before the full story was unfolded, it involved Minnesota health authorities and resulted in new plumbing regulations for the state.

Bundesen went into action swiftly. Hotel registers were combed for

[1] Rosenau, *Preventive Medicine and Hygiene*, 139–141.

names of guests, and questionnaires were sent to them. Every suspected or actual case was followed up. Physicians were warned not to confuse the dysentery symptoms with those of appendicitis and, above all, not to operate for appendicitis on any patient who had recently visited the fair until all necessary laboratory work had been done to rule out amebic dysentery. Then began a searching investigation into the origin of the epidemic. By that time some fourteen hundred persons had contracted the disease. Public health officials from many parts of the nation, including Chesley and Dr. Thomas B. Magath from Minnesota, were invited to Chicago to assist in the investigation. They found that when water pressure was reduced by the tremendous demand during the late afternoon a back suction was created in plumbing systems. In one hotel this reduced pressure pulled water in toilets into a water pipe that leaked into a primitive icebox from which bellboys filled pitchers to supply room calls. Thus guests were receiving ice contaminated with dysentery. The identical result would have been accomplished had they dipped drinking water from sewer pipes. Further investigation revealed faulty cross-connections and other plumbing deficiencies.[2]

Although this epidemic of amebic dysentery, like all epidemics, spread far and wide from its source, there were few, if any, cases in Minnesota. The importance of the outbreak to Minnesota lay in the realization it brought of the necessity for plumbing systems and fixtures that would prevent a similar experience there. A revised Minnesota plumbing code was adopted by the state health board on July 20, 1937. Later, bulletins were issued showing the relationship of plumbing to public health and indicating how plans for plumbing systems for public buildings should be prepared. The board also began to give examinations to individuals who wished to become either journeymen or master plumbers. Applicants were asked such questions as: "What Section of the Code protects the drinking water in a plumbing system from unsafe water?" and "Before a plumbing installation for any public building is started, what state control is carried out to protect the public health?" In 1945 the legislature authorized cities, villages, and boroughs to adopt the plumbing code "by reference" in a local ordinance.[3]

[2] United States Public Health Service, *Epidemic Amebic Dysentery — The Chicago Outbreak of 1933*, pp. v, 72–74, 89, 140, appendix B2 (National Institute of Health, Bulletin no. 166 — Washington, D.C., 1936).
[3] State Board of Health, *Minnesota Plumbing Code* (St. Paul, 1947), and *Plumbing in Relation to Public Health* (Minneapolis, 1942); Minnesota Department of Health, *Information Relative to Preparation and Submission of Plans and Specifications on Plumbing in Public Buildings or Buildings for Public Use* ([St. Paul?], 1946); Section of Environmental Sanitation, Plumbing Unit, "Examination Questions, September 17, 1947," Minnesota Department of Health, Minneapolis; *Laws*, 1945, p. 312.

The basic regulation upon which Minnesota's protection rests, stemming in part from the Chicago dysentery epidemic, is relatively simple, but it marks a milestone in the state's public health progress: "No system of plumbing for a building shall be installed, nor shall any such existing system be materially altered or extended by any person, corporation or public agency in case any such plumbing system is for public use or for the use of any considerable number of persons, or in case any such plumbing system affects or tends to affect the public health in any manner, until complete plans and specifications for the plumbing installation, alterations, or extensions, together with such information as the State Board of Health may require have been submitted in duplicate and approved by the Board insofar as any features thereof affect or tend to affect the public health, and insofar as these features conform to the provisions of the Minnesota Plumbing Code, as amended. No construction shall take place except in accordance with approved plans. Provided that this regulation shall not apply to cities of the first class, except for plumbing installations in hospitals or in buildings in such cities owned by the Federal Government or the State." Regulation 201 says: "There shall be no physical connection between water supply systems that are safe for domestic use and those that are unsafe for domestic use."[4]

Bacillary dysentery, like many another infectious disease, was well known in Minnesota. Isolated cases were reported throughout the state during the 1870s, and during the following twenty years it reached epidemic proportions in various communities and institutions. A severe outbreak, caused by faulty plumbing and drainage, was reported at the St. Peter State Hospital in 1893. Other contagious diseases, of course, also existed in Minnesota. Some of them reached epidemic proportions, while others did not. Cholera was present in many communities and always was feared.[5]

The great epidemics which caused consternation among health officials were not always water-borne as was the outbreak of dysentery at Chicago. But sanitation demanded that all possible sources of contamination be controlled, including water and sewerage systems. It was believed that contamination might also result if proper care was not taken in the handling of dead bodies. Bracken was tremendously concerned about

[4] *Minnesota Plumbing Code*, [1]; *Minnesota State Health Laws and Regulations*, 89 (January 1, 1948).
[5] *Pioneer-Press and Tribune*, July 11, August 29, 1876; *Pioneer Press*, September 26, 1875, July 13, November 18, 1884, September 5, 1885, August 17, 1892; *St. Paul Daily Press*, August 10, 1872; John M. Armstrong, "The Asiatic Cholera in Saint Paul," in *Minnesota Medicine*, 25:994–996 (December, 1942); 26:108–113, 192 (January, February, 1943); letters to Hewitt from H. A. Tomlinson, January 10, 1893, and from D. B. Collins, January 10, 1893, Minnesota Department of Health, St. Paul.

this, although today it is not so important as he thought. Embalming was not always adequate and sometimes the bodies of persons who had died from infectious diseases were not prepared and shipped in a sanitary manner. Indeed, Minnesota cemeteries, during the early period, sometimes offered no permanent resting place for the dead. Frequently, as cities and towns grew, bodies had to be removed to make land available for other uses. After the Civil War complaint was made that the system of burial permits was not being enforced. The remains of a Duluth child had to be taken to Minneapolis in 1872, said an editor, because Duluth "with all her boasted growth and advancement does not possess a cemetery." A few years later a St. Paul newspaper complained that "there should be some means of preventing doctors giving courtesy certificates of death" because "the public health is jeopardized by it." It seemed that people would not take ordinary health precautions when death entered a household where an infectious or contagious disease existed. Dr. C. H. Boardman sternly warned the St. Paul public not to attend funerals of those who died from contagious diseases.[6]

The public was antagonistic in 1886 when railroads adopted strict rules regarding the shipment of dead bodies. These regulations required not only a health officer's certificate but also a certificate from the attending physician giving the cause of death. Undertakers were to issue a statement showing that a corpse had been prepared according to definite rules. In case of an infectious disease the mortician's certificate had to be sworn to before a notary public. Transportation of the bodies of persons who had died of smallpox, cholera, typhoid fever, or yellow fever was forbidden. Local health officers had the greatest difficulty in enforcing proper sanitary requirements at private funerals, although now and again advice was sought from the state health board. Fortunately a legislative act of 1883 had given the state board authority to inspect corpses which had been prepared for transportation in cases of death resulting from contagious diseases. But not until 1898 did Minnesota adopt specific rules and regulations for the transportation of the dead.[7]

The regulations of 1898 were revised by the state health board on July 9, 1901, after consultation with the Conference of State and Provincial Boards of Health, the General Baggage Agents Association of America, and the National Funeral Directors Association. Stating that these regu-

[6] *St. Anthony Express*, May 21, 1852; *St. Paul Pioneer*, November 22, 1866; *Minneapolis Tribune*, February 19, 1868; *Duluth Tribune*, July 24, 1872; *St. Paul Daily Globe*, April 26, 1879; *Pioneer Press*, January 20, 1880.
[7] *Tribune*, January 28, 1886; *Laws*, 1883, p. 178; H. N. Avery to Hewitt, October 29, 1896, Bracken to H. W. Childs, January 1, 1898, and to E. S. Wishard, December 31, 1900, and Childs to Bracken, January 15, 1898, Minnesota Department of Health, St. Paul.

lations were passed in the interest of public health, the board specified that after January 1, 1902, "all non-licensed embalmers shipping remains into or from the state of Minnesota . . . be required to furnish an affidavit to the railroad receiving the remains to the effect that the death of the individual was not due to a communicable disease and that the Minnesota regulations relating to the preparation of the remains of those that have not died of a communicable disease, have been complied with; such affidavit to be forwarded at once to the Secretary of the Minnesota State Board of Health"; and that "shipment of remains by non-licensed embalmers into or from the state of Minnesota, must always be made in hermetically sealed caskets, unless said remains can reach their destination within thirty hours from the time of death of the individual." By 1948 these regulations had been considerably revised, as a result of increased knowledge of embalming techniques, of educational work done by Bracken, and of epidemics.[8]

Health officers were fully aware that old plagues never die. They knew that only constant watchfulness and preventive treatment kept epidemics at arm's length, and they also realized that public ignorance and indifference could lead to a new outbreak at any moment. Such an outbreak — one of Minnesota's most severe smallpox epidemics — swept the state between January 1, 1899, and July 1, 1900. During that period 1,164 cases were reported with 28 deaths. The disease occurred in 114 different localities in 48 counties. This epidemic started, explained Bracken, early in 1899 when a railroad porter carried the disease to St. Paul from the Pacific Coast. Later an immigrant from one of the Scandinavian countries brought smallpox to Minneapolis. Within a few months Minneapolis had reported 296 cases. The disease was taken to Duluth from both St. Paul and Texas. Indeed, seventeen cases in four different communities were traced to the Lone Star visitor. In June smallpox was imported from Montana into Grand Forks, and from there it was taken to Albert Lea. In the summer of 1899 a man returning from California introduced smallpox into Worthington, and a little later it spread to near-by Round Lake. Minnesota, in turn, sent the disease to Wisconsin, Iowa, and South Dakota.[9]

The state health department fought this epidemic by championing

[8] State Board of Health, "Regulations Governing the Transportation of the Dead, August 10, 1901," Minnesota Department of Health, St. Paul; *Minnesota State Health Laws and Regulations*, 132–135 (January 1, 1948); N. C. Pervier and F. Lloyd Hansen, *Report and Review of Research in Embalming and Embalming Fluids by Minnesota State Department of Health* (n.p., n.d.); Bracken Papers, 3:194, 201, 214, 221.

[9] Form letter by Bracken, July 23, 1900, and [Bracken?], "History of Smallpox in Minnesota since January 1, 1899, to May 10, 1900" (typescript), Minnesota Department of Health, St. Paul.

vaccination, even though the state had no compulsory vaccination law, by issuing special circulars, and by distributing a pamphlet which said: "Every one must be on guard against this disease from now on. Railroad officials should notify their ticket agents, especially at small stations, to guard against selling tickets to persons with suspicious eruptions on the face, or with suspicious histories, unless the suspicious party can bring a certificate from a physician, known by the agent to be a reliable man, stating that the party under consideration has neither smallpox nor chicken-pox. School teachers must guard against receiving scholars with any suspicious eruption or history. Schools are probably the means of causing the spread of infectious diseases to a greater extent than any other one agent." [10]

These warnings had their effect. Infected tramps were quarantined, depots were closed and quarantined, and disinfection was carried out whenever possible. Attending physicians took unusual care not to expose themselves. A slightly illiterate citizen of Austin described precautions taken by a local doctor: "The attending Physician has a tent 300 ft. from the house occupied by the patient, he goes there to sleep and once daily removes his outer clothing in a shed near by dons a gown covering all his clothes and goes to see his patient, on coming out of the house he removes his gown washes his hands and face in an antiseptic solution puts on his clothes and comes away from the premisis, he has given up his practice seeing no patients whatever never goes near his office or his house." [11]

Other physicians, however, were not so cautious. All through the epidemic Bracken complained of negligence in reporting cases. He charged that Minneapolis health authorities had been "reversing the diagnosis of able men and claiming that there was no smallpox in the city." He was told that the mayor of Winona did not report contagious diseases, saying that "he had not reported or quarantined them, and that he has told them to stay at home and keep neighbors away simply. He said that it was all nonsense causing people so much expense and trouble for so simple an illness, and asked me what I was going to do about it, with a laugh." But it was against the Minneapolis health officers that Bracken directed his heaviest attack. He charged time and again that the health

[10] State Board of Health, "Regulations . . . Relating to Smallpox, [1899]," (broadside), "Special Circular No. 2, Relating to Smallpox — Resolutions Adopted October 8, 1901," and "Special Smallpox Circular, August 1, 1899," Minnesota Department of Health, St. Paul; H. M. Bracken, "Variola," in American Medical Association, *Journal*, 37:307–310 (August 3, 1901).

[11] *Pioneer Press*, September 16, 1899; H. D. Quarry to Bracken, July 25, 1899, Bracken to W. L. Hollister, January 24, 1900, and John L. Gulden to Bracken, July 25, 1899, Minnesota Department of Health, St. Paul.

commissioner was diagnosing smallpox as chicken pox and that he "does not report the occurrence of infectious diseases to me, as required by law. Minneapolis is the only city in the state that neglects its duty." Later Bracken said bluntly that he could not trust the health commissioner's judgment and, still later, after Bracken attended a meeting of the Minneapolis health board, he wrote the mayor: "I cannot see that your commissioner of health is doing much to control the spread of smallpox. I have no reason to think that vaccination is required of exposed persons; that quarantine is at all strict, that quarantine is long enough for safety, that any effort is made to take a list of exposed persons; that disinfection is at all thorough. . . . In fact, so far as I can determine, the whole affair is handled in a most slipshod manner." Finally, going over the heads of mayor and health commissioner, Bracken requested certificates of successful vaccination from both pupils and teachers in Minneapolis schools.[12]

A special health agent, Dr. Charles H. Norred, then was sent by the board to investigate smallpox in Minneapolis. His candid reports graphically picture the Minneapolis situation. "One of the most serious propositions I have to handle here is the cheap lodging houses," wrote Norred. "A fellow will turn up on the street somewhere, go to some doctor's office for advice and that fool doctor will send him all over town with a card to hunt me and I will finally round him up in some 15c lodging house, hasn't touched anybody, no one has seen him, but there he is. All I can do with that man is to send him to quarantine hospital and fumigate his room — one room." A few days later Norred continued his description: "I believe that there has never been a time, since the appearance of this epidemic, at which we needed a wide awake energetic quarantine officer worse than we do at the present time. The quarantine officer is looked upon something after the style of a dog catcher and as soon as the people were made aware of the fact that a quarantine would be made and maintained, they have even refused to call a physician and have been hiding their cases away in the home and as many members of the family as had any business out or down town, regardless of the vocation, have been going out and in as if nothing had occurred."[13]

Meanwhile Minneapolis city authorities attempted to justify their actions. The mayor told Bracken that he had investigated complaints

---

[12] Bracken to U. O. B. Wingate, February 5, 1900, to Joseph E. Porter, February 6, 1900, to James Gray, January 18, 22, 31, 1900, and to Thomas F. Quinby, February 11, 1900; E. O. Keyes to Bracken, February 24, 1900. Minnesota Department of Health, St. Paul.

[13] Norred to Bracken, March 19, April 22, 1900, Minnesota Department of Health, St. Paul.

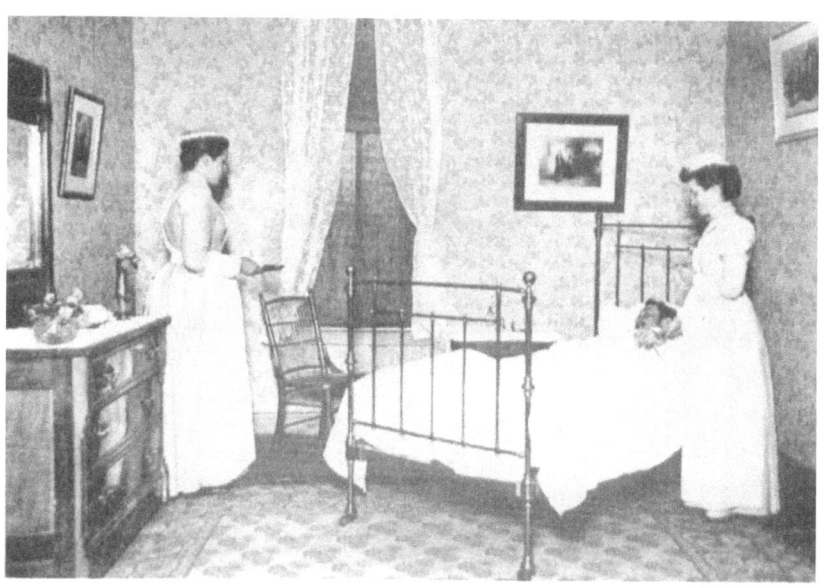

ST. LUKE'S HOSPITAL, DULUTH, IN THE 1880S
Courtesy Minnesota State Medical Association

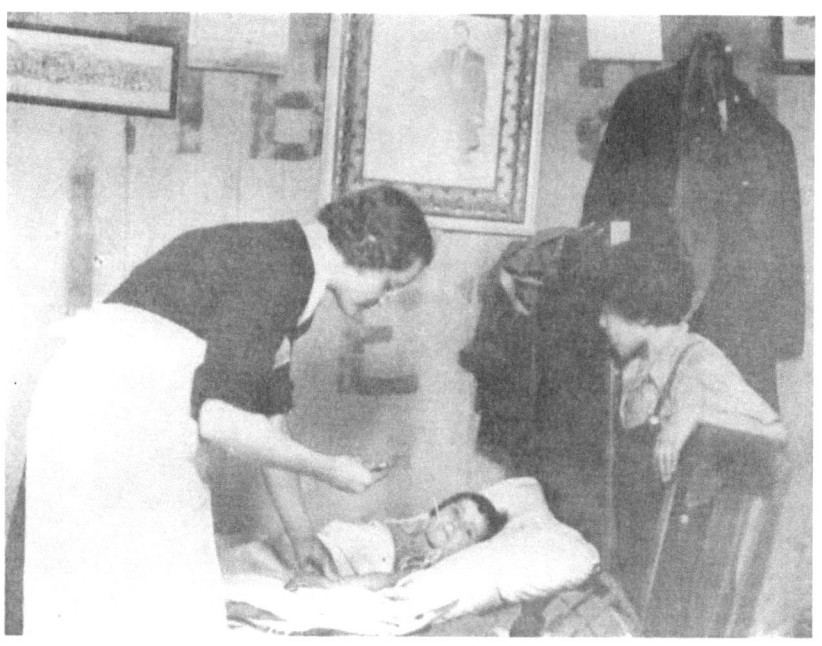

A VISITING NURSE OF YESTERDAY
Courtesy Minnesota Department of Health

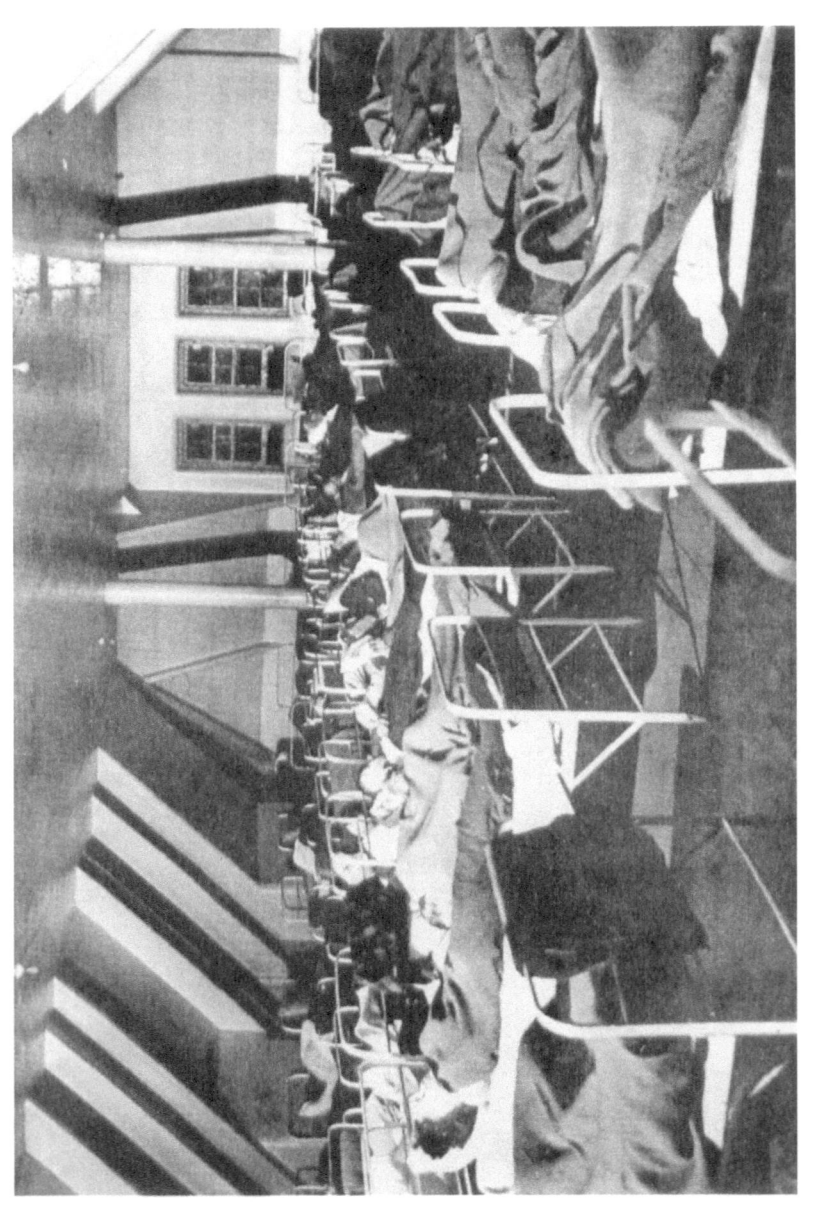

CROWDED CONDITIONS IN A STATE HOSPITAL
Courtesy Minneapolis Star-Tribune

and had found that the "Minneapolis department has complied with the law regarding the reporting of infectious diseases just as the same has been interpreted for several years." Then the mayor deplored a "feud" between the two health officers, Bracken and the Minneapolis commissioner, which, he said, was "not merely unfortunate, it is criminal and if persisted in to the detriment of the health of the state and the safety of our citizens should subject you both to all the penalties that attach to such unmanly behavior." A special investigation of the Minneapolis health department was held in August, 1900. By then few new cases were being reported, and the Minneapolis crisis was over.[14]

The epidemic itself, however, was not ended. Despite Bracken's best efforts, he could not prevent infected individuals from traveling about the state and spreading infection. Dr. Justus Ohage, St. Paul's health officer, was particularly incensed about this, and he wrote Bracken that he strongly objected to having St. Paul "made a dumping ground" of contagious diseases from the neighborhood and especially from Winona. Bracken himself visited Winona and reported to the United States Marine Hospital Service the presence of several hundred cases, many among the Polish population.[15]

When, at the close of 1900, it seemed that the epidemic had exhausted itself, the disease again appeared. It seems to have been carried throughout the state by a traveling orchestra and by the Uncle Tom's Cabin Troop, a theater company. Bracken said definitely that smallpox was "peddled out" by Cosgrove's Orchestra, whose members fondled lasses "so that they now have the eruption nicely developed." The orchestra left smallpox cases behind them at Benson, Wheaton, Lake Crystal, and Wahpeton, North Dakota. Bracken was so worried that he sent out a public "wanted" notice, beginning: "The State Board of Health is anxious to learn the whereabouts of Cosgrove's Orchestra." The traveling players also left smallpox behind them. By April, 1901, many cases were being reported in Lac qui Parle County, and several communities there were quarantined. Quarantine against Yellow Bank and Agassiz townships in that county was raised in the middle of May.[16]

[14] Gray to Bracken, January [no date], 1900, and Norred to Bracken, August 6, 1900, Minnesota Department of Health, St. Paul; *Times* (Minneapolis), August 21, 1900.
[15] Ohage to Bracken, December 7, 1900, and Bracken to Walter Wyman, December 17, 1900, Minnesota Department of Health, St. Paul.
[16] Bracken to the health officer, Brookings, South Dakota, undated, 1901, to F. Norrish, April 3, 1901, to John J. Whyte, May 6, 1901, to F. A. Hudson, May 6, 1901, to Reuben D. Hill, May 8, 1901, and to Nels Lundberg, May 16, 1901; letters to Bracken from Holbrook, January 29, 1900, from S. M. Granger, January 21, 1901, and from Hill, May 14, 1901; State Board of Health, "Wanted-Notice, 1901." Minnesota Department of Health, St. Paul.

More than 8,000 smallpox cases were reported in Minnesota in 1901, and the following year the number jumped to 8,666. It dropped in 1903 to 4,502 and in 1904 to 2,343. The total number of cases from the beginning of the epidemic in 1899 to March 26, 1906, was 27,876, and deaths numbered 208. Bracken told Dr. William J. Mayo that the great expense to communities was in the "care of the cases and the demoralization of business." He spoke also of opposition to vaccination and of the need for strong quarantine laws.

Here Bracken was touching a delicate point, for public opposition to quarantine was decidedly strong. Local newspapers roared against the practice, and families disliked it intensely. From Brainerd a worried woman wrote Bracken: "After reading over your State board of health laws in regards to smallpox i find that our county bord of helth doctor did not treat me quite rite he closed my house for too weeks for a cas of what he called the smallpox and would not furnish us any thing to live on and he never came near the house to us to see of corse he took the man away that had it and thare was one more had it while the house was closed. . . . I am a poor widow woman trying to make a living. I had just began to do quite well had not ben at it long I had 24 men boarding and when the house was quarntuned they let 16 of the men that were exposed go and left the rest shut in the house. . . . now Doctors plese do not cast my letter aside for this has ben a grate damage to me." Some physicians also thought that strict quarantine was too severe.[17]

After careful consideration, Bracken himself concluded that old quarantine regulations were largely a failure. In 1905 he suggested certain revisions to the Conference of State and Provincial Boards of Health, but they were not approved. The following year he recommended changes in Minnesota's quarantine regulations, and these were passed by the state health board at a meeting in July. The board's action was as follows: "It having been established that smallpox will not spread in a well vaccinated community, and believing that all attempts to restrain smallpox in a community not protected by vaccination, by means of quarantine, will fail; that quarantine in a well vaccinated community is unnecessary, that attempts to control the spread of smallpox by quarantine is unscientific, irrational, expensive, and misleading, that authorities are favoring unscientific and illogical methods for its control, and are conveying false ideas as to the safety of the public, the Minnesota

---

[17] Bracken to Mayo, March 29, 1906, and to the editor of the *Odessa Tribune*, April 24, 1901, and letters to Bracken from Norred, April 22, 1900, from Mrs. L. J. Guyett, May 14, 1901, and from A. W. Allen, May 2, 1901, Minnesota Department of Health, St. Paul; *Pioneer Press*, April 10, 1894.

State Board of Health advises that after January, 1908, further attempts to control smallpox in Minnesota by means of quarantine shall be abandoned."[18]

Bracken's joy in the new regulation, which placarded a house and kept the patient quarantined but put no restraint upon the healthy people in the home, was short lived. Dr. W. A. Evans, Chicago health commissioner, was not friendly to the new procedure, nor was the secretary of Iowa's health board. "I admit," said the latter, "that suppression of smallpox by means of quarantine is unscientific, irrational, and expensive, but until concerted action is taken by all the states and various National Departments concerned, it would seem suicidal for a single state, or group of states, to attempt anything so radical as the departure contemplated by the Minnesota Board." Bracken penciled across the top of this letter, "*Not answered.*" Criticism came too from Minneapolis, and Bracken wrote that "Minneapolis is not under any obligation to follow the regulations of the State Board in matters pertaining to smallpox, as the ordinances of a city of the first class in this state (and Minneapolis is one of these) take precedence over the regulations of the State Board of Health."[19]

Despite opposition, Bracken held stanchly to his position on quarantine. He explained his stand again and again. "In this State," he wrote, "with such laws as we have, we are compelled simply to take the position of isolating smallpox cases without any quarantine. We placard the house . . . and forbid both the patient and the *unvaccinated* of the household to leave the premises. . . . We put a premium on vaccination by allowing those of the household who are protected by vaccination to go and come as they please, for we do not believe that smallpox is spread to any great extent by the clothing of the healthy people or by the healthy people themselves." He never grew tired of emphasizing the point that the new regulations threw the responsibilities in connection with smallpox upon the people themselves. Vaccination, in Bracken's opinion, was the answer. "I do not believe," he once said, "that a community or the state should be put to great expense handling these cases of smallpox for the protection of people who can protect themselves at a nominal cost, or no cost at all."[20]

[18] Bracken to Charles V. Chapin, March 11, 1907, Minnesota Department of Health, St. Paul.
[19] Bracken to Wyman, January 28, 1908, and to G. B. Young, November 8, 1911; Louis A. Thomas to Bracken, July 8, 1907. Minnesota Department of Health, St. Paul.
[20] Bracken to John B. Anderson, April 17, 1912, to O. B. Lambert, November 25, 1913, and to A. T. McCormack, April 15, 1914, Minnesota Department of Health, St. Paul.

From 1913 through 1917 there were 10,401 smallpox cases and only 40 deaths reported in Minnesota. It seemed as if the new quarantine regulations, accurate follow-up of exposed persons, and a more tolerant attitude toward vaccination had just about conquered one of the state's major diseases. But every health officer knows that no plague is ever really conquered. Ceaseless vigilance and constant precautions are always necessary. One or two infected persons may set in motion a long chain of deadly events. That happened in 1924. A Canadian recently come to the United States died of malignant smallpox in a Duluth hospital. Between the time of his arrival in Minnesota and the day of his death he had exposed a considerable number of persons. As a result 168 cases with 37 deaths occurred in eight sanitary districts in St. Louis County, in three districts in Carlton County, in two in Aitkin County, in four in Lake County, and in one in Lake of the Woods County. In Duluth 54 cases with 15 fatalities were reported. This outbreak was confined to northeastern Minnesota and terminated in July. By that time malignant smallpox was manifesting itself in both Minneapolis and St. Paul. Cases continued to mount throughout the year until 860 cases and 219 deaths were reported in Minneapolis and 197 cases and 13 deaths in St. Paul. The total number of cases for the state in 1924 was 1,345 with 298 deaths.[21]

At a special meeting of the state health board held on November 15 a resolution was passed declaring smallpox epidemic and authorizing local health boards to arrange for free voluntary vaccination of all inhabitants, not only in those health districts where smallpox cases actually existed but also in those where none were yet present. In December Governor J. A. O. Preus called a meeting to consider methods for the control of the disease. Plans were made for co-operation with the United States Public Health Service and for a special investigation of the epidemic in the Twin Cities by the division of preventable diseases. It was found that the St. Paul Bureau of Health was most alert not only in making diagnoses, in searching for sources of infection, and in follow-up work, but also in seeing that quarantine was strictly enforced.

The Minneapolis situation, however, was entirely different. The official report on the activities of health officers in Minneapolis stated:

1. That up to January 16, 1925, when our investigation was begun, the Minneapolis Health Department apparently had put forth but little effort in searching for sources of infection and in following up con-

---

[21] A. J. Chesley, "Smallpox, Benign and Virulent, in Minnesota," in *Minnesota Medicine*, 2:92 (March, 1919), and *Minnesota's Experience with Smallpox*, 5 (n.p., n.d.); State Board of Health, *Minnesota's Experience with Smallpox of the Malignant Type*, 3 ([St. Paul?], February 5, 1925).

tacts to cases. Throughout the epidemic but few reports of persons outside of Minneapolis, exposed in Minneapolis, were received by the State Board of Health from the Minneapolis Health Department.

2. That families living under the same roof and using common halls, and in some instances other common appointments, were not warned or advised following the occurrence of first cases, and that in some instances of this kind secondary cases occurred which apparently might have been averted.

3. That places of business generally, where cases occurred in workers who continued their work for one or more days after onset, were not advised further than to be notified that the individual taken sick should not return to work without a health officer's certificate, and in many places no notification or advice of any kind was received.

4. That in five hospitals investigated in which cases had occurred prior to January 16, no investigation had been made by the health department and no advice or directions were given regarding vaccination of patients, nurses, and employees, terminal disinfection, and the follow-up of visitors and discharged patients.

5. That of three public schools and one parochial school in which cases occurred among pupils who attended school after first symptoms developed, no investigation was made to check up on the vaccination status of those closely associated with the patients and apparently in three instances at least no notice whatsoever was taken of the occurrence of cases within the schools and no disinfection of desks or school books was carried out. In one school upon inquiry by the school nurse, instructions were given regarding disinfection of books, desks, etc.

Six other equally serious findings against Minneapolis health officials were published, but the first five are typical of the others. Fortunately the attitude of Minneapolis was not that of all Minnesota communities. In January, 1925, Minneapolis, perhaps because of its carelessness, had 207 cases and 81 deaths, while St. Paul happily reported only 18 cases and 7 deaths. Here was one sharply etched example of how adequate public health practices pay.[22]

The great epidemic of 1924–25 did not challenge Bracken's concept of quarantine, although a far stricter quarantine was imposed during the emergency than the regulations of 1906 called for. For all practicable purposes, the Bracken-approved regulation still was in force in 1948. The epidemic brought about another forward step. An extensive vaccination program carried on during 1924 and 1925 resulted in a "mass immunity" which gave Minnesota a period of relative freedom from the disease. From 1926 to 1935, for example, an average of only 225 cases were reported annually. During the decade preceding 1926, exclusive of

[22] Chesley, *Minnesota's Experience with Smallpox*, 6, 12; State Board of Health, *Minnesota's Experience with Smallpox of the Malignant Type*, 8.

the epidemic of malignant smallpox, the average had been over 3,000 cases annually. But smallpox again increased from 1936 to 1940. During that period ninety-four per cent of the cases and all the deaths occurred among unvaccinated persons. The Minnesota State Medical Association sponsored an intensive vaccination program during 1940 and 1941, with the result that only ten cases were reported in 1942 and none in 1943. Physicians believe that smallpox — responsible for 44,473 reported illnesses and 619 deaths in Minnesota from 1913 to 1943 — can be completely eliminated by universal smallpox vaccination. To accomplish this means constant watchfulness and education. Smallpox has not become extinct in Minnesota; it is only being held at arm's length.[23]

Diphtheria, like smallpox, is a disease demanding ceaseless vigilance. It manifested itself in severe outbreaks in Minnesota during the 1870s and 1880s and it continues to be a threat to public health. In 1922 the number of cases reported in Minnesota was 4,269, but in 1937 the figure had dropped to 364. Ten years later, in 1947, there were 326 clinical cases, 174 carriers, and 20 deaths. The state health department, beginning in the 1890s, availed itself of modern laboratory methods and made real contributions to the study of diphtheria. Despite this, diphtheria continued to menace children's health and, from time to time, to assume epidemic proportions.[24]

About the time that Hewitt approved a campus laboratory to be used for diphtheria work, the state health board was receiving innumerable queries concerning antitoxin and was hearing reports that as many as forty cases of diphtheria were present in a single small community. The disease appeared among persons living at home, in hotels, and in isolated rural districts. Health officers had difficulty with physicians who diagnosed diphtheria as croup and failed to take proper care of their patients.[25] Citizens themselves sometimes failed to take ordinary pre-

[23] *Minnesota State Health Laws and Regulations*, 62 (January 1, 1948); State Board of Health, *Reports*, 1922–43, p. 38; H. W. Hill, "Smallpox and Chicken-Pox," in *Journal-Lancet*, 32:1–7 (January 1, 1912).
[24] *History of Steele and Waseca Counties*, 280 (Chicago, 1887); Thomas Hughes, *History of Blue Earth County*, 186 (Chicago, [1909]); *St. Paul Daily Press*, January 12, 1872; *Pioneer Press*, May 10, 1880; *Tribune*, January 7, 1878; State Board of Health, *Annual Reports*, 1879, pp. 28–83; *Reports*, 1922–43, p. 210; statistical data from the Minnesota Department of Health, September 24, 1948. See also chapter 6, above.
[25] *Pioneer Press*, January 10, 1895; Kandiyohi and Lyons Counties, "Reports of Infectious Diseases, 1894–1896," Minnesota Department of Health, St. Paul; letters to Hewitt from G. Brandt, January 10, 1896, from [Emil] King, December 30, 1895, from J. Friend Holmes, January 6, 1896, from C. E. Fawcett, October 1, 1895, from Joseph Weinzierl and Edwin A. Dressel, September 28, 1896, and from Dressel, September 30, October 6, 16, 1896, and Hewitt to Dressel, October 1, 1896, Minnesota Department of Health, St. Paul.

cautions when diphtheria became epidemic. "In regard to the Diphtheria in our town," wrote an indignant resident of New Market, "it is getting worse this winter than ever before. We are having it all the time, and it is a hard thing to Keep the people in. They are Keeping Dances, Parties all over the town and go together. I want you to inform me, wheather we can, stop that as Board of Health of the town, by posting up notices." It was not unusual for diphtheria patients to break quarantine, and on one occasion an angry man destroyed quarantine signs because "he had got over it and he was not going to stay in any longer." When diphtheria broke out at Camp Merritt at the time of the Spanish-American War, the charge was made that physicians failed to report cases.[26]

So much confusion was present in the diphtheria situation that in September, 1898, the state board strengthened its regulations. Bracken stipulated that quarantine for diphtheria "shall continue for four weeks from the time of the appearance of the disease in any patient, or, in lieu thereof, that quarantine be regulated by bacteriological examinations. With the bacteriological examinations, there must be two negative reports, from a responsible laboratory, upon smears taken from the throat of the patient by some responsible person." The board emphasized the bacteriological method as the sole means of diagnosing diphtheria, believing that "it is the presence of the diphtheria bacillus which has the dangerous element."[27]

This diagnostic approach put a heavy burden upon the board's laboratory. Throat specimens arrived from almost every section of the state, and 1,721 examinations were made during 1899–1900. Careful emphasis upon the importance of the laboratory and upon educational procedures led to an awakening public interest. Parents and schools began to feel that perhaps something tangible now was at hand to curb a vicious disease. When a school board asked Bracken what might be done to interest householders in protecting their children against diphtheria, he replied in specific terms: "Permit me to state, that if proper quarantine methods are maintained in the city with reference to those who are known to be suffering from the disease, the next most important agent in the control of the spread of diphtheria is to be found in the organized body of School Inspectors. It is my opinion, that before the opening of

[26] Joseph H. Baltes to Hewitt, November 10, 1896, and F. D. Greene to Bracken, July 8, 1897, Minnesota Department of Health, St. Paul; *Pioneer Press*, June 28, 1898.
[27] Bracken to E. P. S. Miller, September 22, 1898, and to J. W. Magelssen, November 8, 1898, Minnesota Department of Health, St. Paul; *Pioneer Press*, September 29, 1898.

school, the school children in those districts in which diphtheria is prevailing, should have cultures taken from both nose and throat, and if the bacillus diphtheriae is found present, such children should be excluded from school, until a negative report is given by proper authorities. . . . In districts where no diphtheria has been reported, it would not be necessary to examine the school children culturally before the opening of school, but cultures should be taken from *all* school children at any early date after the opening of school, in order to exclude from school any who have present in the nose or throat the bacillus diphtheriae." [28]

Until 1911 no adequate disease census of Minnesota school children had been attempted. In that year Rushford asked for state assistance in the control of an epidemic of scarlet fever, and Chesley was sent to investigate. To assist him the school nurse made a disease census of all children in families represented in the schools. This was the beginning. The state board later sent disease census cards to certain selected schools. The cards were filled out by mothers under the direction of teachers and then were returned to the division of epidemiology. Shortly thereafter the census was extended throughout the state. For the first time state health officials were able to get comparatively accurate figures of the number of cases of the common childhood diseases occurring annually. They discovered that these diseases were much more prevalent than official reports indicated. There were, for example, almost ten times as many cases of measles as were reported each year. Then, too, the school census brought parents into closer touch with health authorities and permitted health officers to explain the advantages of laboratory work. During 1910 the laboratory of the Minnesota Department of Health made 11,061 examinations for diphtheria, and in 1914 the estimated number was 24,698.[29]

Beginning in 1906, antitoxin was furnished to physicians at reduced cost. "The cost of antitoxin can no longer be an argument against its use in Minnesota," wrote Bracken. The state board began distributing antitoxin gratis in 1915, and in 1926 free toxin-antitoxin for diphtheria immunization was made available. Between 1926 and 1937 the board distributed material for 345,703 complete diphtheria immunizations.

[28] Wesbrook to A. J. Stoew, January 3, 1900, and Bracken to Wesbrook, November 7, 1900, and to Harrington Beard, August 12, 1901, Minnesota Department of Health, St. Paul; State Board of Health, *Biennial Reports*, 1899–1900, p. 511.
[29] State Board of Health, Division of Epidemiology, *Biennial Reports*, August 1, 1910–August 1, 1912, p. 195 (Minneapolis, 1914); Laboratory Division, *Biennial Reports*, January 1, 1912–January 31, 1914, p. 5 (Minneapolis, 1915).

The effect of years of patient work was demonstrated in 1930, when diphtheria deaths numbered only 32, or 1.2 deaths per 100,000 population, as compared with diphtheria deaths in 1890 totaling 772 with a rate of 58.9 per 100,000. In 1930, the very year that these figures were released, another startling fact was uncovered. Speaking to a group of pediatricians at the Center for Continuation Study at the University of Minnesota, two Minneapolis physicians reported that "Statistical analysis of mortality rates in the State of Minnesota shows a general decline in the deaths from the more common diseases of childhood since 1915." They pointed out that much still remained to be done to reduce preschool age deaths from diphtheria, scarlet fever, and measles. They advocated, as had others, that more attention be given to routine immunization against diphtheria during infancy and said that the best time for this was at the age of six months.[30]

Diphtheria increased in Minnesota in the period from 1940 to 1946, a situation which led Dr. D. S. Fleming, chief of the section of preventable diseases, to say: "Immunization is particularly urgent for young children. Records for ten years show that forty-two per cent of the diphtheria deaths in Minnesota are among children under five years of age, and sixty per cent are among children under ten." Then he added: "Every child should be given immunization against diphtheria during the first year of life, and again just before he enters school. If a number of diphtheria cases occur in the community, physicians may advise 'booster shots' for children under twelve years of age, as an added safety measure." Despite the fact that no one now needs to die from diphtheria, 283 cases and 14 deaths were reported during the first ten months of 1947. Here is another instance of an old disease in Minnesota which continually must be guarded against. It still remains a "treacherous and deceptive disease, killing early by suffocation or later by sudden death, even during apparently well-established convalescence."[31]

Influenza reached epidemic proportions in Minnesota as early as 1882, when so many cases developed near Pleasant Grove that there were "hardly enough well people to take care of the sick." A few years later,

[30] H. M. Bracken, *Antitoxin Furnished by the State Board of Health, July 9, 1907* (St. Paul, 1907); State Board of Health, *Biennial Reports*, 1916–17, pp. 21–31; *Reports*, 1922–43, p. 235; Minnesota Department of Health, *Diphtheria in Minnesota*, [2] (St. Paul, January, 1939); Erling S. Platou and Paul F. Dwan, "Advances in the Prevention and Treatment of Contagious Diseases of Childhood," in *Minnesota Medicine*, 22:71 (February, 1939).

[31] *Minnesota's Health*, vol. 1, no. 1, p. 2 (January, 1947); vol. 1, no. 12, p. 2 (December, 1947); D. S. Fleming, "Diphtheria in Minnesota," in *Journal-Lancet*, 67:32 (January, 1947).

in 1890 and 1891, the disease hit hard at Lake City, Crookston, Minneapolis, and St. Paul.[32] But not until 1918, when Minnesota was busily engaged in the effort to win World War I, did influenza actually interrupt normal activities throughout the state. This epidemic was important not only because of the large number of cases and deaths, but also because it offers a typical example of how public health officials act in an emergency.

Bracken, like health officers in other states, had watched with concern the steadily increasing number of influenza cases developing throughout the nation in 1918. About the middle of September the disease appeared in Minnesota. It was brought to Wells by a soldier from Camp Sheridan in Illinois. Within forty-eight hours after his arrival home there was a general outbreak of the disease. More than two hundred cases of "flu," seven cases of pneumonia, and one death were reported in this town with a population of about 1,755. "We do not like such a record as this from the Army," Bracken wrote the surgeon general. Meanwhile the University of Minnesota reported the illness of sixteen nurses at the University Hospital and closed that institution to visitors. No new patients were admitted. The first death to be reported was at Fort Snelling. A day later St. Paul newspapers indicated that the epidemic was checked and that there were only a few new cases in the Twin Cities.[33]

Within two days after this optimistic announcement Minneapolis civil and military authorities estimated that approximately 1,000 persons were ill in the city, including 510 army cases at Fort Snelling. At this point Bracken began tightening controls. He permitted public funerals for influenza victims only when caskets were closed during services. He also called a special meeting to deal with the situation. Dr. Egil Boeckman, a member of the state health board, was unable to attend the meeting as he was stationed at Camp Grant, Illinois, but he did furnish Bracken with pertinent information. He wrote that twelve per cent of the men in his camp were down with influenza; that it "spreads like fire, very severe in onset and very prone to complications of Lobar Pneumonia, which is liable to set in on the 5 or 6 day and which is very fatal, 33% to 50% at least"; that throat cultures, as well as autopsy findings of lungs, heart's blood, and sinus secretions, showed practically a hundred per cent of pure pneumococcus; that the army treatment con-

---

[32] *Pioneer Press*, April 20, May 5, 1882, January 1, 11, 20, 1890, January 11, March 6, 1891.
[33] Bracken to W. C. Gorgas, October 1, 1918, Minnesota Department of Health, St. Paul; *Pioneer Press*, September 28, October 1, 2, 1918.

sisted of bed rest and the use of aspirin and quinine; and that patients should be kept quiet for three days after their temperatures returned to normal. He said further that the mortality was greater among boys from the country than among those from cities, and he concluded: "The few suggestions are no doubt old to you, but I want to impress upon the Board that you are dealing with the most serious epidemic of any kind you have ever been up against." [34]

Bracken knew that the Minnesota health board could not cope with the epidemic alone. Already he was being besieged with requests for physicians and nurses from all sections of the state. Fortunately assistance came from both the United States Public Health Service and the American Red Cross. The former appointed Bracken its field director for Minnesota, and authorized him to employ assistant surgeons at a salary of two hundred dollars a month and per diem expenses of four dollars. The Red Cross offered to furnish nurses and to pay them seventy dollars a month. A special state appropriation of ten thousand dollars was given the board for influenza work. National Red Cross officials also ordered the organization of local chapter committees on influenza and added: "When local needs are greater than can promptly be provided by the local Health authorities, the Chapters may offer aid at their own expense. . . . When the combined resources of the local health authorities and of the Red Cross Chapter are insufficient to meet the local need, then the local Health Officer should appeal to the State Board of Health. When the State Board of Health cannot meet this need, it will, in its discretion, appeal to the Federal Public Health Service for needed nursing personnel and will apply to the Division Manager directly for needed supplies. The Division Manager will act upon his own judgment in honoring requests for supplies when made by State Boards of Health." Division managers were authorized to purchase emergency hospital supplies for civilian needs.[35]

The United States Public Health Service conducted all necessary dealings with state and local health boards, so that division offices of the Red Cross would be restricted to providing nursing personnel and furnishing supplies. Actually, however, the Red Cross did much more. It prepared and served cooked food to families stricken by sickness and incapable of serving themselves, sent volunteer housekeepers and care-

[34] *Tribune*, October 4, 1918; Boeckman to Bracken, October 5, 1918, Minnesota Department of Health, St. Paul.
[35] State Board of Health, *Biennial Reports*, 1916–17, p. 14; W. Frank Persons to the manager, Northern Red Cross Division, Minneapolis, October 4, 5, 1918 (telegrams), Minnesota Department of Health, St. Paul.

takers for children to homes, and established Red Cross offices to recruit volunteers as nurses' aids.[36]

While these details were being arranged Bracken began to develop stricter controls. He considered getting military camps quarantined, but he was informed by army medical officers that "it does not appear to this office desirable to attempt to limit the movements of the authorized escorts for the dead, or the casual soldier on leave, in view of the fact that hundreds of thousands of civilians who have been equally exposed to the infection are freely travelling about the country." If this could not be accomplished, Bracken nevertheless could insist that:

1. The disease must be reported.
2. The patient must be isolated.
3. The attendants should wear face masks.
4. The children from an infected household should be kept home from school and no permit for their return should be given until after five days after the subsidence of the last clinical case in the family.
5. Wage earners continuing their occupation must stay away from the sick.
6. All well people must stay out of the house.
7. Foodstuffs must not be handled by anyone from the family in which influenza exists.
8. Quarantine may be enforced if necessary, but as a rule it does not work well on account of the rapid contagiousness of the disease.[37]

By October 12 reports of 2,538 cases had come from 125 sanitary districts outside the Twin Cities. Minneapolis reported 1,538 cases, St. Paul 210, and the military posts about 1,000. There were 52 cases on the White Earth Indian Reservation. By that time new cases were developing so rapidly that hospitals were hard pressed for nurses, and all Minneapolis city hospital ambulances were devoting themselves exclusively to influenza calls. The state health board continued its policy of allowing schools to remain open, although Bracken thought that all public gatherings, such as "political gatherings, conventions, church and school associations," should be prohibited. St. Paul kept its schools under close supervision, insisting that any child not feeling perfectly well be examined by a school nurse or else sent home for examination by a physician. Minneapolis, on the other hand, prohibited all public gatherings, including those in churches and schools, beginning at midnight on October 12. "Downtown theatres," said a reporter, "were packed last night with

[36] Persons to all Red Cross division managers, October 5, 7, 1918 (telegrams), Minnesota Department of Health, St. Paul.
[37] W. P. Chamberlain to Bracken, October 7, 1918, Smith to the division of preventable diseases, October 12, 1918, and Bracken to the *Grand Forks Herald*, October 12, 1918 (telegram), Minnesota Department of Health, St. Paul.

persons who took advantage of their last chance to see a performance until the ban is lifted. Long lines of men and women waited in front of the motion picture and vaudeville theaters during the early hours of the evening."[38]

Despite the advice of the United States Public Health Service that all schools, churches, and theaters be closed, and against the recommendation of city health officers, Minneapolis school authorities then decided to open public schools. "Spanish influenza is primarily an adult disease," a member of the school board said. "One of our school physicians reported that in 156 influenza cases he found not a single child of school age. Stores, saloons and street cars have not been closed up. The state university, whose students are all of the age most affected by the epidemic, decided to open." Health officers and parents took no such view. They exerted such pressure that Minneapolis schools were closed after being open only a half day. This was a wise move, for local cases failed to fall off and cases throughout the state continued to mount. On one day alone, October 24, Duluth reported 18 new cases, Milaca 82, Bemidji and Mankato 100, and Dilworth 125. The number of all cases in the state was estimated at 19,000, although figures vary considerably.[39]

Despite public knowledge that this epidemic was most severe and despite the widely publicized activities of local, state, and federal authorities, it was extremely difficult to maintain ideal controls. Bracken, for example, was troubled by the fact that influenza patients were traveling about the state on railroads. Finally an order was issued prohibiting railroads from carrying such patients unless they were properly masked and regulation receptacles were provided to care for sputum. Another thoroughly vexing problem was the shipment of soldier dead to Minnesota from army camps. "Bodies were coming back from the cantonments to Minnesota and going through Minneapolis and St. Paul in such condition that the train crews were unwilling to handle them," complained the state board. "In many instances the odors were terrific and reports are brought to us that some of the bodies were dripping." The Iowa health board explained why this was so. So many deaths occurred at Camp Dodge "that it has been impossible to get caskets of any kind, in fact every casket that could be used was used and sealed cas-

[38] *Pioneer Press*, October 8, 13, 1918; *Tribune*, October 8, 11, 13, 1918; Smith to Bracken, October 12, 14, 1918, Bracken to the Commission of Public Safety, October 12, 1918, and Bracken, "Influenza-Closing of Schools, October 12, 1918," Minnesota Department of Health, St. Paul.
[39] *Tribune*, October 21, 22, 23, 1918; *Pioneer Press*, October 26, 1918; Blue to Bracken, October 17, 1918 (telegram), and State Board of Health, "Reports of Influenza Cases, October 24, 1918," Minnesota Department of Health, St. Paul.

kets were impossible, but all the precautions possible were taken so far as Camp Dodge has been concerned, and all undertakers in the city of Des Moines were busy and many were imported from the outside to assist."[40]

Three events, all taking place in November, complicated the influenza problem further and no doubt helped to spread the disease. The first was a disastrous forest fire in northern Minnesota, the second was an increase of cases in the Twin Cities, and the third was the Armistice Day celebration. The blaze, hitting in the vicinity of Cloquet, drove many influenza victims from their homes. Nine senior medical students from the University of Minnesota were sent to the fire-swept area. So many influenza refugees flocked into Floodwood that a hospital was established there. Minnesota military officers, sent to the fire district on the Iron Range, found an urgent need for doctors and nurses and feared that the epidemic might "flare up" almost anywhere in the vicinity. Therefore the Red Cross, upon request, moved in. During the next month so many cases filtered into Duluth that its health officer described the city as a "dumping ground" for patients from Knife River, Lawler, Moose Lake, Cloquet, Crookston, and the Iron Range.[41]

Only a few days after St. Paul put drastic restrictions upon all places of amusement, schools, churches, soda fountains, and saloons, an armistice to end the war was announced. Governor Burnquist and the Minneapolis health department ordered all public places closed in that city for the duration of the celebration. As a result people milled about on the streets in such crowds that an increase of influenza cases was predicted. This was particularly unfortunate since the disease had been on the increase in Minneapolis. Shortly after the wild hysteria of November 11, Bracken described the geographic path of the epidemic. It traveled, he said, "from the southern portion of the state up the western boundary and a little more slowly up the eastern boundary. It has been prevalent in St. Paul and Minneapolis to a certain degree since the last week in September. The progress in these two cities is slow, first one district and then another is involved. It gradually extended into the center of the state and now is raging most severely in the northeast portion about Duluth where the tremendous forest fires were." He added that the

[40] C. B. Cooper to Bracken, October 28, 1918; Bracken to Cooper, October 29, 31, 1918; Smith to Guilford H. Sumner, November 4, 1918; Sumner to Bracken, October 30, 1918. Minnesota Department of Health, St. Paul.
[41] *Pioneer Press*, November 1, 1918; Henry A. Bellows to the adjutant general, November 12, 1918, J. T. Gerould to R. D. Gardner, November 14, 1918, and Bracken to E. F. Heffelfinger, December 28, 1918, Minnesota Department of Health, St. Paul.

situation in the north and northeastern portions of the state was still serious.[42]

Although deaths in Minneapolis still averaged eleven daily, the city after thirty-six days opened its schools, churches, and places of amusement. The total number of cases throughout the state to November 15 was 75,110, and Bracken believed that the final total would be very much higher. For the first time in nearly three months less than a hundred new cases were reported to the state board on December 30. The crisis was passed, and from then on the disease slowly subsided. But hundreds of persons, lay and professional, had learned what an epidemic meant and had realized the tremendous importance of state and federal agencies when the public health was seriously threatened. They knew, too, that Minnesota had been drawn into a pandemic of influenza, which had scourged Europe and South America and then had invaded the United States. In Minnesota 7,521 persons had died from influenza in 1918, and 2,579 in 1919. A secondary outbreak in 1920 caused nearly 1,700 deaths, and subsequent outbreaks in 1928 and 1929 resulted in about a thousand deaths in each of those years. In 1937 the state health department received a grant from the Rockefeller Foundation to establish a virus laboratory for the study of influenza.[43]

Brucellosis is another example of the longevity of disease. Its more common name is undulant fever, although frequently it is referred to as Malta fever, Gibraltar fever, Bang's disease, or Bruce's septicemia. Some medical historians say that Hippocrates recognized it. For generations undulant fever raged throughout Europe, but not until 1905 was a case recognized as originating in the United States. Six years later it was endemic throughout the nation. In 1927 the first case recognized as arising in Minnesota was diagnosed. From then until today the medical profession and health officers have sought without too much success to develop a specific remedy.[44]

Undulant fever, Minnesota health officials point out, is essentially the

---

[42] *Pioneer Press*, November 4, 1918; *Tribune*, November 8, 1918; Bracken to Herman M. Biggs, November 13, 1918, Minnesota Department of Health, St. Paul.

[43] *Tribune*, November 16, 1918; *Pioneer Press*, December 31, 1918; Smith to Thomas Hunter, November 26, 1918, Minnesota Department of Health, St. Paul; "The Pandemic of Influenza," in *Minnesota Medicine*, 2:29 (January, 1919); "The Influenza Situation," in *Journal-Lancet*, 38:602 (October 15, 1918); State Board of Health, *Biennial Reports*, 1918–19, p. 37; *Reports*, 1922–43, p. 31. See also chapter 10, above.

[44] Minnesota Department of Health, Division of Preventable Diseases, *Undulant Fever*, 1 ([Minneapolis], May 10, 1929); Section of Preventable Diseases, *Undulent Fever (Brucellosis)*, 1 ([Minneapolis], March, 1948); I. Forest Huddleson, *Brucellosis in Man and Animals*, 65 (New York, 1943); State Board of Health, *Reports*, 1922–43, p. 43; W. L. Boyd, "Minnesota Works on Brucellosis Control," in *Everybody's Health*, vol. 30, no. 5, p. 7 (May, 1945).

same disease in human beings and is caused by the same germ as Bang's disease in cattle, brucellosis in swine and sheep, or fistula of the withers and poll evil in horses. The commonest sources of infection for persons in Minnesota are undoubtedly cattle and swine, and the disease is contracted by drinking raw milk or handling tissue from an infected animal. It is most difficult to diagnose, and it may be confused with influenza, grippe, glandular fever, tuberculosis, typhoid fever, or rheumatism. Although the death rate from undulant fever is slight, cases vary greatly in severity, ranging from a mild, hardly recognizable type to a form, quite rare in Minnesota, which is virulent and rapidly fatal. The usual case is moderately severe but prolonged and very debilitating. It is easier to prevent than it is to treat.[45]

The only real protection against the disease is to pasteurize or boil all milk and cream before it is used. Farmers and others handling livestock are urged to wear rubber gloves. These precautions are particularly necessary, for in Minnesota farm families are those usually exposed. By 1940 brucellosis, far from being a regressive, rare, and self-limited disease, was becoming increasingly common. Eight years later the total number of cases reported in the United States had averaged 4,000 for the preceding two or three years. Minnesota reported 400 cases in 1946, 378 cases the next year, and 203 cases during the first ten months of 1948.[46]

There was real reason, of course, why Minnesota's health department should wish to reduce drastically the number of these cases. In the first place, the brucellosis victim usually is a farmer or a wage earner in a packing plant. Neither can afford to be ill for long, and undulant fever is apt to be a long, drawn-out affair. In the second place, brucellosis causes great discomfort. The common symptoms include weakness, sweating, chilliness, constipation, insomnia, nervousness, and general aches and pains, including headache, backache, and pain in the joints. Added to these are neuropsychiatric symptoms, including a tendency to drowsiness and stupor, loss of memory, irritability of temper, a proneness to shed tears without adequate cause, and an unsteady, timorous, childish manner. The disease is also characterized by an evening rise in temperature, accompanied by weakness and associated with chills and night sweats.[47]

[45] Rosenau, *Preventive Medicine and Hygiene*, 410.
[46] George A. Skinner, "Brucellosis Is a Serious Health Problem," and "Brucellosis in Minnesota," in *Everybody's Health*, vol. 33, no. 2, p. 2 (February, 1948); vol. 33, no. 4, p. 11 (April, 1948); "Beware of Brucellosis," in *Everybody's Health*, vol. 33, no. 3, p. 10 (March, 1948); data from the Minnesota Department of Health, September 27, 1948.
[47] Huddleson, *Brucellosis in Man and Animals*, 89, 93; A. C. Evans, "Brucellosis and Its Implications," in American Medical Women's Association, *Journal*, 3:229–232

Anxious to help control, if not prevent, undulant fever in Minnesota, the state health department in its laboratory and, as a general policy, began taking an active interest in the problem. Staff members did some research with hogs as the probable source of the disease, and some twenty thousand laboratory tests for serum brucella agglutinins were made in 1947. A conference was held in Duluth in July, 1948, to plan a general campaign to wipe out the disease.[48] About the same time Dr. Wesley W. Spink, professor of medicine at the University of Minnesota, reported that a combination of sulfadiazine and streptomycin seemed to be effective in curing patients. Spink also advocated strict legislation requiring the pasteurization of all animal milk. University of Wisconsin scientists announced in July, 1948, that a new drug called "aureomycin" was believed to be effective in treating brucellosis, although it was still in the trial stage. Minnesota legislators were urged by representatives from the state and from Wisconsin and North Dakota to urge Congress to amend current indemnity laws so that the age at which indemnities are paid on infected cattle is reduced from eighteen to twelve months after vaccination. The federal government was asked also to appropriate more money for use in vaccinating cattle against Bang's disease.[49] It seemed, by the close of 1948, that much work still remained to be done before brucellosis, one of man's oldest diseases, was conquered.

(June, 1948); W. H. Hall, "Brucellosis — Clinical Aspects," in *Minnesota Medicine*, 29:679 (July, 1946); T. B. Rice, "Undulant Fever," in *Hygeia*, 25:692 (September, 1947); Smillie, *Public Health Administration in the United States*, 144.

[48] Paul Kabler, Henry Bauer, and C. Barton Nelson, "Human Brucella Melitensis Infection in Minnesota with Hogs as the Probable Source," in *Journal of Laboratory and Clinical Medicine*, 32:854–856 (July, 1947); *Minnesota's Health*, vol. 2, no. 8, p. 3 (August, 1948); information from Paul Kabler, Minnesota Department of Health, September 24, 1948.

[49] *Minneapolis Star*, April 23, July 24, 1948; *Pioneer Press*, March 9, 1948; *St. Paul Dispatch*, March 9, 1948; W. W. Spink, W. H. Hall, J. M. Shaffer, and A. I. Brande, "In Vitro Sensitivity of Brucella to Streptomycin: Development of Resistance during Streptomycin," in Society for Experimental Biology and Medicine, *Proceedings*, 64:403–406 (April, 1947), and "Human Brucellosis: Its Specific Treatment with a Combination of Streptomycin and Sulfadiazine," in American Medical Association, *Journal*, 136:382–387 (February 7, 1948).

21

Adding Life to Years

EVERY YEAR their numbers increase. Some of them have laid by modest savings, a few attempt to live out their declining days on meager pensions, others putter around rest homes, and still more depend on retirement incomes from insurance or from benevolent or charitable organizations. Old men with gnarled hands and seamed faces sit around flophouse stoves. Old ladies knit their lives away in institutions, ranging from those little better than tenements to beautifully managed homes maintained by the King's Daughters or by a church. In homes scattered throughout Minnesota's cities and dotting the countryside reside the aged who, in a very real sense, are the state's forgotten people. Their numbers have increased rapidly during the last half century, but only recently did the public become even faintly aware that a new public health problem was at hand.

Half of the population of the United States was over thirty years old in 1948. In 1800 the median age had been sixteen for the entire country. These figures are surprising enough, but they tell only part of the story. Ten million people were over sixty-five years old when the New Year's chimes rang out in 1948, and it is estimated that that number will have increased to twenty millions by 1975. At that time more than a third of the nation will be forty-five years old or older. Only eighteen per cent of the population had reached this age bracket in 1900. Equally dramatic is the fact that, while three out of every four babies born in 1900 might have expected to live to the age of twenty-five, three of every four born today will reach the age of fifty-seven. In Minnesota today only one-twelfth of all deaths occur in children under five years, one-ninth in persons less than twenty, and two-fifths among persons of seventy or more.[1]

---
[1] Oscar R. Ewing, *The Nation's Health — A Ten Year Program*, 127 (Washington, D.C., 1948); Louis I. Dublin, "Problems of an Aging Population," in *American*

All this means, generally speaking, that Minnesota, like the rest of the nation, must provide for an ever-growing number of older people. The tremendous scope of the problem carries with it social, economic, and psychological implications that eventually will force the attention of public health administrators. It may force the revision of retirement programs now in operation and it may compel the state to recognize the impossibility of discarding a man when he has reached sixty-five. Certainly the entire philosophy of the care of the aged will have to be examined with the greatest care.[2] The division of social welfare of the Minnesota Department of Social Security already has recognized the problem.

"The aging of our population, bringing with it a marked change in our human resources, is the inevitable result of an increase in life expectancy and a less prolific present generation," said a student reviewing Minnesota's human resources in 1943. "Advances in medical technology and extension of medical facilities have carried more and more of the young and middle-aged population inherited from a more prolific generation into the higher age brackets. Seriously emphasizing this shift to the higher age brackets is a lowering of the birth rate, probably only temporarily checked by the present war economy and its accompanying psychology. These two trends affecting the age extremes of the population are certain. Planning for the nation and the state therefore can scarcely ignore them. As a minimum approach they call for the utmost in conservation of our present generation of children together with employment opportunities for more of the older members of the population." [3]

To supply a basis for planning for the care of the aged, a county-by-county survey of Minnesota was completed in 1943. This indicated that from 5.1% to 12.4% of the population of each county was sixty-five years of age or over. In general the southeastern and eastern parts of the state showed the highest proportion of aged people, while the northern and western portions showed the lowest. At least 50% of the aged in several northern counties received assistance in 1943. For the state as a whole 27.5% of those over sixty-five were receiving assistance at the time the study was made. County percentages varied from 11.2 up to 56.3. It was

Journal of Public Health, 37:152–155 (February, 1947); George Lawton and Maxwell S. Stewart, *When You Grow Older*, 5 (Public Affairs Committee, Inc., *Public Affairs Pamphlet* no. 131 — New York, 1947); State Board of Health, *Reports*, 1922–43, p. 27.

[2] United States Department of Labor, Bureau of Labor Statistics, *Care of Aged Persons in the United States* (Miscellaneous Series, *Bulletin* no. 489 — Washington, D.C., 1929).

[3] "Minnesota's Human Resources," in *Social Welfare Review*, vol. 5, no. 5, p. 19 (October, 1943).

predicted that, if the degree of aging found in some counties was to continue until 1955, the case load would exceed ninety thousand and the cost to the state would be more than thirty million dollars annually.[4]

Certain factors, of course, might offset this tremendous financial burden. In the first place, a stable economy might permit old people to live without assistance, as might also retirement insurance or savings. The chances of employment for the older worker in good health also might improve. Then, too, relatives might be able and willing to support older family members. Finally, a new pension philosophy might help solve the problem. Keeping older people well, as the result of an extensive public health program especially designed for the aged, also would play a part in reducing financial assistance.

For many years, when the aged were few in number, Minnesota had little difficulty in caring for them. That, of course, was before older people began to wonder if such a thing as security was possible in a troubled world, particularly a world that felt that a man's usefulness was ended when he reached an arbitrary retirement age. Old age assistance in general has provided little soul balm for the individual forced to retire when he considered himself a useful, wage-earning member of society. Many of these men and women hated the very thought of living out their lives with nothing to do. They looked with distaste upon moving into a home for the aged if they were well or entering a nursing home if they were ill. After attending a farewell dinner given in his honor on his retirement, a thoroughly unhappy businessman described the reactions of hundreds of others in similar circumstances. "At that parting dinner," he said, "they covered me with garlands, then exiled me from the human race, and sent me off into the wilderness."[5]

Yet even in the early period older persons preferred not to enter county homes or even private institutions if they could possibly avoid it. They disliked such institutional names as "Home for the Friendless," "Society for the Relief of the Poor," and "Woman's Christian Home." They privately resented the common knowledge that these institutions were members of the Associated Charities in St. Paul. Not even the Family Service of St. Paul, operated in such an admirable manner, could make the old folks who were visited really happy. Despite the reluctance of older persons to enter homes for the aged, the number of such institutions in-

[4] "Population Aging and Assistance," in *Social Welfare Review*, vol. 5, no. 7, p. 14 (December, 1943).
[5] Lawton and Steward, *When You Grow Older*, 1; Elon H. Moore, "Preparation for Retirement," in *Journal of Gerontology*, 1:202–211 (April, 1946).

creased in Minnesota. By 1945 fifty-four private homes were in operation throughout the state. In addition, there were county-operated homes in about fourteen counties and county-leased homes in nine others, most of them located in the southern and central portions of the state. The Minnesota Soldiers' Home also cared for the aged.[6]

The largest number of privately operated homes were maintained by Lutheran or evangelical church groups and the next largest, by the Catholic church. The total bed capacity of all fifty-four homes was 2,890. Practically all maintained a minimum age limit, most of them setting the limit at sixty-five years, although eight placed it at seventy. Nearly all homes in Minnesota received both men and women. Few accepted persons so helpless that they required nursing or custodial care at the time of admission, although many accepted those with slight infirmities or ailments requiring only a minimum of nursing attention. Most homes numbered among their population, at one time or another, one or more diabetic, blind, or crippled persons, with a larger number of cardiac, arthritic, or nephritic patients. Thirty-six homes were without registered nursing services and twenty-five lacked specifically designed infirmary rooms. Few were equipped with special departments for mental patients, but several had provided segregated rooms for disturbed patients or patients inclined to wander away. A measure of freedom was provided when such rooms had direct access to fenced-in yards.[7]

Summarizing the results of its survey of Minnesota's homes for the aged, the state health department said: "The majority of existing homes for the aged make some provision for the care of sick residents, and approximately one-half of the homes provide this care in the resident's own room. On the whole, facilities for the care of the physically ill are reasonably adequate; provision for the care of the mentally ill or senile is less satisfactory. There appears to be some need for more adequate medical supervision. Pre-admission health investigations should be more generally required for admission to homes of the aged, not necessarily for the purpose of excluding the unfit, but also for planning positively to meet their needs, with pertinent findings made available under medical supervision to the personnel concerned with the care. . . . Few homes for the aged are large enough to employ trained personnel except nursing personnel, and under present conditions it would probably be im-

[6] St. Paul Society for the Relief of the Poor, *Annual Reports*, 1897, p. [20]; [Alice C. Brill], *A History of Family Service of Saint Paul* (St. Paul, 1944); Ethel McClure, *The Care of Sick and Infirm Residents in Homes for the Aged in Minnesota*, map facing p. 4 (Minneapolis, 1945).
[7] McClure, *Care of Sick and Infirm Residents in Homes for the Aged*, 19–25.

possible to secure specialists in such fields as dietetics, mental hygiene or physical therapy, even on a consultation basis." [8]

Speaking before a south-central Minnesota group interested in public health, Dr. R. N. Barr, chief of the section of special services of the state health department, said that the old who were afflicted with chronic diseases were not getting adequate care in the state and added that conditions for them were "atrocious." He also pointed out that Minnesota lacked sufficient beds to provide for the chronically ill in the old age group. This situation, however, was not peculiar to Minnesota. At least 375,000 of those in the United States who receive old age assistance are bedridden or in need of considerable care. Another 25,000 are in public medical institutions. "There are far too few public and private nursing homes," said a national survey, "and few have adequate standards of care; nor has money been made available to assure or maintain quality. The failure of many states to bring such homes under adequate licensure is another factor that impairs quality." It was estimated that the nation desperately needs some 430,000 more beds in qualified nursing and convalescent homes, that at present it has not more than two-thirds of that number, and that the deficit is somewhere between 125,000 and 150,000 beds.[9]

Minnesota, however, was not among the states lacking legal powers to license hospitals, including sanatoriums, rest homes, nursing homes, and boarding homes. In 1941 the legislature passed an act stipulating that no institution for the hospitalization and care of human beings could be established without first being licensed by the state health department. This act also provided that the department should inspect such institutions periodically and establish regulations under which they should operate. A code of standards also was to be established. The act made no significant exception when it stated: "No regulation nor requirement shall be made, nor standard established, under this act for any sanatorium, nursing home, nor rest home conducted in accordance with the practice and principles of the body known as the Church of Christ Scientist, except as to the sanitary and safe condition of the premises, cleanliness of operation, and its physical equipment." Some doubt was felt that the 1941 act extended to public corporation hospitals, and the attorney general ruled that it did not.[10]

[8] McClure, *Care of Sick and Infirm Residents in Homes for the Aged*, 27.
[9] R. N. Barr, "Health Problems of Our Aging Population," an address delivered at the South-Central Minnesota Health Day, Mankato, October 13, 1948; Ewing, *The Nation's Health*, 141.
[10] *Laws*, 1941, pp. 1149–1153; State Board of Health, *Reports*, 1922–43, p. 173.

In order to bring public corporation hospitals within the scope of the hospital licensing law, the legislature in 1943 amended the act as follows: "No person, partnership, association, or corporation, nor any state, county, or local government units, nor any division, department, board or agency thereof, shall establish, conduct, or maintain in the state of Minnesota any hospital, sanatorium, rest home, nursing home, boarding home or other institution for the hospitalization and/or care of human beings without first obtaining a license therefor in the manner hereinafter provided." After the passage of the federal Hospital Survey and Construction Act of 1946 the Minnesota legislature amended the state hospital law to designate the state health department as the state agency charged with the responsibility for the administration of grant-in-aid hospital allotments.[11]

Meanwhile, acting under the provisions of the act of 1941, the state health board, in co-operation with the Minnesota Hospital Association and the Minnesota State Medical Association, prepared a set of standards for hospitals and related institutions and abridged standards for homes for chronic and convalescent patients. Both sets of standards were adopted on December 29, 1941.[12] Thus, for the first time in Minnesota's history, institutions designed especially to care for the aged were brought under a specific code of standards. These standards, revised from time to time, included special provisions to meet the needs of ill or incapacitated aged residents, and were designed to eliminate conditions especially hazardous to them.

In the first place, the state health board required that plans and specifications be submitted to it before building was begun. The department insisted also that all systems of water supply, plumbing, sewerage, and garbage and refuse disposal be approved before installation. Location and communication requirements, such as those for good roads and telephone service, were covered. Adequate lighting in every room and emergency lighting facilities were demanded. Provisions for the care of sick residents included those for beds of household height, for storage space for personal belongings, and for bedside signals. It was stipulated also that "No resident shall be restrained except on written order of a physician; provided that if a resident becomes suddenly disturbed so that he becomes a menace to himself or others, restraint may be applied by the person in charge, but the physician's order should be obtained at

[11] Minnesota, *Laws*, 1943, p. 1030; 1947, p. 763; United States, *Statutes at Large*, vol. 60, part 1, pp. 1040–1049; *Minnesota State Health Laws and Regulations*, 39–42 (January 1, 1948).
[12] State Board of Health, *Reports*, 1922–43, p. 173.

the earliest possible opportunity. In applying restraints, careful consideration should be given to the methods by which they can be speedily removed in case of fire or other emergency." Other sections recommended that homes for the aged should arrange for one or more duly licensed practitioners of the healing arts to be called in emergencies and for at least one person to be in charge of the nursing service. Monthly reports of all deaths and communicable disease reports were mandatory. Provisions referred to the use of narcotics and to the general sanitary condition of the physical plant.[13]

Many aged persons, of course, either did not care to enter homes or were not qualified. Others could get along if they received financial assistance. A few old people found that their own savings, "securely" invested in the period from 1919 to 1929, had depreciated in value or had disappeared altogether. A survey in 1927 by the Minnesota legislature revealed clearly that the "old man or old woman with no means to provide for his or her own support is an actual condition confronting us, as the inevitable result of the great changes in industrial operation." After much debate a pension system was recommended as the best way to take care of the aged poor of Minnesota. Here then was the beginning of Minnesota's old age assistance program, a radical departure from the previous policy of county poor farms and a policy that was to include attention to unemployment compensation, aid to dependent children, maternal and child welfare, aid to the blind, and public health.[14]

By 1937, after the Social Security Act had been passed by the federal government, a special legislative interim committee on social legislation and relief was attempting to co-ordinate national assistance programs with Minnesota policies. This was somewhat difficult, for an act of 1935, providing that not more than seventy-five thousand dollars might be spent for administration of the old age assistance plan up to July 1, 1937, was opposed by the Social Security Board in Washington. In order to remove this objection, the legislature in 1937 amended the previous act. Both acts were designed to promote the public health and welfare by establishing a state-wide system of assistance to aged persons in need. The legislature also provided for appropriations and for penalties for certain violations of the act.[15]

[13] Minnesota Department of Health, *Licensing Laws and Standards for Hospitals and Related Institutions of Minnesota*, 39–48 (Minneapolis, 1944).
[14] Minnesota Legislature, Senate Interim Committee on Old Age Pensions, *Report*, 1929, p. 3.
[15] Minnesota Legislature, Interim Committee on Social Legislation and Relief, *Reports*, 1937, pp. 2–9; *Laws*, 1935, pp. 643–652; 1937, pp. 39, 168; State Board of Control, *Old Age Assistance Act* (Minneapolis, 1937).

A person, said the act, must be sixty-five years old in order to be eligible for old age assistance and he must either be a citizen of the United States or have resided continuously in the United States for twenty-five years. An applicant must have resided in Minnesota for at least five of the preceding nine years. Assistance was to be based upon need, and county agencies were to determine the need. The amended act stipulated that both husband and wife were eligible to receive assistance. The law did not require applicants to assign property holdings, but it did indicate specifically that a claim would be made upon an estate after the death of the recipient of assistance. County agencies were permitted to allow up to one hundred dollars for burial purposes.[16]

In 1936, between March and June inclusive, recipients of old age assistance numbered 102,702. The total amount expended was $1,859,070.-15. The number receiving aid gradually increased until World War II, when increased opportunities for wartime employment made it possible for older persons to remove themselves from state relief. Yet in June, 1943, there were 60,490 old persons on relief rolls throughout Minnesota. Three years later, in June, 1946, the number stood at 54,177.[17]

Death of the recipient has been the major reason for closing old age assistance cases. While almost 75% of cases have been terminated in this manner, only 5.5% have been closed because the recipient found gainful employment. By 1945 the legislature recognized that old age assistance must be extended to provide medical care. The public health problem of the aged, of course, had been in the minds of social workers since the program first was inaugurated. In a very real sense, the entire program was designed to conserve human life. Recognizing this, the legislature amended the old age assistance act to allow for medical, dental, surgical, hospital, and nursing or licensed rest-home care in excess of the forty-dollar maximum that had prevailed up to then. The act also provided that state and county should share equally the expense of any grant in excess of forty dollars.[18]

Minnesota public health officials know, of course, that death is the inevitable end of the aging process, but they also realize that old age can be made happier and healthier for both those on relief and those who are caring for themselves. The problems of aging that are attracting the attention of health administrators are three: (1) the biology of senes-

---

[16] State Board of Control, Division of Old Age Assistance, *A Digest of the Old Age Assistance Act*, 3–6 (St. Paul, 1938).
[17] Minnesota Department of Social Security, Division of Social Welfare, *Annual Reports*, 1942–43, p.13; 1944–45, p. 16; 1945–46, p. 18.
[18] Division of Social Welfare, *Annual Reports*, 1945–46, p. 18; *Laws*, 1945, p. 532.

cence as a process; (2) the human clinical problems of aging and of diseases characteristically associated with advancing years, which include both the mental and the physical changes of senescence and senectitude; and (3) the socioeconomic problems of a shifting age distribution in the population.[19] A distinguished national committee already is at work investigating each of these three aspects. In Minnesota the state health department has taken active interest in chronic diseases and in a program of mental health applicable to the old as well as to the young.

Other agencies and institutions have developed specialized attacks upon the great killers that threaten life in older age. These include cancer, heart disease, cerebral hemorrhage, and nephritis. Today the degenerative diseases make up the vast majority of the total deaths in Minnesota.[20] Of the diseases that attack older persons, two deserve special consideration. They are cancer and heart disease. Both are frequently misunderstood by the public, but each may be controlled to a certain extent if people will heed the warnings and instructions of private physicians and health officials.

In 1937 cancer claimed the lives of 3,789 Minnesotans. Of these, 245 were between the ages of thirty-five and forty-four; 559 were between forty-five and fifty-four; 845 were between fifty-five and sixty-four; and 1,975 were sixty-five and over. During the 170 years from 1776 to 1946 the United States fought seven wars and lost about 575,000 men in battle. The American Cancer Society says that at the present rate, it takes cancer less than three and a half years to kill that many people. Cancer kills one person in every eight in the United States. It kills sixty per cent more people than are killed by all the communicable diseases combined. On the other hand, a great proportion of deaths from cancer may be delayed or avoided.[21]

Approximately one half of all cancer is found in the digestive tract and one third of all cancer is found in the stomach. But certain other body sites also are recognized as danger zones for cancer. Among men these danger zones are lips, throat and mouth, lungs, stomach, prostate gland, and intestines and rectum; among women they are breast, intes-

[19] Edward J. Stieglitz, *Report of a Survey of Active Studies in Gerontology*, 12 (New York, 1942); J. F. Norman, "Our Aging Population," in *Minnesota Medicine*, 24:1066–1071 (December, 1941).
[20] Schmid, *Mortality Trends in the State of Minnesota*, chapter 3; State Board of Health, *Reports*, 1922–43, p. 53; Minnesota Department of Health, "Thirty Years of Health Progress in Minnesota."
[21] State Board of Health, *Reports*, 1922–43, p. 229; American Cancer Society, *The Big 3* (New York, 1946).

ADDING LIFE TO YEARS

tines and rectum, stomach, and genitourinary organs.[22] In their crusade to guide the public toward a better understanding of cancer as a public health problem, the Minnesota division of the American Cancer Society lists seven cancer danger signals:

1. Any sore that does not heal, particularly about the tongue, mouth or lips.
2. A painless lump or thickening, especially in the breast, lip or tongue.
3. Irregular bleeding from any natural body opening.
4. Progressive change in the color or size of a wart, mole or birthmark.
5. Persistent indigestion.
6. Persistent hoarseness, unexplained cough, or difficulty in swallowing.
7. Any change in the normal bowel habits.[23]

Fortunately cancer research and knowledge have grown considerably since a St. Paul physician in 1914 described cancer as a public health problem. After World War I a program of cancer control was worked out with emphasis on education, research, and service. These are the guiding principles of the American Cancer Society, an organization which has branches in many states. The Minnesota division, with representatives in every county, takes as its motto the slogan "Fight Cancer with Knowledge." During 1947 this division made a second contribution of $75,000 toward the completion of the Cancer Research Institute at the University of Minnesota, continued a $5,000 cancer research fellowship at the university, contributed $15,000 toward a cancer detection center at the university, financed follow-up services to cancer patients at the university, and gave the American Cancer Society forty per cent of the gross campaign contributions amounting to approximately $103,000. But this was not all. The Minnesota division has held three continuation study courses in cancer education for practicing physicians; has distributed 900,000 pieces of cancer educational literature to the general public, to schools, and to industry; has placed educational cancer exhibits at conventions and fairs and in hospitals, industrial centers, and schools; and, through motion pictures and addresses in the state's eighty-seven counties, has presented the hopeful message that daring advances in surgery and radiology have saved thousands of potential cancer victims. In ad-

[22] American Cancer Society, Minnesota Division, *Who, What, Why, Where, When of Cancer* (New York, n.d.).
[23] American Cancer Society, Minnesota Division, *What Most People Don't Know about Cancer* (New York, n.d.); Herbert L. Lombard, "Problems of an Aging Population," in *American Journal of Public Health*, 37:170–176 (February, 1947).

dition it has furnished approximately 70,000 dressings for cancer patients and has helped with funds for the transportation of needy cancer patients.[24]

Both the national and state cancer organizations have aided the public's health by telling in laymen's language exactly what cancer is and how it affects man. "Cancer," they say, "is a disorderly growth (increase in numbers) of cells of the patient's own tissues. This growth does not correspond to the laws that control activities of normal cells, it never ceases during the life of the individual, and the tissue so formed never functions as does the normal tissue in the same individual." [25]

Hundreds of school children throughout Minnesota are told that cancer has many recognized causes. Perhaps the most common is some form of chronic or prolonged irritation. Charts demonstrate that this irritation may be of several kinds — chemical, thermal, or mechanical friction. More than two hundred chemicals are capable of producing cancer when introduced into laboratory animals. Children also learn, and carry home to their parents, elementary lessons in the development of body cells. They are told, too, that constant friction of a mole or wart or of an old burn scar may produce cancer in such tissue.

Steadily holding to the thesis that the more the public knows about cancer the more opportunities there are to avoid it, cancer associations and others divide tumors into benign and malignant. A vast mass of free literature describes how cancer may be treated by surgery, X ray, or radium and explains the technique of each. Again and again motion pictures and booklets drive home the fact that most cancers can be cured if they are treated early. Public health nurses are told that they must disseminate information about cancer to the general public; they must themselves keep in touch with current advances and must know how to care for cancer patients. They are urged to stress the importance of periodic physical examinations among the people with whom they work. Special manuals have been prepared for high school students and for college and university undergraduates. The Metropolitan Life Insurance Company has distributed thousands of leaflets telling how cancer deaths can be prevented if only simple rules are followed. Other educational literature includes study outlines for pupils and texts for teachers.[26]

[24] Minnesota State Sanitary Conference, "Minutes," September 30, 1914, pp. 3–19 (typescript), Minnesota Department of Health, Minneapolis; American Cancer Society, Minnesota Division, *Annual Reports*, 1947; *Minnesota's Health*, vol. 1, no. 2, p. 1 (February, 1947).
[25] American Cancer Society, Minnesota Division, *Answers to Common Questions about Cancer*, 3 (Minneapolis, 1947).
[26] American Cancer Society, Minnesota Division, *How Your Doctor Detects Cancer* (New York, 1947), *Cancer and Its Care*, 31 (New York, 1946), and *Cancer: A*

The Minnesota Department of Health, in co-operation with the Minnesota State Medical Association, established a program of cancer control within the section of preventable diseases, which hopes to develop a series of clinics where diagnoses may be made. Early in 1948 a University of Minnesota Cancer Detection Center was opened. This center offered complete physical examinations to men and women over forty-five years of age. About the same time, the American Cancer Society granted the University of Minnesota $44,770 for cancer research. Dr. H. S. Diehl, dean of the university's medical school, announced that cancer research at the university had grown in twelve years from a $2,000-a-year activity to a highly organized project that cost $109,866 during 1946–47. Governor Luther Youngdahl proclaimed April, 1948, as Cancer Control Month and said: "Research at the University of Minnesota made possible through grants of the American Cancer Society already has produced beneficial returns in the search for knowledge that will conquer the disease. The Minnesota Division of the society has given $150,000 toward the establishment of a cancer research center at the university and is now financing a cancer detection center there which will serve all the people of the state." Mayors of Minnesota cities supported drives for funds, and newspapers published stories and photographs of work at the university's detection center. Public interest increased when it became known that nearly half of the first 108 persons examined in the detection center had defects requiring medical attention.[27]

Prompted by additional grants of $88,038 from the United States Public Health Service and $135,888 and, later, $28,398 from the National Cancer Institute, the university was able to launch a program whose full effects would not be apparent for several years. All these activities were designed to catch cancer before it developed to a place where treatment was impossible, and thus to reduce the tremendous cancer death rate among all age groups, but especially among older persons. Public health officers know that cancer is neither inherited nor incurable. The only thing to fear about cancer is neglect. The University of Minnesota wishes to prevent this neglect. Indeed, every agency is working toward that end. They cannot repeat frequently enough that "When cancer is detected in

Study Outline for Secondary Schools (Minneapolis, 1948); Westchester Cancer Committee, *Youth Looks at Cancer* (Bronxville, 1948); Dallas Johnson, *Facing the Facts about Cancer* (Public Affairs Committee, Inc., *Public Affairs Pamphlet* no. 38 — New York, 1947); Metropolitan Life Insurance Company, *There Is Something You Can Do about Cancer* (New York, 1946); New York City Cancer Committee, *Cancer: A Manual for High School Teachers* (New York, 1947).

[27] *Minneapolis Tribune*, February 22, March 25, 1948; *Pioneer Press*, February 22, April 7, 1948; *St. Paul Dispatch*, March 24, 29, 1948; *Minneapolis Star*, April 1, May 8, 1948; *Minnesota's Health*, vol. 2, no. 2, p. 2 (February, 1948).

its early stages and treatment is begun at once, life can be saved and suffering prevented." Thus, for many, old age without cancer is no longer an impossible goal.[28]

Before maturity, the two heart conditions that impair health are congenital defects and rheumatic diseases. From maturity to middle age and beyond, hypertensive heart disease and coronary heart disease account for far too many deaths. As a matter of fact, heart disease is now the number one cause of death in the United States. It is on the increase because more people each year reach the age at which the heart is most likely to get into trouble. But, like those from cancer, many untimely deaths from heart disease can be prevented. From 1914 to 1947, with the exception of 1918 when influenza struck, heart disease has been the leading cause of death in Minnesota. In 1948 Dr. Ancel Keys, director of the University of Minnesota's laboratory of physiological hygiene, boldly said that half the people in the Twin Cities who pass the age of twenty-one are likely to die from heart disease and stated that such diseases would claim the lives of 1,200,000 people a year in the United States by 1960. A survey of Twin City businessmen revealed that ten per cent of those between the ages of forty-five and fifty-four had definite signs of diseases of the heart and blood vessels. During 1947 heart disease caused the death of 8,972 individuals in Minnesota. The tremendous increase may be seen dramatically in other figures. In 1942 the death rate from heart disease was 274.1 per 100,000 population; in 1948 it had jumped to 309.7 per 100,000 population.[29]

Although heart disease is a major killer in Minnesota, the public health committee of the Minnesota State Planning Board which in 1936 recommended a long and detailed program for the control of cancer paid relatively little attention to heart diseases. Saying that heart diseases represent to a large extent the terminal phase of a series of degenerative processes, the committee continued: "They are obviously amenable only to preventive measures and to such alterations in the hygiene of the individual as will permit him to function and exist with a radically altered amount of vital tissue in his body. It becomes overwhelmingly apparent that for age to attempt to simulate youth is a folly that can have only one conceivable result, namely an early death. By some authors the whole subject is dismissed fatalistically as nature's method of removing in-

[28] *Pioneer Press*, June 21, September 26, 1948; *St. Paul Dispatch*, September 30, 1948; "Cancer Is Curable," in *Everybody's Health*, vol. 31, no. 4, p. 10 (April, 1946).
[29] State Board of Health, *Reports*, 1922–43, p. 48; *Pioneer Press*, February 8, March 10, August 15, 1948. Information concerning the death rate from heart disease was obtained from the division of vital statistics of the Minnesota Department of Health on October 23, 1948.

dividuals no longer of biologic value, namely, individuals no longer capable of reproduction. . . . Regardless of how the individual may react to his changing physical capacities, they must be met. They represent the field of adult hygiene, a field of medicine the interest of which to both the individual and the state must be, for some time to come, a matter of increasing concern and importance."[30]

Old people with heart conditions could draw small comfort from such words. Fortunately other organizations in later years said bluntly that it was not true that nothing could be done about heart disease. The verdict of heart trouble in most cases, said the Metropolitan Life Insurance Company, does not mean death overnight. The company points out that thousands of persons with damaged hearts are living comfortable, happy, useful lives because they are co-operating with their doctors in giving their hearts a chance. Many of them may live as long as they could reasonably expect to live without heart trouble. Some of them even have a chance of complete recovery.[31]

Among the most common of the degenerative diseases affecting Minnesota's elderly population is hardening of the arteries. Walls of the arteries harden and narrow and thus reduce the blood flow through them. When the blood supply to the heart itself becomes insufficient, a condition known as "angina pectoris" may appear. Many of the sudden deaths or "heart attacks" among middle-aged persons are due also to coronary thrombosis. These deaths result from the sudden closing of a coronary artery by a clot. With proper care, many persons with these types of heart disease can live nearly normal lives.[32]

Minnesota public health authorities have done little, relatively speaking, with the problem of heart disease among either the young or the old. Certainly they have not paid as much attention to heart disease as they have to tuberculosis or cancer. The bulk of the work in Minnesota has been accomplished by the Minnesota Heart Association, a branch of the American Heart Association, and by the University of Minnesota. These organizations have been tremendously concerned over the rapid increase of heart disease throughout the state and have taken active, positive steps to make the public aware of what heart disease is and how it should be handled. Supported by the Junior League, the Alpha Phi sorority, and the American Legion, the Minnesota Heart Association set

[30] Minnesota State Planning Board, Committee on Public Health, *Report*, 16 ([St. Paul?], December, 1936).
[31] Metropolitan Life Insurance Company, *Your Heart*, 3 (New York, 1946).
[32] E. V. Cowdry, *Problems of Aging*, chapter 7 (Baltimore, 1942); Arlie R. Barnes, "Coronary Heart Disease; Prognosis and Life Adaptation," in *Minnesota Medicine*, 29:886–889 (September, 1946).

out to "spread information about the knowledge and treatment of heart diseases and the need for research funds to combat these diseases, which cause more than one death an hour in Minnesota alone — 8,872 during 1947."[33]

On May 6, 1948, Dr. Paul Dwan, president of the Minnesota affiliate of the American Heart Association, announced that his organization would provide funds to construct and equip a research electrocardiography developing laboratory at the University of Minnesota. A heart research project, the beginning of a ten-year investigation into the causes of high blood pressure and hardening of the arteries, was begun at the university under the direction of Dr. Ancel Keys in January, 1948. Five hundred men, it was announced, volunteered as human guinea pigs for this experiment. Their ages ranged from eighteen to fifty-four and they were from all walks of life. When plans were made by the university for the construction of a heart hospital, said to be the first in the nation, response was immediate and enthusiastic. The American Legion Foundation, in fitting ceremonies, offered $50,000 for the establishment of a heart research professorship. The Variety Club of the Northwest raised $300,000 and application was made by the university for $241,731 of federal funds under the terms of the Hill-Burton Hospital Construction Act. To be located on the east bank of the Mississippi River and close to the university hospitals, the new heart hospital, according to the original plans was to be a three-story structure containing eighty beds, and was to cost $731,195 equipped.[34]

Meanwhile the university continued its heart research program. In September, 1948, Dr. Otto H. Schmitt announced to the American Physiological Society that he had discovered how to make three-dimensional electrocardiograms, a new technique which Dr. Maurice B. Visscher called "amazing" and "absolutely new." The American Heart Association, acting in co-operation with the United States Public Health Service, offered a new technique for treating patients suffering from coronary thrombosis. New drugs, the anticoagulants dicumerol and heparin, were said to be so effective in preventing blood clotting that "one person in three who was expected to die from a specific attack of coronary occlusion will survive that attack."[35]

[33] *Minnesota's Health*, vol. 2, no. 2, p. 3 (February, 1948); *St. Paul Dispatch*, May 20, 1948; "Minnesota Heart Association Program," in *Minnesota Medicine*, 31:79 (January, 1948).
[34] *Minneapolis Star*, May 6, 1948; *Tribune*, November 15, 1947, January 5, October 17, 1948; *Pioneer Press*, April 18, 1948; "The Hill-Burton Bill," in *Minnesota Medicine*, 29:1252 (December, 1946).
[35] *Tribune*, September 17, 1948; *St. Paul Dispatch*, May 10, 1948.

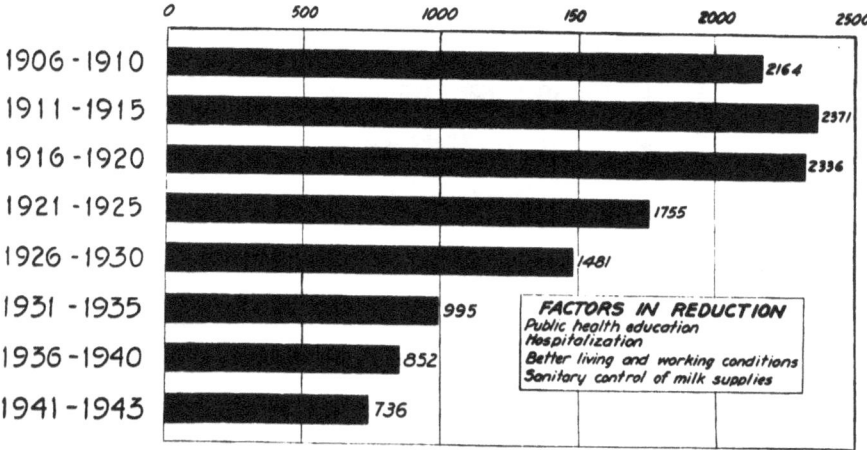

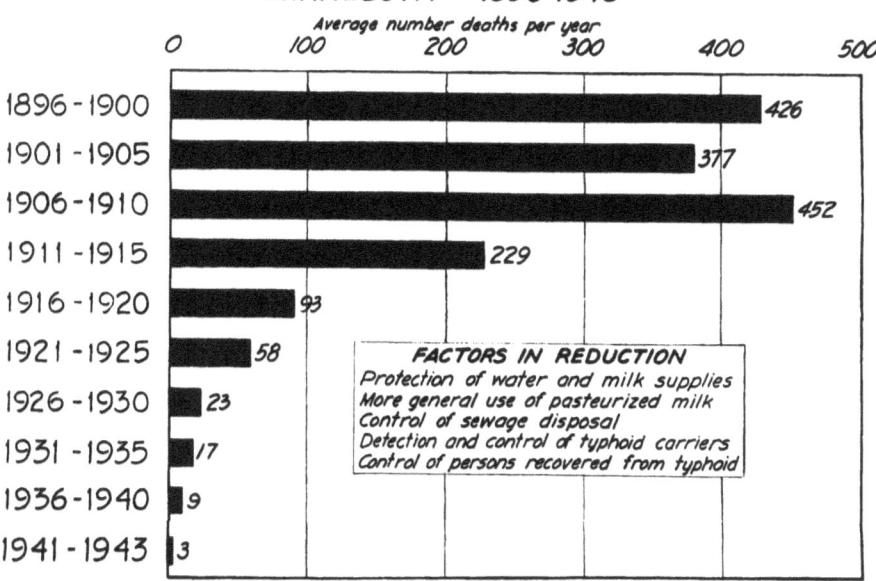

MORTALITY RATES
Courtesy Minnesota Department of Health

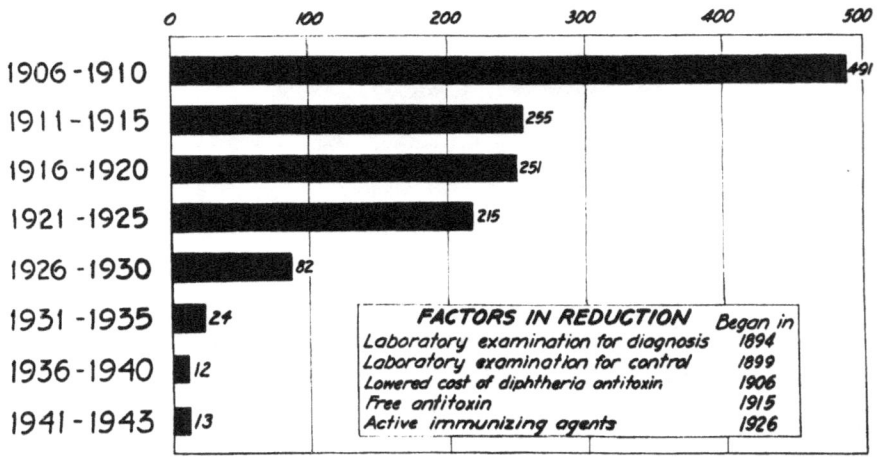

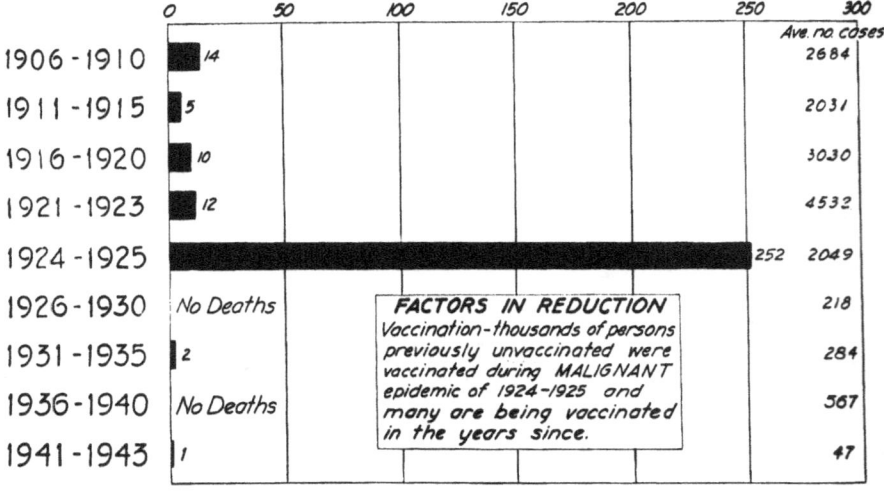

MORTALITY RATES
Courtesy Minnesota Department of Health

By the beginning of 1949 Minnesota's aged were receiving the attention of agencies and benefiting from types of treatment that had not existed only a few years earlier. They could begin to feel that heart disease in old age was not a calamity, if only they learned additional lessons in nutrition, availed themselves of a new screening method for blood glucose, co-operated with their physicians, and took advantage of still newer techniques that were sure to come.[36]

The state's care of its older population, however, entails more than an adequate cancer program sponsored by the Minnesota Department of Health or research in heart diseases by the University of Minnesota and the Minnesota Heart Association. Old age carries with it all too frequently mental disturbances, some of them the unavoidable results of senility and others the results of worry over loss of a job, premature retirement, or a sense of lack of security. Public health officials eventually will realize that these disturbing problems are as real to people as are their aches and pains. How to grow old successfully is a challenge that most persons cannot face alone. But old age can be a relatively rich period if older persons co-operate in aiding one another. Today the goal of those interested in old age is not so much to add years to life as it is to add life to years.[37]

Gerontologists — specialists in the problems attendant upon old age — are vitally concerned with caring for persons past middle age and with making them happy. "What are we to do about the aged and the partially disabled?" asks one of these distinguished specialists. "We cannot plow them under as we used to plow under corn, potatoes, tobacco, and little pigs. And I am equally certain that we cannot just turn them out to pasture and expect them to enjoy life. People are not happy when they are idle, and this is particularly true of older individuals. . . . Age plays for real stakes, not pastime. It wants something to do and it must be real." [38]

Mental hygienists believe that one of the major services that a forward-looking public health program can provide for older men and women is that of giving them something *real* to do. Again and again the point is made that people should retire to something and not from something. Everyone needs to engage in purposeful activity as long as he lives. It is

---

[36] Irving S. Wright, *Diseases of the Arteries: Their Significance, Recognition, and Treatment*, a pamphlet published by the American Heart Association (New York, n.d.).

[37] E. V. Cowdry, "The Broader Implications of Aging," in *Journal of Gerontology*, 2:277–282 (October, 1947).

[38] Theodore G. Klumpp, "Problems of an Aging Population," in *American Journal of Public Health*, 37:157 (February, 1947).

no help to an older person to insist that he live out the remainder of his life without anything to do.[39] A busy, happy oldster is apt to be better both physically and mentally than one with nothing to do but sit drearily and ponder his aches and pains. The time may come when purposeful programs will be an essential part of every home for the aged and when private and public health clinics will exist to help Minnesota's aging population fill its days with worth-while activity.

Indeed, suggestions already have been made on the national level for the creation of departments of gerontology, either independently endowed or affiliated with established centers of learning, which would undertake research in all the sciences related to aging, biologic and sociologic, and would also plan and execute programs to activate elders both mentally and physically. Such departments would plan ideal living environments for them, where they could live active and useful lives. In addition, they would provide geriatricians to attend and rehabilitate the aged ill and to provide care for the truly senile. Contemporary thinking, although approving of sheltered care of the aged, does not condone the old idea of the "retreat," where they are given food and lodging but not what they so desperately need — a purpose in life as manifested in something worth while to do.[40]

The philosophy underlying the newer approach of health authorities to old age is not as yet in operation in Minnesota; nevertheless it must be adopted if the North Star State is to handle successfully its increasing number of oldsters. Today a bill of rights has been enunciated for them by geriatricians. This bill lists ten rights for the nation's aged: (1) the right to be treated as persons; (2) the right to be treated as adults; (3) the right to a fair chance on their merits; (4) the right to a say about their own lives; (5) the right to a future; (6) the right to have fun and companions; (7) the right to be romantic; (8) the right to others' help in becoming interesting to others; (9) the right to professional help whenever necessary; and (10) the right to be old.[41]

Fortunately these rights are being recognized at least on a small scale in Minnesota. Duluth, for example, became conscious of its lack of recreational facilities for the aged. Its Council of Social Agencies, as the result of a survey of other cities throughout the United States, decided that a recreational center for the aged be established. Plans call for a building

[39] George Lawton, *Aging Successfully*, chapter 8 (New York, 1947).
[40] Frank Hinman, "The Story of Old Age," in *Journal of Gerontology*, 2:103–109 (April, 1947); Joseph H. Kinnaman, "Problems of an Aging Population," in *American Journal of Public Health*, 37:163–169 (February, 1947).
[41] George Lawton, "A Bill of Rights for Old Age," in *Journal of Gerontology*, 2:1–10 (January, 1947); Lawton, *Aging Successfully*, chapter 14.

and a paid recreational worker, with activities offered for both men and women. A kitchen was planned where older people might prepare lunches for their friends. Afternoon coffee or tea parties could be arranged. Games, dancing, amateur movies, crafts — all these were provided for. Oldsters could bring mending and sewing to the center. The entire project was developed to suit the particular needs of older persons and to provide for adventures in leisure time. Dr. E. L. Tuohy of Duluth took great interest in this project. He hopes that the Minnesota health department, like the Massachusetts and Indiana state boards of health, may some day organize a department of adult hygiene and geriatrics.[42]

Le Mont Crandall, Minnesota supervisor of old age assistance, knows that the perfect design for a happy, useful, and active old age may not be possible for a large number of people. "However," he says, "it is possible through study and planning to improve the living conditions of the aged, to furnish them with some outlet for their leisure time, to supply adequate care for their mental and physical health problems, and to better their employment opportunities." Crandall warns, too, against foolish planning. "As the average age of the population goes up," he continues, "this aged group influences legislation to a marked degree; and as in the past many ill-advised plans will be advanced to pacify them. In the future this group will exercise significant strength in the political field: there is usually much sentiment connected with any program proposed for the aged. It would be wise, therefore, to consider needs of our aged population and to make adequate plans before ill-advised schemes are proposed by unscrupulous persons, taking unfair advantage of present conditions."[43]

[42] Le Mont Crandall, "Retirement — What Then?" in *Minnesota Welfare*, vol. 4, no. 2, pp. 6–10 (August, 1948); E. L. Tuohy, "Adult Hygiene and Geriatrics," in *Minnesota Medicine*, 31:1013 (September, 1948), and "Geriatrics: The General Setting," in *Minnesota Welfare*, vol. 2, no. 1, pp. 7–9 (July, 1946).
[43] Crandall, "The Aged Face Many Problems," in *Minnesota Welfare*, vol. 3, no. 9, p. 9 (June, 1948). A detailed study on Minnesota's aged who are receiving old age assistance appears in *Social Welfare Review* (now *Minnesota Welfare*) for April, 1945, August–November, 1945, April–June, 1946, and August, 1946.

22

Wanted: More Hospital Beds

THE NORTH STAR STATE is known the world over for its great Mayo Clinic and historic St. Mary's Hospital. The hundreds of patients who go annually to Rochester are seldom aware that Minnesota, like many another state, has insufficient hospitals to meet contemporary needs. Minnesotans, trying to get friends and relatives admitted to either private or public institutions, realize the inadequacies of the state's hospital program only too well. Both physicians and hospital administrators in 1948 complained of crowded wards and of increasing costs which made additions to existing institutions and the building of new ones almost prohibitive. A score of communities felt that they were too far from the nearest hospital and they were searching diligently for ways and means to bring hospital services closer. Public health administrators, doctors, and nurses were all concerned with Minnesota's need for additional hospital beds.

They agree with a national report that the "importance to better health conditions of close working relationships among the hospitals of a region or State can scarcely be over-emphasized." [1] Health officers realize, too, that today's system of hospitals and health centers covering an entire region and offering citizens all types of service is a far cry from the old individualistic philosophy that prompted the establishment of hospitals in early Minnesota. Until very recently the average citizen thought of a hospital as an independent healing institution having little or no relationship to other hospitals or to public health.

Indeed, half a century ago well-intentioned and able individuals seriously challenged the entire hospital idea. A Ramsey County resident, for example, complained bitterly in 1855 when the idea of a county hospital was being considered. On the other hand, innumerable people

[1] Ewing, *The Nation's Health*, 174.

WANTED: MORE HOSPITAL BEDS 437

praised St. Joseph's Hospital in St. Paul after it was once begun. Sponsored by nuns of the order of St. Joseph of Carondelet, this institution ministered to sixty-eight charity patients in 1855, a year after its opening. Its rate to private patients was eight dollars a week, which included a private room "furnished with the careful attendance of the Sister, a doctor, medicine, lights and fuel." Pioneers marching into Minnesota sometimes were treated at army dispensaries, including those at Forts Snelling, Ridgely, and Ripley.[2]

It was not until after the Civil War, however, that hospital construction really boomed in Minnesota. Once started, it moved ahead swiftly. A city hospital was operating in Minneapolis in 1871; two years later a committee of St. Paul residents planned for a municipal hospital; and in 1873 the Minneapolis Cottage Hospital, later St. Barnabas, made its second annual report. Stillwater was planning for a public hospital about the same time. The 1880s witnessed the opening in Minneapolis of the Minnesota College Hospital, Northwestern Hospital, Maternity Hospital, General Hospital, and St. Mary's Hospital. St. Luke's Hospital in Duluth opened in 1882 and St. Mary's Hospital at Rochester, toward the close of the decade. Cottage Hospital built an addition in 1882 and assured the public that it would "always be open to the sick and suffering from all parts of the state."[3]

These institutions and others, although frightfully primitive in some instances, were crowded almost from the time their doors opened. Dr. Arthur B. Ancker, superintendent of St. Paul's city hospital, took great pains in 1886 to describe lack of space in that hospital. He said that the general hospital was taxed to its utmost capacity and pleaded for the erection of additional buildings. With the admission of more than five hundred patients annually, Ancker felt that physical expansion was im-

[2] *St. Paul Daily Pioneer*, January 26, March 23, 1855; Nathaniel W. Faxon, "A History of Hospitals," in American Hospital Association, *Bulletins*, 3:20–26 (January, 1929); Theodore C. Blegen, "Hospitals on the Western Frontier — A Backward Look Through 124 Years," 75, in *Hospitals*, vol. 17, no. 8, pp. 73–75 (August, 1943); Coolidge, *Sickness and Mortality in the Army, 1855–1860*, 57–75; Harvey E. Brown, *The Medical Department of the United States Army* (Washington, D.C., 1873).

[3] *St. Anthony Falls Democrat*, March 23, 1871; *St. Paul Daily Press*, May 3, 1872, April 13, March 15, 1873; *Pioneer Press*, August 5, 1882; John E. Ransom, "Beginnings of Hospitals in the United States," in *Hospitals*, 15:68–71 (December, 1941); 16:74–79 (January, 1942); Theodore C. Blegen, "Frontier Days — When the Hospital Rated as an Acceptable Substitute for Home Care," in *Hospitals*, vol. 17, no. 9, p. 71 (September, 1943); Henry A. Castle, *History of St. Paul and Vicinity*, 1:344 (Chicago, 1912); Isaac Atwater and John H. Stevens, *History of Minneapolis and Hennepin County*, 1:252 (New York, 1895); Atwater, *History of the City of Minneapolis, Minnesota*, 865–870 (New York, 1893); Marion D. Shutter, *History of Minneapolis — Gateway to the Northwest*, 505–512 (Chicago, 1923); Maternity Hospital, Inc., *Maternity Hospital*, [1887–1937], ([Minneapolis, 1937]).

perative. "It must be borne in mind," he said, "that these improvements are asked for in the name of the destitute, sick and injured, that there is no greater charity, no charity that it is more our duty to bestow, than that of caring for our helpless fellow creatures." In Minneapolis, Dr. Charles A. Chase urged construction of a new city hospital because the old one was both crowded and outdated. Northwestern Hospital had outgrown its original quarters by 1885, and it was planning to build on a new site.[4]

Despite the utmost efforts to give competent care to the sick, Minnesota hospitals all too frequently were handicapped by lack of funds and inadequate facilities. After inspecting St. Paul's general hospital, a grand jury committee reported that twenty-three patients were housed in two rooms, that the rooms were warmed by wood stoves, that "neither the hall nor any room in the house has any means of ventilation but by doors and windows," that the dining room was used as a general washing and bathing room, that the entire water supply came from a nearly dry well and from a small cistern which was filled from water carts every three weeks, and that "there are no water closets in or near the house and two small privies at a considerable distance across the open yard are resorted to by all the inhabitants of the house."[5]

Similar charges were brought against St. Joseph's Hospital. Dr. A. B. Cates testified that the institution was dirty, that patients were not washed, and that physicians' orders were ignored. Dr. J. C. Cochran, St. Paul health officer, said he could not learn from nurses the pulses or temperatures of patients because no records could be found. Patients also affirmed that mistakes were made in treatment and that nursing service was indifferent and careless. After describing beds that crawled with vermin, a patient continued: "The beds were generally changed every week, but once in a while they were not. Think I was in the hospital six weeks, sick with typhoid fever. When I convalesced, they gave me tough beefsteak. Another patient had pains in his limbs: heard the doctor give orders to rub them; they were never rubbed. The nurses came between 8 and 9 in the evening and covered us with blankets, when they went away and would not come again unless called until the next morning. The Sisters treated the patients pretty well; occasionally a Sister would speak unkindly; we were in pain, and would sometimes groan, and the Sister would say 'hush, or you will have to leave the hospital.' When I had occasion to call a nurse she would come sometimes in half

[4] St. Paul City Officers, *Annual Reports*, October 31, 1886, p. 492; Minneapolis City Officers, *Annual Reports*, 1889, p. 418; Northwestern Hospital, *Annual Reports*, November 1, 1885, p. 7.

[5] *Pioneer Press*, January 16, December 6, 1877.

an hour: had no way of judging except it seemed so long. The clothes were usually clean, but if one spilled food on them they were not changed." After more than a month of taking evidence and after nuns at St. Joseph's had described in detail how the institution was administered, the hospital was cleared of the charges brought against it by Cates and others.[6]

St. Mary's Hospital at Rochester, opened in 1889, was a typical institution of the times. A three-story brick building, it contained three wards and one private room. Water came from a basement reservoir, while a cesspool took care of sewage. The building was lighted by kerosene lamps, and nurses on night duty carried lanterns to light their way. Another lantern hung from a tree in front of the building to guide physicians or others who might come to the hospital during the night. When a doctor was needed at the institution, someone walked half a mile to town to call him. Like other Minnesota hospitals, St. Mary's grew rapidly, caring for 301 patients in 1890 and for 1,220 ten years later. By that time two additions had been opened.[7]

During the early years of hospital growth considerable apprehension existed among people who believed that hospitals were places to die in and that their chief purpose was to treat charity patients. The latter was especially true of city institutions. In 1877, for example, there was not a single paying patient in St. Paul's general hospital. The patients included nine laborers, twelve servants, two farmers, "together with a soldier, a carpenter, clerk, cigar maker, printer, barber, and one dead beat." Rules were rather strict for both private patients and charity cases. The sick were required to submit quietly to doctors' treatments and directions, were forbidden to use profane or indecent language, to gamble for money, to smoke tobacco, to procure intoxicating liquors, or "to circulate any book, print, pamphlet, or newspaper of a vulgar, immoral or indecent character." Men were not permitted to visit women's wards, and women were not permitted to enter the rooms of men patients. Convalescents were required to assist in any light work around the hospital which was approved by their physician. They also were responsible for the neatness of their beds and bedside tables. At Northwestern Hospital patients rose at six o'clock during the summer and at six-thirty in winter. No patient could take meals in bed without special permission.[8]

Menus, of course, varied from institution to institution, but in almost

[6] *Pioneer Press*, July 21, 26, 31, August 1, 4, 14, 18, 1883.
[7] *A Souvenir of St. Mary's Hospital*, 15, 18 ([Rochester?], 1922).
[8] *Pioneer Press*, December 14, 1877; St. Paul City Officers, *Annual Reports*, 1886, p. 503; Northwestern Hospital, *Annual Reports*, 1900, p. 56.

every hospital emphasis was placed on starchy foods and proteins. Breakfast consisted of coffee or tea with milk and sugar, bread and butter, and meat hash. For lunch patients were served boiled corned-beef hash, turnips, cabbage, potatoes, and bread. Supper was a light meal of coffee or tea and bread and syrup. Special diets, to be ordered by the surgeon in charge, offered milk, chocolate, cocoa, beef tea, chicken broth, mutton broth, gruel, oatmeal mush, cornstarch, boiled rice, eggs, beefsteak, mutton chops, and chicken.[9]

Ancker reported in 1886 that the average number of days in the hospital for each patient was twenty-seven. The mortality rate in the city hospitals of both Minneapolis and St. Paul was ten per cent. "In considering the death rate," explained Ancker, "it should be borne in mind that the greater proportion of our patients come from a class that is composed largely of persons hard-worked and poorly nourished, many of them the victims of intemperance and vicious habits, unable to resist the inroads of disease and the effects of injury. In addition to these facts, so strong is the unreasonable prejudice existing in the minds of the ignorant and uninformed to a public hospital, that they only seek its shelter when the effects of serious disease or the results of severe injury make it their last resort." [10]

Ancker was not as callous as he sounded. He deplored the fact that, because the city hospital had only fifty-two beds, he was obliged to reject four-fifths of those who applied for admittance. Believing that St. Paul must increase its hospital facilities, in 1886 Ancker made a five-weeks tour of eastern institutions in order to gather ideas for a new St. Paul hospital. Upon his return home he asked for additional ground upon which to erect an entirely new, modern building. He defined the modern hospital as one "perfect in heat, ventilation and hygienic qualities, with pleasant surroundings, plenty of light and air." Ancker also deplored the prevailing idea that a hospital was an institution only for paupers. He spoke vigorously on this point: "Statistics show that a large proportion of those who go to a hospital are hard-working, honest and respectable citizens. The benefits they receive are their rights. It is not charity. While they are well the city extends certain rights of citizenship, and these rights are more valuable when a poor man, unable to pay board and doctor bills, can receive attention in a good hospital. The charity idea is a wrong one entirely." [11] Although it was to be many years before

[9] St. Paul City Officers, *Annual Reports*, 1886, p. 501.
[10] St. Paul City Officers, *Annual Reports*, 1886, p. 490.
[11] *Pioneer Press*, January 12, 1885, December 24, 1886.

hospitals were considered public health centers, Ancker's point of view certainly marked a forward step.

Ancker's new viewpoint was apparent also when he insisted that hospital architecture possessed a distinctive individuality and that attempts to convert old structures into hospitals could result only in inefficiency. He told the St. Paul City Council that a modern hospital should contain an administrative unit large enough to accommodate comfortably resident physicians, administrative officers, and nurses. He proposed the inclusion of startling innovations, such as a drug room and a library. He insisted also upon isolated pavilions for the treatment of infectious diseases, and for the insane. With competent knowledge of engineering requirements, he described water supplies and sewerage systems. Finally, he estimated the cost of an ideal institution to be in the neighborhood of a hundred thousand dollars.[12]

So well did Ancker present his recommendations that in 1887 the legislature authorized St. Paul to issue fifty thousand dollars' worth of bonds with which to begin the new hospital. Two years later St. Paul was permitted to issue a hundred thousand dollars' worth of bonds. These sums not only purchased additional land, but also financed the construction of an administration building. This building, which followed in general the plan proposed by Ancker in 1887, marked such an advance in hospital construction that it was said to be second to none in the country. A unit of fifty rooms, it contained offices, reception rooms, family dining rooms, a library, a museum, and a "germ-proof" operating room. The institution, described as a general hospital in the broadest sense of the term, was maintained by municipal tax levy for the benefit of the sick and injured. It was emphasized that this was not a pauper hospital.[13]

By 1892 Ancker, as chief of staff, had established eleven services. These included surgery, deformity surgery, general medicine, obstetrics, pathology, and treatment of nervous diseases, skin and venereal diseases, and diseases of women, of children, of eye and ear, and of nose and throat. More than a thousand patients were treated by Ancker and his staff that year. The gross cost per patient per week was $5.12, while the net cost per patient per week including employees was $3.75. Yet, even with the additional building, the hospital remained so crowded that in 1894 as many as forty patients were sleeping on the floors. By then Ancker was thinking of his institution as something more than a hospital. He was

[12] *Pioneer Press*, January 3, 1887.
[13] Minnesota, *Special Laws*, 1887, pp. 1011–1013; 1889, p. 919; *Pioneer Press*, May 29, 1892; St. Paul City Officers, *Annual Reports*, 1893, p. 877.

reaching out to grasp the idea that a hospital might be a medical center and that St. Paul itself might assume a regional leadership in medicine. Ancker was most explicit on this point, saying: "That a well equipped and well managed hospital must in some measure contribute to the substantial wealth of the community in which it is located, no one familiar with the facts can deny. With St. Paul's excellent hospital accommodations; the well known high standard of professional talent of its physicians and surgeons, and the proximity of the medical department of the University of Minnesota, there is no reason why it should not soon become the medical center of the great Northwest." Then he continued: "Even now are the students of the university and medical men from smaller towns of the surrounding territory seeking clinical instruction in our wards. Patients of means who under other circumstances would go East for relief, now come to St. Paul knowing that they can find here, not only the skill their disease or injury requires, but also the proper hospital accommodations." [14]

Ancker, believing also that safety to public health demanded the transportation of patients with contagious diseases in vehicles other than public hacks, recommended a city ambulance service. Charitable women raised sufficient funds in 1892 to purchase the "latest and most improved" type of ambulance, which entered service in the late autumn. Three years later St. Joseph's Hospital also inaugurated an ambulance service.[15]

Meanwhile other hospitals had remodeled their buildings or had erected entirely new ones. All strove to increase efficiency. The Minnesota Hospital, resulting from a combination of the medical and dental college departments of the Minnesota College Hospital with the Minneapolis Dispensary, announced in 1885 that it would construct a new three-story building at a cost of about twenty-five thousand dollars. St. Luke's Hospital purchased additional space in 1887, and a year later it laid the foundation for a brick building with stone trimmings. This seventy-two bed institution had the most modern sanitary facilities and ventilating system.[16]

St. Anthony Hospital in Minneapolis, organized in 1886, stood at 418 Second Avenue South and offered a unique hospitalization program

[14] *Pioneer Press*, March 31, 1892, April 4, 1894; St. Paul City Officers, *Annual Reports*, 1891, p. 620; 1893, p. 877.
[15] *Pioneer Press*, July 18, 1892, November 8, 1895. For a description of Ancker Hospital in 1948, see the *Pioneer Press*, October 17, 1948.
[16] *Pioneer Press*, June 18, 1885, April 4, 1887, December 14, 1888. See E. N. Flint, "Hospital Construction," in *Northwestern Lancet*, 14:21-24 (January 1, 1894), for a discussion of contemporary hospital standards.

WANTED: MORE HOSPITAL BEDS 443

somewhat similar to hospital care plans of a future day. It maintained branches at Aitkin and Duluth and at Cumberland, Wisconsin. These were designed primarily for the treatment of lumberjacks. An annual membership ticket costing ten dollars entitled the holder to medical and surgical care and to hospitalization. St. Anthony Hospital also paid an indemnity of five dollars a week in the case of a disabling accident. At the main hospital and its three branches, 253 patients were treated, 2,354 prescriptions were dispensed, and $855 was paid in indemnities during 1887.[17]

By 1900 the earlier hospitals in the state had become well established and a score of new ones had been organized. No general characterization could describe these institutions. Each determined its own policies and each represented a particular public, private, or religious point of view. Hospitals belonged to no association in 1900, and they were unlicensed. Anyone could rent a cottage, paint it white, install two or three hospital beds, put a hospital sign on the front of the house, and begin receiving patients. This was particularly true of maternity hospitals, many of which were run by a single person and operated in a private home. During the 1880s, for example, St. Paul health officers were told that "baby farms" were constantly on the increase and that mortality rates were excessively high. No licensing system for maternity hospitals was attempted in Minnesota until many years later, and then Bracken opposed it.[18]

In 1917 the legislature gave the State Board of Control authority to license maternity hospitals and to prescribe general rules and regulations for their conduct. About ten years after the licensing act was passed the Board of Control, through its children's bureau, published its first regulations for maternity hospitals. These rules covered location, buildings, physical equipment, and fire protection, as well as standards for heating and lighting. Other provisions applied to delivery rooms and nurseries, and still others, to the keeping of records. The Reorganization Act of 1939 removed licensing of maternity hospitals from the Board of Control and transferred it to the director of the division of social welfare of the Department of Social Security. On June 30, 1940, there were 267 hospitals in the state licensed to care for maternity patients. Of these, 7 were specialized hospitals caring for unmarried mothers, 55 were ma-

[17] *Pioneer Press*, January 1, 1888.
[18] "Why License Hospitals?" in *Minnesota Hospitals*, vol. 1, no. 4, p. 3 (January, 1937); "Pioneer Nursing," in *Minnesota Nurse*, vol. 1, no. 3, pp. 6, 22 (December, 1927); *Pioneer Press*, July 27, 1886; Bracken to John S. Fulton, February 4, 1918, Minnesota Department of Health, St. Paul.

ternity homes, and 205 were general hospitals, of which 21 were operating under temporary or provisional licenses.[19]

A new set of standards, prepared by Ethel McClure, supervisor of maternity hospitals, and John O. Hedwall, institutional inspector, appeared in 1941. The far-reaching public health aspect of these regulations is indicated by the number of organizations that offered advice and suggestions. These included not only the Minnesota Department of Health, but also the Minnesota Hospital Association, the Minnesota State Medical Association, the Minnesota Nurses' Association, the Minnesota State Board of Nurse Examiners, the Twin Cities Obstetric Round Table, and the Department of Obstetrics and Gynecology and the Department of Pediatrics of the University of Minnesota. Certain of the regulations were reviewed by representatives of the Maternity Home Council, an organization composed of superintendents and social workers in institutions for unmarried mothers.[20]

Results of the licensing of maternity hospitals demonstrated clearly the need for a similar system for other nursing institutions. Physicians and health authorities, therefore, approved an act passed by the legislature in 1941 which transferred the licensing of all hospitals, including maternity hospitals and related institutions, to the Minnesota Department of Health. Two years later the act was amended to include state and local governmental institutions. Having broad application, the hospital licensing law covered all places providing hospitalization for the sick or injured or care for chronic or convalescent aged and infirm persons, including those residing in homes for the aged.[21]

On April 20, 1944, the State Board of Health adopted elaborate standards for Minnesota hospitals, which, generally speaking, fell into the following groups: standards for general and specialized hospitals, for homes for unmarried mothers, for homes for the aged, for maternity homes, and for homes for chronic or convalescent patients. Special fire protection requirements established by the state fire marshal were also included. Regulations were drawn up covering admission and death rec-

[19] Minnesota, *Laws*, 1916–17, pp. 301–308; 1939, p. 946; State Board of Control, Children's Bureau, *Standards for Maternity Hospitals of Minnesota*, 9–16 (St. Paul, 1928); Division of Social Welfare, *Annual Reports*, 1939–40, p. 51.

[20] Division of Social Welfare, Medical Unit, *Standards for Maternity Hospitals of Minnesota*, [5] (St. Paul, 1941).

[21] *Laws*, 1941, pp. 1149–1153; 1943, pp. 1030–1032; [American Hospital Association], Commission on Hospital Care, *Hospital Care in the United States*, 594–596 (New York, 1947); Howard Burrell, "Looking into the Future — Legislation," in *Hospitals*, vol. 14, no. 6, pp. 52–55 (June, 1940); McClure, *Care of Sick and Infirm Residents in Homes for the Aged*; American Hospital Association, *Incorporation, Taxation, and Licensure of Hospitals in the United States* (Chicago, 1937).

WANTED: MORE HOSPITAL BEDS 445

ords, ophthalmia neonatorum, and conduct of visitors.[22] In addition to the development of hospital standards, state health officials planned for an environmental sanitation survey of all institutions. The survey was to cover the water supply; plumbing and disposal of sewage and garbage; food sanitation, including storage, refrigeration, and handling of food and dishwashing and handling of dishes and utensils; and insect and rodent control. By 1947 either complete sanitation surveys or plumbing inspections had been made in 125 hospitals. A nutritionist on the staff of the division of child hygiene visited a number of institutions in order to advise on menu planning and to investigate complaints.[23]

In 1947 licenses were issued to Minnesota institutions through the hospital licensing unit of the division of hospital service of the Minnesota Department of Health. At that time the professional staff consisted of three registered nurses with hospital and public health backgrounds. This group, together with others, classified the hospitals of the state to cover practically every type of institution, including state and private mental and epileptic hospitals, tuberculosis sanatoriums, and nursing homes. The number of these institutions at the close of 1947 was approximately 451, with a total of 34,286 beds. During that year 471 applications for licenses were received and 465 licenses were granted.[24]

The Minnesota Department of Health carried out this broad program with the assistance of an advisory board composed of four representatives of the Minnesota Hospital Association, two representatives of the Minnesota State Medical Association, and the state director of public instruction. The purposes of the program were to "ensure in the light of existing knowledge safe and adequate care for patients in places other than their own homes or those of relatives." This was to be effected in three ways: (1) by preventing the establishment of substandard places; (2) by maintaining and improving the standards for care in existing institutions; and (3) by serving as a source of information on hospital facilities and needs and on the newer developments in the field of hospital care.[25]

[22] Minnesota Department of Health, *Licensing Laws and Standards for Hospitals and Related Institutions of Minnesota*. The state health department was first given authority to designate a prophylactic to prevent infant blindness in 1917. Minnesota, *Laws*, special session, 1916–17, p. 489.
[23] Division of Child Hygiene, *The Minnesota Hospital Licensing Program, 1942–46*, p. 2 (Minneapolis, 1947).
[24] Minnesota Department of Health, *The Minnesota Hospital Licensing Program — Annual Reports*, 1947, p. 2, and *Minnesota Directory of Licensed Hospitals and Related Institutions*, 1947 (Minneapolis, 1947).
[25] Viktor O. Wilson and Ethel McClure, "Complete Coverage Is Feature of New License Regulations in Minnesota," in *Hospitals*, vol. 18, no. 5, pp. 40–43 (May, 1944.)

State medical and public health administrators did not stop with a licensing law for institutions, even though it was the first of its kind in the United States. There was still another gap that needed plugging. This was the licensing of superintendents and administrative heads of hospitals and sanatoriums. It was as much in the interest of public health, argued supporters of this view, to license the heads of hospitals as it was to license the institutions themselves. Therefore the legislature in 1947 passed another act, which once more made the state a pioneer in hospital legislation. This law stipulated that no person can act as the head of a hospital without being registered with the state health department. It said further: "No person shall be granted any such registration unless such person be at least 21 years of age, of good moral character and has had at least two years' experience in an administrative position in such an institution in this state, or one of equal standing in another state, or has successfully completed one year of formal training in an approved course in hospital administration, together with one year internship therein." Fortunately for those who wished training, the University of Minnesota in 1946 had established a program of graduate study in hospital administration.[26]

Passage of legislative acts, admirable as they were, did not automatically solve Minnesota's hospital problems. In 1942 patients admitted to hospitals numbered 308,304, comprising 11% of the state's population. Of the patients admitted, 44.6% underwent surgery. The average percentage of autopsies in the nation was 23.2, and Minnesota stood near the top of the list with 33.8%. Among the vexing problems during the years of World War II was lack of personnel in hospitals and difficulty in keeping costs down. Administrators were resentful of a public that felt that hospitals were making money when, in reality, it was difficult for institutions to break even. The average patient in 1944 could not be given good care, it was said, for less than from four and half to five dollars a day.[27]

Minnesota, like many another state, lacked sufficient hospital beds after World War II. Indeed, the nation at large needed an additional 195,000 general hospital beds in 1947 to bring the level of available hospitalization up to the average considered necessary to maintain good public health. A Minnesota survey showed the need for 4,746 additional general hospital beds, 6,905 mental hospital beds, and 5,427 chronic

[26] "License Law Amended," in *Minnesota Hospitals*, vol. 9, no. 6, p. 2 (May, 1945); *Laws*, 1947, pp. 394–396.
[27] Paul H. Fesler, "Hospital Services in Minnesota," in *Minnesota Municipalities*, 29:3 (January, 1944).

WANTED: MORE HOSPITAL BEDS

hospital beds. All in all, the state lacked 17,078 beds of all types on August 24, 1948. Certain areas, particularly in the north, had no local hospital service whatever, and patients were obliged to drive many miles to reach the nearest institution. Many communities were eager for the construction of hospitals close to them. They wanted residents to have good hospital care and they believed also that a hospital would stimulate local business.[28]

Yet these same communities frequently failed to realize the many problems attendant upon hospital construction. In the first place, many of them had no clear conception of what size an institution should be to best meet their needs. They did not know, for example, that an institution does not operate economically and efficiently until it has between twenty-five and thirty beds. Indeed, fifty beds is set by the United States Public Health Service as the efficiency figure.[29] Even the most enthusiastic supporters of new hospitals were aghast when they learned the cost of construction. In 1948 the per-bed cost ranged between $13,000 and $16,000. Using the minimum figure, this meant that a Minnesota town would have to spend at least $390,000 for a thirty-bed institution. This was expensive enough, but there was more to consider. The annual operating cost of such an institution is one-third of its construction cost. Thus, a thirty-bed hospital would cost $130,000 a year to operate. Few communities in Minnesota could by themselves swing that type of program. Yet, in some instances, local pride interfered with one possible solution: the merging of several communities for the building of a hospital within a reasonable distance of each. But not even a pooling of municipal resources could have financed all the hospitals needed in Minnesota.

Fortunately the federal government in 1946 provided means to help finance hospital construction throughout the nation. The Hospital Survey and Construction Act not only provided an over-all plan for the establishment of different types of institutions, but also stipulated that federal funds would be available for the construction of hospitals. If local communities could raise two-thirds of the completed cost of a hospital, including the equipment, the federal government would contribute one-third. Important as this financial aid was, it by no means constituted the entire program. In the first place, responsibility for the conduct of the program rested largely with the individual states. The Minnesota

[28] Commission on Hospital Care, *Hospital Care in the United States*, 412; Minnesota Department of Health, Division of Hospital Services, *The Minnesota Hospital Program*, August 24, 1948, a mimeographed report.
[29] Interview of the author with Dr. Helen L. Knudsen, November 3, 1948.

Department of Health, therefore, became responsible for the administration of the program in Minnesota. The department was to acquaint citizens with the details of the federal plan as it applied to Minnesota and was to secure public co-operation. Secondly, the federal survey and construction program established a system of progressive steps which must be met by any community seeking aid under the act and it set forth in elaborate detail general standards of construction and equipment. A State Advisory Council was appointed to assist the health department in the development of the program. Between May, 1946, and March, 1947, a survey of Minnesota's hospital facilities was made in order that the health department would know the state hospital situation and could report it to the United States Public Health Service, the federal agency charged with administering the provisions of the Hospital Survey and Construction Act.[30]

The federal law required planning for facilities in five types of institutions: general and allied special hospitals, mental disease hospitals, tuberculosis hospitals, chronic disease hospitals, and public health centers. In the general and allied special hospital group, the federal law considered facilities adequate if beds were provided at the ratio of four and one-half beds per one thousand population. This ratio allowed 12,681 beds for Minnesota on the basis of an estimated population in 1946 of 2,817,972. These beds, however, must be distributed in accordance with the standards of at least four and one-half beds, four beds, and two and one-half beds per one thousand of population, respectively, in each of the following three types of areas: base area, intermediate area, and rural area.

A base area was defined as a community containing a teaching hospital of a medical school prepared to give care to every kind of acute illness. The intermediate area was a community with a population of at least twenty-five thousand containing a hospital with approximately a hundred beds or more which was equipped for the diagnosis and treatment of all but the most specialized types of acute illness. The rural area, as might be expected, was defined as a community not designated as a base or intermediate area and containing an institution for the care of common illnesses and injuries and for obstetrics.

Results of the hospital survey begun in 1946 by the state health de-

[30] *Statutes at Large*, vol. 60, part 1, pp. 1040–1049; Minnesota, *Laws*, 1947, p. 763; Commission on Hospital Care, *Hospital Care in the United States*, 11; *Minnesota's Health*, vol. 1, no. 1, p. 3 (January, 1947); "Plan for Hospitals, Public Health Centers in Minnesota Submitted," in *Minnesota Municipalities*, 33:35–47 (February, 1948); Ray M. Amberg, "Progress in State-Wide Hospital Facilities Survey," in *Minnesota Hospitals*, vol. 2, no. 5, p. 1 (September, 1946).

partment revealed that there were in Minnesota 190 general and allied special hospitals with a normal total bed capacity of 10,331. These figures did not include federal hospitals nor specialized wards of ten beds or less in general hospitals for the care of tuberculosis or chronic or mental disease patients. They excluded also institutions that had closed since the time of the survey. The hospital situation in Minnesota showed further that in ninety-nine instances buildings or parts of buildings having a total normal capacity of 2,396 beds should be replaced. In these cases buildings either were not fire resisting or they were not adaptable to hospital service because they had been built for other purposes. Of the ninety-nine condemned buildings or parts of buildings, seventy-three were judged eligible for replacement at their present location.

Minnesota was divided into eleven regions, and specific areas and communities were designated within them in which acceptable hospitals existed or proposed ones would be located. General hospital projects were given priority ratings and classified in four groups, beginning with locations that had no hospitals and ending with thirty-five existing hospitals. This priority program, of course, did not mean that every community in the first priority group would automatically have a new hospital within any stipulated time. It meant only that if communities within the first priority group could raise sufficient funds and fulfill other requirements they would receive consideration before communities in other groups. It meant also that it would be possible for communities in other groups to have hospitals before all locations in group one had them. In other words, the program was a flexible one.

By the close of 1948 ten communities had met preliminary requirements and were started on new hospital programs. Of the ten, three had awarded contracts. They were the Baudette Municipal Hospital, the Greenbush Community Hospital, and the Rochester Health Center. Seven other institutions nearing the contract stage were Wells Municipal Hospital, St. Luke's Infirmary at Duluth, Renville County Hospital at Olivia, St. Michael's Hospital at Sauk Centre, Worthington Municipal Hospital, Community Memorial Hospital at Blue Earth, and St. John's Hospital at Red Lake Falls. Of the ten, six were in the first priority group and two were in the last group. In addition to these ten communities, some twelve others in the second priority group were showing interest in improving their hospital facilities. These included such towns as Bagley, Anoka, and Pine City.

Minnesota public health engineers know how slowly a modern hospital moves to completion. Not only applications, but also architect's drawings must be approved by both the state and the United States Public Health Service. Checking of final plans, for example, involves a detailed review of the heating, ventilating, lighting, and plumbing and of the explosion hazards of the operating room and the hot water system. Review of the plumbing installation is concerned with the sanitary features of the equipment, including sterilizers and the waste and water piping. Other hospital facilities reviewed by the state health department from a public health standpoint include such items as sewage disposal systems and water systems where required, food handling facilities, garbage and waste disposal, and facilities for general cleanliness.

Not until all these details were checked was the Baudette Municipal Hospital contract awarded on August 9, 1948, three months after the state had approved the initial application step. The Baudette hospital is fairly representative of the size and cost of smaller institutions being built in Minnesota under the terms of the Hospital Survey and Construction Act. Plans called for a twenty-four bed hospital of fire-resistant construction with fireproofed structural steel skeleton and floor assembly, exterior walls and interior partitions of masonry, and concrete floors with asphalt or rubber tile, or terazzo on cement finish. The building consists of a basement and two stories. A small chapel and quarters for six nurses are located on the main floor. The total cost was estimated at $316,546.62, which means a cost of $13,189.44 per bed.[31]

Although Minnesota plans for other institutions similar to the Baudette Municipal Hospital, its over-all program is far more extensive. Under the federal program the state hopes to build thirty-four general hospitals, four chronic disease units, one mental disease hospital, and two public health centers. The total number of beds in these groups will number about 1,822. Federal funds allocated in 1948–49 for these purposes amounted to $1,655,175. In 1949–50 total federal funds were $1,725,122. The total federal grant for a five-year program is estimated at $8,555,663.[32]

Despite the tremendous financial assistance from the federal government, Minnesota could not hope, with these grants alone, to bring its hospital program into line with contemporary needs. Therefore, to supplement the work of federal agencies, the state itself has developed an extensive hospital building program. These nonfederal projects include

[31] Minnesota Department of Health, Division of Hospital Services, "Hospital Construction Program — Summary of Low Bids on Baudette Municipal Hospital, 1948" (mimeographed report); Graham L. Davis, "Planning the Hospital for Community Service," in *Minnesota Medicine*, 29:1112–1116 (November, 1946).

[32] Division of Hospital Services, *The Minnesota Hospital Program*, table 1.

WANTED: MORE HOSPITAL BEDS 451

the construction of fifty-six general hospitals, two chronic disease units, seventeen mental disease hospitals, and thirty homes for the aged. The aggregate number of beds is nearly six thousand. Although such an extensive program will take years to complete and will cost a fantastic figure, it is necessary if the health of Minnesota's citizens is to be cared for properly. The legislature in 1947 appropriated funds for the construction of geriatric hospitals of 161 beds each at Fergus Falls, St. Peter, and Moose Lake. Another is planned as an addition to the state hospital at Rochester. The Virginia General Hospital built a 125-bed addition for chronic patients in 1948, and the Crookston General Hospital with 142 beds was under construction. At International Falls a health center was opened, and at both Eden Prairie and South St. Paul plans were under way for new hospitals. Bethesda Hospital in St. Paul announced a $1,500,000 building program, and the Jewish Hospital Association planned to construct Mount Sinai Hospital in Minneapolis at an estimated cost of $2,500,000. The University of Minnesota requested federal aid to help build its Mayo Memorial Medical Center. These are only a few of the many plans materializing throughout Minnesota since the passage of the Hospital Survey and Construction Act.[33]

If the Minnesotan, observing unusual hospital construction activity through the state in 1948, was confused by complicated procedure and bewildered by the definitions of the several types of hospitals, he need not have worried overmuch. Whether he realized it or not, a general pattern was slowly emerging. The final goal was a system of co-ordinated institutions designed to provide complete care for all patients. In this plan the Twin Cities and adjacent tributary communities are designated as the base area. In this area the University of Minnesota Hospitals with their medical school connections are the base hospital. The Elliot Memorial Hospital, the first unit of the university hospitals, was formally dedicated and opened to receive patients on September 5, 1911.

Other hospitals in the Twin Cities may serve as base hospitals in accordance with the development of their facilities and services. In addition to the base area, the state has been divided into eleven regional hospital locations which were chosen because of their development as major trading centers and major traffic flow centers and because of the character of existing hospital and medical consultation services. Seventy-five area hospitals and thirty-nine rural hospital locations have been dis-

[33] *Laws,* 1947, p. 1285; *Tribune* (Minneapolis), June 16, 22, September 30, 1948; *St. Paul Dispatch,* July 27, 1948; *Minneapolis Star,* May 20, September 10, 1948; *Pioneer Press,* May 20, September 14, 1948.

tributed in the eleven regions outside of the Twin Cities. The thirty-nine existing and proposed rural hospitals of approximately thirty-five beds or less are made tributary to the adjacent area hospitals.

The citizen wishing to make Minnesota's hospital plan even more specific might imagine that he lives at Deer River, which has a rural hospital and is in Region V. He becomes ill and first is treated at the Deer River rural hospital. Physicians there, however, feel that he needs attention in a large institution; so he is transferred to Grand Rapids, where the services of an area hospital are available to him. From there he may be removed to a regional hospital at Duluth. If his case demands more expert attention than a regional institution can offer, the patient would be taken to the base hospital at the University of Minnesota. This could occur in any one of the eleven areas in which the state is divided. The state plan contemplates locating hospitals in such a manner that an institution will be not more than twenty miles away from any resident.[34]

"In the development of a coordinated system of hospitals," said the Minnesota Department of Health, "it is thought that the base hospitals and their medical staffs can provide educational, diagnostic and treatment facilities and services to the physicians and patients of the regional hospitals. These in turn can provide area and rural hospitals with such services as they are unable to provide for themselves. It is proposed that the mechanics of this type of cooperation among hospitals be developed around interlocking medical staffs, the referral of patients as the needs of the cases require, and the provision of laboratory, x-ray, and medical consultation services. For the mutual benefit to the patient, the physician and the hospital, this type of cooperation may also extend to the administrative matters of service planning, financing and superintendency. As logical as this proposal may seem, it will not be possible to establish it immediately, but it may be evolved over a period of years through area and regional cooperation in planning by medical societies, hospital boards of directors and hospital administrators." [35]

Minnesota health authorities look forward to more than a co-ordinated system of general hospitals. The Hospital Survey and Construction Act also provided for 5,636 chronic disease hospital beds, 1,838 beds for the care of the tuberculous, and 14,090 beds in mental disease hospitals. Chronic disease hospitals, providing medical treatment for the

[34] *St. Paul Dispatch*, January 27, 1948; *Minneapolis Star*, February 5, 1948; Ewing, *The Nation's Health*, 174–178.

[35] Division of Hospital Services, *Minnesota Plan for Hospitals and Public Health Centers*, 15 (Minneapolis, 1948).

WANTED: MORE HOSPITAL BEDS 453

cure or rehabilitation of chronic conditions, including the degenerative diseases, have been planned for thirty-seven communities. Their geographic spread covers the state most adequately. In 1948 Minnesota had more than 2.5 beds per death for tuberculosis patients. Many authorities believed that numerous small sanatoriums were not the most desirable facilities and that they should be replaced in the future by larger institutions.

The federal program called also for the establishment of public health centers. On the basis of one center per thirty thousand of population, Minnesota was entitled to ninety-four centers. Although the establishment of centers cannot be undertaken until the Minnesota statutes are modified to allow for the development of local health jurisdictions, the state health department has made a preliminary assignment of centers throughout the state. Under 1948 conditions of organization, however, Minnesota did have fourteen existing health units in need of acceptable physical plants. These included the three metropolitan health departments of Minneapolis, St. Paul, and Duluth; the St. Louis County Health Department; and the Rochester-Olmsted Health Department. In addition, there were the eight existing and contemplated district health units of the Minnesota Department of Health. Finally, there was the University of Minnesota's students' health service, which provided a rather complete health program for students, nonacademic employees, and faculty.

A health center, generally speaking, is a physical plant housing the various departments and activities of a health unit or units. It is proposed that, when the headquarters of more than one unit are located in the same community, one health center be constructed to house the facilities of all. This, said the Minnesota health department, should be done in the interest of economical and efficient operation. Duluth affords a typical example. In that city on Lake Superior, a public health center, constructed with the assistance of a federal grant, should house the Duluth City Health Department, the St. Louis County Health Department, the district office of the Minnesota Department of Health, and the branch laboratory operated jointly by the three agencies. Consideration should also be given to providing office space and facilities in this health center for other public and private health agencies in Duluth.[36]

[36] Division of Hospital Services, *Minnesota Plan for Hospitals and Public Health Centers*, 17–21. Maps showing the distribution of the several services face pages 11, 15, 18, 21. See also Michael M. Davis, *Clinics, Hospitals, and Health Centers* (New York, 1927).

23

The Mentally Ill

TODAY Minnesota spends more than five million dollars annually to care for the mentally ill.[1]

Seventy-six years ago, when Hewitt was involved in a score of perplexing health problems, only the violently insane were committed to institutions. Little was known of the psychology of maladjusted persons. Indeed, the very term "neurotic" had not come into the national vocabulary. And the idea of preventive treatment had not yet developed. Yet, during the early years of Minnesota's health board, attempts were made to see that inmates of mental hospitals lived in a sanitary environment. The second section of the act establishing the board of health said specifically: "The State Board of Health shall place themselves in communication with the local boards of health, the hospitals, asylums, and public institutions throughout the State, and shall take cognizance of the interests of health and life among the citizens generally." This section also instructed state health officers to act in an advisory capacity to the State of Minnesota in all hygienic and medical matters, "especially such as relate to the location, construction, sewerage, and administration of prisons, hospitals, asylums, and other public institutions."[2]

During the autumn of 1872 Hewitt and Dr. A. W. Daniels, acting as a committee from the health board, arrived at St. Peter to investigate conditions at the State Hospital for the Insane. This relatively new institution had been incorporated by a legislative act in 1866. Commissioners and trustees had been appointed, and they quickly selected 210 acres one mile south of St. Peter and located the hospital there. The asylum

[1] Minnesota Department of Health, Mental Health Unit, *A Program of Preventive Treatment for the Mentally Ill in Minnesota*, 1 (Minneapolis, 1948).
[2] Minnesota, *Laws*, 1872, pp. 64–66. See also the *St. Paul Daily Press*, February 29, March 1, 1872, February 7, May 7, 1873, February 27, 1874.

was opened for patients and the first case was admitted on December 12, 1866. When Hewitt arrived at the hospital, he saw a confusion of temporary buildings surrounded by jerry-built shelters for horses, Durham bulls, two yoke of working oxen, thirteen cows, and twenty-one fat hogs. Chickens scratched at manure piles. He learned that 160 acres of land were under cultivation to furnish hay and oats for livestock and to provide inmates with beans, onions, potatoes, and turnips. Although the permanent building was not yet completed, two sections and a basement were in use. The institution, in 1872, could accommodate about 150 patients, but when Hewitt visited the place 247 were already confined.[3]

Dr. Cyrus K. Bartlett, brought from Northampton, Massachusetts, as superintendent in 1868, seemed enthusiastic over progress both in building and in treating patients, but he warned: "Until civilization changes in its effect on the mental and physical constitution of man from what it has done in the past, or education is so conducted as to increase, rather than impair the brain power of each individual, insanity will be frequent and probably increase, and hospitals and asylums must be built and sustained." Like other superintendents before and after him, Bartlett deplored the small amount of money spent for the care of mental patients. He thought that a contribution of one dollar from every Minnesota citizen and a yearly tax of "one mill on the dollar of valuation" would build an institution large enough to provide amply for the wants of every insane person in the state. "Small as these amounts seem," he concluded realistically, "no State in the Union has taxed itself to that extent in behalf of this christian charity."[4]

Bartlett listed the patients in his care under twelve headings: acute mania, chronic mania, monomania, puerperal mania, paralytic mania, epileptic mania, periodical mania, nymphomania, melancholia, dementia, senile dementia, and idiocy. The greatest number fell in the first category. Although Hewitt was interested in these diagnoses, his primary duty was to inspect the hospital's sanitary environment. He did say, however, that the only hope of cure, in a large proportion of cases, was in prompt and suitable treatment in a hospital. Neither Hewitt nor Bartlett described treatment being given to patients.[5]

[3] State Board of Health, *Annual Reports*, 1873, pp. 85, 91–93; Minnesota Hospital for Insane, *Annual Reports*, 1872, pp. 9, 20; Cyrus K. Bartlett, *A Brief History of the Minnesota Hospitals for Insane* (n.p., 1893).
[4] Hospital for Insane, *Annual Reports*, 1872, p. 26.
[5] Hospital for Insane, *Annual Reports*, 1872, p. 40; State Board of Health, *Annual Reports*, 1873, p. 93; Minnesota State Conference of Charities and Correction, *Proceedings*, January 14–16, 1895, pp. 62–67.

Hewitt contented himself with approving generally the plan and accommodations of the permanent building, but he condemned without qualification the temporary structures. The ventilation was only passable, there was no drainage, and the privies were wretched; halls were narrow, ceilings low, rooms small, and floors, doors, and windows were in a dilapidated condition. Although Hewitt could not know it, similar conditions were to continue in state mental hospitals for years. He wrote a blistering report, saying: "Your committee are compelled to declare the temporary hospital for the insane a disgrace to the State. Nothing but the watchful care of the medical officers, under so unfavorable circumstances, has prevented a fearful rate of sickness and mortality, — the legitimate consequence of such wretched provisions for the insane poor of the State. No where else, except in the crowded tenement houses of our great cities are the same number of people crowded into so limited space."[6]

When Hewitt again visited the St. Peter asylum, he noted two evils that needed correction. In the first place, crowded conditions delayed the admittance of patients who, if they could have received treatment earlier, might have been cured. In the second place, Hewitt said that patients were not sent to the hospital until relatives had despaired of their recovery at home. He recommended, as a true economy on the part of the state, that ample provision be made for hospital treatment at the earliest possible moment after attack and urged that the legislature appropriate additional funds to be used to extend hospital facilities.[7]

Bartlett agreed with him, but the superintendent had his own troubles. Even though the south wing of the permanent building had been completed and patients had been moved there as fast as rooms became available and even though the worst portion of a temporary building had been abandoned, Bartlett was still faced with an overcrowded institution. He had planned for a hospital population of 247 patients, but he actually had 303 under his supervision. Admissions offered another problem. Friends sometimes insisted that patients be admitted at improper times; courts were committing more and more individuals; intemperance seemed to be swelling the number of inmates. More and more old folks, too, were coming under Bartlett's care, so that he wrote with wry humor: "But we sometimes suspect the aged and feeble, exhausted by the struggles of life, fretful and troublesome from increasing senile dementia, not inaptly termed the 'second childhood,' are 'hurried

[6] State Board of Health, *Annual Reports*, 1873, p. 92.
[7] State Board of Health, *Annual Reports*, 1875, p. 9.

over the hill to the poor house' and the insane asylum, without due consideration."[8]

The three major causes, said Bartlett, which brought patients to his hospital were ill-health, intemperance, and epilepsy. He pointed out that insanity was often, and perhaps generally, the result of a combination of causes and that the term "ill-health" probably approximated as true a reason for insanity as any other. "Whatever has reduced the vitality, whether hard work, sickness, poor and insufficient food, and air, unhealthy location or employment, hereditary weakness, bad habits, nostalgia, exposure to extremes of heat and cold, severe and prolonged mental effort, or any other depressing cause, becomes an agent of disease and contributes to the final overthrow of mental balance," Bartlett said.[9]

Bartlett also believed, not without some reason, that epileptics very generally became insane, but he was not quite positive that intemperance was a cause of insanity. He knew that intemperance often existed with insanity, but he believed that it might be either a cause or a result. Hewitt had been interested in this problem for some years. Indeed, Governor Horace Austin in 1873 had directed Hewitt to visit both the Massachusetts State Inebriate Asylum at Boston and the New York State Inebriate Asylum at Binghamton. Before Hewitt returned to Minnesota he had studied eight eastern institutions and had attended a meeting of the American Association for the Cure of Inebriates in New York City. He had even corresponded with an inmate of an inebriate asylum and had gathered testimonials from a number of distinguished workers in the field, including Dr. N. S. Davis, president of the Chicago Washingtonian Home.[10]

Hewitt's trip resulted in the establishment of an inebriate asylum in Minnesota, although such an institution was opposed by several elements throughout the state. An act to "establish a fund for the foundation and maintenance of an Asylum for Inebriates" had become law in 1873 but had been challenged because it imposed a special tax on liquor dealers. When twenty thousand dollars had been accumulated in this manner, the governor was empowered, with the advice of the Senate, to appoint a five-man commission to establish an inebriate asylum. Funds came in so slowly, however, that the Minnesota State Medical Association formally asked legislators to take immediate action to provide

[8] Hospital for Insane, *Annual Reports*, 1873, p. 25; *St. Paul Daily Press*, February 27, December 5, 1874.
[9] Hospital for Insane, *Annual Reports*, 1873, p. 26; Minnesota State Conference of Charities and Correction, *Proceedings*, October 29–31, 1895, pp. 37–42.
[10] State Board of Health, *Annual Reports*, 1874, pp. 19, 39, 42.

for the hospital. At the same time legislation was introduced calling for repeal of the law. When that failed an attempt was made to have the Minnesota Supreme Court declare the act unconstitutional, but the court declared it valid on November 25, 1876.[11]

Once it became known that Minnesota actually was to have an inebriate asylum, several communities sought to have it located near them. The three major rivals were Rochester ("where there are twenty saloons"), High Forrest ("quiet town"), and Worthington ("where no liquor is sold"). Rochester was selected, and the executive board of the Minnesota Inebriate Asylum on August 24, 1876, met to make plans for a building program. Governor John S. Pillsbury told legislators when they convened on January 4, 1877, that a farm of 160 acres had been purchased for nine thousand dollars and that foundations for two buildings had been laid. Perhaps Pillsbury was a trifle skeptical about the project, for he said that this beginning would "demonstrate by experiment whether such an institution in our State is as needful, and will be as valuable as many believe."[12]

Hewitt believed with W. L. Wilson, president of the board of the inebriate asylum, that "inebriety" — the uncontrollable propensity to get drunk — was a disease akin to, though differing widely from, other forms of insanity. He agreed that, like other forms of insanity, inebriety could be treated and that the treatment must be partly physical and medical and partly mental and moral. Hewitt was perfectly willing to take an active part in the asylum's program, but Staples, a member of the state health board, thought that the board should not concern itself with it in any way. Hewitt knew perfectly well that this was impossible, if for no other reason than that the state board was bound by law to inspect such institutions. He realized, too, that the active interest of the board might very well furnish much-needed moral support to a hospital that was almost constantly under fire during the early years of its existence.[13]

No sooner had plans been made for the Rochester inebriate asylum than clamor arose to have it changed to an institution for the care of the insane. Bills to accomplish that purpose were introduced in the legislature, and some citizens of Rochester supported the move provided they could keep a state institution close to the town. "An institution for reclamation of inebriates," wrote an open enemy, "is an impracticable

[11] *St. Paul Daily Press*, February 21, 27, March 1, 4, 6, 7, 18, 23, May 7, 1873, February 8, 1874, February 3, 11, 1875; *General Laws*, 1873, pp. 119–121; State of Minnesota v. John Klein, 22 *Minnesota*, 328–336.
[12] *St. Paul Daily Press*, February 18, 1875, August 25, 27, 1876; Pillsbury, *Annual Message*, 25 (St. Paul, 1877).
[13] Minnesota State Inebriate Asylum, *Annual Reports*, 1877, p. 10; Staples to Hewitt, December 7, 1876, Minnesota Department of Health, St. Paul.

THE MENTALLY ILL 459

humbug, which has proved an expensive failure in every State where it has been tried, and which will sooner or later be abandoned in Minnesota. Let us profit by the experience of other States, and make our new building at Rochester available for practical purposes instead of a towering monument of extravagance and imbecility." [14]

Hewitt said flatly that inebriate asylums had proved to be the only means of care and cure for drunkards. The Minnesota Temperance Union plead with the legislature not to convert the Rochester asylum into a hospital for the insane, saying that "the care of inebriates very largely depends upon the will of those who are to be saved as well as upon pleasant surroundings during their hospital life," and that no patient of his own free will would enter the ward of an insane hospital for treatment. Despite these protests the legislature in 1878 transferred all the property of the inebriate asylum to a new institution which became Minnesota's second hospital for the insane. Provision was made, however, that the newly created asylum care for inebriates. There was such a small balance remaining in the account of the inebriate asylum that only $389.91 was transferred.[15]

Treatment of patients in hospitals both at St. Peter and at Rochester was criticized again and again. In 1878 the legislature was told that the St. Peter hospital was grossly mismanaged, that cruel practices prevailed, and that a patient had been strangled to death by a keeper. A Senate investigating committee found that finances were handled in an inept manner and that patients had received cruel treatment. Hewitt observed such crowded conditions that he recommended that a commission of thoroughly competent men be appointed to investigate. Asylum superintendents admitted that such conditions existed, but they maintained stoutly that no complaints from any quarter had reached them. About 79 patients were being treated at the Rochester hospital and 648 at St. Peter. Near the close of 1879 medical commissioners for the two insane asylums made their report. They found nothing to say regarding either management or discipline, but they, like everyone else, spoke of overcrowding and said that patients were sleeping on improvised beds upon the floor. Perhaps it was not within the commissioners' jurisdiction to speak of the sudden and unexplained death of Terence McDonough.[16]

Not until ten years later was public mention made of how patients ac-

[14] *Pioneer Press*, January 13, 23, 1877, January 31, 1878.
[15] State Board of Health, *Annual Reports*, 1876, p. 5; *Pioneer Press*, January 30, 1878; *Laws*, 1878, p. 153; State Treasurer, *Annual Reports*, 1878, p. 9; State Auditor, *Annual Reports*, 1878, p. 28.
[16] *Pioneer Press*, February 21, November 24, 1878, January 1, December 16, 1879; State Board of Health, *Annual Reports*, 1878, p. 11; Hospitals for Insane, *Annual Reports*, 1878, p. 4.

tually were handled. Then an inspection committee reported merely that "in about 1 per cent of the cases some form of restraint is used." The following year a committee, throwing caution to the wind, said with great emphasis and deliberation that Minnesota's asylums were firetraps and a disgrace to the state. The committee's description of how inebriates were handled certainly justified Hewitt's stand against the closing of the Rochester inebriate hospital. "The house is so full," said the inspectors, "that it is impossible to give them [*inebriates*] separate quarters, and as a consequence they are kept in the wards with other patients. As a rule they are wholly lost to all sense of honor; they take special delight in imposing upon the unfortunates around them, and oftentimes resort to acts of cruelty, simply to hear their victims rale [*sic*] and swear." The committee also spoke of the inferior quality of the attendants.[17]

The *Pioneer Press*, which for years had been interested in the problem of the inebriate as well as that of the insane, devoted a long editorial to conditions in Minnesota institutions. Immediate action was demanded from the legislature. "The insane asylum at Rochester," exploded the *Pioneer Press*, "was created by an act which transformed an inebriate retreat into a refuge for the insane. Both classes are now subject to detention there, and they are, it appears, confined together. That a victim to the passion for drink, otherwise in the possession of his natural faculties, should be confined with the insane is not creditable to our civilization or in accord with the high reputation of this state in the matter of care for the defective and dependent classes; and it is certainly no less revolting that the insane should be made victims of the brutal element among the confirmed inebriates, who amuse themselves by arousing passions which an unhinged mind can no longer control. The separation of these two classes should be provided for at once." [18]

Once again a committee investigated conditions and once more made recommendations to improve management. Little good resulted, primarily because the legislature was loath to undertake any reforms. It had, however, authorized the creation of a third insane hospital at Fergus Falls, and one detached wing had been built and was ready for use in 1890. This new institution had been approved in order to reduce the population load on the older asylums, but little had been done to improve conditions at either Rochester or St. Peter. Meanwhile the number of insane had been increasing rapidly throughout the nation. Minnesota was not an exception to this trend. The proportion of inmates of Minnesota insane hospitals in 1870 was 1 in 2,136 inhabitants; in 1875, 1 in

[17] *Pioneer Press*, November 17, 1887, July 20, 1888.
[18] *Pioneer Press*, July 21, 1888.

1,375; in 1880, 1 in 1,078; in 1885, 1 in 845; and in 1890, 1 in 666. For the ten-year period ending on July 31, 1888, the average increase of insane patients under state care was more than 10% yearly. During the year ending on July 31, 1888, it was 11.2%, and in the year ending on July 31, 1890, it was 6.7%, a considerable drop.[19]

By that time a radical change had come about in the supervision of state institutions. Asylum superintendents no longer were absolute dictators. In 1883 a legislative act established a State Board of Corrections and Charities. This act was amended in 1885 and again in 1887. Provision was made for a nonpartisan board consisting of six persons, who were to serve without compensation. A paid secretary was to administer the board's affairs. The board was to "investigate the whole system of public charities and correctional institutions, examine into the condition and management thereof, especially of prisons, jails, infirmaries, public hospitals, and asylums. . . ."[20]

The Board of Corrections and Charities might have been just another political agency had it not been for the selection of an unusually honest and astute man as secretary. Hastings H. Hart, a humanitarian like Hewitt, had no formal training for the work which faced him. He was graduated from Oberlin College and, before assuming his duties as secretary, was pastor of a Congregational church in Worthington, Minnesota. He brought to his new position high ideals, tempered with a sense of realism, that resulted in reforms not only for mental patients, but also for inmates of other state institutions. His work in Minnesota became so well known nationally that in 1898 he was called to the staff of the Russell Sage Foundation. From there he progressed to even wider fields and, before his death, he was recognized not only at home but abroad.[21]

Among Hart's distinguished contributions to the care of the insane were several asylum investigations which he urged upon incumbent governors. Results of these inspections undoubtedly improved the physical and sanitary environment of patients and also assured them better treatment from attendants. In 1889, for example, a committee investigating the Rochester asylum said that "the supervisors and attendants have been grossly negligent in the matter of reporting to the superintendent, or any of the assistant physicians, cases of ill treatment of patients by the attendants. This neglect arises largely from the fact, that there is, and has been an unspoken agreement among the attendants that none of them should make report of any wrongful acts committed by an asso-

---
[19] State Board of Corrections and Charities, *Biennial Reports*, 1889–90, p. 13.
[20] *Laws*, 1883, p. 171; 1885, p. 45; 1887, p. 144.
[21] William W. Folwell, *A History of Minnesota*, 4:407–413 (St. Paul, 1930).

ciate. . . . That the discipline of the attendants has not been as strict as should have been enforced by the Superintendent, and that there has not been that amount of immediate supervision by the Supervisor as might have been performed by him. . . . That there have been cases of abusive and inhuman treatment of patients by attendants."[22]

The Rochester investigating committee sat for fifteen days and examined 138 witnesses. The outcome was of vital concern to inmates not only at Rochester, but also in institutions elsewhere in the state. The major criticism concerned brutal practices of attendants. Hart's committee recommended nine ways to remedy this abuse. Trustees of three hospitals adopted three of these entirely and others in part. The three recommendations adopted were: (1) that there should be an increase in the number of assistant physicians, one of whom should be a woman; (2) that additional supervisors should be appointed from among the attendants, who should patrol the wards to promote efficiency and to prevent or report abuses; and (3) that attendants' training schools be established.

Hart was disappointed that all nine recommendations were not adopted. He thought trustees of asylums were neglecting "some of the most important suggestions of the committee, namely, those in the direction of improving the *morale* of the service, and creating a stronger sentiment of fidelity among the attendants. There is, as yet, no sufficient incentive to attendants to do the best possible work. Many take it up as temporary employment. They do their duty because they are closely watched and know they will be discharged or otherwise punished if they do not. There is very little *esprit de corps!*"[23]

Despite improvement, conditions in Minnesota asylums were far from ideal. Mechanical restraints still were being used and, in some instances, were sanctioned by superintendents. The criminal insane were not segregated from the "innocent and honest" insane. Crowded conditions resulted in epidemics of various types. During an epidemic of dysentery at the asylum at St. Peter in 1893, a physician told Hewitt that faulty plumbing and drainage was the cause. The acting superintendent was even more outspoken, saying that there was not a single trapped closet in the wards. "For some reason," he continued, "Dr. Bartlett never paid any attention to the sanitary condition of the house and resented any suggestion as to the necessity for better plumbing and drainage. The trustees of course think only of the expense involved because it is so difficult to get money from the legislature for the different institutions.

---

[22] State Board of Corrections and Charities, *Biennial Reports*, 1889–90, p. 260.

[23] State Board of Corrections and Charities, *Biennial Reports*, 1889–90, p. 20; Hospitals for Insane, *Biennial Reports*, 1889–90, pp. 20, 21, 71.

THE MENTALLY ILL 463

... Erysipelas is endemic in the house and has made its appearance in the fall and staid until spring, for several years past. Its spread is due to want of proper personal sanitation, but that cannot be entirely overcome so long as we are so over crowded and do not have efficient trained help." [24]

Asylum populations remained fairly static. In 1892, for example, there were 1,043 patients at the St. Peter hospital; two years later, however, the number had fallen to 980. The Rochester institution had a population of 1,137 in 1892 and 1,166 in 1894. At the turn of the century these figures were about the same as they had been six years earlier. Scarcely a year went by that hospital superintendents did not plead for better sanitary conditions and increased appropriations. They said it was impossible to ventilate wards well, complained of defects in plumbing, and maintained that ceilings and floors were unsafe.[25]

One definite improvement, however, was noted. This lay in the field of diagnosis and treatment. Although there was no notion of preventing mental illness, there was increasing knowledge of how to care for it after it appeared. More attention was being paid to case histories and to individual treatment. Better nursing took the place of mechanical restraints. "The disturbed and violent patients are more tractable," said Dr. G. A. Chilgren at the St. Peter State Hospital, "and we were long ago able to discontinue the use of all forms of mechanical restraint, the trained nurse at the bedside taking the place of the restraint sheet, camisole, or crib.... Mechanical restraint seems but a confession of weakness, an acknowledgment of one's inability to do anything for the patient, as it is perfectly evident that a patient tied down in bed cannot even be kept clean." [26]

Medical baths, hot packs, hot and cold baths were all in use by 1900. Massage, both manual and electrical, was given by six operators at the Rochester institution. Turkish baths were being introduced. Another innovation was the establishment of a diet kitchen which furnished special menus. A training school for nurses was under way. The Drs. Mayo directed and assisted in surgery. On the other hand, not too many recreational activities were provided in any asylum. The chapel and amusement hall at Rochester were without seats and stage scenery. Reading material was scarce and, at Fergus Falls, for example, it in-

[24] Minnesota State Conference of Charities and Corrections, *Proceedings*, 1898, pp. 73–85; letters to Hewitt from Collins, January 10, 1893, and from Tomlinson, January 14, 1893, Minnesota Department of Health, St. Paul.
[25] Hospitals for Insane, *Biennial Reports*, 1893–94, pp. 7, 79; 1895–96, pp. 3, 6, 7, 17, 83; State Board of Corrections and Charities, *Biennial Reports*, 1899–1900, p. 21.
[26] Hospitals for Insane, *Biennial Reports*, 1895–96, p. 22.

cluded only one copy each of eight such magazines as the *Cosmopolitan* and the *Ladies' Home Journal*.[27]

Although superintendents of insane hospitals frequently were willing to point out sanitary defects, they were not so apt to be completely frank concerning administrative problems. Most superintendents spoke glowingly of the substitution of nurses for mechanical restraints, but few, if any, told of growing dissatisfaction among the nurses themselves. Nurses believed, of course, with their superintendents, that they were dealing with a specific public health problem, for the state committed most of the patients cared for in the mental institutions. But nurses felt that they themselves were being treated like laborers instead of professionals. It remained for the Board of Corrections and Charities to point out the "continuous change" in the nursing personnel in mental institutions and to recommend building nurses' homes and increasing salaries. Ten years later nurses' homes at both Fergus Falls and St. Peter were nearing completion, and it was hoped that the legislature soon would provide for a dormitory at Rochester.[28]

The year 1901 marked a radical change in the management of mental hospitals and other state institutions. The legislature then abolished the Board of Corrections and Charities and created a Board of Control to provide for the management and control of the charitable, reformatory, and penal institutions of the state. In addition to its general duties, the new board was to "encourage and urge the scientific investigation of the treatment of insanity and epilepsy by the medical staffs of the insane hospitals, and the Minnesota Institute for Defectives." Transfer of mental patients from one hospital to another also was in the hands of the board, as were all questions as to the propriety of commitment.[29]

Other reforms, in line with national trends, provided more privileges for patients. Inmates were permitted to correspond freely with persons outside the institution's walls. A patient also could write to either the governor or the Board of Control. Superintendents were required to furnish writing paper and stamped envelopes for this purpose. Provision was made also for the parole of patients, and they were to receive suitable clothing and money to pay expenses home when they were discharged. To stop innumerable complaints from relatives and friends that they did not receive reports of patients' conditions, superintendents

[27] Hospitals for Insane, *Biennial Reports*, 1895–96, pp. 87, 210.
[28] Hospitals for Insane, *Biennial Reports*, 1893–94, p. 21; State Board of Control, *Biennial Reports*, 1905–06, p. 69.
[29] *Laws*, 1901, p. 133. For a brief history of the Board of Control and the institutions under its management from 1901 to 1922, see Minnesota Board of Control, *History of the State Board of Control* ([St. Paul, 1922]).

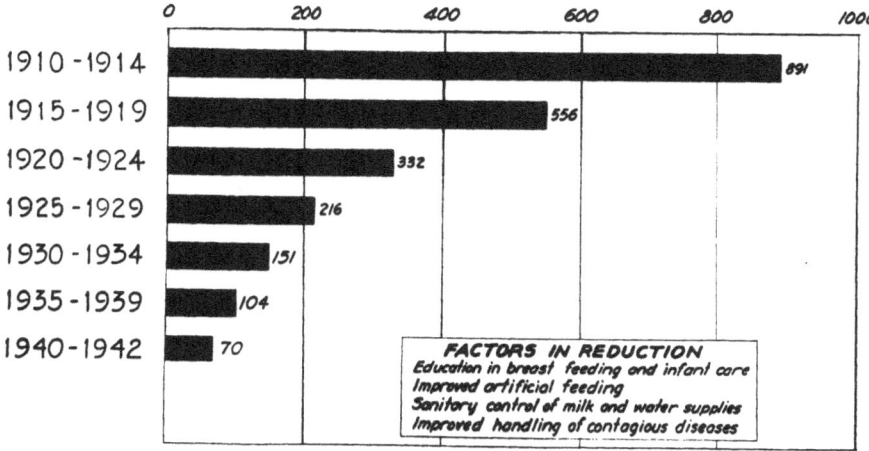

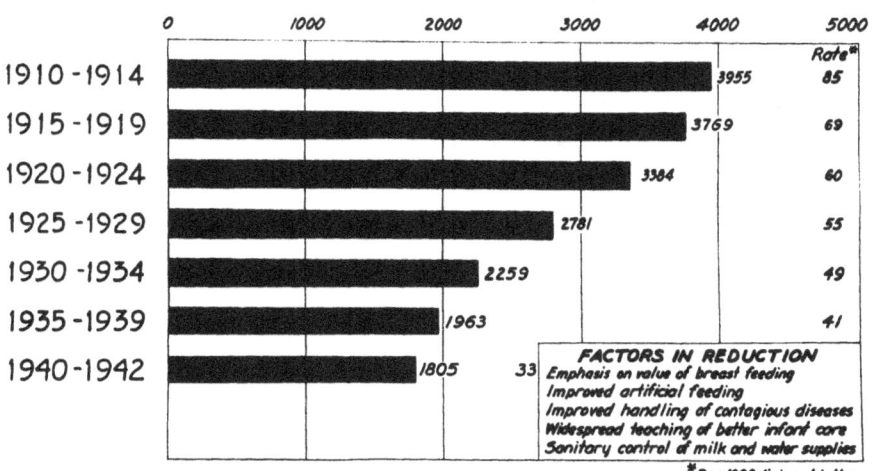

MORTALITY RATES
Courtesy Minnesota Department of Health

NOTICE

BOIL YOUR DRINKING WATER.

The supply of Good Drinking Water having become exhausted water is being pumped through the mains from the old station at the creek.

As this water is **Unfit** for domestic use unless boiled we would suggest that you boil the water at least twenty minutes before using it.

It is expected that there will be an abundant supply of pure water within the next ten days.

C. W. MORE, Health Officer,
JOHN J. MURNIK,
J. C. POOLE,
Members Board of Health.

Dated, Eveleth, Minn., June 23d, 1900.

NOTICE

To all Persons, owning or occupying any property within the Village of Eveleth.

You are hereby notified to remove all filth, rubbish and foul matter from your lots and yards; to provide proper drainage for carrying off water from beneath the houses and from the premises.

Burn all you can safely of the rubbish, garbage, etc., and place the rest in piles in the adjoining alleys and it will be removed by the village scavenger.

The privy vaults and water closets emptied of their contents and the vaults thoroughly disinfected. For this purpose we would recommend the free use of lime or copperas. The contents of the privy vaults must be taken to the dumping grounds.

You are also notified to provide a proper and suitable receptacle as a barrel, keg or box which must be water tight, and keep it in a place convenient for the scavenger to remove the contents every day or two as may be required as provided in Section 1, Ordinance No. 23.

These receptacles shall be placed on a platform about three (3) feet high. All garbage, slops and refuse matter must be deposited in them, and under no circumstances thrown on the ground.

For penalty for failure to comply with this notice within ten days see Section No. 10, Ordinance No. 23, Village of Eveleth.

By order of the Board of Health,

P. E. DOWLING,   C. W. MORE, M. D.,
JOHN J. MURNIK,   Health Officer.
Members Board of Health.

NOTICE

The Board of Health have hired a scavenger to remove slops, offal and refuse matter from your premises.

The only requirements being asked of you is that you place all slops etc., in a barrel located in a convenient place, on a platform sufficiently high to enable the scavenger to empty the contents into his slop box without having to dip it out with a pail.

There are too many barrels to be emptied in a day for him to do this properly unless these requirements are complied with, and he has been given orders not to empty any barrels not so placed.

The Board of Health asks you to aid them in keeping the village in a clean and healthy condition.

C. W. MORE, Health Officer,
JOHN J. MURNIK,
J. C. POOLE,
Members Board of Health.

Dated, Eveleth, Minn., June 23d, 1900.

Sanitation Notices Issued by the Eveleth Board of Health
From the author's collection

were ordered to give immediate notice to next of kin of the death, serious illness, or special change of any inmate.[30]

This new emphasis on "altruistic, humanitarian, and scientific" programs did not suddenly correct evils in Minnesota's mental hospitals, but it did pave the way for gradual improvement. A marked step forward was a program to provide for the aftercare of the insane. This was most significant, for never before had patients received any state attention after they were discharged. By 1906 the Board of Control had succeeded at least in raising doubts in the minds of superintendents at the Anoka State Hospital, the Hastings State Hospital, the School for Feeble-Minded and Colony for Epileptics, and the hospitals at St. Peter, Rochester, and Fergus Falls that old ways were good enough.

Generally speaking, the Board of Control, although dissatisfied with sanitary conditions, was pleased with the work of medical staffs and with their attention to new developments in the care of the mentally ill. No longer were mental diseases classified as crudely as they had been a quarter of a century earlier. In 1906 staff physicians were using such terms as "acute melancholia," "senile dementia," "dementia praecox," and "manic-depressive insanity." More and more attention was being paid also to the physical health of inmates. Pointing out that there is always physical deterioration in mental cases, the superintendent at St. Peter said that it was necessary that the "hospital for the insane should be as thoroughly equipped as the general hospital with the facilities for the study and treatment of physical ailments. It has been our experience that the chance for mental restoration is always dependent upon the extent to which physical regeneration is possible."[31]

This certainly was a progressive attitude and it led eventually to the idea of the prevention of mental disorders. For decades all thinking had been based upon the idea of taking into custody and treating the insane, and practically no serious thought had been given to preventing mental disorders that were increasing as Minnesota's population grew larger. Indeed, many physicians felt that insanity was an act of God and could not be prevented. The change came about 1910. Then the Board of Control published a statement that set in motion a whole new train of thought and that was to lead eventually to the development of a mental hygiene program by the state health department.

"As time goes on," the Board of Control reported, "and the accumulation of unfortunate wrecks of humanity continues to increase in our state institutions, the question of the causes which are primarily responsible

[30] State Board of Control, *Biennial Reports*, 1905–06, p. 19.
[31] State Board of Control, *Biennial Reports*, 1905–06, pp. 230, 260.

for this condition becomes more and more acute. It is a short-sighted policy for the state to load itself with this constantly increasing burden of disease and misery without making some systematic and intelligent effort to determine the causes which operate to bring about these results. The rule that an ounce of prevention is worth a pound of cure is peculiarly applicable here. A careful study of the history of each case that comes to be treated at each of the hospitals for the insane, the School for Feeble-Minded and penal institutions carried on systematically and persistently for a considerable period of time, would, we believe, form the basis of future legislative action along the lines of prevention which would be of incalculable and permanent value to the state and all its people."[32]

Fortunately the legislature saw the wisdom of this point of view and appropriated five thousand dollars for research. A special committee, the first in Minnesota to deal with the causes and prevention of insanity, went to work. Members were Henry Wolfer, warden of the State Prison at Stillwater; Dr. Harry A. Tomlinson, superintendent of the St. Peter State Hospital; and Dr. Arthur C. Rogers, superintendent of the School for Feeble-Minded at Faribault. The Carnegie Institute furnished a trained investigator. Later the Eugenics Record Office of New York underwrote the salary of a field worker.[33]

Investigation began on this public mental health project with the tracing of pedigrees of families who had one or more members in the school for feeble-minded. A total of 377 families having 477 children in the Faribault institution were studied. The total number of individuals charted was 30,273. The most important conclusion reached was that "there are distinct strains of mental defect from which a large percentage of the cases come that require public care and support not only in institutions for feeble-minded, but as paupers in the general community, and delinquents and criminals before our courts." In one family, for example, in which data were found for 187 individuals, 21 were feeble-minded, 3 epileptic, and 2 insane, and 11 were notorious sex offenders. Another family of 112 persons produced 21 feeble-minded individuals, 5 insane, 2 criminals, 18 sex offenders, 2 tramps, and 14 alcoholics.[34]

Sensing the importance of this study in determining the causes and consequences of mental deficiency and the need for identifying the more important lines of descent responsible for mental defectives in Minnesota, the Board of Control organized a bureau of research with offices in

[32] State Board of Control, *Biennial Reports*, 1909–10, p. 20.
[33] *Laws*, 1911, p. 325; State Board of Control, *Biennial Reports*, 1911–12, p. 25.
[34] State Board of Control, *Biennial Reports*, 1913–14, p. 205.

St. Paul. The bureau in 1920 began a systematic mental examination of individuals in mental hospitals and in public schools. These examinations were extended to cover the state reformatories, the state schools at Faribault and Owatonna, the State Hospital for Crippled Children, the State Department of Education, county welfare boards, orphan asylums, maternity hospitals, workhouses, and general hospitals. Summer courses in mental deficiency also were given at the University of Minnesota. The purpose behind this program, of course, was to try to determine the cause of mental instability in order to devise ways and means to prevent it.[35]

By 1924 the bureau of research consisted of a director, three mental examiners, and a stenographer. The intelligence of inmates of four institutions had been studied by the examiners and the findings published:

	Feeble-minded	Below average	Above average
State Reformatory	24	72	19
State Training School for Boys	28	73	17
State Reformatory for Women	38	81	13
Home School for Girls	29	80	7

In addition, special group intelligence studies were made, educational tests for individual examination were devised, and a rating scale was developed. It is significant, too, that in 1924 the director of the bureau of research pointed out the necessity for mental clinics throughout the state.[36]

The Minnesota Department of Health was not unaware of what was being done to care for the mentally disabled. Bracken had spoken of mental diseases that warped the mind and judgment of individuals.[37] For many years the board, as required by law, had made annual sanitary inspections of asylums. Indeed, at the regular meeting of the board on April 16, 1901, an engineer was employed for the specific purpose of visiting state institutions. By 1906 the state health board was advising state officials in hygienic and medical matters pertaining to asylums and other public institutions. Two years later the board passed the following regulations: "A successful vaccination must be required of all officers and employees in state institutions when such individuals are brought into contact in any way whatever with the wards of the institution." Superintendents were ordered to report "each and every case" of contagious disease to the state board and to the local health officer within twenty-

[35] State Board of Control, *Biennial Reports*, 1921–22, pp. 57–61.
[36] State Board of Control, *Biennial Reports*, 1923–24, pp. 57–61.
[37] "The Future Population of the United States," in the Bracken Papers, 3:12. This article is bound at the back of the book following the index.

four hours after the disease was discovered.[38] Epidemiologists and sanitarians frequently had investigated specific outbreaks in mental hospitals. Chesley knew of the work of the bureau of research of the State Board of Control. World War I, however, gave impetus to consideration of the problem of mental disabilities, not only among troops, but also among civilians. As psychology and psychiatry developed, public health officers gradually realized that there were fields which might properly be of concern to them. Visiting nurses, in both urban and rural communities, were almost constantly finding maladjusted individuals and families. Social workers, too, were reporting that the congestion and tempo of modern life were resulting in serious personal and family problems.

The State Board of Control recognized the complicated pattern of life in Minnesota early in the 1920s. "A tremendous burden has been placed upon the community in its attempt to meet the demands placed upon it by the changing times," it said. "The process of absorbing so large a share of the energy of a people, and of providing recreational outlets for them, has gone on in a half conscious and wholly ineffective way. . . . The public dance halls which are springing up at every crossroad in the state, where the most obnoxious forms of dancing take place without restraint and where moonshine is frequently sold in flagrant violation of law, are cesspools of the most infectious character and are contributing in large measure to delinquency and immorality."[39]

In addition to this growing realization that the cultural climate of Minnesota was fostering behavior problems, there developed — slowly at first, but then more rapidly — the idea that persons committed to asylums constituted only a fraction of the individuals who needed guidance and perhaps care.

Dr. M. L. Stiffler, director of St. Paul's Child Guidance Clinic, outlined a mental hygiene program in 1927, which paved the way for future work. Stiffler maintained that mental hygiene should be of community concern and divided the work of such a program into the specific treatment of the insane and feeble-minded and, secondly, into preventive work. Yet, he said, prevention was considered a novelty by many and a fad by some. "It was not so long ago," Stiffler continued, "that periodic physical examinations, the summer round-up of children about to enter school in the fall, and inoculation against contagious diseases, were con-

[38] State Board of Health, *Biennial Reports*, 1901–02, p. 272, and "Minutes," July 14, 1908; Bracken to O. B. Gould, August 6, 1906, Minnesota Department of Health, St. Paul.
[39] State Board of Control, *Biennial Reports*, 1921–22, p. 58.

sidered innovations and yet this preventive program of physical hygiene is now quite generally accepted and practiced. . . . A mental health study is very essential for children who through force of circumstances must spend their childhood in an environment which is a substitute for their own home." Then he indicated again the need for psychiatric study of children.[40]

By 1928 the term "preventive psychiatry" was beginning to replace the older words "mental hygiene." Dr. E. M. de Berry, University of Minnesota psychiatrist, wrote: "With the realization that mental illnesses, personality defects, social maladjustments, etc., were due not to anything inherited by the patient but to experiences of early childhood, adolescense, etc., psychiatry began to take a real and intense interest in the therapy and prevention of these conditions. This attitude was revolutionary." A year later, health officers and social workers heard detailed discussion of the psychiatric and mental hygiene needs of a city. They were told, for almost the first time, that it was not enough to provide for maladjusted children; it was equally imperative that the needs of adults be met.[41]

The economic depression, beginning in 1929, emphasized the increased necessity for all forms of social work and renewed focus upon problems of the mentally unfit both in and out of state institutions. These problems were not only educational, medical, economic, and industrial, but, as Mrs. Blanche L. La Du, chairman of the State Board of Control, said, they were also "the human problem of adjusting the individual to life as he must meet it, and with his rehabilitation if he is unable to meet it." The depression, even if it curtailed funds for mental programs, certainly stimulated interest in them. Professor E. D. Monachesi, for example, was studying juvenile delinquency, and Dr. H. S. Lippman was evaluating the contributions of psychiatry to children's case work. Adult delinquency became increasingly important.[42]

The state health department, of course, had developed a child hygiene program during the depression period and members on its staff had watched with intense interest the very evident trend toward the prevention of mental diseases, whether they were slight personality defects or more serious maladjustments. One fact stood out crystal clear: Minneso-

[40] Minnesota State Conference and Institute of Social Work, *Proceedings*, 1927, pp. 215–219.
[41] State Conference and Institute of Social Work, *Proceedings*, 1928, p. 91; 1929, p. 12; William A. O'Brien, "Mental Hygiene in the Schoolroom," in *Everybody's Health*, vol. 30, no. 5, p. 11 (May, 1945).
[42] State Conference and Institute of Social Work, *Proceedings*, 1933, p. 2; 1934, pp. 29–43, 127–130; 1935, pp. 116–119.

ta's asylums were overcrowded and there was desperate need for a statewide mental hygiene program. By 1947 there were 1,340 patients in the Anoka State Hospital; 1,433 in the Willmar State Hospital; 1,621 in the Rochester State Hospital; 1,930 in the St. Peter State Hospital; 944 in the Moose Lake State Hospital; and 2,544 in the School for Feeble-Minded and Colony for Epileptics at Faribault. No one knew how many citizens at large needed mental guidance. However, on a national basis, it was estimated that at least thirty million Americans needed mental therapy.[43]

Conditions in Minnesota's mental hospitals had been suspect from the time when Hewitt made his first inspection of the asylum at St. Peter. Late in 1947 and early in 1948 several Minnesota groups began to think of making independent investigations. The Minnesota Unitarian Conference made a report which the *Minneapolis Tribune* called a "sobering" document. "Until the privations and inefficiencies described in this report are eliminated," said the *Tribune,* "Minnesota must have an uneasy conscience, not alone with respect to the thousands of patients in those institutions, but to their anguished families." The Unitarian report, delivered to Governor Luther W. Youngdahl on April 26, 1948, declared that no Minnesota hospital met the minimum standards of the American Psychiatric Association; that the average operating cost allowed for Minnesota hospitals was one-fifth of the amount required; that the hospitals had 38 doctors, 340 nurses, 591 attendants, and 30 social workers fewer than were required by the American Psychiatric Association; that restraints, including mitts, cuffs, sheets, shoulder straps, and, in one hospital, chains, were substituted for treatment; and that livestock owned by institutions received better care and treatment than did patients.[44]

At the time this report was being made, a staff writer and photographer on the *Minneapolis Tribune* visited all seven state hospitals and published a series of shocking stories, documented by photographs of almost unbelievable barbarity, describing conditions. Despite this visual evidence that Minnesota's mental institutions needed correction, a legislative research committee was reported to have said that salaries of attendants were not out of line when compared with other institutions, that all hospitals were suffering from a lack of trained employees, that mental patients in Minnesota were being given good treatment in nearly

[43] Minnesota, *Legislative Manual,* 1947, pp. 158–160; *Minneapolis Star,* April 27, August 2, September 10, 1948.
[44] *Tribune,* April 27, 1948; *St. Paul Dispatch,* April 26, August 16, 1948; "Mental Hospital Figures Released," in *Minnesota Medicine,* 31:677 (June, 1948).

all cases, and that the use of restraints was limited. Whatever the facts in the matter were, the various reports renewed interest in the care of the mentally disabled and led to further activity. Governor Youngdahl appointed a Citizens' Mental Health Committee, the Minnesota district of the Missouri Lutheran Synod asked the support of all civic and church organizations to bring conditions in mental hospitals to public attention for public action, representatives from Minnesota's hospitals visited similar institutions in other states, and a newspaper poll revealed that eighty-five per cent of those interviewed favored increasing funds for the care of the mentally sick. These and other activities paved the way for the legislature to consider the problem in 1949.[45]

Fully realizing the need both for better treatment of the mentally ill and for the prevention of mental diseases, the Minnesota Department of Health in 1948 created a mental health unit under the supervision of William Griffiths. This unit not only distributed literature prepared by such institutions as the New York Committee on Mental Hygiene and the National Committee for Mental Hygiene, but also sent to interested persons nontechnical and easy-to-read pamphlets. For parents wishing to know more about the mental growth and problems of infants, the state health board distributed a packet of eight pamphlets with such titles as *When a Child Hurts Other Children, When a Child Uses Bad Language,* and *When a Child Has Fears.* Another pamphlet for free distribution was concerned with the behavior problems of older children.[46]

Distribution of free literature, important as it is, is only the beginning of the planned work of the mental health unit. In 1948 extensive plans were being made for a program of preventive treatment for the mentally ill in Minnesota. This was the first time in the history of the state that such an over-all program was conceived. Pointing out that, with the exception of a very few private, nonprofit mental hygiene clin-

---

[45] *Tribune,* May 13, 14, 15, 17, 18, 20, 22, 24, 25, August 18, 19, 1948; *Minneapolis Star,* April 27, August 2, 1948; *St. Paul Dispatch,* August 16, 1948; *Minnesota's Health,* vol. 2, no. 6, p. 4 (June, 1948); vol. 2, no. 7, p. 3 (July, 1948). See also Arthur T. Laird, "Three Months in a State Mental Hospital," in *Minnesota Medicine,* 31:376–380, 677 (April, June, 1948).

[46] Edith M. Stern, *The Mental Hospital: A Guide for the Citizen* (New York, 1947); George K. Pratt, *Your Mind and You* (New York, n.d.); National Association to Control Epilepsy, *Are Epileptics Employable?* (New York, 1948); Lawrence S. Kubie, *Psychiatry and Industry* (New York, 1945); Lawton and Stewart, *When You Grow Older;* Evelyn Millis Duvall, *Building Your Marriage* (Public Affairs Pamphlet 113 — New York, 1946); Herbert Yahraes, *Alcoholism Is a Sickness* (Public Affairs Pamphlet 118 — New York, 1946); George Thorman, *Toward Mental Health* (Public Affairs Pamphlet 120 — New York, 1946); New York Committee on Mental Hygiene of the State Charities Aid Association, *Some Special Problems of Children* (New York, 1947); United States Children's Bureau, *Helping Children in Trouble* (Publication 320 — Washington, D.C., 1947).

ics in the state, there were no mental hygiene clinics to which a mentally ill person could go for treatment, the mental health unit proposed the establishment of at least twenty-eight full-time mental hygiene clinics. The Minnesota Department of Health planned, therefore, to ask the legislature in 1949 for a grant-in-aid program for seventy thousand dollars to be used for the subsidization of community mental hygiene clinics.

This request, said the state health board, was fully justifiable. "The sum of $70,000 for operating the two proposed clinics may at first appear great. When this figure is compared with the sum of more than $5,000,000 that is spent annually for institutional care, however, it is insignificant. The establishment of these mental hygiene clinics in this state would constitute a great advancement toward prevention, in which direction we must eventually go. It has been estimated that each commitment to a state mental institution costs the state $5,000 to $7,000 when direct costs for care and related costs for assistance to families are considered. . . . While great savings would result from the establishment of this program, the financial aspect of our proposal must not be the primary consideration. Our first reason for urging such a program lies in our regard for the mentally ill as individuals. Our efforts must be directed toward attacking this problem at its beginning, when there is still a possibility for cure. In getting at this problem at its source, we help the individual to help himself. We also help him to avoid the prolonged treatment that would be necessary if his condition were allowed to become progressively worse." [47]

If Minnesota should adopt this proposal for the establishment of mental health clinics, the action would be directly in line with national thinking and would carry on work already begun with funds furnished by the federal government under the terms of the National Mental Health Act passed in 1946. The purpose of this act was the "improvement of the mental health of the people of the United States through the conducting of researches, investigations, experiments, and demonstrations relating to the cause, diagnosis, and treatment of psychiatric disorders; assisting and fostering such research activities by public and private agencies, and promoting the coordination of all such researches and activities, and the useful application of their results; training personnel in matters relating to mental health; and developing and assist-

[47] Minnesota Department of Health, *A Program of Preventive Treatment for the Mentally Ill*, 8.

THE MENTALLY ILL 473

ing States in the use of the most effective methods of prevention, diagnosis, and treatment of psychiatric disorders." [48]

A National Advisory Mental Health Council was created, health conferences were provided for, and an appropriation of $7,599,000 was made to carry out the provisions of the act. A portion of this total was earmarked for the use of the several states. Under the terms of the act, Minnesota for the fiscal year 1948–49 received $68,000. These funds were used to subsidize existing mental hygiene clinics, to give demonstration projects in mental hygiene, to train personnel for service in the field of mental health, to further professional training, and to study state statutes. The Duluth Mental Health Clinic, for example, received $3,000 with which to pay the salary of a psychiatric social worker. Other grants were made to the St. Paul Wilder Child Guidance Clinic and to the Rochester Counseling Clinic. Acting as the state mental health authority, the health department also granted the Minneapolis public school system $6,000 to support, in part, a mental health demonstration program. Other agencies receiving assistance were the Institute of Child Welfare and the School of Public Health at the University of Minnesota and the Governor's Advisory Committee on Mental Health.[49]

With the active interest and participation of the state health department, with the assistance of a governor's committee, and with the enthusiastic support of innumerable religious and civic organizations, Minnesota in 1949 at last seemed ready to embark on a really modern, intelligent program for the care of the mentally sick. But everyone knew that this scientific and humanitarian planning could materialize only if the legislature realized its tremendous significance.

[48] *Statutes at Large*, vol. 60, part 1, pp. 421–426.
[49] Minnesota Department of Health, *A Program of Preventive Treatment for the Mentally Ill*, 10–13.

24

Patterns for Tomorrow's Health

ALTHOUGH details are blurred and the general outline shifts constantly, perhaps the patterns of tomorrow's health programs may be discerned today. All over the nation there is a growing awareness of the need for greater health protection for the people. Perhaps never before have men and women been quite so exercised over preserving their own health and that of their children. All this, of course, is a part of their quest for security. Yet, much as they desire the very best in health protection, many people seem unwilling to extract the cost of it from their own purses. Some are afraid of private medical practice and others fear the intervention of government in health affairs. A middle group believes that insurance or group hospitalization programs offer the only satisfactory solution. The truth is that the United States is in the midst of a transitional period, which may modify radically the practice of both private medicine and public health. But out of the welter of debate that so frequently carries more emotionalism than objectivity, one fact emerges strong and clear: public health problems will assume new forms and will have to be met with new techniques. Many of the vexing questions which faced Hewitt already have disappeared and have been replaced by situations never dreamed of by the first secretary of the state health board.

Through the years the Minnesota Department of Health has become more and more a consulting agency, ready to give advice and service to communities in need. It has sought, although sometimes vainly, to place responsibility upon the shoulders of local health officers rather than to dominate community action. Its policy has been to co-operate, not to coerce. The future may witness an intensification of planning toward the division of Minnesota into health districts, with each district financing its own health program and employing its own staff of physicians, nurses, and engineers. But in 1948 this plan was hung on two pickets. First, legislative action was needed to permit the creation of districts. Second, rural areas must want a district program badly enough to pay for it. And even if the first requirement was met, it would be some years, perhaps, before the entire state could be thus organized. A war or a business recession, of course, might set back such a program indefinitely. Yet independent health districts, comprising one or more counties, is one of the plans for the future.

The procurement of competent public health nurses for rural areas is another problem whose answer lies in tomorrow. In 1948 there were insufficient nurses to fill Minnesota's need. It was true, of course, that trained public health nurses were being graduated from the University of Minnesota's School of Public Health. But graduate public health nurses were not going into rural areas to practice in sufficient numbers. The reasons for this seem obvious once they are explained. Nurses say candidly that salaries are low, but they are quick to point out that that is not their major objection to public health work in country districts. They complain that all too frequently counties will not hire a nurse unless she has an automobile of her own. Girls say frequently that they cannot afford a car. They point out also that their allowance for mileage does not begin to pay the cost of operating an automobile. They say, too, that industrial nurses and other public health nurses in urban areas are not required to furnish their own automobiles and that the advantages of living in a city far outweigh those of living in a single room in an isolated village. Another objection — and this seems to be a major one — is that the rural public health nurse, if she is to operate at all effectively, must bend her program to suit the idiosyncrasies of physicians engaged in private practice. If she is lucky, she may work with an admirable group of men; if she is unfortunate, her entire program may be ruined by one doctor who does not believe in vaccination or pasteurization or mental hygiene. It is frequently said that the success or failure of Minnesota's rural health program depends altogether too much upon men in private practice.

Regardless of the reasons why Minnesota has a shortage of nurses, limited health programs, and poorly paid health officers, the fact remains that in 1948, according to Dr. A. B. Rosenfield, director of the sixth district of the Minnesota Department of Health, twenty-four counties had no nursing service and seventy-five per cent of them had only part-time health officers and nurses. "There should be one nurse for every 5,000 people," Dr. Rosenfield said. "But in Minnesota we have only one nurse for 11,000 to 15,000 people. Health programs are limited to maternal and infant care and to communicable diseases. The largest problem — adult hygiene — is ignored."[1]

This situation, of course, is not unique to Minnesota. In 1948 a federal program called for increasing the nation's supply of 190,000 active physicians to 227,000 by 1960, the present supply of 75,000 dentists to 95,000, the present number of 318,000 nurses to 443,000, and the supporting personnel by comparable numbers. In addition, it was proposed to double the number of acceptable hospital beds as rapidly as possible, certainly within fifteen years, and by 1960 to have added 600,000 beds to the nation's hospitals. The final goal was twofold: to establish and maintain adequate local health units everywhere, and to increase and improve the training of public health workers to the end that their numbers would be doubled. This meant, of course, that all persons then would have access to the health and medical services they required.[2]

Recommendations such as these were only a portion of a significant report on the nation's health transmitted to President Truman on September 2, 1948, by Oscar R. Ewing, federal security administrator. Assisted by more than eight hundred professional and community representatives who had met in Washington earlier in the year, Ewing prepared a program that reflected the thinking of some of the nation's most distinguished leaders, representing such organizations as the Federal Council of the Churches of Christ in America, the National Association of Manufacturers, the American Federation of Labor, the American Hospital Association, the American Medical Association, and the Chamber of Commerce of the United States of America. Among the distinguished Americans on the executive council were Dr. Paul R. Hawley, Philip Murray, and President James L. Morrill of the University of Minnesota.

Despite the fact that the report was not received favorably in all quarters, one thing was certain — it would do much to emphasize the necessity for a better public health program throughout the nation and thus might have a very definite influence in Minnesota.[3] The report assumed, rightly or wrongly, that only a combination of the efforts of local, state, and federal units could possibly result in a major improvement in public health. This implied, of course, that a truly efficient health program no longer can be financed satisfactorily without federal funds. In 1948 Minnesota was receiving such money under the Hospital Survey and Construction Act and from other grants.

[1] *Pioneer Press*, March 18, 1948.
[2] Ewing, *The Nation's Health*, 15–17.
[3] *Minneapolis Tribune*, November 8, 1948.

PATTERNS FOR TOMORROW'S HEALTH

The report also emphasized nine services that were imperative if the level of public health throughout the nation was to be raised. These were:

1. Medical and dental care: The primary requirement is that every area should have enough medical manpower of all kinds to meet local needs and that their essential services should be available to everyone in a health center or hospital clinic, in offices, the home, or wherever care is needed.

2. A healthful community: Every town, city, rural area should be guarded by a well-staffed public health department against the spread of diseases through sewage, water, milk, food, insects, animals, poisonous fumes, and other environmental hazards.

3. A community clinic: The need for community clinics will vary with the facilities that exist in the area, and with the access that all people have to its services. It will be particularly important for smaller towns and rural areas to have a publicly owned facility in which both private medical workers — physicians, dentists, nurses, and supporting personnel — and public health workers can have offices and work together for the provision of full preventive, diagnostic, and consultation services.

4. A community hospital: This type of hospital is just what its name implies, a hospital fitted to community needs, large enough to care for all births and other ordinary hospital needs among the population it serves. Such a hospital will be most important in rural areas, or small towns such as county seats, and should be so placed that no one in the county is more than an hour's easy travel from such a hospital; clinics, of the type described above, should be even more conveniently placed.

5. A district hospital: Urban centers should have larger hospitals to which local residents have direct access, and to which people from smaller surrounding communities or rural districts can be referred to receive services not available in community hospitals — the services of surgeons, pediatricians, orthopedists, obstetricians, radiologists, and of the clinical laboratory. In the district hospital, complete diagnostic services would be available, as would treatment for serious pathological conditions.

6. Special hospitals: Under this heading fall a wide variety of health facilities, institutions for all types of chronically ill patients, closely associated with general hospitals. Special home care for invalided and aged persons should be provided. Rehabilitation, including vocational training, also should be available in general hospitals, special centers, and related institutions.

7. A medical center: There should be at least one medical center in every State, preferably associated with a medical school. In the center, medical research would be carried on and medical personnel trained. It would provide refresher courses for doctors of the region and provide extension training to keep them abreast of medical science and latest techniques. The center, moreover, should work with other hospitals and local doctors to make available the latest knowledge, equip-

ment and methods, and would receive patients from surrounding communities for highly specialized care and study.

8. Coordination: Even a full range of the essential services and care outlined here will fail in its total purpose of improving health unless all of them are organized for the closest teamwork to achieve the best possible services for the community as a whole.

9. A prepayment plan: A system of insurance should make it possible for everyone to have comprehensive care without worrying about meeting sudden bills out of current pay, without exhausting savings or going into debt, and without being dependent on charity care.

In addition to these special efforts to attain health, the report assumed certain other contemporaneous and parallel steps. These included attempts to raise standards of living so as to assure better nutrition, recreation, and other similar contributions to healthful living; efforts to increase benefits for the aged and permanently disabled so that their minimal essential economic needs might be provided for; attempts to secure better educational systems in both number and quality; efforts to secure adequate housing for the people of the nation — a fundamental requirement; and, finally, an increased understanding on the part of the people of the benefits to be derived from scientific medicine and public health methods.[4]

This ambitious proposal is bolstered by evidence showing that in the nation as a whole there is much unfinished public health business. The report points out, for example, that the United States has one of the highest accidental death rates of any nation. As a cause of death, accidents are surpassed only by heart disease and cancer. Accidents disable tens of thousands annually and are responsible for about 10,400,000 injuries. The cost to the injured in medical treatment and lost wages amounts to $3,000,000,000 annually. Property damage, overhead costs of insurance, and indirect costs incidental to these accidents add another $3,400,000,000. In 1946 there were 98,000 deaths in the United States from all types of accidents. The list was headed by motor vehicle accidents, and falls came second, followed in order by drowning, burns, conflagrations, and railway accidents. Although Chesley in 1924 spoke of the automobile as a public health hazard, citing increasing mortality rates and implying that drivers should be careful, the Minnesota Department of Health has not put into practice an accident-prevention program.[5] In 1948 Minnesota public health officials spoke of an

[4] Ewing, *The Nation's Health*, 4–6.
[5] Chesley, "The Automobile as a Public Health Hazard," in *American Journal of Public Health*, 14:917–920 (November, 1924).

PATTERNS FOR TOMORROW'S HEALTH 479

accident-prevention program as an activity that the future was almost sure to bring.

Much work still remains to be accomplished in the field of sanitation, not only in Minnesota but also throughout the country. The problem of safe milk has not been completely solved in the state. Indeed, during 1948, milk shipped from Minnesota was rejected by Texas. In the country at large twenty per cent of fluid milk sold was not pasteurized. The increase in the number of cases of brucellosis in Minnesota in 1948 caused Dr. Wesley W. Spink, professor of medicine at the University of Minnesota, to ask for strict legislation requiring pasteurization of milk. Spink added that he expected such laws would meet strong opposition from many quarters, "particularly from the hundreds of small dairy operators who are selling raw milk." [6]

A vast amount of education, planning, and construction must take place before Minnesota has adequate water protection and scientific sewerage systems. A two-year survey of sanitation needs throughout the United States revealed that over 2,000,000 persons in 5,700 communities with populations of over 200 had no public water supply system, and that 79,000,000 in 15,000 towns and cities had systems needing extension or improvement. In rural areas only 12,000,000 persons are adequately served and 27,000,000 need new or improved water supplies. These figures, impressive as they are, do not tell the complete story. Some 9,000 towns and cities, with a total population of 6,000,000, need complete sewerage systems, and nearly 10,000 cities and towns with nearly 80,000,000 persons need improved systems. In the entire nation only 6,500,000 persons live in places where systems need no improvement or expansion. The homes of 33,000,000 persons living in rural areas require new or improved systems. These sanitary needs are enormous. Complete protection throughout the country would require an expenditure of $7,700,000,000 at 1948 prices. Of this total amount, $2,200,000,000 would be spent for waterworks, $3,700,000,000 for sewage disposal systems, $166,000,000 for garbage disposal facilities, and $1,600,000,000 for all other types of sanitation facilities, such as septic tanks, privies, and pure-water sources for rural homes.[7]

The specific needs for Minnesota, according to the report, include the construction of 217 new waterworks and improvements in 420 existing systems at an estimated cost of $45,805,000. The state also needs 552 more wells and 605 more pumps. To satisfy Minnesota's needs for sewage treat-

[6] *Pioneer Press*, April 23, 1948.
[7] Ewing, *The Nation's Health*, 23.

ment plants, some 351 communities will have to build entirely new systems, while 316 will have to make improvements in existing systems. Only fourteen communities reported no needs. To care for garbage adequately, Minnesota would have to have an additional 397 garbage trucks, 2 incinerators, and 191 land fill installations. These would care for the needs of 210 communities at an estimated cost of $4,214,000, or a per capita cost of $2.80. Throughout the state's rural areas some 151,200 new or repaired water supply systems, 215,200 new or repaired privies, and 16,100 new or repaired septic tanks are needed. These needs are challenged by sanitary engineers, but nonetheless they indicate that the state could well expand its facilities.[8]

The United States Public Health Service, although it pointed out that death rates from filth-borne diseases such as typhoid fever, dysenteries, and diarrhea-enteritis have declined through the years, said emphatically that Americans "must not lose sight of the fact that our fight against the diseases of insanitation is a continuing one." It warned that protective barriers already erected must be maintained and reinforced. "We have come to realize," it continued, "that health is not the mere absence of disease but a positive state of body and mind which is conducive to a full and productive life. This concept of health requires that environmental sanitation include more than the mere prevention of disease by measures directed at man's environment. It must also include those measures which tend to improve positive health even though they may not be concerned directly with disease prevention."[9]

Closely allied to problems of waterworks and sewage disposal plants is the problem of stream pollution. Minnesota, of course, had been concerned with this for many years, and in 1945 the state created a water pollution control commission. The Eightieth Congress recognized that states might very well further their water pollution control activities with the assistance of federal funds. Therefore it passed a law providing for loans to local governments — $22,500,000 a year for each of five years — to assist in building treatment plants to reduce the pollution of rivers and other streams. "This act," said the federal security administrator, "makes only a beginning upon the total sanitation job that remains to be done, but in view of the inflationary pressures which exist in this country today, and the shortages of manufacturing services and trained

[8] Federal Security Agency, *Nation-Wide Inventory of Sanitation Needs*, tables 5–12 (United States Public Health Service, *Public Health Reports, Supplement* 204 — Washington, D.C., April, 1948).
[9] Federal Security Agency, *Nation-Wide Inventory of Sanitation Needs*, 1; Samuel W. Abbott, *The Past and Present Condition of Public Hygiene and State Medicine in the United States* (Boston, 1900).

PATTERNS FOR TOMORROW'S HEALTH

personnel, it probably represents the most that is feasible at this time." It was hoped that in the future, certainly by 1960, loans and grants for elimination of water pollution, for garbage disposal, and for rural sanitation would total about $400,000,000 a year. Minnesota might be expected to receive its share of that amount.[10]

Other problems that exist today, but whose answers lie in tomorrow, concern such illnesses as tuberculosis, venereal diseases, heart diseases, rheumatic fever, and poliomyelitis. Curiously enough, few persons realize that rheumatic fever snuffs out the lives of more children than does polio. As early as 1908 epidemic anterior poliomyelitis was the subject of a regulation passed by the State Board of Health, and a year later the board discussed the wisdom of excluding children from school because of polio. Polio caused over 200 deaths in 1910. By 1916, when 343 cases, including 32 deaths, were reported in a period of seven and a half months, and the year's total reached 912 cases with 105 deaths, the board had developed a series of regulations, one of which made polio a reportable disease. Previously Hill and others had published epidemiologic studies of polio in the state. In 1917 cases reported numbered 75, with 10 deaths, and the state health board sent a form letter to physicians saying that the board wished to make a thorough examination of every survivor of the 1916 epidemic. Free clinics for examination and treatment of infantile paralysis were conducted throughout the state by Dr. A. J. Gillette, professor of orthopedic surgery at the University of Minnesota, and by Dr. Willard P. Greene of the state health board.[11]

From 1916 through 1945 Minnesota had some infantile paralysis cases annually, with a peak in 1925 of 955 cases and 145 deaths. In 1946 the disease appeared in severe epidemic form, with 2,903 cases reported among Minnesota residents. Minneapolis was hardest hit, but polio cases were reported from eighty-six of the state's eighty-seven counties. More than seventy-two per cent of the cases occurred among children under

[10] Minnesota, *Laws*, 1945, pp. 761–770; United States, *Statutes at Large*, 62:1155; Ewing, *The Nation's Health*, 24.

[11] State Board of Health, "Minutes," October 20, 1908, October 5, 1909; Bracken to C. A. Harper, August 17, 1916, Minnesota Department of Health, St. Paul; "Poliomyelitis," in *Journal-Lancet*, 36:487–489 (August 15, 1916); "Some Figures on Poliomyelitis in Minnesota," in *Journal-Lancet*, 36:520 (September 1, 1916); H. W. Hill, "The Epidemiology of Anterior Poliomyelitis," in *Northwestern Lancet*, 29:369–374 (September 1, 1909); H. W. Hill, *Epidemiologic Study of Anterior Poliomyelitis in Minnesota*, (Chicago, 1910); W. H. Frost, Samuel G. Dixon, and H. W. Hill, "Report of Committee on Methods for the Control of Epidemic Poliomyelitis," in American Medical Association, *Journal*, 57:1275–1278 (October 14, 1911); A. S. Hamilton, "Epidemic Poliomyelitis in Minnesota in 1908," in *Northwestern Lancet*, 30:2–9 (January 1, 1910); W. P. Greene, "Poliomyelitis: An Epidemiological Study with Summary of After-Care Treatment in Minnesota," a paper read before the Minnesota State Medical Association at Duluth in September, 1918.

fifteen years of age, and more than half the total deaths occurred in that same age group. By the time the 1946 epidemic was virtually over, the National Association for Infantile Paralysis had spent more than a million dollars to pay for emergency hospital space, respirators, hot pack machines, and other equipment, and for nurses, physical therapists, and epidemiologists. Chesley pointed out that the 1946 epidemic was noteworthy because of the manner in which local, state, and national resources were mobilized to provide adequate diagnostic facilities.[12]

Polio was relatively dormant in 1947, but the following year it swelled to such proportions that it gave Dr. Harry M. Weaver, research head of the National Foundation for Infantile Paralysis, grave concern. By November 10, 1948, 1,236 cases had been reported in Minnesota, with 81 deaths. All authorities on polio agreed that the solution to the mystery of how the tiny, invisible virus gets into the human body, how it travels inside the body, how it does damage, and what makes it grow and develop must be solved by research done in the future. Sister Elizabeth Kenny, Australian nurse and crusader, had her method of treating polio recognized in Minnesota on December 17, 1942, when the Elizabeth Kenny Institute was established in Minneapolis with the help of funds from the National Foundation for Infantile Paralysis. This action followed clinical investigations begun two years earlier at the Minneapolis General Hospital with funds and facilities made available by the Board of Public Welfare. Despite later controversy that developed over the Kenny treatment, Sister Kenny's work did much to help center national attention on Minnesota and on polio. As the result of the work of several agencies — the Kenny Institute, the Mayo Clinic, and the University of Minnesota Medical School and Hospital — Minnesota was declared to be among the best-equipped states in the nation to fight an epidemic.[13]

Not all future problems, of course, are as widespread as that of polio. Yet they are equally significant to patients concerned and should be given the same intensive research. In 1947 the state health department

[12] "Polio Breaks All Records," in *Minnesota Health*, vol. 1, no. 2, p. 3 (February, 1947); Section of Preventable Diseases, "Poliomyelitis in Minnesota in 1946," a mimeographed tabulation dated January 3, 1947.
[13] *Tribune*, October 31, 1948; "Minnesota Mobilizes All Forces to Fight Polio," in *Everybody's Health*, vol. 31, n. 7, p. 8 (September–October, 1946); Edward C. Rosenow, "A Study of the 1946 Poliomyelitis Epidemic by New Bacteriologic Methods," in *Journal-Lancet*, 68:265–277 (July, 1948); Elizabeth Kenny and Martha Ostenso, *And They Shall Walk*, chapter 12 (New York, 1943); Elizabeth Kenny Institute, *A Brief Résumé of the Story of Sister Elizabeth Kenny and the Elizabeth Kenny Institute for Infantile Paralysis* (Minneapolis, [1944]); John F. Pohl, "The Kenny Concept and Treatment of Infantile Paralysis," in *Journal-Lancet*, 65:265–271 (August, 1945); Maurice B. Visscher and Jay A. Meyers, "Sister Kenny — Five Years After," in *Journal-Lancet*, 65:309 (August, 1945). Statistics were obtained from the Minnesota Department of Health, November 16, 1948.

warned Minnesota physicians of the possibility of poisoning in young infants by nitrates in well water. Two cases had been reported from western Minnesota, and others had been reported from Iowa and Kansas. Although most babies recovered if they were given water from a different source, the state health department wished to learn, if possible, something more about the problem. Studies of the nitrate problem began shortly after the first poisonings were reported and will continue into the future. A controlled study of nitrate poisoning by well water was undertaken in six southwestern counties by health engineers. Engineering angles of the nitrate problem were studied by a public health engineer, and Dr. John Stam, pediatrician of Worthington, was retained on a part-time basis to take charge of the medical aspects of the survey. This is only one of a number of situations on which work will be projected into the future.[14]

Health administrators speak of other situations which they feel belong to the field of public health. They speak of air pollution, pointing out that here is an area of investigation that as yet has been scarcely touched except as a phase of industrial health. Little has been done to assure the general public that it will have clean air to breathe. Dust, pollen, fog, smoke, and "smog"—all these are worthy of additional attention. Although some cities do have local ordinances prohibiting excessive chimney smoke, few communities have thought in terms of prohibiting other polluting agents. Countless hay fever victims, for example, would benefit from a pollen control program. Air pollution has countless ramifications, all of which impinge directly upon the public's health.

Forward-looking public health officials say, too, that their interest in the future might very reasonably extend to the home environment. To what extent such a program might go, no one could say for certain in 1948. Yet the thinking along these lines is intriguing and seems to possess a certain logic. One argument might run as follows: Today the state health department approves the plans of public buildings before construction is begun. After construction is under way, health engineers inspect plumbing and other facilities to see that the safety of citizens using that structure is assured. If such inspection is good for a public building, why should it not be good for a private dwelling? Most people spend more time in their homes, by and large, than they do in public structures

[14] "Babies Poisoned by Well Water," in *Minnesota's Health*, vol. 1, no. 5, p. 4 (May, 1947); "Nitrate Problem Studied," in *Minnesota's Health*, vol. 2, no. 6, p. 3 (June, 1948); Hunter H. Comly, "Cyanosis in Infants Caused by Nitrates in Well Water," in *American Medical Association, Journal*, 129:112–116 (September 8, 1945); R. L. Faucett and H. C. Miller, "Methemoglobinemia Occurring in Infants Fed Milk Diluted with Well Water of High Nitrate Content," in *Journal of Pediatrics*, 29:593–596 (November, 1946).

such as office buildings or hospitals. If a restaurant is told by competent inspectors how to wash dishes and prepare food in a sanitary manner, why should not the housewife be taught the same lessons? Should not tenements, apartment houses, and single dwellings be offered the same services that hotels, taverns, and cafes are?

Still another vexing problem that some health authorities feel might come within their province in the future concerns nutrition. The widespread effect of inadequate diets, says the federal security administrator, is evident in lowered resistance to disease. An integral function of a public health program in nutrition, therefore, would be to develop satisfactory methods of appraising the nutritional status of representative population groups, in order to discover human nutritional requirements and to identify more clearly the effect of different levels of nutrition upon the degenerative diseases. Improved methods need to be developed for measuring nutrients and additional research remains to be done if the functioning of nutrients within the body is to be understood.[15]

The future should see expansion in programs already under way — in industrial health, in maternal and child welfare, in dental health, in school health, and in the care of Minnesota's Indians. Late in 1948, there were insufficient funds to provide hospitalization for all tuberculous Indians, and in November it was said that at least $200,000 would be necessary in 1949 to meet Indian relief and medical costs.[16] Hospital construction and care of the aged, as has been indicated, both have a long way to go before a satisfactory solution is achieved. Much remains to be accomplished by inspectors of hotels and resorts. Food handling in a proper manner is a lesson yet to be learned by far too many. War or business depressions would bring health problems peculiar to these conditions, including those resulting from a decrease in the standard of living and an increase in the number of unmarried mothers. The diseases of rural life, including the occupational diseases of agriculture, are going to demand more attention. If the United States Department of Agriculture is concerned with rural nutrition, sanitation, and health services for migratory workers, state health departments will have to bend a portion of their program, at least, to supplement this work of the federal government.

Tomorrow's health problems, even when they are viewed generally, are so vast, so complicated, and so expensive that they are puzzling both to professional health administrators and to laymen. It is easy enough to recommend that the most elementary requirement for the improve-

[15] Ewing, *The Nation's Health*, 25.
[16] *Tribune*, November 16, 1948.

ment of rural health services is the extension of health departments to serve every rural community in the nation. The American Public Health Association has proposed that this be done and that the 3,071 counties in the nation be grouped into fewer than 1,200 units of local health administration.[17] It is fairly simple to say that all eating places should be inspected frequently enough to guarantee that they consistently maintain sanitary conditions, yet such a program cannot possibly be carried out unless there is sufficient money to finance it and sufficient trained personnel to operate it. The casual commentator may be correct when he deplores the lack of adequate sanitary facilities in either urban or rural areas, but his words avail little unless both money and talent are available to bring about the needed reforms.

Unfortunately, too many health officials, especially in the past, have made the serious mistake of failing to launch an educational program which would acquaint the public with what public health stands for and what specifically the health department is doing in the interests of the people. Citizens cannot be expected to support a health program if they know nothing about the department's activities. A sound program of public relations is needed desperately if public support is to be won. There is no justification for health administrators to ignore the newspaper press for months on end and then suddenly to ask that same press to support a public health measure. Too many citizens in too many states are ignorant of public health because public health administrators have not tried to keep the work of their departments in the minds of the people. The New York City Health Department supplies an excellent example of how dignified promotion can be handled.[18]

If people know what their money is being spent for, they are more apt to support measures that result in increased taxation. It is generally said that a per capita expenditure of two dollars would result in a program of conventional public health activities. If a more elaborate program, including cancer control or mental hygiene, is desired, the per capita cost would be $2.50. And if public health nursing should be broadened to include bedside care of the sick, the per capita cost would increase to $3.50. These figures, of course, are only approximations.[19]

A public health program may be financed in several ways: It may receive funds only from the political unit in which it operates — township, county, state, or municipality; it may draw funds from several of these

[17] Haven Emerson and Martha Luginbuhl, *Local Health Units for the Nation* (New York, 1945).
[18] *New York Times*, November 6, 1948.
[19] Frederick D. Mott and Milton I. Roemer, *Rural Health and Medical Care*, 540 (New York, 1948).

units; or it may receive funds from any one of these units plus grants from the federal government. It may also receive subsidies from private agencies. Minnesota for many years has received grants from federal sources. Indeed, some of the activities of the state health board would not have been possible without these funds. The total government expenditures — federal, state, and local — for civilian health in the United States in 1947 was $1,962,000,000. This included the medical care of the needy not in institutions, community health protection, rehabilitation, hospital construction and maintenance (training), health man power, and research. Yet this sum, vast as it was, did not begin to cover the cost of a really adequate health program.

Such a program, projected for the year 1960 and covering the same items as those listed above, has been estimated at $4,107,000,000. Of this total, the federal government would contribute $2,312,000,000 and state and local organizations $1,795,000,000. Such an investment, advocates of the program say, would ultimately produce an annual return in national wealth of several times that amount, not only in terms of cash, but also in terms of human welfare and of added national strength and vitality. Ewing, in his report, explained at length the potential returns expected from the expenditure of such a large sum of money on a nationwide public health program.

"Through this program," said Ewing, "we can expect to reduce deaths from preventable causes — those we have the knowledge and skills to prevent — by almost one-fourth in the next 10 years. We should be able to eliminate most deaths and sicknesses from malaria, typhoid, dysentery, undulant fever and typhus; from smallpox, diphtheria, whooping cough, tetanus and measles. We should be able to spread throughout most of the country the benefits of child and maternal health work and, by this means, sharply reduce the needless deaths of infants and mothers that occur each year by at least 45,000.

"A concerted attack upon the problems of old age, and of chronic diseases, should at the very least delay the disability of tens of thousands of people, and reduce our national losses from these causes in terms of human lives, national productivity, and personal suffering. Rehabilitation will help many of those who are now dependent on others to lead independent and more active lives. We can place no top estimate on the things that can be achieved by future developments in the promotion of mental health as we overcome the severe shortages that now limit all progress in this field." [20]

[20] Ewing, *The Nation's Health*, 28, 30, 34. For a discussion of contemporary health legislation, see Joseph H. Ball, "National Health Legislation," in *Minnesota Medicine*, 31:977–980, 1015 (September, 1948).

In order to help meet the expenses of such an extensive program, the federal security administrator recommended a government insurance plan as opposed to a voluntary plan. He pointed out that a satisfactory system of health insurance should provide that: (1) everyone have ready access to adequate health and medical services, (2) everyone have the kind of services, and all the services, he needs to promote better health, and (3) everyone be able to obtain these without regard for the level of his personal income. He concluded that voluntary insurance plans, such as the Blue Cross, cost too much for many citizens to join them. Only about half the families in the United States, said the federal security administrator, can afford "even a moderately comprehensive health insurance plan on a voluntary basis," and he added: "It is apparent that the Blue Cross plans are not supplying, in the lower-income areas, the extra purchasing power that is necessary to increase their supply of health services and resources appreciably." Minnesota, with an average per capita income of $1,090 in 1946, had 29.4% of its population enrolled in the Blue Cross in 1948. For the United States, whose average per capita income in 1946 was $1,200, only 19.2% of the population was enrolled.[21]

Those supporting government insurance say that such a program would eliminate the financial barrier between any person and the services needed to promote better health, and that government insurance would improve the health of the people by stimulating the development of more nearly adequate supplies of health resources — doctors, nurses, hospitals, and other services — and their equitable distribution throughout the country, through the assurance that there will be a steady and effective demand for them. Advocates of the program propose the passage of a federal law containing twelve points. Despite the fact that a government insurance program has been bitterly opposed, no discussion of the nation's future health would be complete without an examination of the proposed act.

The law, say its advocates, should determine who would make prepayments and who would receive benefits. Coverage should be as broad as practicable, and benefits should be available to all gainfully employed persons who are covered and to their dependents. The act should also provide for health services to noninsured groups for whom public responsibility already is acknowledged, through special premiums paid by public and private agencies on their behalf. It should specify the size of insurance payments, and rates should be based on individual ability to pay; that is, they should be established as a percentage of earnings instead of as a flat rate irrespective of income. Benefits should be as

[21] Ewing, *The Nation's Health*, 36.

comprehensive as possible with only such limitations as may be unavoidable at the beginning. Administrative authorities should have power to extend services as rapidly as practicable. "It should be clearly specified that the benefits are to be administered through Federal-State-local cooperation, with the major emphasis on administration at the State and local levels, so that the keynote is decentralization and local participation. It should be equally clear that payment for services provided through physicians, dentists, nurses, laboratories and hospitals would be made at rates and by methods mutually agreeable to them and the insurance system."

The law would give explicit guarantees to insured persons and their dependents, including guarantees as to their rights to benefit solely by reason of their insurance; their right to make a free choice, individually or in association with other insured persons, of physician, dentist, hospital, etc., and to make a change in that choice; their right to have their personal records kept confidential, to be protected against discrimination, to make complaints or appeals before appropriately constituted committees, and to have recourse to court review of administrative decisions which they believe are unfair. With such guarantees, insured persons would know that they would get what they are entitled to receive from the insurance system, and that the doctor-patient relationship would be maintained.

The proposed act would also explicitly guarantee to the members of the professions providing services the right to participate in the plan or not, to act individually or in groups, to accept or reject patients who choose them, to retain control of professional aspects of professional service, to choose the method of payment for services rendered, to negotiate rates or amounts of payment and other matters through representatives of their own choosing, to make complaints or appeals before appropriately constituted committees, and to turn to the courts for review of administrative decisions.

It is recommended also that the law make special provisions to meet the needs of rural areas and the urban centers that serve them. This, it is maintained, is essential if modern health services are to be brought to those who live far away from the large cities and if patients are to be able to travel to distant medical centers when necessary. Provision should be made, too, to furnish financial aid for professional education and research, including postgraduate training, refresher courses, and research technique.

State and local administration of the law, it is recommended, should be as follows: "Since the benefits would be provided in local areas under State plans, the law should state the minimum conditions to be observed by States and localities in administering the benefits on a decentralized basis. This would meet the insurance obligations of the Federal Government, and the rights of insured persons and the providers of service. The condition should include legal authorization for a State agency, performance of a State-wide survey and development of a State plan, observance of requirements and guarantees in the Federal law, use of State and local advisory councils with broad civic, consumer, and professional representation, merit system administration, allocation of funds to localities on a fair basis, and delegation of substantial administrative authority to local areas as mapped out by the State plan."

Federal administration should be assigned to a small board of fulltime members including both professional and nonprofessional representatives and should be so constituted as to co-ordinate this insurance system with other social security and public health programs. The act should also establish an advisory council, "with members representing the interested public, consumer and professional groups, and with responsibility to advise the Federal board on all important decisions made within the framework laid down by Congress."[22]

A three-year interval would have to elapse between the passage of such a law and the actual beginning of a government insurance program. This period would be used to increase medical resources, to set up administrative and operating machinery, and to make certain that insured persons and providers of services knew their rights and were ready to exercise them. At the end of three years those insured and their dependents would be able to obtain the health and medical services needed up to the capacity of the personnel and facilities existing at that time and the limits of local availability. The ultimate goal — that a hundred per cent of the population be insured — would take somewhat longer. This, in brief, summarizes a problem that the people of Minnesota surely will have to consider in years to come.

The estimated cost of such a government insurance program, although it would vary to reflect current economic conditions, would be about three per cent of annual earnings up to $4,800 a year, probably divided between subscriber and employer. It is said that "If the dental and home-nursing services start on a limited basis and develop gradually, it will be difficult to fix a contribution schedule that would not require several changes. The cost might amount to an additional 0.5 per cent of annual

[22] Ewing, *The Nation's Health*, 94.

earnings at first and rise to about one per cent when these services became more adequate. The Federal Government might consider paying for these services out of general revenue."

Advocates of the program insist that these expenditures would represent only limited new burdens on the economy or on the contributors. What new costs arose, they say, would be for the most part substitutes for expenditures already being made, without insurance, for the same kinds of services. Under government insurance, expenditures would be made "out of earnings all the time, when the people are well, working and earning — not merely when they are ill. They would be made by all the people who work and earn, and not merely by those who happen to be sick. They would be made in fixed and budgetable percentages of earnings, regardless of how often illness strikes, how severe it is, and how much care is needed or how expensive it is." [23]

Whether or not compulsory government health insurance is socialized medicine depends to a large degree on definitions. It certainly is true that such a program is opposed on the grounds of socialization, although the federal security administrator on several occasions has stated definitely that no system of socialization is proposed under the plan for government insurance. Thomas A. Hendricks, secretary of the council on medical service of the American Medical Association, told a Minnesota audience that government health insurance would be the equivalent of federal regimentation of doctors and added that such a program would be opposed by the American Medical Association. During the Eightieth Congress the Wagner-Murray-Dingell bill, which provided for compulsory health insurance, was defeated, although it was backed by President Truman. Hendricks said the American Medical Association objected to national health insurance because it believed such a plan would lower the quantity and quality of medical services and would cost a tremendous amount. He denied that most "ordinary" physicians in the United States favored government insurance, said that the same type of program in England was not working out well, and declared that the best method of medical care can be had when the American is independent and when his doctor is independent. These statements all were denied by Ewing, who was speaking at the same time before the Co-operative Health Federation of America in Minneapolis.[24]

It must not be thought, however, that medical associations are the

[23] "National Health Programs," in *Ohio State Medical Journal*, 44:1035–1044 (October, 1948).
[24] Ewing, *The Nation's Health*, 105; *Tribune*, November 8, 1948; *Pioneer Press*, November 8, 1948.

PATTERNS FOR TOMORROW'S HEALTH

only groups opposing a government health insurance plan. In 1948 the Brookings Institution, at the request of Senator H. Alexander Smith, chairman of a Senate health committee, published one of the strongest arguments against government health programs. Briefly summarized, the conclusions said that the United States is among the healthiest nations in the world; that the United States, under a voluntary system of medical care, has made greater medical and scientific progress than any other nation; that nonwhites in the United States have poorer health than whites, but that this is not due mainly to inadequacy of medical care; and that health advances among whites and nonwhites during the past forty years do not indicate fundamental defects in the American system.

The report next says that statistics drawn from draftees have been used unreliably to demonstrate that there is bad health among the people and that there is need for a radical change in medical care for individuals. It points out that medical care in the United States compares favorably with that in other nations before World War II. The report maintains that health work in extremely poor rural areas cannot be solved satisfactorily by the use of subsidies, but must come from improving economic activities or getting people to move to other areas. It admits frankly that there are some individuals and families in the United States who cannot pay for adequate medical care and says that in the future, as in the past, these people will be cared for by philanthropy or public funds. The statement is made that some of them could not afford even to pay government insurance premiums.

When it discussed compulsory health insurance, the Brookings Institution spoke with extreme candor. It said that such a program would result in a high degree of government regulation and control over physicians, dentists, nurses, and others engaged in giving medical care. Such regulation would be most difficult to administer. The institution also suggested that politics might interfere with the successful administration of a program of compulsory insurance. But it pointed out that, whether or not politics became a factor, the government would stand between practitioner and patient and thus might impair a normal relationship. It stated also that the sheer administration of government insurance would result in a great increase in government employees to keep records and accounts and to make investigations. Thus the cost of medical care to the average citizen would increase because of administrative expense, because insured persons would make unnecessary and unreasonable demands upon medical facilities, and because some physicians and agencies might use the system to their own advantage. Near the close of its recommendations, the Brookings Institution maintained that, even if a government insurance plan were put in operation, it could not possibly care for all the people requiring attention at the beginning of the program, because there are not enough physicians, dentists, and nurses in the United States.

The last point read: "Proposals for compulsory insurance provide for payment of practitioners under one or all of three methods: (a) fee for service, (b) per capita, or (c) salary. Use of the fee-for-service device represents the minimum degree of socialization, but it is administratively difficult. Administrative difficulties would probably result in the adoption of the per-capita system which represents practically complete socialization. It seems questionable whether a country which once embarks on compulsory insurance can turn back but must attempt to remedy defects by more complete government control and administration."

Yet the Brookings Institution, although it condemned in no uncertain terms national health insurance, did suggest that both the national government and state governments might appropriately devote money and energy to research and developments in public health, to health education at the school level, to the teaching of preventive medicine, to the acquisition of physical facilities and the training of personnel, and to the provision of systematic care for the indigent and the medically indigent.[25]

Somewhere, of course, between the report of the Brookings Institution and the plan proposed by the federal security administrator lies a middle ground of truth. Unfortunately, in 1948, this truth was obscured by flames of passion that enveloped it in such fire that the public was confused. Misunderstandings existed on both sides. Dr. John Peters, professor of medicine at the Yale University School of Medicine, said that the chief sources of controversy within the medical profession and between physicians and the public arose from two misconceptions. "The first of these," said Peters, "is the general opinion that the chief function of medicine is distribution. The second is the failure of the medical profession to appreciate fully that medicine is intended primarily for patients, not for physicians."[26]

A somewhat similar point of view was expressed in public opinion polls, one of which showed fifty-nine per cent in favor of expanding the social security program to include benefit payments for sickness, dis-

[25] George W. Bachman and Lewis Meriam, *The Issue of Compulsory Health Insurance*, chapter 3 (Washington, D.C., 1948).
[26] Peters, "Medical Care," in *Consumer Reports*, 9:270 (October, 1944); "Committee Holds Line on Health Insurance," in *Minnesota Medicine*, 31:913 (August, 1948).

ability, and doctor and hospital bills, while the other indicated that sixty-eight per cent favored having the Social Security Act broadened to pay both doctor and hospital care. Two distinguished medical authorities indicated in 1948 that rural health needs could not be met adequately without national health insurance. At the same time that Dr. Leonard A. Scheele, surgeon general of the United States Public Health Service, was telling the National Committee for Mental Hygiene that failure to apply known methods to control infectious diseases results in many preventable deaths annually, Basil O'Connor, president of the American Red Cross and of the National Foundation for Infantile Paralysis, declared that the nation's health was being threatened by the "machinations" of short-sighted individuals working for national health legislation.[27]

Public health and preventive medicine, despite their astonishing progress, still have a long way to go. In 1876, the year of the nation's great centennial festival at Philadelphia, Dr. Henry I. Bowditch spoke truly when he told the International Medical Congress that public hygiene was the most important matter with which any community could concern itself. Yet, continued Bowditch, little attention had been given public health, except when "under the influence of some frightful epidemic, the panic-struck nations have been aroused from their usual apathy, and have then vainly tried to resist the pest by drugs, by appeals to the gods whose laws they have never studied, or finally, perhaps, by legal enactments, after the days of suffering have passed." [28]

Much the same point of view was expressed at the American Public Health Association meeting in Boston in November, 1948. Delegates from Minnesota and elsewhere heard Lemuel Shattuck praised as the "pathfinder" of public health in the United States and as the author of the "bible of public health in America." Shattuck's report to the Massachusetts legislature in 1850, a document that Hewitt studied assiduously, was said to be so far ahead of his time that some of the ends he proposed have still to be achieved.[29]

Certainly Shattuck's declaration of faith not only has profoundly influenced the inception and growth of the public health movement in

[27] American Institute of Public Opinion (Gallup Poll), Princeton, New Jersey, Release of August 14, 1943; National Opinion Research Center, Denver, Colorado, "Special Report on Federal Health Insurance," October, 1944; *New York Times*, November 4, 6, 1948; Mott and Roemer, *Rural Health and Medical Care*, 562. See also J. S. Jones, "What the Farm Communities Expect of Hospital and Medical Care," in *Minnesota Hospitals*, vol. 11, no. 5, p. 2 (September, 1946).
[28] Bowditch, *Public Hygiene in America*, 1 (Boston, 1877).
[29] *New York Times*, November 7, 1948.

Minnesota, but it also serves as a reliable guide to future activities. Shattuck said: "We believe that the conditions of perfect health, either public or personal, are seldom or never attained, though attainable; — that the average length of human life may be very much extended, and its physical power greatly augmented; — that in every year, within this Commonwealth, thousands of lives are lost which might have been saved; — that tens of thousands of cases of sickness occur, which might have been prevented; — that a vast amount of unnecessarily impaired health, and physical debility exists among those not actually confined by sickness; — that these preventable evils require an enormous expenditure and loss of money, and impose upon the people unnumbered and immeasurable calamities, pecuniary, social, physical, mental, and moral, which might be avoided; — that means exist within our reach, for their mitigation or removal; — and that measures for prevention will effect infinitely more, than remedies for the cure of disease." [30]

[30] Commonwealth of Massachusetts, *Report of a General Plan for the Promotion of Public and Personal Health*, 10.

Index

ABATTOIRS. *See* Slaughterhouses
Abbott, William H., Indian health survey, 232
Abbott Hospital, Minneapolis, 355
Accidents, domestic, 189; factory workers, 311; hazards, 311, 316; industrial: *1890s*, 311, *1909–10*, 317, *1900*, 319; miners, 314–317; railroad employees, 318, 319; prevention: 391, instruction, 189, legislation, 311, 312, 318, 319, campaign, 317
Actinomycosis, 71, 72
Ada, sewerage system, 144
Adams, Harold S., heads hotel inspection division, 339, 340
Adams, J. L., Morgan physician, 288
Adenoids, school children, 379
Adulteration. *See* Drugs; Food; Liquor; Medicines
Aged, the, problems and care, 418–435; per cent U.S. population, 418; reasons for increase, 419; Minnesota survey, 419; retirement, 419, 420, 433; homes, 420–424, *see also* Homes for the aged; diseases and infirmities, 421, 426–433, *see also* Cancer, Heart diseases; care of chronically ill, 422; problems, 425; need for purposeful activity, 433–435; rights, 434; in mental hospitals, 456; home care proposed, 477; increased benefits proposed, 478; need for expanded program, 484. *See also* Old age assistance
Agnes, Lake, sanitary survey, 295
Ah-Gwah-Ching, state sanatorium, admits Indian patients, 238; act providing for, 270; described, 280
Air pollution, problems, 483
Aitkin, meat inspection, 154; health board, 200; smallpox, 201, 202, 229, 230; hospitals, 201, 443; nurse, 366
Aitkin County, smallpox, 214, 229, 230, 404
Albert Lea, smallpox, 49, 398
Alden, John, Ely physician, 314
Alger, Smith Lumber Co., 207, 210, 214

Allen, Robert M., Indian agent, 227
Allotment Act, *1887*, 234
Alpha Phi Sorority, supports heart program, 431
American Assn. for the Cure of Inebriates, 457
American Cancer Society, 426, 427, 429
American Child Health Assn., 195
American Fur Co., 15, 221
American Health Resort Assn., 269
American Heart Assn., 431, 432
American Hospital Assn., 476
American House, Minneapolis, 199
American Legion, supports heart program, 431
American Legion Auxiliary, 183
American Legion Foundation, gift for heart research professorship, 390, 432
American Meat Packers Assn., 157
American Medical Assn., 34, 476; *Transactions*, 37; committee on state health boards, 41, on health problems in education, 195; preventive medicine section urged, 84; medical legislation and education conference, 321; recommends school eye and ear examinations, 377; opposes government health insurance plan, 490
American Nurses Assn., 353, 365
American Physiological Society, 432
American Psychiatric Assn., 470
American Public Health Assn., 67, 80, 84, 165, 195, 237, 350, 493; engineering section, 169; milk supply committee, 172; health survey, 194; rural health services proposed, 485
American Red Cross, 383, 493; commission to Poland, 177; home nursing program, 192; furnishes sanitary unit, 255, 256; relations with state board, 275–277; tuberculosis work, 275, 277; Christmas Seals: 284, controversy over, 278; aids in nurses' training, 358; nursing service, 360, 361, 366; maternity care, 363; aid in influenza epidemic, 366, 411, 412, 414

495

American Red Cross Nursing Service, 365
American Social Hygiene Assn., 195
Ames, A. A., Minneapolis health officer, 49, mayor, 108, 109
Ames, A. E., Minneapolis physician, 33; on medical society committee, 41
Anatomical specimens, difficulty of obtaining, 12
Ancker, Arthur B., hospital superintendent, 354; urges new city hospital, 437, 440; views on hospitals, 440–442
Ancker Hospital (St. Paul city hospital), X-ray unit, 284; nursing school, 353; crowded conditions, 437, 438, 440, 441; new building, 437, 440, 441; described, 438; charity patients, 439, 440; average days per patient, 440; cost per patient, 441; services, 441, 442; ambulance, 442
Anderson, Gaylord W., heads public health school, 350
Andrews, C. C., 269
Anesthetics, use in frontier surgery, 10
Animal diseases, relation to human welfare, 70; laboratory work, 70–72, 83. *See also* Cattle; Horses; Livestock; Sheep; Swine
Anoka, lumber production, 197; venereal disease problem, 252; hospital facilities, 449
Anoka County, industrial accidents, 311; swimmer's itch, 348
Anoka State Hospital, 291, 465; sewage disposal, 290; population, *1947*, 470
Anthrax, investigated, 83; rules for reporting, 179
Antitoxin, prepared and distributed, 69, 178, 185, 408
Antituberculosis movement, 94. *See also* Tuberculosis
Archibald, R. W., dairy inspector, 168
Are You Livin'?, health dept. booklet, 193
Armstrong, John, conducts clinic, 258
Army camps, sanitation, 22, 27; venereal disease problem, 184, 254, 256, 258, 259, 262, 263; water supplies investigated, 194; influenza, 410–413
Arsenobenzol (salvarsan), distributed, 256
Arsphenamine (salvarsan), distributed, 257, 261
Asbury Hospital, Minneapolis, 355
Ashbrook, Charlotte G., social worker, 256
Associated Charities, St. Paul, 354, 420
Asylums. *See* Mental hospitals
Aureomycin, for brucellosis, 417
Austin, Gov. Horace, 457
Austin, sewage disposal, 138; sewerage system, 144; physician, 399
Autopsies, 446

"BABY-FARMING," St. Paul, 385, 443
Baby Welfare Service, St. Paul, 365
Bagley, hospital facilities, 449
Bakeries, legislation, 312; sanitary program, 341
Baldwin, William O., speaker, 34
Bang's disease, 415, 416. *See also* Brucellosis
Barbers, legislation, 350
Barbour, N., pioneer physician, 13
Barnard, A., Indians' physician, 223
Barr, R. N., heads administration section, 196, special services section, 422
Bartlett, Cyrus K., hospital supt., 455–458
Barton, Clara, visits Minnesota, 3
Barton, E. R., Indians' physician, 231
Basic Science Act, 350
Bass, Frederic H., 381; directs engineering division, 88, 89; biographical sketch, 89; leaves health dept., 96; on engineer board, 146
Bassetts Creek, Minneapolis, pollution, 107, 108
Bathing, endangered by stream pollution, 293, 300, 303
Bathing beaches, sanitary surveys, 194
Battle Lake, sanatorium, 281
Baudette, chlorination plant, 113; sewage treatment plant, 144, 304, 306; water pollution, 299; Rainy survey laboratory, 302; hospital, 449, 450
Baudette Municipal Hospital, 449, 450
Baum, A. Clark, army physician, 23
Baumann, Fritz, chemist, 79
Bayliss, Mrs. Willard, 166
Beauticians, legislation, 350
Beltrami County, in health district, 189; smallpox, 212; nurse, 362, 363
Beltrami County Welfare Board, 363
Belyea, E. H., health officer, 200, 203
Bemidji, headquarters health district, 189; smallpox, 208, 212; hospital, 215; restaurant surveys, 341; swimmer's itch, 348; nurse, 362; influenza, 413
Bemidji State Teachers College, 193, 264
Bennett, Russell H., 144, 145
Benson, typhoid fever, 121; sewerage system, 144; smallpox, 401
Berg, E. H., heads hotel inspection division, 339
Berry, A. E., Rainy survey report, 303
Berry, Charles, New Ulm physician, 101
Bethany Home, Minneapolis, 246
Bethesda Hospital, St. Paul, 451, 453
Bilious diseases, 14
Births, Minnesota, *1886*, *1887*, 68; registration, 178; among Indians, 241; illegitimate, *1947*, 365; laxity in reporting, 385
Bixby, Tams, relations with Hewitt, 74
Blue Cross, enrollment, 487

INDEX 497

Blue Earth, hospital, 449
Blue Earth County, smallpox, 49; in health district, 189; nursing, 362; schools, 375
Blue Earth County Council on Intergovernmental Relations, 195
Blue Earth County Medical Society, 377
Boarding homes, legislation, 422
Boardman, C. H., St. Paul physician, 397
Boats, inspected, 331; legislation, 349
Boeckman, Egil, 410
Bois des Sioux River, water analyzed, 115
Bois Fort, Indian agency, 224. See also Nett Lake Indian Reservation
Bonne & Howe, lumber co., 213
Borup, Charles W. W., pioneer physician, 14
Bosch, Herbert M., heads health dept. section, 196, 348
Botulism, reporting rules, 179
Bovey De Laittre Lumber Co., 202
Bowditch, Henry I., speaker, 493
Boy Scouts of America. See Scout camps
Boynton, Ruth E., director child hygiene division, 235; heads maternity and infancy program, 387
Bracken, Henry M., 75, 84, 91, 136, 321, 354, 467; vice-president state health board, 77; named secretary state board, 77; biographical sketch, 77, 78; expands laboratory, 79, 81; personality, 79, 84, 92, 94; opposes creation of livestock board, 83; inspection trips, 84; author, 84, 85, 86; speaker, 84, 85, 87, 162, 321; interest in public health education, 84, 191; views on sanatoriums, 86; studies abroad, 87; interest in vital statistics, 91; political difficulties, 92–98; attitude toward efficiency commission, 95; dropped from state board membership, 95; relations with Burnquist, 96; resignation, 96, 98, 176, 274, 277; district supervisor U.S. health service, 98; work evaluated, 98; water analyses circular, 117; urges vaccination, 119, 210, 319, 400; efforts for sanitary sewage disposal, 139, 142, 143; concern with meat inspection, 153, 154, 156, 157, 314; campaign for pure milk, 162, 164, 167; campaign against smallpox, 208–214, 227–230, 399–403, 405; interest in lumber camp sanitation, 214; concern with Indian health, 227, 232, 233, 233n.; relations with Indian agents and physicians, 228, 229, 230; concern with venereal diseases, 252–256; on social hygiene commission, 255; requests Red Cross sanitary service, 255, 256; campaign against tuberculosis, 269–277; controversies with tuberculosis agencies, 274–277; efforts for stream pollution control, 288–291; concern with iron range health and sanitation, 313, 315–317; interest in railroad sanitation, 319–321, 322n.; proposes nurses' supervisory staff, 357; urges care in measles cases, 376; concern with child health, 377, 378, 381, 383, 384; concern over handling of dead bodies, 396; relations with Minneapolis health officials, 401; views on quarantine, 402, 403, 405; directions for diphtheria control, 407; efforts for influenza control, 410–415
Brackett, A. P., lumber co. physician, 202
Brainerd, 246; chlorinates and filters water, 113; sewers, 134, 143; meat inspection, 154; lumber production, 197; smallpox, 202, 402; switchmen's strike, 318; swimmer's itch, 348
Breckenridge, water supply, 113, 115, 120; physicians, 120; typhoid fever, 120
Brimhall, S. D., heads veterinary section, 83
Brink, Frances V., supt. nurses, 357, 358
Bronchitis, among Indians, 221
Brookings Institution, arguments against government health insurance plan, 491
Brophy, William A., 242
Brower, J. W., vii
Browersville, milk-processing plant, 172
Brown, Edward J., investigates smallpox outbreak, 205–207
Brown, Robert L., health officer, 314
Brown, Rome G., 289
Brownell, O. E., sanitary engineer, 179
Brucellosis, control measures, 174, 416, 417; prevalence, 415; cases, *1940s*, 416; symptoms, 416; treatment, 417. See also Undulant fever
Bruno, F. J., Red Cross official, 276
Buena Vista Sanatorium, 281
Bundesen, Herman, health officer, 394, 395
Burnquist, Gov. J. A. A., 414; urges larger health dept. appropriation, 96; plan for health dept. reorganization, 97; asks Bracken's resignation, 98; asked for aid for child hygiene division, 384
Burns, Mark L., 235
Butcher shops, inspected, 150, 151; sanitary conditions, 152
Butler Ship Building Corp., cafeteria surveyed, 341
Butter, early production, 158; recommendations for production, 159; substitutes opposed, 175. See also Oleomargarine

CALDWELL, JAMES, lumberman, 203
Calhoun, Lake, Minneapolis, 108

Camden, pumping station, 112
Camp, George A., lumberman, 202
Camp and Walker, lumber co., 202
Camp Grant (Ill.), influenza, 410
Camp Ripley, health program, 194; venereal disease control, 262, 263
Campbell, S. W., Indian agent, 230
Campbell (Minn.), 115
Camps, defined, 216. *See also* Army camps; Children's day camps; Indians, health camps; Lumber camps; Mining camps; Railroad construction camps; Scout camps; Summer camps; Tourist camps; Trailer camps
Canada, protests against smallpox spread, 212; co-operates in boundary pollution studies, 296
Canada Dept. of Health, represented at Rainy pollution conference, 300
Canby, sewage treatment plant, 144; asks aid for infant clinic, 384
Cancer, deaths, 180, 426; control program, 196, 427–430; nursing services, 368; danger zones, 426; among old people, 426–430; symptoms, 427; causes, 428; research: 429, grants, 427
Canning factories, waste disposal, 147
Cannon Falls, sanatorium, 281
Cannon River, pollution: 286, study, 297
Cappelen, F. W., engineer, 111
Capser, Henry C., 336
Carey, William N., 146
Carli, Christopher, pioneer physician, 15
Carlton, smallpox, 207
Carlton County, influenza, 186; in health district, 189; nursing service, 368; smallpox, 404
Carman, J. B., vaccinates Indians, 231
Carriers, typhoid fever, 118, 119, 121, 180, 194, 199, 343, 363; tuberculosis, 283; diphtheria, 406
Cass County, smallpox, 213
Cass Lake, smallpox, 227, 229; Indian agency, 235; health unit, 238; hospital, 240
Cataract House, Minneapolis, 100
Catarrh, at Fort Ripley, 10
Cates, A. B., 438, 439
Cattle, diseases: laboratory work, 69–72, actinomycosis, 71, 72, anthrax, 83, hemorrhagic septicemia, 83, "lumpy jaw," 154, Bang's disease, 415, 416, *see also* Brucellosis; tuberculosis tests, 71, 72, 83, 153, 154, 163, 170; inspected, 71, 72, 153, 154, 163; slaughtering of diseased, 155, supervised, 154; endangered by water pollution, 286, 293; sanitation of shipping pens, 320. *See also* Animal diseases; Dairy herds; Livestock
Cedar Lake, Minneapolis, 2, 108

Centerville, 116
Centerville Lake, 106
Century of Progress, Chicago, dysentery epidemic, 394
Cerebral hemorrhage, 426
Cesspools, condemned, 128; St. Paul ordinances, 131; source of water contamination, 286, 287
Chalybeate Springs, St. Anthony, 2
Chamberlain-Kahn Act, 255
Chancroid, cases reported, *1918*, 257, 258, *1919–21*, 261. *See also* Venereal diseases
Chapin, Charles V., 334
Chase, Charles A., 438
Chase and Miller, lumber co., 202
Chatfield, cholera infantum, 376
Cheese, early handling methods, 158; impure, 159. *See also* Dairy products
Cheese factories, waste disposal, 293
Chesley, Albert J., 118, 144, 187, 317, 337, 468, 478; on epidemiological division staff, 89, director, 95; biographical sketch, 89, 176; field trips, 90; refuses state board secretaryship, 96; director preventable diseases division, 96, 357; calls attention to Mississippi pollution, 144; efforts for sanitary milk standards, 165; named secretary state health board, 176; with Red Cross Commission to Poland, 177; outlines health dept. work, 177; administrative policies, 178, 196; reorganizes health dept., 178, 196; concern with disease reporting, 179, 180, 253; lists leading death causes, 180; urges county diphtheria immunization work, 180; efforts for federal aid for public health, 181; concern with child health program, 182; duties compared with Hewitt's, 183, 184; aids in developing influenza laboratory, 186; concern with trachoma, 186, 232; endorses district health units, 188; health surveys, 193, 194; interest in army sanitation, 194; venereal disease program, 194, 253; personality, 195; honored by medical assn., 195; public health professor, 195; official positions in health organizations, 195; concern with Indian health, 237, 238; on social hygiene committee, 255; efforts for water pollution control, 293, 294, 302, 304; report on occupational diseases, 323; advocates field nurse corps, 357; sets up maternal and child welfare program, 386; investigates dysentery outbreak, 395; scarlet fever epidemic, 408; comments on poliomyelitis epidemic, 482
Chicago (Ill.), smallpox, 49; milk handling methods, 164; fire, *1871*, 243; dysentery epidemic, 394

INDEX 499

Chicken pox, investigated, 179; reporting rules, 180; epidemic among Chippewa, 203; quarantine, 377
Child conservation, advisory committee on, 384
Child-health days, 387
Children, relation of scholastic methods to health, 57; deaths: noninfectious diseases, 66, Minneapolis, 109, decrease, 373; crippled: care of, 189, 364, 390, hospital, 273, 364, 467, *see also* Gillette State Hospital for Crippled Children, nursing services, 367, 368, clinics, 368, 390, orthopedic plastic program, 390; Indian, 227, 239; diseases: 227, 373, 375, 376, noninfectious, 66, immunization and inoculation, 189, 486, tuberculosis, 282, adenoids, 379, communicable, 384, 386, infectious, 386, poliomyelitis, 481; health camp, 239; day camps, 273; hospital for tuberculous, 282; in industry, 310–313; illegitimate, 364; preschool nursing services, 371; handicapped: 377, 379, 380, instruction in care of, 364; courses in physical observation of, 380; physical examinations, 384, 468, urged, 378; pamphlets on behavior problems, 471. *See also* Maternal and child health program; School health program
Children's Bureau, U. S. Dept. of Labor, 181, 384, 391; co-operates in state child health program, 182, 386, in maternal deaths survey, 388
Children's Protective Society, Minneapolis, 383
"Children's Year Campaign," 383
Childs, J. A., engineer, 179
Chilgren, G. A., 463
Chippewa Health Unit, 238
Chippewa Indians, diseases: smallpox, 203, 225, 227–231, measles, 203, 227, 231, contagious, 220, 222, treatment, 222, syphilis, 223, statistics, 224, trachoma, 232, 234, 235, 236, 240, tuberculosis, 234, 235; population, *1881*, 224; vaccination, 225, 228, 231; economic conditions, 226, 369; health surveys, 232, 234; sanitary conditions, 234–236; nursing service, 237; hospitals, 238, 240; relief, 239; health camp, 239. *See also* Indians
Chiropody, legislation, 350
Chisago County, swimmer's itch, 348; nursing service, 368
Chisholm, milk pasteurization, 169
Chisholm Creek, sanitary survey, 295
Chlorination. *See* Water supplies
Cholera, 396; St. Paul, 6; brought by steamboats, 6, 33; Ft. Ripley, 10; early prevalence, 11; lumber camps, 15, 16; Red Wing, 33; reporting rules, 179; among Indians, 221; shipment of victims' bodies forbidden, 397
Cholera infantum, among Indians, 222; prevalence, *1870s, 1880s*, 376
Christ Episcopal Church, Red Wing, 33, 34, 35, 40, 60, 80
Christian, Mr. and Mrs. George H., 272
Christianson, Gov. Theodore, 145
Christmas Seals. *See* American Red Cross
Cincinnati Reformed College of Medicine, 13
CIO. *See* Congress of Industrial Organizations
Citizens' Mental Health Committee, 471
Civil War, Hewitt's service, 17–29
Civil Works Administration, establishes nursing service, 182
Clague, Frank, state senator, 93
Clark, Taliaferro, 232, 256
Claussen, Oscar, 144
Climate, Minnesota, relation to health, 1–16; comments of travelers and settlers, 1; attracts invalids, 1–4; benefits investigated, 6, 7; survey in relation to epidemics, 37; relation to tuberclusosis investigated, 266–268
Climatotherapy, vogue of, 6
Clinics, Indians' diagnostic, 239; venereal disease, 256–258, 262, 263; tuberculosis, 283, 360; immunization, 360; child guidance, 373, 468; children's, 384, 385, 390, crippled, 360, 364, 368, 390; prenatal, 387; rheumatic fever, 390; mental hygiene, proposed, 472; community, proposed, 477; infantile paralysis, 481
Cloquet, hospital, 369; influenza, 414
Cloquet Lumber Co., 214
Clough, Gov. David M., fails to reappoint Hewitt, 74–76
Cochran, J. C., health officer, 438
Coleman, Anna Mae, nurse, 357
Communicable diseases, reporting rules, 180; change in rank as death cause, 181; control in rural areas, 189; work of public health nurses, 359, 361, 367; regulations, 364; children, 384; immunization and vaccination, 391. *See also* Contagious diseases; Diseases; Infectious diseases; specific diseases
Community Health Service, Minneapolis, 390
Community Memorial Hospital, Blue Earth, 449
Conference of State and Provincial Health Authorities, 84, 195, 321, 397, 402
Conference of State Sanitary Executives, 85
Congress of Industrial Organizations

(CIO), protests lumber camp conditions, 218
Consolidated Chippewa Agency, 235, 237
Consumption. *See* Tuberculosis
Contagious Disease Hospital, Minneapolis, 273
Contagious diseases, 220; control, 180, 181; among Indians, investigated, 234; spread by railroad passengers, 319; innoculation, 468. *See also* Communicable diseases; Diseases; specific diseases
Cook County, in health district, 189
Coonan, Mrs. Daniel, 165
Co-operative Health Federation of America, 490
Corbett, J. F., bacteriologist, 290, 291
Corey, Sir Robert, directs calf-vaccine station, 52; provides Hewitt with vaccine, 54
Coronary thrombosis, 431, 432
Corpses. *See* Dead bodies
Cottage Grove, tuberculosis survey, 283
Cotton, C. E., meat inspector, 155
Council of Jewish Women, 383
Council of National Defense, women's division, 383
Country clubs, sanitary investigations, 346
Craig, Charles P., 95
Crandall, Le Mont, supervisor old age assistance, 435
Crawford, Dean W. H., 393
Creameries, waste disposal, 172, 293
Crooks, Ramsay, 221
Crookston, sewers, 134; hotel, 205; smallpox, 205; sanatorium, 281; influenza, 410, 414; hospital, 451
Crookston General Hospital, 451
Croup, children, 376
Crowell, N. S., Ft. Ridgely physician, 11
Crozier, A. W., hotel inspector, 333, 334
Crystal, Lake, smallpox, 401

DAIRIES, inspected, 83; sanitary conditions, 83, 158; improvement in methods, 163, 164; oppose pasteurization, 165; sanitary surveys, 168; requirements, 168
Dairy herds, tested, 160, 163, 168. *See also* Cattle
Dairy products, adulteration protested, 149, 158; efforts for pure, 157–174; early handling methods, 158; legislation, 160
Daniels, Asa W., 42n., 223, 454
Davis, E. J., Mankato physician, 33, 48
Davis, Theodora, nurse, 237
Day, David, Indians' physician, 221
De la Barre, W., Soudan physician, 315
Dead bodies, preparation and transportation, 86, 396, 397, 413; regulations, 397, 398

Deaths, Minnesota, *1875*, 6, *1887*, *1891*, 68; causes: analyzed, 57, leading, 69, 180, 426, 430; better classification urged, 66; typhoid fever, 106, 110, 118, 121, 376; diarrheal diseases, 106, 376; cancer, 180, 426; smallpox, 199, 200, 398, 402, 404–406; Indians, 222, 241; tuberculosis, 272, 274, 279, 285, *1875*, 6, *1870s*, 267; mines, 316; infant, 373, 376, 383, 391; children: rheumatic fever, 390, decrease, 409; maternal: 391, decrease, 373, causes, 388, surveys, 388; diphtheria, 406, 409; influenza, 410, 415; age proportions, 418; heart diseases, 430, 432; accidents, 478
Deerwood Sanatorium, 281
Defense plants, sanitary investigations, 324, 325. *See also* individual plants
Degenerative diseases, 421, 426; increase, 180; reasons for change in rank as death cause, 181. *See also* Aged, the; Cancer; Heart diseases
Dental health, education, 386; programs, 391–393; problems investigated, 392; courses, 392; extension of state aid urged, 393; flouride treatments, 393; expanded program recommended, 484
Dental practice, legislation, 350
Dentists, co-operate with dental health division, 183; ratio to state population, *1940*, *1944*, to school population, *1944*, 392; shortage, 392; courses for, 392; contribute to research program, 393; needed, 476, 477
Detroit (Mich.), Rainy pollution meetings, 302, 303
Detroit Lakes, sanitary survey, 295
Dewey, John J., pioneer physician, 13
Diarrheal diseases, Ft. Ripley, 10; St. Paul, 106; deaths, 106, 376; Minneapolis, 109; investigated, 179; Indians, 221; decrease, 480
Diehl, H. S., 429
Dilworth (Minn.), nurse, 366; influenza, 413
Diphtheria, early prevalence, 7, 11, 16; lumber camps, 15; Dodge County, 59; laboratory work, 80, 81, 91, 192, 406, 407, 408, in England, 52; from impure water, 109, 129, 141, milk, 165, 173; reporting rules, 180; immunization: advocated, 180, 409, children, 389, 390; Indian treatment for, 227; iron range, 314, 315; carriers, 406; *1870s*, *1880s*, 406; statistics, 406, 409; regulations, quarantine, diagnosis, 407; *1940s*, 409. *See also* Antitoxin; Toxin-antitoxin
Diploma law, 62
Diseases, theories as to causes, 50; waterborne, 111, 117, 133, 394, 396; from faulty waste disposal, 139; reporting

INDEX

rules, 179; Indians: 220, 221, 229, 231, increase with contact with whites, 223, statistics, *1881*, 224, investigated, 234; from impure food, 343; school census, 408. See also Animal diseases; Communicable diseases; Contagious diseases; Degenerative diseases; Endemic Diseases; Epidemic diseases; Infectious diseases; Occupational diseases; specific diseases
Disinfection, better apparatus urged, 66
Dock, George, 79
Dodge, James A., 110
Dodge County, diphtheria, 59
Drake, Daniel, 5, 11
Drew, Charles W., 161
Drugs, early scarcity, 12; adulteration prohibited, 45; purity standards set, 350; sale of harmful, prohibited, 350
Dukelow, Donald A., public health educational director, 192
Duluth, 202, 246; health resort, 2; water supplies, 113, 114, 123, 126; sprinkling system, 127; privies, 138; sewage disposal, 144, 290; food poisoning, 152; diseased cattle slaughtered, 154; meat inspection, 154, 157; dairy herds tested, 163; milk pasteurization, 166, 170; trachoma clinic, 185; nurses, 187, 278, 357; state dept. laboratories, 188; lumberjack mecca, 199; smallpox: 204, 208, 210, 398, 404, patients treated, 199, 200, conference, 210, cost of epidemic, 211; typhoid fever, 290, 314; harbor survey, 295; co-operates in pollution study, 297; factories inspected, 312; restaurant survey, 341; food handlers' courses, 341; swimmer's itch, 348; cholera infantum, 376; child health program, 379, 384; infant welfare organization, 383; influenza, 413, 414; brucellosis conference, 417
Duluth City Health Dept., 453
Duluth Council of Social Agencies, 434
Duluth Mental Health Clinic, 473
Duluth, Missabe, and Iron Range R.R., 212, 329
Duluth-Superior Harbor, pollution, 297
Dwan, Paul, 432
Dysentery, Ft. Ripley, 10; Hibbing, 113, 115; from faulty waste disposal, 139, impure milk, 165; investigated, 179; reporting rules, 179; Indians, 221, 222; amebic, from impure water, 315, 394, 395; iron range, 317; Chicago, 394–396; bacillary, 396; decrease, 480

EAGLE BEND, meat inspection, 154
Ear examinations, in schools, 377, 378
East Grand Forks, filter plant, 90; chlorination plant, 113

Eberhart, Gov. Adolph O., 233; appoints efficiency and economy commission, 95
Eberth, Karl Joseph, describes typhoid bacillus, 100
Eden Prairie, hospital, 451
Eggestine, Adelia, nurse, 263, 279
Elbow Lake, diphtheria investigation, 377
Elizabeth Kenny Institute, 482
Elk River, physician, 201
Elliot Memorial Hospital, University of Minnesota, 451
Elmo, Lake, health resort, 2
Ely, sewerage system, 144; smallpox, 230; physician, 314; swimmer's itch, 348
Embalmers, licensed, 178
Embalming, 397; fluids examined, 91
Emergency Maternal and Infant Care Program, 363
Emerson, Haven, 194
Employers, attitude toward workers' health, 308; liability, 311
Encephalitis, epidemic, reporting rules, 179
Encephalomyelitis, equine, virus laboratory, 186
Endemic diseases, survey, 35, 36
Engineering Club, Minneapolis, 144
Engineers, public health, 188; district, 189
Engineers' Society, St Paul, 144
Epidemic diseases, survey, 35, 36; instruction, 62. See also Epidemics; specific diseases
Epidemics, scarlet fever, 6; surveys, 35, 36, 37; smallpox, 48, 49, 75, 199–204, 227, 398–402, 404, 405; typhoid fever, 91, 101, 117–123, 314, 315; influenza, 97, 176, 180, 186, 366, 384, 385, 387, 410–415; chicken pox, 203; measles, 203, 221, 314; dysentery, 394. See also specific diseases
Epilepsy, 457, 464
Erysipelas, lumber camps, 202; state hospital, 463
Evans, W. A., Chicago health commissioner, 403
Eveleth, sewerage system, 144; hospitals, 186, 209; typhoid fever, 315
Ewing, Oscar R., reports on nation's health, 476–481, 486–490, 492
Eye examinations, in schools, 189, 377, 378

FACTORIES AND SHOPS, sanitary surveys, 183, 324; ventilation, 309; inspection laws urged, 311; safety hazards, 311; inspected, 312; orders for safety devices and sanitation, 312. See also Industrial health
Fagan Brothers, lumber co., 215

Fair Oaks Lodge Sanatorium, 281
Fairs, sanitary conditions and inspections, 337. See also Minnesota State Fair
Family Nursing Service, St. Paul, 365
Family Service, St. Paul, 420
Faribault, 116; dry-earth closets, 138; meat poisoning, 156; diphtheria investigation, 377
Farmington, sewage disposal, 286n.
Farrell, L. S., engineer, 294
Fergus Falls, sewers, 134; sewerage system, 144; restaurant owners' and employees' school, 341; geriatric hospital, 451
Fergus Falls State Hospital, 465; established, 460; reading materials, 463; nurses' home, 464
Fever and ague, among Indians, 222
Filtration. See Water supplies
Financial depression, *1930s*, affects Indians, 239; effect on venereal disease program, 262; stimulates interest in mental programs, 469
Finch, J. E., 4
Fire escapes, legislation, 332
Fish, endangered by water pollution, 145, 286, 293, 297, 300, 302, 303
Flagg, S. D., 41
Flandrau, Charles E., 223
Fleming, D. S., heads preventable diseases section, 196, 409
Floodwood, hospital, 414
Florida, competition with Minnesota for invalids, 2
Flouride treatments, dental, 393
Foker, Leslie W., heads industrial health division, 324, 330
Folwell, William W., university president, 22; in Civil War, 25; characterizes Hewitt, 27; relations with Hewitt, 31, 65; offers Hewitt public health professorship, 61; on medical college committee, 62; urges medical teaching dept., 63; views on medical dept. reorganization, 65
Fond du Lac, Indian agency, 224
Fond du Lac Hospital, Cloquet, 369
Food, impure: legislation forbidding sale, 45, Minneapolis ordinance, 151, diseases from, 343; adulteration: 57, 148, 149, 175, legislation, 45, 175; handlers and handling: 148, legislation, 312, 335, courses, 341, need for further education, 484; program for pure, 148–175, 194, 340–344; poisoning cases, 152, 340; Indians, 227; in hospitals, surveyed, 445. See also Butter; Cheese; Dairy products; Meat; Milk
Ford, Mrs. Marie, vii
Forest fires, 9, 79, 176, 414

Forest Lake, 104; septic sore throat epidemic, 173
Fort Frances (Ont.), smallpox, 225; paper mill, 299; dam, 303; Rainy pollution hearing, 304
Fort Ridgely, physicians, 10, 11, 221, 222; dispensary, 437
Fort Ripley, described, 9; physicians, 9, 221; illness among troops and civilians, 10; dispensary, 437
Fort Snelling, 222, 243, 245, 257, 264; physician, 9; Veterans' Hospital, 146; vaccination, 194; venereal disease problem, 256, 258; swimming pool investigated, 349; influenza, 410; dispensary, 437
Fosston, smallpox, 205, 206
Fox, Carroll, surgeon U.S. health service, 95; surveys Minnesota public health administration, 382
Freeborn County, in health district, 189
Fridley, purification plant, 122; pump company, 345
Frontenac, health resort, 2

GARBAGE DISPOSAL, recommendations, 137; resorts, 346; Scout camps, 348; homes for aged, 423; hospitals, investigated, 445; equipment needed, 480
Gastroenteritis, at university, 173
Geriatric hospital, 451
Geriatrics, need for division of, 485. See also Aged, the
Gerontology, creation of departments suggested, 434
Gibraltar fever. See Brucellosis
Gilbert, D. C., Mountain Iron physician, 314
Gilfillan, Joseph A., 225, 227
Gillette, A. J., poliomyelitis clinics, 481
Gillette State Hospital for Crippled Children, 364; mental examinations, 467
Glanders, control program, 70; investigated, 83; reporting rules, 179
Glen Lake Sanatorium, described, 281; nurses, 366
Gonorrhea, 260, 262; among Indians, 221, 236; cases reported: *1918*, 257, 258, *1919–21*, 261. See also Venereal diseases
Goodhue, schools, 377
Goodhue County, disease survey, 35, 36
Goodhue County Medical Society, 35, 36
Gopher Ordnance Works, sanitary investigations, 324, 325; trailer camps, 345
Gould, J. F., 295
Governor's Advisory Committee on Mental Health, 473
Grand Forks (N. D.), typhoid fever, 118; smallpox, 398
Grand Portage, Indian agency, 224

INDEX

Grand Rapids, physician, 13; lumber camp, 199; health officer, 200; smallpox, 201; quarantine hospital, 201
Granite Falls, sanatorium, 281; asks aid for infant clinic, 384
Grave-robbery, acts to prevent, 12
Gray, R. & Co., lumber co., 209
Great Lakes Board of Public Health Engineers, 298
Great Lakes Drainage Basin Sanitation Agreement, 296, 298
Great Northern R.R. Co., 316
Greenbush Community Hospital, 449
Greene, Willard P., 481
Greenleaf, Col. H. S., Ft. Snelling surgeon, 256
Griffin, Ezra, supplies vaccine, 49
Griffiths, William, public health educational director, 192, 193; heads mental health unit, 471
Gronvold, Charles, author, 56
Gunn, John C., 9

HACKNEY, JOSEPH M., state senator, 93, 166
Hallock, sewage treatment plant, 144
Hamline University, at Red Wing, 32; social hygiene courses, 264
Hammond, Gov. Winfield S., suggestion re hotel surveys, 334
Hand, Daniel W., on state board, 42n., president, 100, 104; author, 55; surgery professor, 62; comments on St. Paul water, 104; ventilation report, 309
Hanks, Stephen, steamboat captain, 15
Harmony, typhoid fever, 123
Harriet, Lake, Minneapolis, 108
Harrington, Francis E., health officer, 171
Harris, starch factory, 289
Hart, Hastings H., secretary corrections and charities board, 461, 462
Hartley, E. C., 387
Harwood, W. E. hospital head, 15
Hasson, Alexander B., Ft. Ridgely physician, 10, 222
Hastings, water pollution, 293
Hastings State Hospital, 465
Hawley, Augustine B., Red Wing physician, 30-34
Hawley, Paul R., 476
Hay fever, victims attracted to Minnesota, 2, 3
Head, J. Frazier, army physician, 9, 221
Health agencies and officers, local, legislation, 44, 45; school sanitary surveys, 58; number, *1889*, 59, *1895*, 73; medical training, 73, 82, 84; place in public health program, 78; conference of state and, 101; functions, 127; accused of laxity, 139; relations with state dept., 149, 179, 188; jurisdiction over meat, 157, dairy products, 158; diseases reported to, 180; confusion over jurisdiction, 188; bill to authorize county, 190; stream pollution control, 288

Health boards, state, functions, 81-83. See also Minnesota State Board of Health

Health insurance, proposed government plan, 478, 487-490; opposed, 490-492; public attitude toward, 492

Health units, district, 188-190; federal aid, 189; co-operation advocated, 476

Heart diseases, leading cause of death, 180, 430; nursing, 368; from rheumatic fever, 390; hospital, 390, 432; among aged, 426, 431; deaths, *1942*, *1948*, 430, *1947*, 430, 432; public education program, 431; research, 431, 433; problems, 481

Heating, instruction, 62; legislation, 334; schools, 373-375, 377

Hedwall, John O., 444

Hendricks, Thomas A., 490

Hennepin County, tuberculosis deaths, *1875*, 6; milk dealers indicted, 161; tuberculosis survey, 283; swimmer's itch, 348; nursing services, 357, 366; survey, 367; dentists, 392

Hennepin County Fair, sanitation, 337

Hennepin County Graduate Nurses Assn., 355

Hennepin County Medical Society, 162, 262; milk commission, 166; co-operates in x-ray project, 284

Hennepin County Public Health Service, 368

Hennepin County Tuberculosis Assn., 284

Hewitt, Charles N., 12, 44, 92, 159, 183, 313, 406; Civil War service, 17-29; Geneva (N. Y.) practice, 17, 20; education and training, 18-20; personal appearance, 21; personality, 27, 30, 33, 36, 40, 42, 43, 65, 74; receives citation, 28; Potsdam (N. Y.) practice, 30; visits Red Wing, 31, 32; church work, 33, 40, 60, 80; Red Wing practice, 33, 35, 36, 37, 38, 40, 76; activities for state medical society, 33, 41, president, 65; views on preventive medicine, 33, 63; marriage, 34; library, 35; secretary county society, 35, on committee, 36; Red Wing home, 35, 40; sued, 36; criticizes medical profession, 36; advocates statewide disease prevention program, 36; survey of climate and epidemics, 37; public health precepts, 37; speaker, 37, 50, 65, 101, 109, 116; author, 37, 56, 57, 59; views on immigrant inspection, 39; concern with railroad sanitation,

39; government medical examiner, 40; hospital, 40; laboratory, 40, 50, 67, 69–73; efforts to establish state health board, 41, 224; named secretary state board, 42; works for co-operation of local and state agencies, 44; publication program, 44; campaign against smallpox, 44, 46–51, 57, 200–206, 225, 226; studies abroad, 44, 51–53; urges vaccination, 47, 48, 204, 206, 376; contagious diseases circulars, 48; vaccine station, 53–55, 73; edits state board publications, 55–60; outlines state board work, 56; state water survey, 57; efforts for pure water supplies, 57, 100, 101, 105, 106, 109, 111, 115; removes state board office to St. Paul, 60; professor public health, 60, 61; role in medical college organization, 62; professor preventive medicine, 62; chairman medical examining board, 63; plans for medical teaching dept. at university, 63; opposition to, 64, 65; attitude toward homeopaths, 65; dean medical examining faculty, 65; presidential address American Public Health Assn., 65; views on national health organization, 67; interest in vital statistics, 68; diphtheria and antitoxin work, 69; work with animal diseases, 70–72; campaign against infectious diseases, 73; plans for rural health services, 73; views on functions of state board, 74; attitude toward politics, 74; dismissal, 74–76, 77; urges courses for health officers, 82, 84; views on local health board functions, 127; interest in sanitary sewage disposal, 135, 136, 137, 139; efforts for pure food, 149, 152, 153, 155; lists leading death causes, 180; duties compared with Chesley's, 183, 184; interest in public health education, 191, 350; concern with Indians' health, 222, 224, 227; interest in venereal disease, 252; survey of tuberculosis in relation to climate, 266, 267; comments on tuberculin, 268; advocates isolating tuberculosis patients, 269; concern with stream pollution, 286–288; industrial health policy, 309; criticizes factory law, 312; stresses need for public health nurses, 354; introduces maternal and child health program, 373, contribution to, 375; concern with school health and sanitation, 374, 375, 377; investigates St. Peter hospital, 454–456; interest in problems of inebriates, 457, 458, 459; asks state hospitals investigation, 459

Hewitt, Mrs. Charles N., 34, 51, 53, 74

Hibbing, chlorination plant, 113; dysentery, 113, 315; sewer system, 144; lumber co., 210; smallpox, 212; water supply, 313; miners' health, 314

Hill, C., 41

Hill, Hibbert W., 176; directs epidemiology division, 88; biographical sketch, 89; field trips, 90; investigates poliomyelitis epidemics, 91; typhoid epidemics, 91, 119, 120; personality, 92; program for support of health dept., 92; resigns, 95; executive secretary public health assn., 98, 274; aids in trachoma survey, 232; comments on tuberculosis death rate, 274; poliomyelitis studies, 481.

Hill, Nathan B., 42n.

Hill-Burton Hospital Construction Act, 423. *See also* Hospital Survey and Construction Act

Hillary, Michael, army physician, 23

Hinckley, forest fire, 79; meat inspection, 154

Hoag, Earnest B., supervises Minneapolis hygiene dept., 379; director school hygiene, 380, 381

Hoffman, Marie Broker, nurse, 237

Hog cholera, 72; investigated, 83

Holley, Frances, nurse, 370

Holton, H. D., 252

"Home doctor" books. *See* Medical books

Home environment, sanitary inspections proposed, 483

Home Hotel, Minneapolis, 199, 200

Homeopathic Hospital, Minneapolis, 251

Homeopaths, opposition to Hewitt, 65

Homes for the aged, attitudes toward, 420; number, *1945*, 421; described, 421; survey, 421; regulations and standards, 423, 444; plans for construction, 451

Hookworm, reporting rules, 179

Hopewell Hospital, Minneapolis, 273

Hormel, George A., 157

Horses, diseases, 70; glanders, 70, 83, 179; encephalomyelitis, 186; fistula of the withers and poll evil, 416

Hospital Survey and Construction Act, 432, 447, 448, 476; state program under, 449–453

Hospitalization programs, for lumberjacks, 215, 443; St. Anthony Hospital, 442. *See also* Health insurance

Hospitals, army in Civil War, 18, 21, 23, 25, 26; Indian, 238, 240; venereal disease clinics, 258; nurses' training schools, 355; maternity, 357, 386, 443, 444, *see also* Maternity hospitals; naval station, 365; licensing laws, 387, 422, 443, 446; legal responsibility of state board, 387, 454; heart, 390, 432; beds needed: 422, 476, *1947*, 446, *1948*, 447;

standards, 423, 444; early and modern systems compared, 436; crowded conditions, 436, 437, 438, 440, 441, 456, 459, 460; early attitude toward, 436, 439, 440; early, described, 437–440; growth, 437, 439, 441–443, 449, 451; construction: recommendations, 441, per bed cost, 447, federal aid, 447, 450, problems, 447, 449, 450, state program, 450, 451; sanitary surveys, 445; number and capacity, *1947*, 445; licenses granted, *1947*, 445; advisory council, 445, 448; patients admitted, *1942*, 446; program under federal act, 448–453, see also Hospital Survey and Construction Act; number and condition, *1946*, 448, 449; survey of state facilities, 448, 449; general, 450, 451; chronic disease, 450, 451, 452; mental disease, 450, 451, 452, see also Mental hospitals; geriatric, 451; area and regional, 451, 452; bids for tuberculous, 452, 453, see also Sanatoriums: inebriate, 457–460, see also Minnesota State Inebriate Asylum; mental examinations, 467; special district and community, proposed, 477; need for additional, 484. See also individual hospitals

Hotels, legislation, 312, 332–335, 339, 340; inspections and inspectors: 332–337, 339, transferred to health dept., 336, need for further work, 484; sanitary conditions, 332, 333; affected by modern transportation, 335. See also Fairs; Resorts; Restaurants; Summer camps; Tourist camps; Trailer camps

Houghton, Douglas, 220

House of the Good Shepherd, St. Paul, 250

Houston, school, 377

Hoyt, Henry F., health officer, 151

Hubbard, Gov. Lucius F., confers with Hewitt on smallpox emergency, 201

Hubbard County, smallpox, 213

Hunekens, E. J., heads child conservation division, 384

Hunt, T. W., Lanesboro physician, 71

Hunt, W. A., author, 59

Hutchinson, Robert, iron mine physician, 314

Hutchinson, sewerage system, 144; meat poisoning, 152

ICE, cutting prohibited in Mississippi River, 105; pollution investigated, 105n.; concern over purity, 174

Ickes, Harold, approves engineer board appointment, 146

Immigrant ships, health conditions, 38; better sanitation urged, 67

Immigrants, health conditions, 38

Indian Reorganization Act, 234, 238

Indians, diseases: 6, 7, 203, 220–236, statistics, *1881*, 224, treatment, 227, investigated, 232, 233, 234, 274, see also specific diseases; joint responsibility of U.S. and state for health, 181; health problems and control, 220–242; vaccination, 220, 223, 225, 228, 231; deaths: infant, 221, 240, leading causes, 222, *1881*, 225, rate, 241; births: proportion to population, 221, *1881*, 225, rate, 241; medicine men, 222; government physicians, 223; Minnesota agency created, 223; reservations and communities, *1948*, 223, area, 224; sanitary conditions, 223–225, 227, 234–236; agencies, *1872*, 224; allotments, 226, 227; economic conditions, 226, 239, 241; spread disease, 229, 231; quarantine, 230, 231; health surveys, 232, 234; liquor: sale to, prohibited, 232, legalized, 240; federal aid for health program, 234, 238; schools, 235; health recommendations, 236; nursing services, 237, 279, 369; hospitals, 238, 240; health camps, 239; homes and living conditions, 241; expanded health program recommended, 484. See also Chippewa Indians; Sioux Indians; Winnebago Indians

Industrial camps, regulations, 216; sanitary investigations, 322; dispute over jurisdiction, 322. See also Lumber camps; Railroad construction camps

Industrial health, lumberjacks, 6, 197–214, 225, 230; program: 187, 308–330, transfer to health dept. advocated, 97, expansion recommended, 178, 484; serological examinations, 264; legislation, 310, 311, 312, 318, 319, 324; miners, 314–318; occupational hazards and accidents, 316–319, 324, see also Accidents; railroad employees, 318–322; vaccination, 319; physical examinations, 323; investigations, 324, 328; nursing services, 370. See also Factories and shops; Industrial camps; Workers

Industrial wastes, starch factory, 116; pollutes public waters, 116, 286, 288, 289, 293, 298–305; stockyards, 129; slaughterhouses, 129, 136, 142; canning factories, 147; creameries and cheese factories, 293, 298; systems investigated, 296; problems studied, 297; paper mills, 299–305; projects for improved facilities, 306

Inebriate hospitals, 457–459, 462; treatment recommended, 458. See also Minnesota State Inebriate Asylum

Infant mortality, 57; among Indians, 221, 240; efforts to reduce, 365, 391; causes, 383

506 THE PEOPLE'S HEALTH

Infant Welfare Society, Minneapolis, 365
Infantile paralysis. *See* Poliomyelitis
Infectious diseases, among children, 386; reporting: laxity, 400, law, 401. *See also* Communicable diseases; Diseases; specific diseases
Influenza, research in England, 52; *1918* epidemic, 97, 176, 180, 186, 357, 366, 384, 385, 410–415; laboratory, 185, 186, 415; nursing, 186, 357, 366; control measures, 186, 410–415; in *1880s, 1890s*, 409, 410; symptoms and treatment, 410; army camps, 410, 411, 412, 413, statistics, 410, 412, 413, 415; among Indians, 412
Insanity. *See* Mental diseases
Instruments, early surgical and clinical, 11; furnished Indian physicians, 232
Intemperance, believed insanity cause, 457
International Boundary Commission, jurisdiction over Rainy River, 301; Rainy survey, 303; hearing on Rainy pollution, 305
International Congress on Tuberculosis, 273
International Falls, paper mill, 299, 302, 306; dam, 303; sewage treatment urged, 304, plans for, 306; water pollution, 304, 305; health center, 451
International Hotel, St. Paul, 33
International Medical Congress, 493
Iowa Dept. of Health, 403, 413; agreement with Minnesota and Wisconsin depts., 297
Iron ranges. *See* Mesabi Iron Range; Vermilion Iron Range
Irvine, H. G., heads venereal diseases division, 179, 256; describes division's work, 256, 257; biographical sketch, 257; summarizes results of venereal disease program, 259–261; comments on suggested venereal disease law, 264; author, 327
Irwin, Vern D., heads dental health education section, 391; lists problems, 392; surveys dental health literature, 392
Isanti County, nursing services, 360, 370
Isanti Public Health Assn., 360
Itasca County, trachoma, 186; in health district, 189; lumber camps, 197; smallpox, 225, 226
Izaak Walton League, interest in sewage treatment project, 144, in water pollution control, 292–295

JACKSON COUNTY, in health district, 189
Janssen, C. A., meat inspector, 156
Jaundice, reporting rules, 179
Jewish Hospital Assn., 451
Johnson system, water purification, 112
Johnston, Mrs. D. S. B., 246
Jones, Talbot, health officer, 104, 129, 133
Jordan, W. A., directs dental health division, 391
Journal-Lancet, article on venereal diseases division, 256
Junior League, Minneapolis, raises heart hospital funds, 390, 431

KABLER, PAUL, heads medical laboratories section, 196
Kanabec County, dentists, 392
Kaposia, Indian village, diseases, *1845*, 222
Keene, Charles H., 379
Kenny, Sister Elizabeth, 482
Keyes, C. F., 144
Keys, Ancel, directs physiological hygiene laboratory, 430, heart research, 432
Kimball, Anne, vii
Knife River, smallpox, 214; influenza, 414
Knights of Pythias, St. Paul, sponsors prostitution lectures, 247
Knudsen, Helen L., vii
Koch, Robert, 50, 53; discovers tubercle bacillus and develops tuberculin treatment, 268
Koivunen, Ilmar, union president, 217
Koochiching County, in health district, 189
KOST, JOHN, *Domestic Medicine,* 9
Kutz, C. W., 146

LAC QUI PARLE, 222
Lac qui Parle County, smallpox, 401
Lake City, influenza, 410
Lake County, smallpox, 404
Lake Julia Sanatorium, 281
Lake Michigan Sanitation Congress, *1928*, 298
Lake of the Woods, affected by Rainy pollution, 303
Lake of the Woods County, smallpox, 404
Lake of the Woods Sportsmen's Assn., petitions for Rainy pollution control, 301
Lake Park, sanatorium, 281
Lakes, source of water supplies, 102, 103; pollution, 143, 293; investigations and surveys, 295, 297. *See also* Public waters pollution control
Lakeville, meat poisoning, 156
Lanesboro, physician, 71
Lawler, influenza, 414
Laws. *See* legislation under various subject entries
League of Minnesota Municipalities, interest in milk campaign, 166, 171

INDEX

Lee, John T., meat inspector, 152
Leech Lake, lumber camp, 199
Leech Lake Indian Reservation, 223, 224; smallpox, 225, 229; measles, 227; agent, 231; trachoma surveys, 232; tuberculosis rate, 234. *See also* Chippewa Indians; Indians
Legislation. *See* legislation under various subject entries
Lennon, B. M., hotel inspector, 333
Leonard, William H., 62, 206
Leprosy, reporting rules, 179; diagnosed as syphilis, 252
Lexington (Ky.), medical instruction center, 5
Licensing, scavengers, 132; embalmers, 178; rendering plants, 178; rental boats, 349; healing practices, 350; barbers, beauticians, chiropodists, 350; nurses, 355; hospitals and related institutions, 386, 387, 422, 443, 444, 446
Lighting, instruction, 62; legislation regulating, 334; regulations for homes for aged, 423
Lincoln, Abraham, reviews troops, 28
Lind, Gov. John, 255
Lindberg, A. W., heads hotel inspection division, 339
Lippman, H. S., 469
Liquor, law prohibiting adulteration, 45; sale to Indians prohibited, 232, legalized, 240
Little Falls, chlorination plant, 194; laboratory for milk and water analyses, 194; lumber co., 213; state health dept. branch, 263; infant welfare organization, 383
Litzenberg, J. C., 384
Livestock, regulations re diseased, 157; endangered by stream pollution, 296, 303. *See also* Animal diseases; Cattle; Dairy herds; Horses; Sheep; Swine
Lumber, production, *1848–99*, 197
Lumber camps, tuberculosis, diphtheria, scarlet fever, 15; typhoid fever, 15, 199, 202; vaccination, 59, 206; smallpox, 197–214, 225, 230; described, 198; sanitary conditions, 198, 202, 203, 214–216, 218, 308; accidents, 202; erysipelas, 202; quarantine, 206; sanitary regulations and recommendations, 211, 212, 216; first aid facilities, 215; surveys, 215, 216, 218; water supplies, 216; food, 216; termed health menace, 230. *See also* Lumber companies; Lumberjacks
Lumber companies, attitude toward employee's health, 201, 208, 215, 216, toward vaccination, 202, 203, 205–207, 209, toward quarantine, 209; employ physicians, 207, 208; laxity in smallpox outbreaks, 209, 212, 213; represented at smallpox conference, 210; cost of smallpox to, 211; employee medical and hospital plans, 215; commissary prices, 216. *See also* Lumber camps; Lumberjacks
Lumberjacks, smallpox, 6, 197–214, 225, 230; vaccination: urged, 203, 204, 206, attitude toward, 205, compulsory, proposed, 210, certificates required, 212; pay withheld in smallpox cases, 210; medical and hospitalization plans, 215; wages, 216. *See also* Lumber camps; Lumber companies
"Lumpy jaw" cattle, 154, 156
Lymanhurst School for Tuberculous Children, described, 282

MACALESTER COLLEGE, sewage disposal, 131
McClure, Ethel, supervisor maternity hospitals, 444
McDaniel, Orianna, 323; biographical sketch, 79; on health dept. staff, 79–81, 83, 84; diphtheria research, 80; directs Pasteur institute, 88, 91, 96, preventable diseases division, 179; diphtheria surveys, 377
McGillivray, Helen, nurse, 389
Magath, Thomas B., 395
Malaria, in early Minnesota, 7; Ft. Ripley, 10; Winona, 14; reporting rules, 179
Malta fever. *See* Brucellosis
Mankato, 246; physician, 33, 48, 101; smallpox, 48, 49, 75; water supply, 101, 113; typhoid fever, 119; health district headquarters, 189; health survey, 195; sanitary conditions on fairgrounds, 337; restaurant surveys, 341; diphtheria investigation, 377; influenza, 413
Mankato Daily Review, comments on Hewitt's dismissal, 75
Mankato State Teachers College, 192, 264
Mantoux tests, 185, 283, 368, 369. *See also* Tuberculin tests; Tuberculosis
Marcley, Walter J., 280
Marden, Charles S., state senator, 93
Mark, Hilbert, 283
Martin County, in health district, 189
Maryland Public Health Assn., 272
Maryland State Board of Health, 272
Maryland Tuberculosis Commission, 272
Massachusetts, labor laws, 310; child conservation division, 384
Massachusetts State Board of Health, 41
Massachusetts State Inebriate Asylum, 457
Maternal and child health program, 189, 373–393; federal aid, 181, 182, 183, 385,

386; services to expectant mothers, 189, 387, 390; nursing services, 359, 363, 365, 367, 368, 387, 389; personnel trained, 386; prenatal clinics, 387; literature distributed, 387; obstetrics and pediatrics courses, 388; recommendations, 388; maternal deaths surveys, 388, efforts to reduce, 391; industrial maternity policy, 390; infant vaccination and immunization, 390; care of soldiers' wives, 390; manual for physicians, 390; expanded program recommended, 390. *See also* Child health program; Children; Emergency Maternal and Infant Care Program; Maternity homes; Maternity hospitals; Sheppard-Towner Act
Maternity Home Council, 444
Maternity homes, admissions, *1947*, 365
Maternity Hospital, Minneapolis, 390, 437
Maternity hospitals, 437; investigated, 357; legislation, 386; licensing, 387, 422, 443, 444, 446; classes for expectant mothers, 390; number, *1940*, 443, 444; standards, 444; mental examinations, 467
Mattocks, Brewer, 4; health officer, 102, 248, 249
Mayo, Charles H., advocates pasteurization and low milk bacterial count, 171; Rochester health officer, 172; surgery at state hospital, 463
Mayo, William J., 12, 401; criticizes Bracken, 94; surgery at state hospital, 463
Mayo, William W., 33; on state health board, 77; reports on impure foods, 148
Mayo Clinic, Rochester, 436; poliomyelitis work, 482
Mayo Foundation, sanitary emgineering fellowships, 296
Mayo Memorial Medical Center, 451
Measles, cases reported, *1927*, 180; pamphlets on, 192; among Indians: 203, 221, 222, 224, 227, 231, surveys, 232, 233; epidemics, 203, 221, 314; iron range, 314, 315; children, 375, 376, 408, 409. *See also* Epidemics
Meat, laboratory investigations, 81; efforts for pure, 149–157; peddlers, 150; ordinances, 151, 152; poisoning cases, 152, 156, 314; inspection, 150, 154, recommendations, 153; legislation, 153, proposed, 156; instructions to inspectors, 155; sale of diseased, 156
Medical books, in pioneer homes, 5, 8; Hewitt's library, 35
Medical centers, proposed, 477
Medical practice, legislation, 62, 64, 350
Medical schools, early, 5, 11, 20

Medical service organizations, incorporation act, 350
Medical students, examinations, 62, 63
Medicine, adulteration prohibited, 45
Medicine men, Indian, methods, 222, 241
Meningitis, in domestic animals, investigated, 83; epidemic, investigated, 179
Meningococcic serum, distributed, 185
Mental diseases, annual cost, 454; causes, 457; treatment investigated, 464; committee on causes and prevention, 466. *See also* Mental health; Mental hospitals
Mental health, programs: 196, 465, 471–473, outlined, 468, aftercare program, 465, need for, 470, federal aid, 472, *1948–49*, 473; early hospital treatment recommended, 456; trend toward preventive treatment, 465, 468, 469; courses in, 467; renewed focus on problems, 469; literature distributed, 471; clinics proposed, 471, 472. *See also* Mental diseases; Mental hospitals
Mental Health Act, federal, 472, 473
Mental hospitals, investigated, 454, 456, 459, 460, 461, 462, 470; jurisdiction over, 454, 461, 464; early conditions, 455, 456, 459, 460; care and treatment of patients, 455, 456, 460, 462, 463, 464, 465, 470; management, 459, 461, 462; proportion of inmates to population, 460, 461; crowded conditions, 462, 470; sanitary conditions, 463, 465; nurses and nurses' homes, 464; mental examinations, 467; number of patients, *1947*, 470; report on, 470; operating costs, 470; conditions, *1948*, 470; need for larger staffs, 470; campaign for support, 471. *See also* individual state hospitals
Mercer, W. A., Indian agent, 231
Merchants Hotel, Crookston, 205
Merchants Hotel, St. Paul, 251
Merriam, Gov. William R., praises state health board, 116
Merrill, B. J., health officer, 59, 206
Mesabi Iron Range, physicians, 15, 314; sanitary conditions, 140, 308, 314, 315, 317; trachoma surveys, 232; prostitution, 252; health conditions and control measures, 314–318; influenza, 414
Metropolitan District Planning Assn., 144
Metropolitan Drainage Commission, 136, 144, 145
Mettle, Meta, nurse, 356
Miasma, defined, 5; believed to cause typhoid fever, 100
Michael Dowling cerebral palsy project, 364
Michaelsen, George S., 326, 329

INDEX

Michelet, Simon, Indian agent, 231
Michigan State Dept. of Health, 210
Midwives, 385, 387
Milaca, influenza, 413
Milk, investigations, 81, 179; diseases from impure, 100, 118, 121, 165, 173; early handling methods, 158; adulterated, 158, 159, 161, 163; program for pure, 159–174, 194; fat content: tests, 159, standards, 160; dealers indicted, 161; Twin Cities consumption, *1888*, 161; analyzed, 161, 163, 194; municipal ordinances, 165; certified: 167, 172, regulations, 168; bacterial count standard, 171, 174; Minnesota consumption, *1930*, *1933*, 173; production standards, 174; sale of substandard prohibited, 174; Scout camps, 348; problems to be solved, 479. See also Dairy products; Food; Milk pasteurization
Milk pasteurization, 71; advocated, 162; Chicago and Toronto, 164; standards, 165; program, 165–174; opposed, 165, 166, 170; defined, 169; effects, 171; public demand, 172; health dept. requirements, 172; legislation, 174, urged, 417, 479; plants: 180, courses for operators, 169, number, *1945*, 174, act regulating, 174, investigated, 194; for prevention of undulant fever, 416. See also Milk
Millard, Perry H., anatomy and physiology professor, 62; supports medical practice act, 64; medical school dean, 65, 76; opposes Hewitt, 76
Mille Lacs band, Chippewa Indians, agency, 224; economic conditions, 226, 369; smallpox, 229, 231
Mills, Fred C., heads Scout committee, 347
Mineral Springs Sanatorium, 281
Miners, health conditions and control measures, 314–318
Mines, safeguards, 316; accidents, 316, 317; sanitary conditions, 316, 317, 318; inspected, 316, 318. See also Industrial health
Mining camps, water pollution from, 289; sanitation, 314; sanitary conditions, 317
Mining companies, attitude toward health inspector, 316
Minneapolis, hotels, 2, 100, 199, 200, see also individual hotels; vital statistics returns, 68; hospitals, 79, 121, 161, 239, 251, 258, 273, 353, 355, 364, 365, 390, 437, 438, 439, 440, 442, 443, see also individual hospitals; typhoid fever, 91, 100, 101, 107, 109, 110, 118, 119, 122; water supplies: 91, 100, 105, 106, efforts for pure, 107–113, 122, 124; compared with St. Paul as to health, 105; death rates, 106, 109; diarrheal diseases, 106, 109; scarlet fever, 109; diphtheria, 109; early sanitary conditions, 125, 134–136; sprinkling system, 127; sewage disposal, 134–136, 144–147, see also Twin City sewage treatment project; milk-borne epidemics, 173; state health dept. quarters, 184; public health nurses, 187, 356, 379; health surveys: 194, schools, 378, 379; smallpox, 199, 204, 212, 399–401, 404, 405; prostitution and control measures, 243, 245, 247, 251, 257, 262; venereal disease clinics, 258; health authorities: 262, first, 127, criticized, 400, see also Minneapolis Dept. of Health; tuberculosis: care of patients, 271, 273, 278, 282, surveys, 284; trade, *1870s*, 308; factories inspected, 312; food sanitation: hotels and restaurants, 341, milk, 159, 161, 162, 163, 170, 171, meat, 150–154; public baths surveyed, 349; cholera infantum, 376; influenza, 385, 410, 412–414; quarantine rules, 403; poliomyelitis, 481. See also Twin Cities
Minneapolis Associated Charities, 214, 271, 356, 379
Minneapolis Board of Education, 379
Minneapolis Board of Public Welfare, 482
Minneapolis City Council, investigates water supply, 109; waterworks committee, 111; authorizes chlorinating plant, 112; approves "night-soil" dump, 136; meat ordinances, 151; prostitution ordinance, 246
Minneapolis City Dispensary, 271, 272
Minneapolis Community Health Service, 365, 390
Minneapolis Cottage Hospital. See St. Barnabas Hospital
Minneapolis Daily News, co-operates with health dept., 257
Minneapolis General (City) Hospital, 121; venereal disease clinics, 258; nurses' training, 355, 364; opened, 437; mortality rate, 440; poliomyelitis investigations, 482
Minneapolis Health Dept. (Board of Health, Division of Public Health), 453; inspects dairy cattle, 153; venereal disease control, 258; co-operates in X-ray project, 284; food sanitation program, 340; investigated, 401; efforts to control smallpox, 404, influenza, 414
Minneapolis Journal, prints venereal disease pamphlet, 262; comments on care of tuberculous, 271
Minneapolis Restaurant Assn., 341
Minneapolis-St. Paul Sanitary District, act providing for, 145

Minneapolis Tribune, comments on meat inspection, 152; describes mental hospitals, 470
Minneapolis Woman's Club, urges school physical examinations, 379
Minnesota, climate: relation to health conditions, 1–16, travelers' and settlers' comments, 1, benefits investigated, 6, 7; as a health resort, 1–4, 38, 85; water surveys, 57, 115, 286, 289; population and vital statistics, *1880s*, 68; rank in public health work, 96; public waters, 99, 287; resort business, 335; state government reorganized, 336
Minnesota Academy of Medicine, 84
Minnesota Academy of Natural Sciences, 110
Minnesota Advisory Commission, 97; tuberculosis work, 275–277; relations with health dept. 275; repudiates contract with Red Cross, 276; supervises county sanatoriums, 281
Minnesota and Ontario Paper Co., waste disposal, 302-305
Minnesota Assn. for the Prevention and Relief of Tuberculosis, 273, 274
Minnesota Bureau for Crippled Children, 364
Minnesota College Hospital, Minneapolis, 161, 437
Minnesota College of Homeopathic Medicine, 64
Minnesota Dental Assn., 183, 248, 393
Minnesota Drainage Commission, 90
Minnesota Efficiency and Economy Commission, 95; recommendation *re* hotel inspector, 333
Minnesota Farm Bureau Federation, public health exhibit, 192
Minnesota Federation of Women's Clubs, supports sanitary milk movement, 165, creation of child hygiene division, 383
Minnesota Heart Assn., 431, 432
Minnesota Home School for Girls, 467
Minnesota Hospital, Minneapolis, 442
Minnesota Hospital Assn., prepares hospital standards, 423; advises on maternity hospital regulations, 444; represented on advisory board, 445
Minnesota Hospital College, 64
Minnesota Industrial Commission, surveys logging camps, 218
Minnesota Institute for Defectives, 464
Minnesota Institute of Governmental Research, Inc., analysis of public health expenditures, v
Minnesota Junior Chamber of Commerce, interest in restaurant sanitation, 341
Minnesota legislature, interim committees: on Twin Cities sewage treatment project, 144, on boundary waters pollution, 292; authorizes development of maternal and child welfare program, 386. See also legislation under various subject entries
Minnesota Magdalen Society, 246
Minnesota Nurses Assn., 444
Minnesota Public Health Assn., 96; supports creation of public health commission, 97; nurses, 186; incorporated, 274; Christmas Seals agent, 275; tuberculosis policy, 275; relations with health dept., 275–277; repudiates contract with Red Cross, 276; part in tuberculosis work, 277; co-operates in nurses' training, 358; child health work, 385, 386
Minnesota Public Health Seal Fund, 360
Minnesota Public Safety Commission, 383
Minnesota Railroad and Warehouse Commission, regulates station facilities, 322
Minnesota Resources Commission, 304
Minnesota River, sanitary survey, 306
Minnesota Sanitarium Assn., 279
Minnesota Social Hygiene Commission, 254, 255
Minnesota Society for the Prevention of Blindness, 326
Minnesota Soldiers' Home, Minneapolis, 354, 421
Minnesota State Board of Control, 290; co-operates in venereal disease control, 261; supervises sanatorium, 281; investigates maternity hospitals, 357; represented on child conservation committee, 384; licenses maternity hospitals, 386, 443, prescribes rules, 443; jurisdiction over state institutions, 464, over mental hospitals, 465; recommendations *re* prevention of mental disorders, 465; research bureau, 466, 467, 468
Minnesota State Board of Corrections and Charities, 461, 464
Minnesota State Board of Health, v, 48, 62, 65, 76, 77; committee on epidemics, climatology, and hygiene, 4; established, 41, 42, 224, 454; functions, 42, 43, 74, 78; legislation concerning: act establishing, 42, 454, infectious diseases of animals, 83, quarantine, 127, jurisdiction over meat, 157, water pollution control, 287–290, 294, 297, 305, industrial health hazards, 324, hotel inspection, 336, 340, rental boat licensing, 349, county nurses, 358, 371, school water supplies and sewage disposal, 381, 382, maternal and child health, 386, hospitals, 387, 422, 423,

444, 446, public institutions, 454, 458; publications, 55–60, 193, 326, 389; program outlined, 56; program for political support, 92–95; political difficulties, 93–97; abolishment recommended, 96; plan for reorganization, 97; relations with physicians, 98. *See also* Bracken, Henry M.; Chesley, Albert J.; Hewitt, Charles N.; Minnesota State Dept. of Health; Smith, Charles
Minnesota State Board of Nurse Examiners, 444
Minnesota State Board of Pharmacy, 350
Minnesota State Bureau of Criminal Apprehension, 263
Minnesota State Bureau of Labor. *See* Minnesota State Dept. of Labor and Industry
Minnesota State Bureau of Labor Statistics, 308, 312
Minnesota state commissioner of education. *See* Minnesota State Dept. of Education
Minnesota state commissioner of labor. *See* Minnesota State Dept. of Labor and Industry
Minnesota State Conference for Social Work, 192
Minnesota state dairy and food commissioner, office created, 175; investigates liquor, 174
Minnesota state dairy commissioner, milk investigations, 159, 162; office established, 160; inspects herds, 160, 167; warns milk dealers to clean premises, 161; convictions for adulterated milk sales, 163; supports sanitary milk campaign, 166
Minnesota State Dept. of Agriculture, Dairy, and Food, recommendations *re* milk bacterial count, 171; control of pasteurization plants, 174; co-operates in water survey, 296, in hotel surveys, 334; represented at Rainy River hearing, 304
Minnesota State Dept. of Conservation, surveys of streams, 294, of summer camps, 347; interest in Rainy pollution control, 300–302, 304
Minnesota State Dept. of Education (Public Instruction), 378, 380, 382, 445; aids dental program, 183, 393; co-operates in social hygiene courses, 264; health division, 364; vocational rehabilitation division, 390; mental examinations, 467
Minnesota State Dept. of Health, prepares and dispenses vaccines and serums, 48, 49, 184, 185; quarters, 60, 184; collects vital statistics, 68, 91; divisions and sections: laboratories, 69–73, 79–83, 88, 91, 101, 184–186, 253, 406–408, veterinary, 79, 83, engineering, 88, 90, Pasteur institute, 88, 90, 91, epidemiology, 88, 408, venereal diseases, 98, 176, 178, 179, 255–262, tuberculosis, 98, 176, 178, 277, child conservation, 98, 384, sanitation, 166, 168, 172, 178, 180, 218, 293, 299, 323, 338, 346, 349, records, 178, vital statistics, 178, supt. of nurses, 178, preventable diseases, 178–180, 185, 186, 194, 196, 264, 306, 327, 404, 429, educational agent, 178, 191, dental health, 183, 196, 391–393, child hygiene, 187, 196, 237, 380, 383–391, 445, industrial health, 187, 196, 314, 318, 323–330, 339, educational, 191–193, 196, hotel inspection, 194, 196, 337–349, departmental administration, 196, medical laboratories, 196, rural health service, 196, public health nursing, 196, 327, 363, 364, 370, 371, environmental sanitation, 196, 339, 350, special services, 196, 422, mental hygiene, 196, 471, 472, water pollution control, 339, municipal water supply, 339, general sanitation, 339, 344, hospital service, 445; work with animal diseases, 70, 72, 88; jurisdiction over meat, 81, 83, 153, 154, 157; tuberculosis work, 81, 83, 179, 185, 266–269, 272–278, 283; efforts for pure water supplies, 81, 90, 105n., 113, 116, 117, 124, 179, 395, 423; diphtheria work, 81, 91, 406–409; pure milk program, 81, 158, 162–174, 179; typhoid fever work, 81, 179; history, 86; organization, 88, 96, 178, 179, 196; appropriations, 94, 95, *1915*, 383; growth, 98; public waters pollution control, 134, 146, 183, 287–305; efforts for sanitary sewage disposal, 137, 139–141, 143–147, 423; relations with local health agencies, 149, 179, 188, 474; hotel and restaurant program, 149, 337–350; maternal and child health program, 158, 373–393, 408, 469; work outlined, 177; smallpox control, 179, 200–214, 228, 398–404; poliomyelitis work, 179, 481; Indian health work, 181n., 227, 232, 236–240; concern with nurses and nursing, 182, 183, 186, 356–358, 360, 366, 368, 372, 445; pneumonia program, 185; influenza control, 185, 186, 410–415; program for district health units, 188–190; educational literature and exhibits, 192, 193, 204, 399; venereal disease control, 194, 252, 253, 255–265; Camp Ripley health program, 194, 263; cancer control, 196, 429; industrial health program, 197, 200–214, 216, 315–330; trachoma recommendations,

233; hospital program, 357, 423, 444–453, 467; administration surveyed, 382; regulations *re* shipment of corpses, 397, 398; quarantine regulations, 402–404; program for aged, 419, 421–423; mental health program, 426, 465, 467, 471–473; need for geriatrics and adult hygiene division, 435; lacks accident prevention program, 478; nitrate poisoning studies, 483. *See also* Bracken, Henry M.; Chesley, Albert J.; Hewitt, Charles N.; Minnesota State Board of Health; Smith, Charles E.

Minnesota State Dept. of Labor and Industry, inspects railroad and lumber camps, 214, 215, mines, 316, railroad switches, 319, industrial camps, 321, 322; industrial safety campaign, 317; interest in railroad employees' welfare, 318

Minnesota State Dept. of Social Security, social welfare division, 364, 387, 419; services to crippled children, 390; licenses maternity hospitals, 443

Minnesota State Emergency Relief Administration, 182, 239

Minnesota State Fair, public health exhibits, 192; sanitary conditions and inspections, 331, 337

Minnesota state game and fish commissioner, 299, 293

Minnesota State Inebriate Asylum, 457–460

Minnesota State Library Commission, 280

Minnesota State Live Stock Sanitary Board, established, 83; jurisdiction over meat, 157; supports milk campaign, 166; tuberculin tests, 168; recommendations *re* milk bacterial count, 171; tuberculosis and brucellosis program, 174; water survey, 296; represented at Rainy pollution hearing, 304

Minnesota State Medical Assn. (Society), 37, 50, 65, 195, 256; reorganized, 33; committee on legislation, 41, on epidemics and hygiene, 100; supports county health bill, 191; radio program, 192; favors establishment of sanatorium, 270; endorses school eye and ear examinations, 377; sponsors maternal mortality survey, 388, vaccination program, 406; cancer control program, 429; advises on maternity hospital regulations, 444; represented on advisory board, 445; asks action for inebriate hospital, 457

Minnesota State Medical Examining Board, 62, 63, 350

Minnesota State Oil Inspection Dept., 334

Minnesota State Planning Board, 323, 430

Minnesota State Prison, Stillwater, typhoid fever, 100; water supply, 113; convict labor regulated, 310

Minnesota State Reformatory for Men, results of mental tests, 467

Minnesota State Reformatory for Women, mental tests, 467

Minnesota State Reorganization Act, *1939*, 443

Minnesota State Sanitary Conference, 381

Minnesota State School for Feeble-Minded and Colony for Epileptics, 465, 470

Minnesota State Training School for Boys, mental tests, 467

Minnesota Supreme Court, upholds legislation *re* milk, 160, *re* inebriate hospital, 458

Minnesota Temperance Union, 459

Minnesota Unitarian Conference, reports on mental hospitals, 470

Minnesota Water Pollution Control Commission, 305–307

Minnesota's Health, health dept. bulletin, 193

Minnetonka, Lake, health resort, 2

Minnewaska, Lake, sanitary survey, 295

Mississippi River, source of water supplies, 91, 99, 106, 107; ice cutting prohibited, 105; pollution: 105, 107, 125, 132, 136, 144, 145, 292, 293, by sewage, cause of typhoid, 121, condemned, 134, 145, hearing, 290; sanitary investigations and surveys, 108, 110, 145, 291, 295, 298; drainage system, 287

Mitchell and McClure, lumber Co., 207

Monachesi, E. D., 469

Moorhead, W. P., on health dept. laboratory staff, 79

Moorhead, sewer system, 144; restaurant surveys, 341

Moorhead State Teachers College, 264

Moose Lake, influenza, 414; geriatric hospital, 451

Moose Lake State Hospital, number of patients, *1947*, 470

Moose River, lumber camp, 202

Morgan, water supply, 288

Morrill, James L., university president, 476

Morrison, John, Indian-school teacher, 231

Morrison County, children examined, 384

Mount Sinai Hospital, Minneapolis, 451

Mountain Iron, 208; smallpox, 214; physician, 314; health board, 314

Mower County, in health district, 189; rural school described, 389

INDEX 513

Mullin, R. J., heads health dept. laboratory, 95
Murphy, Ignatius J., 96, 274
Murphy, John H., pioneer physician, 13
Murray, Philip, 476

NAPLIN, MRS. LAURA E., director hotel inspection division, 339
National Advisory Mental Health Council, 473
National Assn. for Infantile Paralysis, 482
National Assn. for the Prevention of Infant Mortality, 383
National Assn, for the Study and Prevention of Tuberculosis, 273, 275, 277, 321
National Assn. of Manufacturers, 476
National Cancer Institute, 429
National Committee for Mental Hygiene, 471, 493
National Education Assn., 195
National Foundation for Infantile Paralysis, 493
National Organization for Public Health Nursing, 350, 356
Nelson, C. B., vii
Nephritis, among the aged, 426
Nett Lake Indian Reservation, tuberculosis rate, 234. *See also* Chippewa Indians; Indians
New Brighton, slaughterhouse waste disposal, 142; cattle slaughtered, 154; stockyards, 155; munitions plant, 325; trailer camp ordinance, 345
New Market, diphtheria, 407
New Orleans (La.), medical assn. meeting, 34; sewage disposal, 131
New Ulm, 306; typhoid fever, 101, 121; sewer system, 143, 144; public abattoir recommended, 156
New York City Health Dept., public relations program, 485
New York Committee on Mental Hygiene, 471
New York Ethical Society, nurses, 353
Newcomb, C. A., Methodist minister, 14
News Letter, state board publication, 389
Nickerson, hospital, 208
Nigg, Clara, heads influenza laboratory, 186
"Night soil," disposal methods, 131–134, 136, 137. *See also* Sewage
Noise, relation to workers' health, 328
Nopeming Sanatorium, 281
Norred, Charles H., 400
North Branch, physician, 116
North Wisconsin R.R., lumber camps, 204, 206, 207
Northern Lumber Co., 209
Northern Pacific R.R., 319, 201
Northern Pump Co., trailer camps, 345

Northfield, dry-earth closets, 138; sewage disposal, 286n.
Northrop, Cyrus, 63; relations with Hewitt, 65
Northwest Airlines, commissary investigated, 340
Northwestern Hospital, Minneapolis, 79; trains nurses, 353, 355; opened, 437; plans new building, 438; rules, 439
Northwestern Pediatric Society, 383, 385
Nurses and nursing, early attitude toward, 352; training programs, 353; controversy over trained and untrained, 354; legislation, 355; in influenza epidemic, 357, 366, 411, 414; old people's homes, 421; mental hospitals, 464; increase in number recommended, 476. *See also* Public health nurses and nursing
Nursing homes, legislation, 422
Nursing in Industry, health dept. publication, 326
Nutrition, program proposed, 484
Nye, Katherine, conducts clinic, 258
Nyquist, Ann, vii, 370n.

OAK GROVE HOUSE, Minneapolis, 2
Oakland Park Sanatorium, 281
O'Brien, C. D., St. Paul mayor, 250
Obstetrics, postgraduate courses, 388
Occupational diseases, prevention program, 323–330; in agriculture, program needed, 484
O'Connor, Basil, 493
Offensive Trades Act, 90
Ohage, Justus, health officer, 212, 401
Old age assistance, *1943*, 419; case load and cost predicted, 420; chronically and mentally ill recipients, 422; legislation, 424, 425; statistics, 425. *See also* Aged, the
Oleomargarine, act prohibiting manufacture and sale, 175
Oliver Iron Mining Co., 141, 208, 315–318
Olivia, hospital, 449
Olson, Floyd B., Hennepin County attorney, 170; governor, 302
Onigum, agency physician, 228; Indian sanatorium, 239
Ontario Dept. of Health, co-operates in Rainy pollution control, 300–304, 306
Orcutt, Wright T., 197
Orphan asylums, mental examinations, 467
Otter Tail City, distance from physicians, 13
Otter Tail County, tuberculosis survey, 283
Otter Tail County Sanatorium, 281, 283
Otter Tail River, water analyzed, 115;

contamination, 120; swimming pool surveyed, 349
Owatonna, diphtheria investigation, 377

PACKING HOUSES, sanitary conditions, 152
Paper mills, stream pollution from wastes, 299, 300, 302, 303, 305
Paratyphoid fever, at university, 121; vaccine, 184. *See also* Typhoid fever
Parisien, Josephine, nurse, 237
Park Palace Hotel, Lake Elmo, 2
Park Place Hotel, St. Paul, 102
Parsons, Louisa, heads nurses' school, 353
Pasteur, Louis, 50; Hewitt's work with, 53
Pasteur Hospital for Infectious Diseases, described, 88
Pasteur Institute (Paris), described, 53
Patent medicines, advertised, 2, 13
Peckham, Stephen F., state chemist, 57; investigates water supplies, 108, 115
Pearce, N. O., vii
Pediatrics, postgraduate courses, 388
Pellagra, reporting rules, 179
Pembina band, Chippewa Indians, 224
Penicillin, for trachoma treatment, 240
Pensions, old age. *See* Old age assistance
Pepin, Lake, pollution, 145; Arese at, 220
Peters, John, professor of medicine, 492
Pettengill, Manasseh, 2
Phalen Creek, pollution, 102, 150
Phalen, Lake, St. Paul water source, 101–104; park, 105
Phalen Park, St. Paul, children's cottages, 273
Pharmacists, legislation, 350
Phelps, E. B., 291
Phelp, R. M., 270
Phlebotomy, practiced by Indians, 222
Phthisis, tubercular. *See* Tuberculosis
Physical examinations, workers, 323; children, 378, 379, 384, 468
Physicians, pioneer: 13, 15. theories on climate and health, 4, 5, on typhoid fever, 100, keep weather records, 5, investigate climate benefits, 6, hardships, 8, 10, 13, 14, training, 11, 13, supplies imported, 15; employed by mining cos., 15, by lumber cos., 15, 207, 208, 212; on iron range, 15, 314; relations with state board, 98; public health district, 188; army, report on Indian health, 221; to Indians; 221, 223, 224, 240, difficulties, 231; osteopathic, 258; urged to co-operate in venereal disease program, 260; favor establishment of sanatorium, 270; increase in number recommended, 476, 477. *See also* individual physicians
Pickands-Mather Mining Co., 318

Pierson, Oscar C., on health dept. staff, 80; vital statistics work, 92; assistant secretary state board, 96; heads records division, 178
Pierson, Mrs. O. C. (Gerda C.), heads vital statistics division, 96, 178
Pillager, school, 380
Pillager band, Chippewa Indians, 224; smallpox, 225
Pillsbury, Alfred F., interest in venereal disease control, 255
Pillsbury, George A., Minneapolis mayor, 152
Pillsbury, Gov. John S., comments on inebriate asylum, 458
Pillsbury Mills, medical services for employees, 324
Pine City, hospital facilities, 449
Pine Tree Lumber Co., 213
Pipestone, Indian hospital, 238
Pitt Iron Mining Co., 316
Pleasant Grove, influenza, 409
Plumbers, examinations, 395
Plumbing, legislation, 334; code, 395; regulations, 396, 423; hospital survey, 445
Plymouth Church, St. Paul, establishes home for prostitutes, 246
Pneumonia, deaths, 69, 180; serum, 185
Pokegama Falls, lumber camp, 199
Poliomyelitis, epidemics: 97, *1910*, 91, *1916*, 186; investigated, 179; reporting rules, 180; convalescent serum, 185; nursing, 186; clinics, 481; regulations, 481; problems, 481; statistics, 481, 482
Polk County, smallpox, 214
Population, Minnesota: *1888*, 68, characteristics affecting public health, 38; aging of, 224; Chippewa: *1881*, 224, at Red Lake, 240; age distribution, 418; trends affecting, 419
Potsdam (N. Y.), 18; Hewitt's practice, 30
Potter, Calvin, Red Wing claim, 32
Potter, Hazard, 19–22
Potts, F. R., health officer, 150
Powell, Thomas T., 232
Powers Dry Goods, Inc., Minneapolis, nurse, 327
Powers-Simpson Pine Lands and Logs Co., 209, 210
Prescott (Wis.), river pollution, 145
Preus, Gov. J. A. O., calls smallpox control meeting, 404
Preventive medicine, early attitude toward, 9; Hewitt's views, 63, 66
Privies, declared health danger, 128, 137; dry-earth, 137, 138; in rural areas, 137–141; instructions for, 139, 140; lumber camps, 216; water pollution source, 286, 287; number needed, 480

INDEX 515

Prostitution, 262; control measures, 243–254, 257, recommended, 244, 247; ordinances, 244, 246, 250, 251, 253; health aspects, 249, 252, 256, 258, 260; legislation, 252, 253; in military areas, 254
Psittacosis, research, 186
Psychiatry, need for preventive, 469
Public health, population characteristics influencing, 38; courses, 62, 182, 192; establishment of university dept. urged, 64; Hewitt's address on, 66; Minnesota administration surveyed, 95, 382; commission advocated, 97; problems of *1872* and *1922* compared, 178; federal aid, 181, 182, 183, 476, 486; new problems, 181, 187; interest of private and public agencies in, 183; educational program, 191–193, 357, 367, 368, need for, 86, 178, 485; surveys, 194; problems and needs for future consideration, 474–494; proposed national program: 476–481, 486–490, 492, opposed, 476, services listed, 477, results to be expected, 486; per capita cost of adequate program, vi, 485; means of financing programs, 485; cost to state, v, vi
Public health associations, county, tuberculosis work, 278
Public health centers, plans for, 450, 453, 474, 475; number, *1948*, 453
Public health districts, plans for, 474, 475; units, 188, 189
Public Health in Minnesota, state board publication, 58–60, 137, 191, 193
Public health nurses and nursing, need for, 73, 354, 367, 370, 475; subsidized, 182; state board, 186; expansion, 186; number, *1930*, *1948*, 187; district units: 188–191, federal aid, 189; county: activities, 188, 189, 358–372, bill to establish county or multiple-county depts., 190, federal aid, 356, number, *1919*, 357, educational work, 357, 367, county budgets, 360, Isanti County, 360, 366, administration, 360, 387, in wartime, 362, 365, in influenza epidemic, 366, recommendations, 367, legislation, 371, state aid, 371; services to Indians, 237; tuberculosis work, 278, 279, 360, 366, 367; work among children, 278, 359, 361, 387, 389; industrial health work, 326, 327; Twin Cities, 356; uniforms, 356; number, *1919*, 357; activities, 357, 359–371; legislation, 358; working conditions, 358, 359; training, 358, 362, 364, 370; in maternal and infant health program, 359, 362, 364, 365, 387, 389; salaries, 360; defined, 364; cooperate with welfare workers, 364; advisory committee, 387; dental health courses, 392; work with cancer, 392; problems in rural areas, 475, 476. *See also* Nurses and nursing

Public waters pollution control, 286–307; surveys and investigations, 57, 146, 183, 288, 290, 291, 293–299, 302, 305, 306; legislation, 287–291, 294, 297, 305; conference, 292; factors involved, 295. *See also* Lakes; Sewage and sewage disposal; Stream pollution; Water supplies; individual rivers and lakes

Public Works Administration, funds for sewage treatment project, 146
Pumping stations, 106, 112
Puposky, sanatorium, 281
Purcell, Edward, army physician, 9
Pure Food and Drugs Act, 175

QUARANTINE, better techniques urged, 66; cattle, 72; tuberculosis, 85; laxness, 85, 163, 164, 400; state board's right to establish, 127; smallpox: hospitals, 201, 209, lumber camps, 206, 209, 212, 214, Indians, 228, 230, 231, by railroads, 399, public attitude, 400, 402, regulations, 402–405; recommended for trachoma, 233; venereal diseases, 257; chicken pox, 377; diphtheria regulations, 407; influenza, 412

RABIES, laboratory work, 81; virus in milk, 161; reporting rules, 179
Railroad construction camps, sanitation, 321, 322
Railroads, sanitary conditions: 39, 319, 320, 322, program for improvement, 318–323, surveyed, 322n.; precautions against smallpox, 49, 319, 399; shipment of corpses: 86, 413, regulations, 397, 398; sell cattle killed on tracks, 146; represented at smallpox conference, 210; rights of way through Indian reservations, 226; accidents and preventive legislation, 318, 319; switches inspected, 319; dangers of infection, 321; water supplies: 321, investigated, 124, regulations, 320, inspected, 322; dust conditions studied, 329. *See also* Industrial health; Workers, railroad
Rainy River, pollution control, 299–307
Ramsey County, early physicians, 13; health survey, 194; swimmer's itch, 348; prostitutes indicted, 250; children examined, 384
Ramsey County Graduate Nurses Assn., 353, 355
Ramsey County Medical Society, 75
Ramsey County Planning Board, 325
Ramsey County Public Health Assn., 284
Ramsey County Tuberculosis Pavilion, 281

Ramsey County Welfare Board, 284
Ranier, water pollution, 303; sewage treatment urged, 304
Red Lake Falls, hospital, 449
Red Lake Indian Reservation, physician, 224, 255; school, 231; tuberculosis rate, 234; living conditions, 235; nurse, 237; X-ray survey, 239; population, 240; venereal diseases, 263; trachma, tuberculosis surveys, 274, 284. *See also* Chippewa Indians; Indians
Red River of the North, sanitary surveys, 15, 115, 298; drainage system, 287; pollution, 307
Red River Valley, water survey, 57, 115; seed treatment plants, 328
Red Wing, 200, 246; described, 31, 32; physicians, 31, 33, 35–40; early sanitary conditions, 32; cholera, 33; Episcopal church, 33, 34, 35, 40, 60, 80; hospital, 40; Hewitt's laboratory, 40, 50, 376; vaccine station, 53–55, 60, 73; prostitution, 245; antipollution conference, 292; industries, *1870s*, 308; cholera infantum, 376
Redwood Falls, sewer system, 144
Reed, James, health officer, 314
Reinhard, E. G., biologist, 294
Remedies, fads in, 4; used by pioneers, 8, 16, by Indians, 222, 227
Rendering plants, licensed, 178
Renfro, William C., pioneer physician, 13
Renville County Hospital, 449
Reservoirs, St. Paul, 106, 107; Minneapolis, 111
Resorts, water supplies inspected, 124; sanitary conditions, 335, 346; inspections, 338, 346; number, *1927*, 338, *1948*, 346; need for further inspection work, 484
Respiratory diseases, at Ft. Ridgely, 11; among Indians, 224
Rest homes, act regulating, 422
Restaurants, legislation, 335, 340; sanitation program, 340–344; employees' schools, 341; sanitary principles, 342
Reynolds, Myron H., on health board, 77; heads veterinary dept., 79, 83, livestock board, 83
Rheumatic fever, control program, 390; cause of heart diseases, 390, 430; children, 390, 481; problems, 481
Rheumatism, among Indians, 221
Rhodes, J. C., Stillwater physician, 33
Rice, W. C., dairy commissioner, 160
Riley, William A., 194
Riverside Sanatorium, 281
Robbinsdale, typhoid fever, 122
Rochester, sewage disposal, 141; diphtheria, 141; impure foods reported, 148; food poisoning, 152; health officer, 172; health district headquarters, 189; sanitary conditions on fairgrounds, 337; clinic, 436; hospitals, 436, 437, 453, *see also* Minnesota State Inebriate Asylum; Rochester State Hospital
Rochester Counseling Clinic, 373
Rochester Health Center, 449
Rochester-Olmsted Health Dept., 453
Rochester State Hospital, 270; sewage disposal, 288; nurses' school, 353, addition planned, 451; care of inebriates, 459, 460; early conditions, 459, 460; investigated, 459, 460, 461, 462; treatment of patients, 459, 460, 461, 462, 463; population: *1878*, 459, *1892*, *1894*, 463, *1947*, 470; management, 461; recommendations for, 462; dormitory, 464
Rockefeller Foundation, 186, 195, 415
Rocky Mountain spotted fever, investigated, 82n.; reporting rules, 179
Roger, E. C., Carver physician, 33
Rogers, Arthur C., 466
Rogers, Harvey G., sanitary engineer, 299, 307; Rainy survey, 300, 305
Rosemount, trailer camps, 345
Rosenfield, A. B., district health director, 475
Rosser, J. C., 100; health officer, 200, 202, 226
Rosser, T. L., engineer, 108
Round Lake, small pox, 398
Roux, Emile, diphtheria antitoxin work, 53
Rum River, lumber camps, 197, 198; pollution hearing, 290
Rushford, sewer system, 144; scarlet fever epidemic, 408
Russell Sage Foundation, 461
Rynning, Ole, comments on climate and health, 7

ST. ANTHONY, health resort, 2; early medical practice, 13
St. Anthony Falls, sprinkling system, 126
St. Anthony Hospital, Bemidji, 215
St. Anthony Hospital, Minneapolis, 442, 443
St. Barnabas Hospital, Minneapolis, 251, 355, 437
St. Cloud, waterworks, 114; water tests, 124
St. Croix Lake, health resort, 2
St. Croix Lumber Co., 15
St. Croix River, early source of municipal water, 99; pollution, 146; surveys, 298, 306
St. Croix Valley, early physicians, 15; lumber production, 197; lumber camps, 197, 201

INDEX

St. James, sewerage system, 144
St. John's Hospital, Red Lake Falls, 449
St. Joseph's Hospital, St. Paul, 7; nursing school, 353; number of patients and rates, *1855*, 437; early conditions, 438; ambulance service, 442
St. Louis County, 315; trachoma, 186; in health district, 189; smallpox, 214, 404; sanatorium, 280; tuberculosis survey, 283; resorts and taverns, 346; nurse, 359
St. Louis County District Court, decision against meat inspection law, 152
St. Louis County Health Dept., 187, 453
St. Louis County Public Health Assn., 278
St. Louis Park, typhoid fever, 122; beet-sugar factory, 289
St. Louis River, drainage system, 287; pollution study, 297
St. Luke's Hospital, Duluth, 437
St. Luke's Hospital, St. Paul, 353, 442
St. Luke's Infirmary, Duluth, 449
St. Mary's Hospital, Duluth, 258
St. Mary's Hospital, Minneapolis, 355, 437
St. Mary's Hospital, Rochester, 436, 437, 439
St. Michael's Hospital, Sauk Centre, 449
St. Paul, 221; cholera, 6; diphtheria, 7; typhoid fever, 7, 100, 106; hospitals, 7, 273, 284, 353, 365, 437–442, 451, *see also* individual hospitals; early physicians, 13, 33; hotels, 33, 102, 251, *see also* individual hotels; smallpox, 46, 398, 404, 405; vital statistics returns, 68; compared with Minneapolis as to health, 105; death rates, 106; diarrheal diseases, 106; water supplies, 101–107, 113, 288; early sanitary conditions, 125–128, 130; sewage disposal, 128–134, 138, 144–147, *see also* Twin City sewage treatment project; engineers' society, 144; food sanitation: flour and liquors, 149, meat, 150–154, milk, 161, 163, 170; state health dept. quarters, 184; public health nurses, 187, 278, 356, 357; health surveys: 194, schools, 379; health officer, 212, 401; prostitution and control measures, 243–251, 257; cigar stores, 249; syphilis, 251; venereal disease clinics, 258; tuberculosis: 278, 284, care of patients, 271, 273, 281, survey, 284; trade, *1870s*, 308; factories inspected, 312; child guidance clinic, 373, 468; cholera infantum, 376; welfare agencies, 383, 420; "baby-farming," 385, 443; influenza, 410, 412, 414; mental research bureau office, 467. *See also* Twin Cities
St. Paul and Sioux City R.R., 49

St. Paul Board of Public Works, 131, 134
St. Paul Bureau (Board, Dept.) of Health, 453; fight for pure water, 105; established, 127; drainage contracts, 131; meat inspection program, 151; proposes medical examinations for prostitutes, 251; efforts to control smallpox, 404
St. Paul Chamber of Commerce, 103, 149
St. Paul City Council, efforts for waterworks, 103; considers sewerage systems proposals, 128; milk ordinance, 163; prostitution ordinance, 244; report on prostitution, 249
St. Paul Globe, comments on Hewitt's dismissal, 75
St. Paul Medical College, 64
St. Paul, Minneapolis, and Manitoba R. R. Co., 226
St. Paul Park, tuberculosis survey, 283
St. Paul Pioneer Press, 148, 158; comments on smallpox rumor, 49, on Hewitt's dismissal, 75, on Minneapolis sewage disposal, 135, on tuberculin treatment, 268, on nurses, 352; reports on sewers, 130; denounces milk adulteration, 161; describes lumber camps, 202; criticizes treatment of inebriates, 460
St. Paul Society for the Suppression of Vice, 248
St. Paul Water Co., 103, 104
St. Paul Water Dept., 107
St. Peter, sewers, 134; geriatric hospital, 451
St. Peter State Hospital, 465; milk supply, 168; dysentery outbreak, 396; incorporated, 454; investigated, 454, 456, 459, 460, 470; opened, 455; early conditions, 455; patients classified, 455; old people, 456; crowded conditions, 456, 459; sanitary conditions, 456, 462; management, 459, 461; treatment of patients, 459, 463; population: *1878*, 459, *1892*, *1894*, 463, *1947*, 470; erysipelas, 463; nurses' home, 464
Salisbury, A. H., health officer, 109
Salvarsan, 254; distributed, 256. *See also* Arsphenamine
Sanatoriums, county: need for competent medical directors, 86; act providing for, 86, 272, 274, established, 277, 281, number, *1946*, 280; effect on tuberculosis deaths, 185; recommended for Indians, 232; Indian patients, *1940–46*, 240; movement for, 269, 270, 272; state: act providing for, 270, described, 280, *see also* Ah-Gwah-Ching; change in populations, 282, 283; attitude *re* functions, 283; act regulating, 422
Sand Beach Sanatorium, 281
Sanitation, U. S. needs, 479. *See also*

sanitary conditions, investigations, surveys, under various subject entries
Sauk Centre, hospital, 449
Sauk City, sewerage system, 144
Sauk Rapids, smallpox, 6
Scarlatina, among children, 376
Scarlet fever, early prevalence, 6, 7; lumber camps, 15; reported by local boards, 46; resulting from impure water, 109, from faulty sewer drainage, 129, from impure milk, 165, 173; among children, 109, 373, 375, 409; investigated, 179, 408; pamphlets, 192; on iron range, 314
Scavingers, 133, 136, 137; licensed, 132
Scheele, Leonard A., 493
Schmitt, Otto H., 432
School buildings, heating and ventilation, 57, 373, 374, 375, 377, 380; surveys, 58, 374, 375; bill to prohibit use of unsanitary, 93; water supply tests, 124; sanitary conditions, 235, 374, 380; construction, 377; legislation *re* jurisdiction over, 381
School Health News, health dept. bulletin, 193
School health program, 373, 374, 375, 377-383, 389; nursing services, 189, 357, 359, 361, 365, 368, 371, 389; eye examinations, 189, 377, 378; physical examinations, 189, 379; rheumatic fever control, 189, 390; health instruction, 193, urged, 373; trachoma surveys, 232; health surveys, 361, 375; diphtheria investigations, 377, immunization, 389, 390; ear examinations, 377, 378; state aid, *1915*, 383; clinics, 385, asked for, 384; expanded, 391; dental program, 391-393; precautions against smallpox, 399; directions for diphtheria control, 407; disease census, 408; closing policies in influenza epidemic, 412, 413; cancer instruction, 428; mental examinations, 467; Minneapolis mental health demonstration program, 473; expanded program recommended, 484. *See also* Children; Maternal and child health program; School buildings
Schoolcraft, Henry R., comments on Indian health, 220
Schulz, C. G., supt. public instruction, 381
Scoboria, C. Q., health officer, 200, 201
Scottish Rites Masons, Duluth, child health program, 384
Scout camps, sanitary supervision, 124, 331, 332, 347, 348
Scrofula, among Indians, 221
Scurvy, among soldiers, 22
Sedgwick, J. P., 384

Septic sore throat, traced to milk, 165, 173; reporting rules, 179
Septic tanks, needed, 480
Septicemia, hemorrhagic, in cattle, 83
Serological tests, of draftees, 263; of civilians, 264
Sewage and sewage disposal, instruction in, 62; purification in England and Germany, 89; inspections, 90; St. Paul, 125-134; sewers and sewerage systems: 126, recommendations, 127, St. Paul, 128-134, construction problems, 130, Waring and New Orleans methods, 131; public opposition, 133, Minneapolis, 134-136, water carriage system, 140, drainage problem, 141, increase in number, 143, state board resolutions *re*, 290, investigated, 296, state fair, 337, hospitals, 441, need for further work and planning, 479; Minneapolis, 134-136; small towns and cities, 137, 141-144; iron range, 140; Rochester, 141; treatment facilities: Hallock, Baudette, and Canby, 144, Twin Cities, 144-147, 298, surveys, 297, 298, state institutions, 298, 306, projects, 306, number needed, 479; Duluth, 290; problems studied, 297; restaurants, 342; tourist camps, 345; resorts, 346; Scout camps, 348; homes for aged, 423; hospitals, survey, 445; pollution of waters by, *see* Public waters pollution control, Streams, Water supplies
Sewall, J. S., 128
Shakopee, smallpox, 46; sewage disposal, 142
Shattuck, Lemuel, 493, 494
Shattuck School, Faribault, meat poisoning, 156
Sheardown, S. B., Stockton physician, 33
Sheep, scabies, 70, investigated, 83; brucellosis, 416
Shepard, George M., 145
Sheppard-Towner Act, *1921*, 181, 182; provisions for Indian nursing, 237; public health nursing, 358, for maternal and child health programs, 386
Sherer, Elizabeth, nurse, 237
Sibley, Henry H., 221, comments on malaria and consumption, 7
Silver nitrate, distributed, 185
Sioux Indians, contagious diseases, 220, 222. *See also* Indians
Sisters of the Good Shepherd, St. Paul, 247
Slaughterhouse cases, hearings, 90
Slaughterhouses, England, 87; waste disposal, 129, 136, 142; removal from cities recommended, 150; inspected, 151, 157; sanitary conditions, 154; public, recommended, 156

INDEX

Slayton, sewerage system, 144
Sleepy Eye, sanitary conditions, 142
Smallpox, among Indians, 6, 203, 220–223, 225, 228–231, investigated, 234; early prevalence, 11, 46; control measures: 46–58, 179, 192, 200–214, 225, 228–231, 398–404, legislation, 45, conferences, 210, 211; epidemics: *1878*, 48, 49, *1899–1906*, 75, 227, 398–402, *1882–83*, 199–204, cost, 203, 204, *1924–25*, 404, 405; railroad precautions, 49, 399; lumber camps, 197–214, 230; spread by lumberjacks, 199, 202, 203, 204, 208, 209, 212, by Indians, 203, by travelers, 398, 401; statistics, 213, 231, 398, 402, 405, 406; decrease, 214; shipment of victims' bodies forbidden, 397; laxity in reporting, 399; diagnosed as chicken pox, 400. *See also* Bracken, Henry M.; Hewitt, Charles N.; Quarantine; Vaccination; Vaccine stations; Vaccines
Smith, Alexander H., 491
Smith, Charles E., assistant secretary state health board, 97, secretary, 176; controversy over tuberculosis work, 275–277
Smith, Edward P., Indian agent, 223
Smith, Harry, vii
Smith, Vespasian, 42n., 226
Social hygiene, training school for women lecturers, 256; courses, 264
Social Security Act, 181, 183, 189; aid available to Minnesota under, 182; provision for Indian health work, 238, for maternal and child health, 386, for dental health, 391, for old age assistance, 424; amendment to cover doctor and hospital care recommended, 493
Solberg, C. F., statistics commissioner, 68
Soldiers' Venereal Disease Fund, 255
Soroptimist Club, Minneapolis, funds for Indian nurses, 239
Soudan, hospital, 15, 315
South International Falls, plans for sewage treatment, 306
South St. Paul, tuberculosis survey, 283; hospital, 451
Southern Minnesota Medical Assn., 85
Southwestern Minnesota Sanatorium, 281
Spanish-American War, typhoid fever outbreak, 118
Sparta, lumber camps, 209; typhoid fever, 315
Spink, Wesley W., 417, 479
Split Hand River, lumber camps, 202
Spooner, sewage treatment plant urged, 304, plans for, 306
"Spotted fever," 7
Sprinkling systems, as means of water pollution, 126

Stam, John, Worthington pediatrician, 483
Stanchfield, Daniel, lumberman, 197
Staples, Franklin, professor medical practice, 62; investigates cattle diseases, 72; surveys tuberculosis in relation to climate, 266–268; on state health board, 458, president, 77
Starch factories, wastes pollute water, 116
Starkey, James, 128, 129
Stassen, Gov. Harold, asked to investigate lumber camp conditions, 217; calls venereal disease conference, 263
State boards of health, duties in and out of states, 66. *See also* Minnesota State Board of Health
State institutions, water supplies inspected, 124; sewage disposal, 143; trachoma survey, 232; tuberculosis survey, 269; appropriation for sewage treatment facilities, 306; responsibilities of health dept. *re*, 454
State Organization for Public Health Nursing, 358
Steamboats, carry cholera, 6, 33
Stephenson, W. J., Indians' physician, 228
Stevens, John H., 13
Stewartville, cattle quarantined, 72
Stiffler, M. L., 468
Stillwater, health resort, 2; scarlet fever, 6; physicians, 15, 33; lumber camps, 59; prison, 100, 113, 310; sprinkling system, 126; sewers, 134; hospital, 437
Stockyards, waste disposal, 129
Stone, A. J., 247
Straight River, sanitary surveys, 295, 297
Stream pollution, by garbage, 101; by sewage, 101, 107, 126, 142, 143, 289, 291, 296, 300, 302, 303, *see also* Sewage and sewage disposal; by dead animals, 107; endangers fish, 145, 286, 293, 296, 297, 300, 302, 303, natural environment, 286, livestock, 286, 293, 296, 303, bathers, 293, 296, 303, ice supplies, 303; state board statement *re*, 172; control program: 286–307, investigations and surveys, 146, 183, 291, 293, 295–298, 302, 305, 306, legislation, 287, 288, 290, 294, 297, 305, public attitude toward, 297, federal aid, 480, 481; by hamlet and farm drainage, 286; from privies and cesspools, 286, 287, *see also* Privies; by industrial wastes, 286, 289, 293, 299, 300–305, *see also* Industrial wastes; effect on recreational activities, 296, 302. *See also* Public waters pollution control; individual streams

Streetcars, ventilation, 321
Streptomycin, brucellosis treatment, 417
Stuart, A. B., chairman medical society committee, 41; president state health board, 42; author, 55
Sulfa drugs, trachoma treatment, 240
Sulfadiazine, brucellosis treatment, 417
Sullivan, Ralph R., epidemiologist, 263, 348
Summer camps, sanitary standards and surveys, 347–349
Sunnyrest Sanatorium, 281
Sunrise River, pollution, 116
Superior (Wis.), smallpox, 212
Superior, Lake, source of Duluth water, 114; pollution, 126, 290; drainage system, 287; sanitary surveys, 295, 297
Surber, Eugene W., biologist, 294
"Swamp fever," in horses, 83
Swan, Mrs. James G., 383
Swan River Logging Co., 210
Swedish Hospital, Minneapolis, 355
"Swimmer's itch" (*schistosome dermatitis*), investigated, 306; in summer camps and resorts, 348; preventive measures, 348
Swimming pools, sanitary surveys, 349
Swine, actinomycosis, 71; cholera, 72, 83; plague, 72, 83; trichinosis, 157; brucellosis, 416
Syphilis, 251, 252, 262, 264; among Indians, 221, 223, 236; discussed by dental assn., 248; early use of term, 248; circulars distributed, 253; cases reported: *1918*, 257, 258, *1919–21*, 261, among soldiers, 263; efforts to control, 323; among industrial workers, 327. See also Venereal diseases

TAVERNS, rural, sanitation, 346
Taylor, H. L., 94
Taylor, W. S., 205, 206
Taylors Falls, smallpox, 199; swimmer's itch, 348;
Tearse, C. D., 145
Thief River Falls, sanatorium, 281; nurse, 357
Thompson, Ashley, 225
Thomsonians, 15
Timber Producers Assn., 217, 218
Tomlinson, Harry A., 466
Toronto (Ont.), milk handling methods, 164; Rainy pollution meeting, 301
Tourist camps, sanitary conditions, 338; investigated, 344; regulations, 345
Tower, 315; physician, 15, 314
Town supervisors, jurisdiction over health matters, 45
Townsend, G. F., health officer, 108
Toxin-antitoxin, 185, 389, 390, 408
Trachoma, clinic, 185; hospital, 185; surveys, 185, 238; among Indians, 221, 232–234, 236, 240; symptoms, 233; treatment, 233, 240; Minnesota's rank, 234; decrease, 240; among school children, 379
Trailer camps, 325; investigated, 345
Trichinosis, investigated, 83; cause, 83; control measures, 157; reporting rules, 179
Trinko, Agnes, nurse, 356
Truman, President Harry, 476; backs compulsory health insurance bill, 499
Tuberculin, for tuberculosis treatment, 268
Tuberculin tests, cattle, 72, 83, 153, 154, 162, 163, 168; branding of cattle reacting to, 154; opposed, 158
Tuberculosis, victims attracted to Minnesota, 1–3, 38, 85; cases and deaths, 6, 68, 69, 180, 185, 234, 267, 272, 279, 283, 285; among Indians: 7, 84, 221, 222, 223, 224, 235, 236, 238, 239, 240, 241, sanitorium recommended, 232, investigated, 234, 274, 284; lumber camps, 15; sputum examinations, 69, 278; of cattle: 71, 72, 269, investigated, 83, control program, 174, see also Tuberculin tests; laboratory work, 81; isolation hospitals urged, 85; recognized as communicable and preventable disease, 85; program outlined, 85; legislation, 86, 272, 274; from impure milk, 165; epidemiological investigations, 185, 278; nursing services, 186, 278, 360, 366, 367, 368; among prostitutes, 246; relation to climate investigated, 266–268; treatment and care, 268, 271, 280, 282, see also Sanatoriums; educational program, 269, 272, 273, 274, 278, 279; surveys, 269, 278, 283–285; conferences, 271; appropriations, 274; controversy of agencies interested in, 275; program for handling cases, 276, 277; tag days, 278; studies of spread, 278; community control, 278; reporting rules, 278; carriers, 283; X-rays, 283, 284; iron range, 315; dangers of infection in transportation, 321; problems, 481. See also Mantoux tests
Tuohy, E. L., Duluth physician, 435
Twin Cities, sewage treatment project, 144–147, 298; declared single sanitary district, 146; meat inspection, 157; milk sources and consumption, 161; dairies inspected, 162; dairy herds tested, 163; opposition to pasteurization, 170; pasteurized milk consumption, *1930*, 173; pasteurization plants, 174; lumberjack mecca, 199; heart diseases, 430; hospital base area, 451. See also Minneapolis; St. Paul

INDEX 521

Twin Cities Obstetric Round Table, 444
Twin City Ordnance Plant, trailer camps, 345
Two Harbors, complains of impure milk, 159
Typhoid fever, 106, 290; early prevalence, 7, 11, 69, 99; lumber camps, 15, 199, 202; laboratory work, 81; transmission: by water, 91, 100, 101, 107, 109, 110, 118–122, 139, milk, 100, 118, 121, 165, 173, flies, 100, 118, 139, 317, food, 118, 119, 122; epidemics, 91, 101, 117–123, 314, 315; theories *re* origin and spread, 100; control methods, 118; decline, 123, 124, 480; investigations, 179; reporting rules, 180; iron range, 314, 315, 317; children, 373, 376; shipment of victims' bodies forbidden, 397. See also Deaths; Paratyphoid fever; Vaccination; Vaccines
Typhus, reporting rules, 179

ULRICH, HENRY D., 256
Ulrich, Mabel S., supervisor social hygiene education, 256
Undulant fever, 415; traced to milk, 173; sources of infection and precautions, 416. See also Brucellosis
Union Gospel Mission, boys' club camp, 348
United Charities, St. Paul, 356
United Commercial Travelers, 336, 337, 338; supports hotel legislation, 333, 334; protests hotel inspection transfer, 336
U. S. Bureau of Fisheries, represented at Rainy pollution hearing, 304
U. S. Dept. of the Interior, appropriations for Indian health, 238
U. S. Dept. of Labor, Children's Bureau. See Children's Bureau
U. S. government, meat inspection, 156; Indian health survey, 232; aid for child health work, 385
U. S. Marine Hospital Service, 85, 401; inspects immigrant ships, 39; investigates diseases among Indians, 234
U. S. Office of Indian Affairs (Dept. of), created, 223, 234; collects statistics on Indian diseases, 224; furnishes vaccine in smallpox epidemic, 228; recommends sanatorium for Indians, 231; trachoma circular, 233; appropriation for Indian health, 234; report on Indian health, 241
U. S. Public Health Service, 181, 255, 259, 302, 339, 340, 382, 385, 404, 447; supervisor, 98; Mississippi survey, 144, 292; investigates sewage treatment project, 145; milk sanitation advisory board, 165; endorses pasteurization, 172; milk ordinance, 174; recommendations *re*: dental health-survey, 183, Indians, 236, 238, serological tests, 263, state sanitary districts, 356; influenza control, 413, protective health measures, 480; trachoma surveys, 186, 232; aids venereal disease program, 194, 262; investigates Indians' diseases, 234; report on Indian health, 234; asked to investigate trachoma and tuberculosis among Indians, 274; co-operates in X-ray project, 284, pollution control, 296, 301, restaurant sanitation, 340, trailer camp surveys, 345; supervises railroad water supplies, 322; restaurant code, 341; sanitary restaurant campaign, 343; interest in dental health, 393; aid in influenza epidemic, 411; cancer research grants, 429; administers hospital act provisions, 448; approves hospital plan, 450
U. S. Veterans Hospital, Ft. Snelling, waste disposal, 146; tuberculosis patients, 280
University of Minnesota, 380; public health professorship, 60, 61, courses, 62, 182, 350, 358, 362, 370; students' physical examinations, 61; regents, 62; assumes medical examining board functions, 62; medical school (college): 73, 76, organized, 62, reorganized, 64, poliomyelitis work, 482; agricultural experiment station, 77, 143; laboratories, 82; paratyphoid fever, 121; hospitals: 121, venereal disease clinics, 258, legislation regulating, 350, nurses' training, 364, army base, 365, influenza outbreak, 410, heart, 432, Twin City area base, 451, poliomyelitis work, 482; sewage disposal, 136, 143; supports milk campaign, 166; pasteurization course, 169; agricultural college, 171; gastroenteritis outbreak, 173; preventive medicine and public health dept., 182, 183, 195, 350; dentistry school, 183; health dept. quarters, 184; influenza, 186, 385; social hygiene courses, 264; botany and zoology depts., co-operate in pollution control, 296; farm school kitchen and cafeteria surveyed, 341; public health school, nursing courses, 350, 358, 362, 370; obstetrics and pediatrics dept., 383, 387; heart research, 390, 431, 432, 433; continuation study center: 409, courses in industrial health nursing, 327, in obstetrics and pediatrics, 388; cancer research institute, 427, detection center, 429, obstetrics and gynecology dept., 444; hospital administration courses, 446; Mayo Memorial Medical Center,

451; student health service, 453; mental deficiency courses, 467; child welfare institute, 473
University of Wisconsin, brucellosis research, 417

VACCINATION, smallpox: urged, 47, 48, 204, 206, 210, 225, 226, 319, 399, 400–403, opposed, 47, 57, 202, 203, 319, in England and Ireland, 51, lumber camps, 59, 201, 203, 204, 206, 210, 211, soldiers, 194, railroad employees, 201, 319, Indians, 203, 220, 223, 228, 231, absence of state law, 205, 212, health dept. regulation, 211, attitude toward compulsory, 376, infants, 390, programs evaluated, 405; typhoid fever, 118, 119; communicable diseases, 391. *See also* Vaccine stations; Vaccines
Vaccine stations, London, 51; Hewitt's at Red Wing, 53–55, 60, 73
Vaccines, dispensed by health dept., 48, 49, 184, 185, 200; "point" defined, 49n.; first Minnesota production, 53; typhoid, 119, 184; paratyphoid, 184; pertussis, 185; smallpox, 185, 200, 228; influenza, 186. *See also* Vaccine stations
Van Cleve, Mrs. Charlotte O., describes domestic workers, *1880s*, 309
Van Dusen, Isaac, pioneer physician, 15, 314
Variety Club of the Northwest, gifts for heart hospital, 390, 432
Variola. *See* Smallpox
Varioloid, lumber camps, 202. *See also* Smallpox
Venereal Disease Control Act, 181, 262
Venereal diseases, early prevalence, 11; federal aid for control, 181, 183, 255, 262; military problem, 184, 254–256, 258, 259, 262, 263; control program, 189, 194, 254–265; Indians: 221, 224, 240, 263, survey, 238; relation to prostitution, 246, 259, 260; recognized as public health problem, 248; lack of control laws and regulations, 253; control bureau proposed, 254; reporting, 255, 258, 259, 260; dispensaries, 256; educational work, 256–259, 261, 262; clinics: 256, 257, 258, 262, 263, statistics, *1919–21*, 261, discontinued, 262; cases reported, *1918*, 257; regulations, 257, 258; social service work, 261; laboratory work, 261; history of health dept. work, 262; treatment, 263; serological tests, 263; nursing service, 368; problems, 481. *See also* Chancroid; Gonorrhea; Soldiers' Venereal Disease Fund; Syphilis; Venereal Disease Control Act
Ventilation, instruction, 62; shops and factories, 309, 312; mines, 316; trains and streetcars, 320; investigations, 328; schools, 373–375, 377, 380
Vermilion Iron Range, trachoma surveys, 232; prostitution, 252
Vermillion River, pollution, 286
Vincent George E., 75
Virginia, flood, 124; venereal disease clinic, 261; illness among miners, 314
Virginia General Hospital, 451
Visiting Nursing Assn., Minneapolis, 365
Visiting Nurse Society, Chicago, 353
Visiting Nurse Society, Philadelphia, 353
Visscher, Maurice B., 432
Vital statistics, analyzed, 57, 91, 92; collected and published, 68; inadequacy of early records, 68; importance to public health, 178
Vocational High School, Minneapolis, 239
Vocational Hospital, Minneapolis, 239

WABASHA, sanatorium, 281
Wade, E. Marion, laboratories chief, 179
Wadena, smallpox, 225; sanatorium, 281
Walker, James R., government physician, 203
Walker, T. B., statement on smallpox outbreak, 205
Walker, sanitorium, 238, 270, 280, 281
Walling, P. A., pioneer physician, 13
Warner, C. F., Mankato physician, 101
Waseca, prostitution, 245
Wassermann tests, 253, 254, 256, 260, 261, 389
Water Pollution Control Act, 305
Water supplies, analyzed, 81, 101, 102, 106, 108, 109, 110, 124, 194, 289, 302; progress in Europe and U. S. compared, 89; surveys and investigations, 90, 108, 115, 124, 179, 194, 318, 322, 325, 445; from streams, 91, 99, 101, 107; in early Minnesota, 99; program for pure, 99–124, 180, 196, municipal systems: 101–114, St. Paul, 101–107, Minneapolis, 107–113, Mankato, Winona, Stillwater, Duluth, 113, St. Cloud, 114; from lakes, 101–104, 106; filtered, 107, 110–113, 120; contaminated, 109, 125, 129, 142, relation to disease, 99–101, 105, 107, 121; causes, 115; bill to prohibit, 116; chlorinated, 112–114, 117, 120, 122, 123; rural areas: 114, surveys, 115; lumber camps, 198, 199, 216; iron range, 315, 317, 318; railroads: 320–322, regulations, 124; state fair, 337; resorts, 338, 346; restaurants, 342, 344; tourist camps, 345; Scout camps, 348; homes for aged, 423; hospitals: 441, survey, 445; need for further work, 479, 480. *See also* Plumbing; Public waters pol-

lution control; Stream pollution; Water Pollution Control Act; Waterworks; Wells
Waterville, water pollution, 289
Waterworks, municipal, 103, 104, 111–114, 120–122; plans approved by health dept., 124; state board resolution *re*, 290; number needed, 479. *See also* Water supplies
Watkins, F. L., 95
Watson, Percy T., 239
Weaver, Harry M., 482
Webster, L. J., 283
Welfare agencies, co-operate in dental health program, 183, with public health nurses, 363, 365; county, mental examinations, 467
Welles, Edward R., Episcopal minister, 33
Wells, condemned, 101; public attitude toward, 104; contaminated, 104, 107, 119, 133, 286, 287; artesian, 106, 110, 110n.; decrease in number, 107; arguments against, 114; chief water source in rural areas, 114; Red River Valley, 115; construction: 115, early, 99, suggestions for, 101, 344; inspected, 344; number needed, 479; nitrate poisoning from, 483. *See also* Water supplies
Wells, (Minn.), sewer system, 144; influenza, 410
Wells Municipal Hospital, 449
Wesbrook, Frank F., 176; biographical sketch, 72; directs health dept. laboratory, 72, 73, 79, 84, 88, 91, resigns, 95; university president, 73; secretary pro tem state board, 77; speaker, 80; diphtheria work, 80; views on functions of health board laboratories, 81–83; urges health officers' training courses, 82; supports public health instruction in medical schools, 84
West, James E., Scout official, 347
Western Hygiean Home for Invalids (Winslow House), St. Anthony, 2
Wheaton, smallpox, 401
Wheeler-Howard Act (Indian Reorganization Act), 234, 238
White Bear Lake, 2, 102, 104
White Earth Indian Reservation, 223, 224; smallpox, 225, 228, 229; Indians vaccinated, 225, 231; population and allotments, *1894*, 227; health survey, 232; trachoma surveys, 232, circular, 233; tuberculosis rate, 234; sanitary conditions, 235; influenza, 412. *See also* Chippewa Indians; Indians
White Oak Point, Indian agency, 223, 224, 225
Whittaker, Harold A., 291; heads chemical laboratory division, 89, water and sewage laboratory, 90, sanitation division, 90, 96, 179, 298, 299, 317, 321, 323, 338, 347; biographical sketch, 90; pure milk campaign, 164, 165, 169; chairman milk sanitation board, 165; Rainy survey, 298–301, 303
Whooping cough, cases reported, *1927*, 180; reporting rules, 180; pamphlet, 192; Indians, 221, 222, 227; children, 373
Wilder Child Guidance Clinic, St. Paul, 468, 473
Wilder Dispensary, St. Paul, 390
Wilder Foundation, St. Paul, 356
Willey, Samuel, St. Paul physician, 33
Williamson, Thomas S., comments on Indian diseases, 222
Willmar, sewage disposal, 142
Willmar State Hospital, influenza, 186; population, *1947*, 470
Wilson, Horace B., 373, 374
Wilson, Louis B., bacteriologist, 79, 81, 82n.
Wilson, Netta W., surveys dental health literature, 392
Wilson, Viktor O., heads special services section, 196, child hygiene division, 390
Wilson, W. L., 458
Winch, George D., on state health board, 42n.; tuberculosis survey, 266, 267
Winchell, N. W., water survey, 115
Winnebago Indians, smallpox, 6; population, birth and death rates, 221; tuberculosis, 223; prostitution, 226. *See also* Indians
Winnipeg, smallpox, 205, 212
Winona, health resort, 2; early physicians, 14; early health conditions, 14; smallpox, 46, 220, 401; slaughterhouse, 72; waterworks, 113; sewers, 134; dry-earth closets, 138; sewerage system, 144; food poisoning, 152; meat inspection, 154, 157; pure milk program, 167, 168; prostitution, 245; restaurant ordinance, 341; laxity in disease reporting, 399
Winona Independent, supports pure milk program, 167
Winslow House (Western Hygiean Home for Invalids), St. Anthony, 2
Wisconsin State Board of Health, represented at smallpox conference, 210; co-operates in pollution control, 292, 297
Wittbecker, W. A., hotel inspector, 334–336; heads hotel inspection division, 337, 338
Wodehouse, R. E., Ontario deputy health minister, 301
Wold, Theodore T., heads hotel inspection division, 339

Wold-Chamberlain Field, commissary investigated, 340
Wolfer, Henry, 466
Women, in industry, 310; unmarried, admitted to maternity homes, *1947*, 365
Women's clubs, support sanitary milk movement, 165, child conservation, 384
Woodward, Frank L., 294, 298
Workers, lumber industry, 6, 197–214, 225, 230, *see also* Lumber camps, Lumberjacks; industrial: employers' attitude toward health, 308, wages, 308, 310, complain of working conditions, 309, hours, 310, women and children, 310, *see also* Factories and shops, Industrial health; domestic, *1880s*, 309; miners, 314–318, *see also* Mesabi Iron Range, Mines, Mining camps, Vermilion Iron Range; railroad, 318–322, *see also* Railroads
Works Progress Administration, nursing and housekeeping aid project, 182; pamphlets on disease control, 192; work among Indians, 239
World War I, 254, 275
World War II, 262, 305, 362, 390

Worthington, 461; privies, 139; sanatorium, 281; smallpox, 398; efforts for inebriate asylum, 458
Worthington Municipal Hospital, 449
Wounds, treatment, 50, 50n.
Wren, John V., Indians' physician, 223
Wulling, Frederick J., 350

X-RAY, mobile units, 183, 185, 283, 284; surveys, 189; of Indians, 239; tuberculosis examinations, 280; public attitude toward, 284

YELLOW FEVER, reporting rules, 179; shipment of victims' bodies forbidden, 397
Yellow Medicine County, asks aid for children's clinic, 384
Yersin, Alexandre, 53
Young, Ruth, assists in clinic, 263
YWCA, St. Paul, 246; Minneapolis, 390
Youngdahl, Gov. Luther, proclaims Cancer Control Month, 429; comments on mental hospitals, 470; appoints mental health committee, 471

ZEIEN, THOMAS, physician, 116

www.ingramcontent.com/pod-product-compliance
Lightning Source LLC
Chambersburg PA
CBHW020911020526
44114CB00039B/132